Other great products from Carbs & Cals

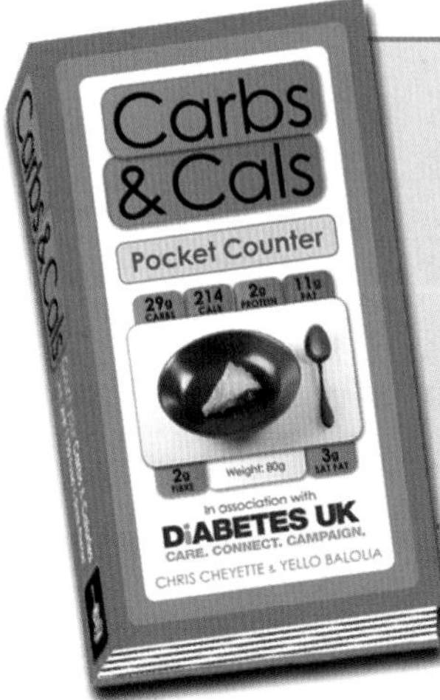

Carbs & Cals Pocket Counter

With over **750** photos, it's a great accompaniment to the Carbs & Cals book. Perfect when out & about!

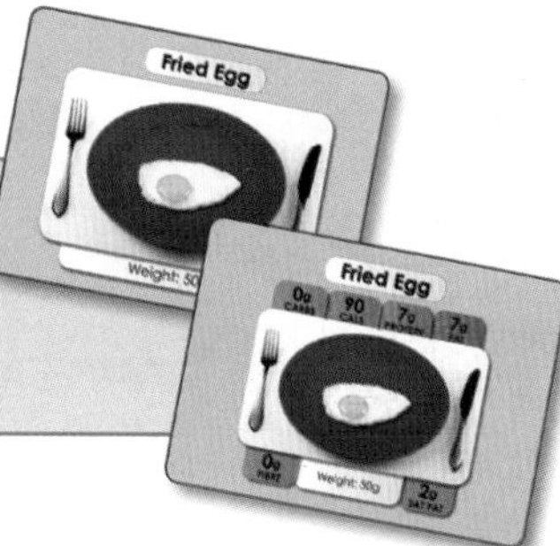

Flashcards

54 cards in each pack

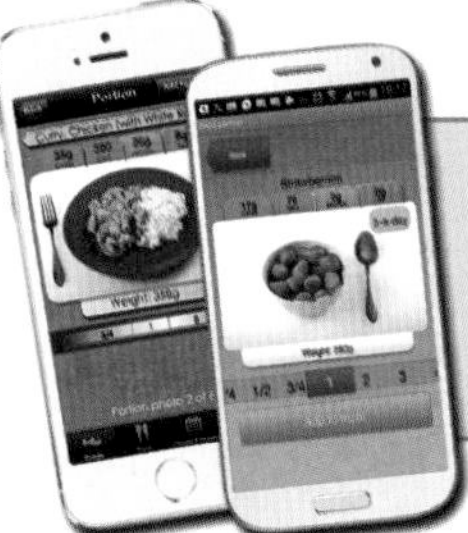

App

Over **3,500** photos

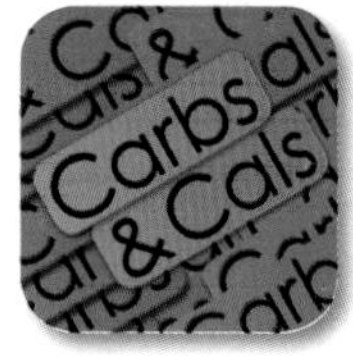

All products available at:

www.carbsandcals.com

Carbs & Cals

Count your **Carbs** & **Calories**
with **over 1,700 Food** & **Drink Photos!**

5TH EDITION

In memory of our dear friend Tom Rawlins

First published in Great Britain in 2010 by Chello Publishing Limited
5th edition published in 2013 by Chello Publishing Limited
Registered Company Number 7237986
www.chellopublishing.co.uk | info@chellopublishing.co.uk

This edition of Carbs & Cals is in association with Diabetes UK.
Diabetes UK is the operating name of The British Diabetic Association.
Company limited by guarantee. Registered in England Number 339181.
Registered office: Macleod House, 10 Parkway, London NW1 7AA.
A charity registered in England and Wales (Number 215199) and in Scotland (Number SC039136).

ISBN: 978-1-908261-06-9

Authors	Chris Cheyette BSc (Hons) MSc RD Yello Balolia BA (Hons)
Research Dietitian	Eleana Papadopoulou MPH MSc (Oxon) RD
Photography	Yello Balolia BA (Hons)
Design & Layout	Lesley Mitchell Yello Balolia BA (Hons)

Printed in the UK 0414

For more information, please visit:
www.carbsandcals.com

With special thanks to Eleana Papadopoulou (Research Dietitian) for her contribution in the making of this book.

Carbs & Cals

FREE Health Resources

Want access to 30 FREE resources for diabetes, weight loss & healthy eating (worth £29.99)?

Simply visit **www.carbsandcals.com/register** and enter the following code:

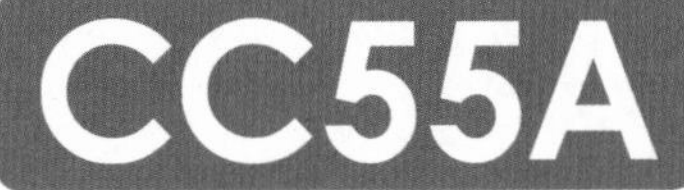

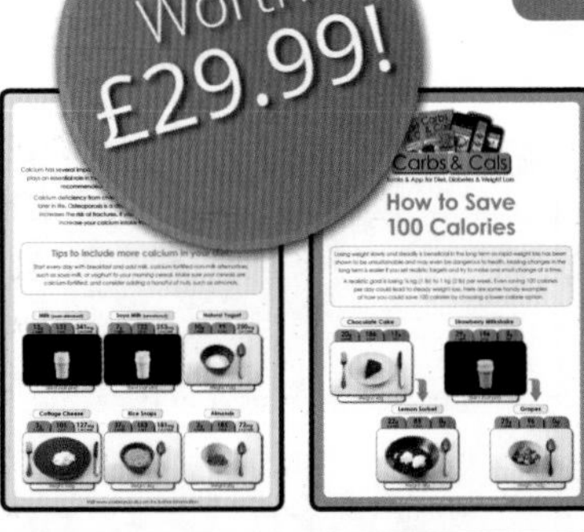

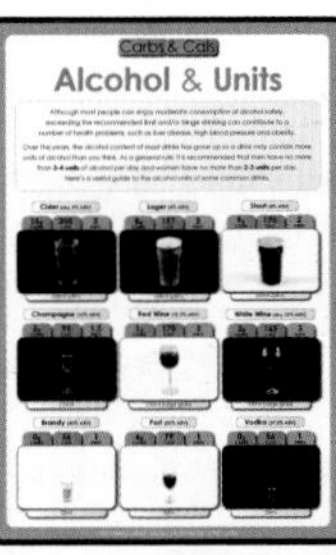

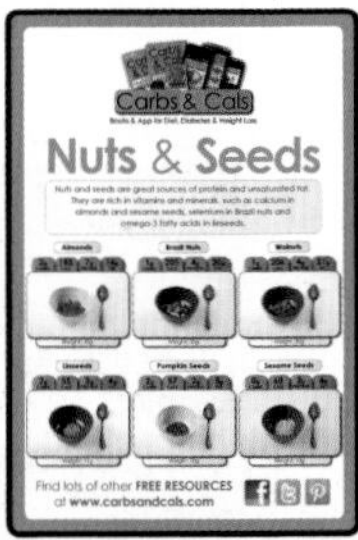

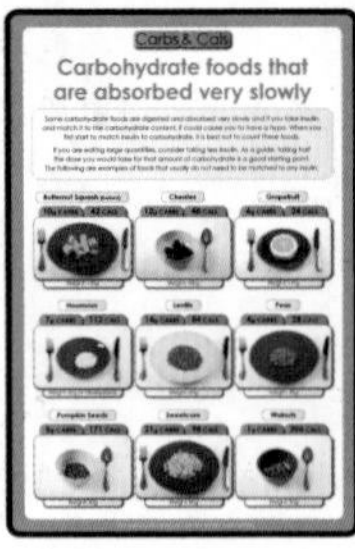

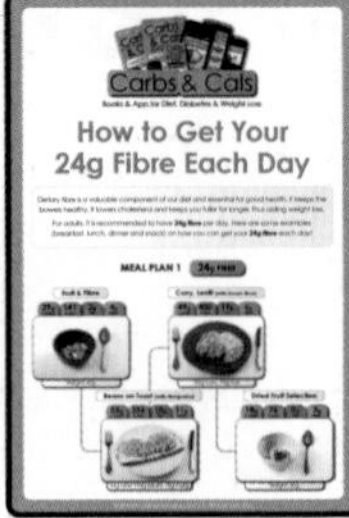

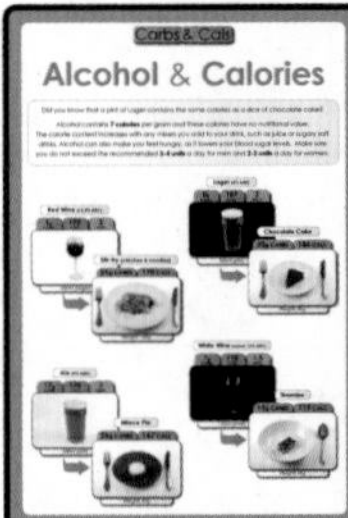

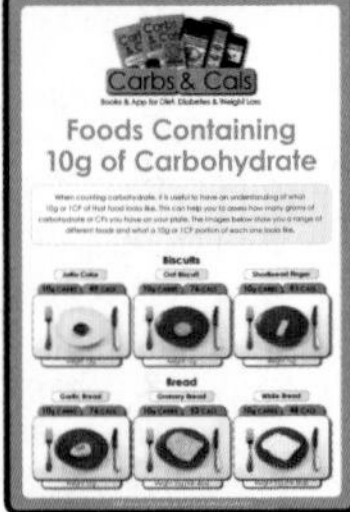

All resources are in printable PDF format. They're only available to registered customers, so don't delay – sign up today!

It's quick, easy and completely free!
www.carbsandcals.com/register

Contents

Foreword

Carbohydrate counting is an important part of diabetes management, especially for people with Type 1 diabetes.

Carbs & Cals is a great tool for those people with diabetes who count carbohydrates as part of the management of their condition. This easy-to-use visual reference guide allows you to compare what is on your plate with the pictures in the book, to find out the amount of carbohydrate and calories in the food you are eating. Knowing how many calories are in a portion of food is also really helpful information for people who are trying to lose weight, and may let you know that you need to eat a smaller portion or opt for something a little healthier.

Having all of this information at your fingertips, in an easy to understand format, will help to give you greater control over your diabetes and also give you the information you need to help you make healthier choices at meal times. Whatever your goals, we are sure that you will find *Carbs & Cals* a great help in achieving them.

Simon O'Neill
Director of Health Intelligence and Professional Liaison
Diabetes UK

DiABETES UK
CARE. CONNECT. CAMPAIGN.

www.diabetes.org.uk

Introduction

Welcome to *Carbs & Cals*. This book contains over 1,700 photos of a wide range of popular food and drink items. The carbohydrate, calorie, protein, fat, saturated fat and fibre values are clearly displayed in colour-coded tabs around each photo. This highly visual approach makes it incredibly quick and easy to see the nutrient content of the food and drink you consume. *Carbs & Cals* is the perfect support tool for carbohydrate counting in diabetes, weight management, portion control and general healthy eating.

Healthy Eating Principles

A healthy balanced diet is important for maintaining good health. It improves general wellbeing, helps with weight management and reduces the risk of long-term conditions such as heart disease, Type 2 diabetes and cancer. But what does 'healthy eating' really mean? Within our diet there are 5 main food groups. The Department of Health's Eatwell Plate shows the proportions of the 5 different food groups, including snacks, that we should eat and drink each day to ensure we meet our nutritional requirements. A healthy balanced diet contains a variety of foods from all food groups.

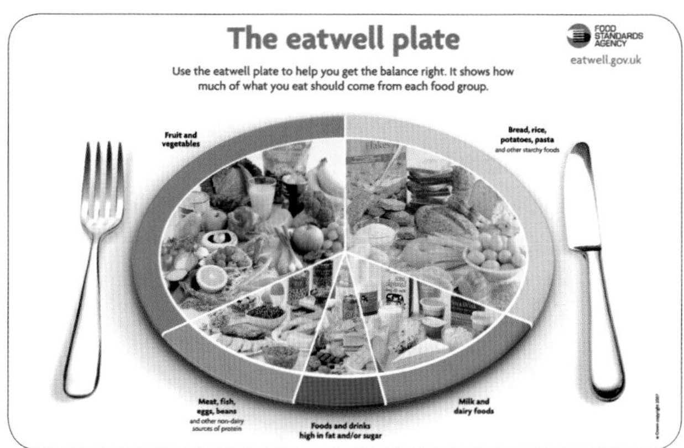

Therefore, try to eat:

1. At least 5 portions of fruit and vegetables each day.
2. Starchy carbohydrates at each meal. Starchy carbohydrates include foods like bread, pasta, potatoes, chapatis, rice and cereals. Choose wholegrain varieties, where possible.
3. Some milk and dairy foods.
4. Some meat, fish, eggs and beans.
5. A small amount of food and drink high in fat and/or sugar.

Top Tips for Healthy Eating

Aim for three meals a day and avoid skipping meals

Have breakfast, lunch and dinner each day. Make sure you space these meals out over the day, as they will provide you with energy and help you avoid snacking in between meals.

Include starchy carbohydrates at each meal

Starchy carbohydrates provide energy, and some are rich in B vitamins, which help release energy from food. Where possible, choose the wholegrain varieties of these foods, as they are high in dietary fibre, which helps maintain the health of the digestive system. Examples of wholegrain foods include wholegrain breakfast cereals, wholemeal and wholegrain bread, and brown rice. It is a common misconception that starchy foods are fattening – it depends on how much is eaten and whether fat is added during preparation and cooking.

Aim for at least 5 portions of fruit & vegetables each day

Fruit and vegetables are packed with vitamins and minerals, they are excellent sources of dietary fibre and are low in fat and calories. The World Health Organisation recommends eating a minimum of 5 portions of fruit and vegetables a day to reduce the risk of long-term conditions, such as heart disease and Type 2 diabetes.

The following count as one of your 5-a-day:

- 80g of fresh, frozen or tinned fruit and vegetables.
- 30g dried fruit.

- A glass (150ml) of pure unsweetened fruit or vegetable juice. This can only be counted once per day.
- Smoothies that contain at least 80g of 1 variety of whole fruit or vegetable.
- 3 heaped tablespoons of beans and pulses.

Most fruit and vegetables count towards your 5-a-day, apart from potatoes, cassava and yam, as they count as starchy carbohydrate. Make sure that you eat a variety of fruit and vegetables, as each type contains different vitamins and minerals. This book includes a yellow border around the portions that count as one of your 5-a-day.

Include more pulses

Pulses include beans, peas and lentils. They count as one of your 5-a-day, they are good sources of protein and are low in fat and calories. They are high in dietary fibre, they improve your cholesterol levels and if you have diabetes, pulses have less of an effect on blood glucose levels.

Aim for at least 2 portions of fish per week

Fish is a good source of protein. It is recommended to have at least 2 portions of fish per week, including 1 portion of oily fish, such as mackerel, salmon, fresh tuna or trout. Oily fish contains a type of polyunsaturated fat called omega-3, which lowers triglyceride levels and helps protect against heart disease. People with diabetes are advised to have at least 2 portions of oily fish per week.

Drink alcohol in moderation

It is recommended that men have no more than 3-4 units per day (e.g. 1½ pints of 4% volume lager) and that women have no more than 2-3 units per day (e.g. a 250ml glass of 12% volume wine). As it is important to avoid binge drinking, it is not advisable to save up your units and have them all at the same time. Over the years, the alcohol content of most drinks has risen and a drink may therefore contain more units of alcohol than you think. The number of units each alcoholic drink portion contains has been included in this book to make it easier for you to monitor your alcohol intake. It is also important to bear in mind that alcohol is high in calories, and that these calories have no nutritional value. Therefore, cutting back on alcohol may help with weight management.

Cut down on fat, particularly saturated fat

Since saturated fat increases the risk of heart disease, choose unsaturated fats and oils instead as they help maintain healthy cholesterol levels and triglyceride levels. See pages 12-13 for more information about the different types of fat. As fat is high in calories, reducing your intake may help with weight loss. Here are some tips to help you cut down on fat:

- Choose lean meat cuts and limit the amount of processed meat, such as burgers and sausages.
- Remove the visible fat from meat and the skin from chicken.
- Grill, steam or bake instead of frying.
- Use less oil, butter and spreads.
- Choose lower fat dairy foods where possible, such as semi-skimmed milk, reduced fat cheese and low fat or fat free yogurts. You can also have milk alternatives, such as soya or rice milk, but choose the low fat/sugar alternatives and make sure they are enriched with calcium.

Limit sugar and sugary foods

This does not mean you should exclude sugar from your diet. Small amounts of sugar can be enjoyed occasionally as part of a healthy diet. However, foods high in sugar are also often high in calories. Choosing sugar free or diet fizzy drinks/squashes instead of sugary versions can be an easy way to reduce your sugar intake. Artificial sweeteners, such as aspartame, sucralose, stevia, acesulfame-k and saccharin contain no calories and have no effect or a minimal effect on blood glucose levels.

Limit salt intake to 6g or less a day

A diet that is high in salt can raise your blood pressure, increasing the risk of stroke and heart disease. Add flavour to your food using herbs and spices instead of salt, and avoid processed foods.

Diabetic products

If you have diabetes, do not use food that is labelled as diabetic or suitable for people with diabetes. Diabetic foods are of no benefit to people with diabetes. They tend to be more expensive than the conventional products, they can be high in fat and calories, they still affect blood glucose levels and they can have a laxative effect.

The Nutrients in our Food

Carbohydrate

During digestion, carbohydrate is broken down into glucose, which is used by the cells of the body as their main source of energy. Carbohydrates can be classified into two main categories: starchy carbohydrates and sugars. Starchy carbohydrates include foods like bread, pasta, chapatis, potatoes, yam, noodles, rice and cereals. Sugars can be categorised as natural sugars and added sugars. Natural sugars include:

- Fruit sugar (known as fructose), present in all types of fruit.
- Milk sugar (known as lactose), present in milk and yogurt.

Added sugar includes table sugar (e.g. caster and granulated), glucose, glucose syrup, invert syrup and honey.

How much carbohydrate should I eat each day?

Carbohydrate requirements vary between individuals and depend on age, gender, weight and physical activity. The Guideline Daily Amount (GDA) of carbohydrate is 230g for women and 300g for men. The minimum carbohydrate intake to ensure proper functioning of the brain and the central nervous system is 130g per day. For a balanced diet, the majority of carbohydrate intake should come from starchy carbohydrates, fruit and vegetables, and some dairy products. Sugary food and drink should be enjoyed occasionally, in small amounts.

Protein

Our body requires protein for cell growth, maintenance and repair, for the production of hormones and enzymes, and for the proper functioning of the immune system. Protein is found in both animal and plant-based foods. Meat, poultry, fish, dairy products, eggs, pulses, tofu and soya are excellent sources of protein.

For most adults, 1g of protein per kg of body weight is sufficient to meet the daily requirements. If you weigh 70kg, for example, a protein intake of 70g is sufficient. In the UK, protein intake is usually in excess of requirements.

Endurance and strength athletes are likely to require higher amounts of protein in their diet (up to 1.7g per kg of body weight per day). Protein acts as an additional source of fuel and also provides the building blocks for muscle repair and development. Eating larger quantities of protein has not been shown to improve sports performance or increase muscle mass. The body is only able to use a certain amount of protein and eating large amounts offers no nutritional benefit.

High protein foods, such as full fat dairy products and meat, are high in saturated fat, which can increase the risk of heart disease. Frequent consumption of red meat has also been associated with colon cancer. In people with kidney disease, high protein intake may worsen kidney function. A registered dietitian can provide further individual advice on protein requirements based on your personal needs.

Fat

Fat is an important part of our diet. It is a major source of energy for the body and is essential for the absorption of the fat-soluble vitamins A, D, E and K. It insulates the body, provides a protective layer around the essential organs and is a structural component of all cell membranes. Of all nutrients, it is the most concentrated source of energy, therefore eating too much fat can lead to weight gain, which increases the risk of heart disease, Type 2 diabetes and some cancers.

There are three main types of fat:

Saturated fat: Mainly found in animal sources, such as meat fat, milk, cheese and butter, and also in vegetable sources, such as coconut oil and peanuts. Saturated fat raises total cholesterol levels and unhealthy LDL cholesterol levels, thus increasing the risk of heart disease. It also impairs blood glucose control by increasing insulin resistance. Information on the saturated fat content of foods and drinks is included in this book to help you to monitor your fat intake and stay within your requirements.

Monounsaturated fat: Usually liquid at room temperature, it is mainly found in olive and rapeseed oil, some nuts and seeds, and in some spreads. It lowers unhealthy LDL cholesterol levels but does not lower healthy HDL levels, thus decreasing the risk of heart disease.

Polyunsaturated fat: Found in some vegetable oils and spreads, nuts and seeds. It lowers unhealthy LDL cholesterol levels, but also lowers healthy HDL cholesterol levels. It is also found in oily fish, as omega-3, which lowers blood triglyceride levels.

The table below shows the Guideline Daily Amounts of fat and saturated fat for men and women. These figures are based on an average person. Your individual needs may be higher or lower, depending on your calorie requirements.

	Men	Women
Calories	2,500	2,000
Fat	95g	70g
Saturated Fat	30g	20g

Fat & weight loss

Evidence shows that in order to achieve successful weight loss, it is important to keep an eye on the overall calorie content of your diet. Per gram, fat contains more than double the calories of carbohydrate and protein, so a low fat diet could potentially lead to successful weight loss. Understanding which foods contribute large amounts of fat to your diet can be an important step in deciding where to make the appropriate changes.

This book makes it easier to see which foods to eat in smaller quantities or avoid altogether if you are trying to cut down on calories or reduce your fat intake. For example, you could consider swapping deep fried chips with oven chips and thus save 187 calories and 16g fat.

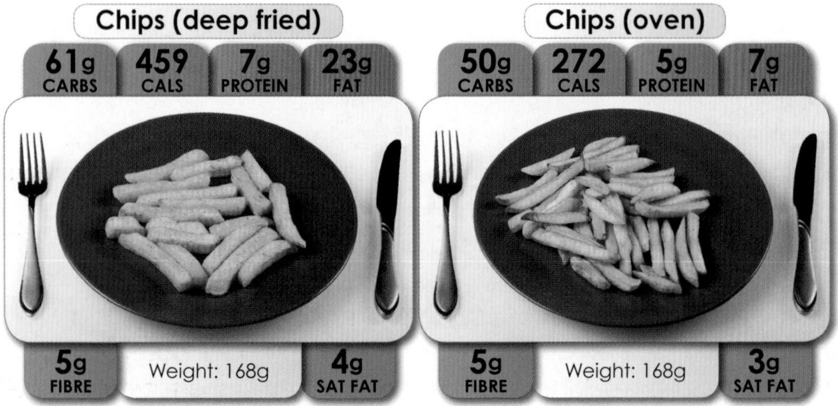

Fibre

Dietary fibre is classified as part of carbohydrate and is only found in foods of plant origin, such as fruit, vegetables, cereals and pulses. It has no calories and it passes through the gut largely undigested. Its many important health benefits make it a valuable part of our diet. There are two types of fibre – soluble and insoluble – and most fibre-containing foods contain a mixture of the two.

Soluble fibre is found in oats, pulses, fruit and vegetables. It decreases cholesterol levels and slows down the rate at which glucose enters the bloodstream. Insoluble fibre is found in fruit and vegetables, pulses and in all wholegrain cereals like wheat, rye and oats. It helps prevent constipation and it speeds up the time it takes for food to travel through the gut, thus reducing the time that waste products linger in the bowel.

The Guideline Daily Amount for dietary fibre intake is 24g for adults. In the UK, however, most people need to increase their dietary fibre consumption by 50% to reach the 24g target. Increasing fibre intake can help with weight loss as it slows down the rate at which the stomach is emptying, helping to keep you fuller for longer. It is important to note that any increase in dietary fibre consumption should be accompanied by an increase in fluid intake. This book can help you work out if you are meeting your daily fibre requirements.

Alcohol

Although most people can enjoy moderate consumption of alcohol safely, exceeding the recommended limit and/or binge drinking can contribute to a number of health problems, such as liver disease, high blood pressure and obesity. As mentioned earlier, the maximum alcohol recommendation for men is no more than 3-4 units per day and for women no more than 2-3 units per day. It is important to keep in mind that per gram, alcohol contains 7 calories, and these are 'empty calories', meaning they are of no nutritional value – an important consideration for weight management. One unit of alcohol provides 56 calories, however, the addition of sugar, sugary mixers, cream or fruit juice increases the calorific content of alcoholic drinks. Cutting down on your alcohol intake could help you to control your weight.

Calories

Calories are the units used to measure the amount of energy in food and drink. The number of calories varies according to the nutritional composition of each item of food and drink we consume. The calorie content per gram of carbohydrate, protein, fat and alcohol is as follows:

1g carbohydrate = 4 calories	1g protein = 4 calories
1g fat = 9 calories	1g alcohol = 7 calories

As seen above, fat has the most calories per gram; therefore, if you eat foods that are high in fat, you are likely to consume more calories and gain weight.

How many calories should I aim for each day?
This depends on a number of factors, including age, gender, physical activity levels and whether you are trying to lose, maintain or gain weight. It is possible to get a more accurate idea of your calorie requirements by speaking to a registered dietitian. The Guideline Daily Amount (GDA) for calories is 2,000 for an average woman and 2,500 for an average man. Sometimes GDAs are labelled 'for adults'; in such cases, these figures are actually based on the GDA for women, in order to encourage men with lower energy requirements to consume fewer calories.

Why count calories?
If you are trying to lose or gain weight, it is useful to have an understanding of the amount of calories in the food and drink you consume. Knowing the calorie content of food helps us to carefully select the types of food we eat so that we can avoid excess, choose healthier options (usually lower fat options) and maintain a healthy weight. If you are currently gaining weight, this indicates that you are consuming more calories than those you burn through physical activity and while doing your everyday activities. This can easily happen: 1 kilogram is 7,000 calories, so if you consume just 100 calories per day more than your requirements (e.g. by eating one or two biscuits each day), in one year this is equal to 36,500 calories. This could mean a weight gain of around 5kg (10lb) in one year, just by having 100 calories per day more than you need.

This book makes it easier to see where you can reduce portion sizes or make lower fat and calorie choices in order to lose weight. It can also help you to identify where you can make small changes that actually make a big overall difference.

Guide to Weight Loss

Before you start making lifestyle and dietary changes to lose weight, it is important to consider the reasons why you want to lose weight and to have realistic expectations about what you hope to achieve.

Making changes in the long term is easier if you set realistic targets and try to make one change at a time. Losing weight gradually is more beneficial in the long term, since rapid weight loss has been shown to be unsustainable and may even be dangerous to health.

Am I a healthy weight?

Calculating your Body Mass Index (BMI), which is a measure of your weight in relation to your height, will tell you whether you are a healthy weight. You can use an online BMI calculator, such as the one at www.carbsandcals.com/bmi, you can ask your healthcare team, or you can work it out yourself using the following equation:

$$\text{BMI} = \text{Weight (kg)} \div \text{Height (m)}^2$$

For example, if your weight is 72kg and your height is 1.68m, then your BMI = 72 ÷ (1.68 x 1.68) = **25.5 kg/m²** . Once you have your BMI, you can see which range it falls into by comparing it to the table below.

BMI (kg/m²)	Category
Under 18.5	Underweight
18.5 – 24.9 Asian: 18.5 – 22.9	Healthy weight
25 – 29.9	Overweight
30 – 35	Obese
Over 35	Morbidly obese

It is important to note that if you have a large amount of muscle, your BMI may be in the overweight range, even though you have little body fat.

Another way to check whether you are a healthy weight is to measure your waist circumference, which gives an indication of your body fat distribution. Waist measurement is taken by measuring the circumference of your waist at the midway point between the bottom of your ribs and the top of your hips. The table below shows the waist sizes that increase the risk of a number of health conditions, such as Type 2 diabetes, cardiovascular disease, cancer and stroke. Having a BMI of 25 or over increases your risk too.

Waist Measurement for:	At Increased Risk	At High Risk
Men	Over 94cm *(37 inches)* Asian: Over 90cm *(35.5 inches)*	Over 102cm *(40 inches)*
Women	Over 80cm *(31.5 inches)* Asian: Over 80cm *(31.5 inches)*	Over 88cm *(34.5 inches)*

Studies have shown that losing 5-10% of your body weight can bring significant health benefits, including a reduction in blood pressure, cholesterol and triglyceride levels and a lowered risk of Type 2 diabetes, to name just a few.

How to lose weight safely

A safe weight loss rate is 0.5-1kg (1-2 lbs) of body weight each week. Losing more weight than this places you at risk of nutrient deficiencies and increases the possibility of putting the weight back on. To achieve the recommended weight loss rate, it is necessary to reduce dietary intake by about 600 calories per day (4,200 calories per week). This reduction could be by diet alone or by a combination of diet and increased physical activity. If 600 calories seems a lot, it may be worth thinking about breaking it up into smaller 100–200 calorie reductions. Eating a smaller portion or choosing a healthier option can be helpful in this process.

On the following page is an example of how you could save 100 calories by choosing a different type of dessert:

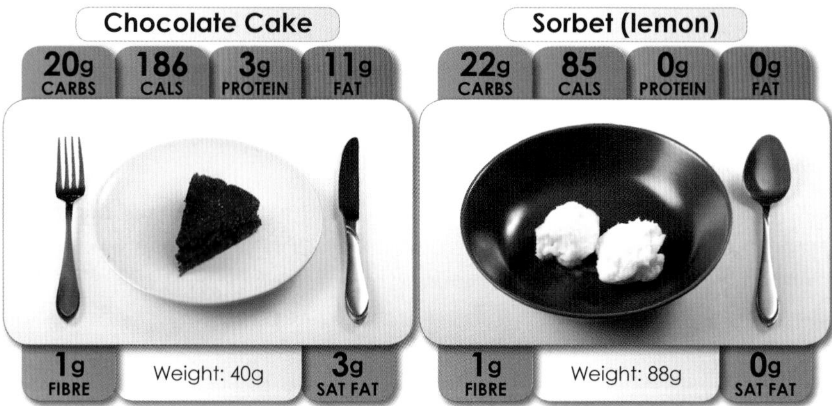

Recently, low carbohydrate diets have attracted significant attention from people who want to lose weight. In the short term, people who follow low carbohydrate diets may lose weight quickly. However, studies that have compared very low carbohydrate diets with conventional low fat diets have found no difference in weight loss between groups at the end of the first year of following the diet, or in the long term. The long-term effectiveness of low carbohydrate diets is still not proven.

Per gram, carbohydrate foods contain less than half the calories of fat, which rules out the common misconception that starchy carbohydrates (such as bread and pasta) are fattening. Foods which are high in fat have a much higher calorie content gram-for-gram:

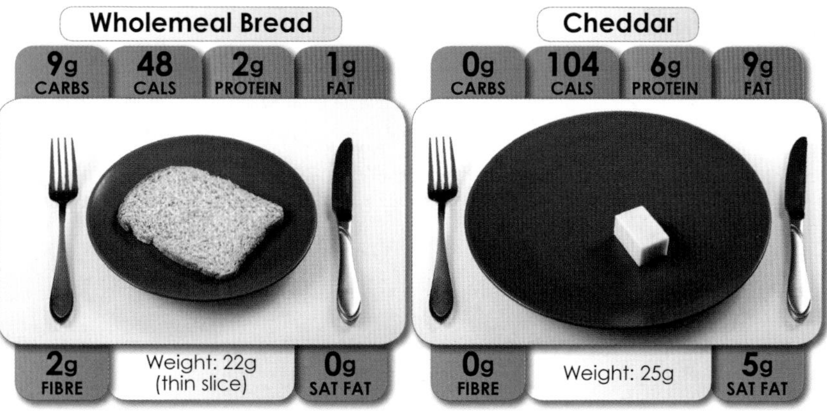

The amount of starchy carbohydrate eaten is still important when considering losing weight. Sugary foods like biscuits, chocolates and cakes are very palatable and are usually high in fat, making it extremely easy to consume too many calories within a small portion.

Losing weight in a healthy way is a big challenge in itself, and keeping it off can be even harder. So if you don't achieve your target or you put on some of the weight you lost, do not despair! Accept the occasional slip up as a learning experience, focus on your aim and always remember your hard work and the progress you have made. Whatever your goals may be, it is important to discuss your diet plan and what you want to get out of it with your healthcare team. Let them know your main aim and they will help you set realistic short-term goals to help you get there.

Diabetes

Diabetes is a condition in which the glucose levels in the blood are too high because the body cannot use the glucose properly. The main aim of diabetes treatment is to reduce the risk of diabetes-related complications, such as heart disease, eye and kidney problems. To achieve this, patients need to keep their blood glucose, blood fats and blood pressure levels within the normal range and to maintain a healthy lifestyle. There are two main types of diabetes: Type 1 and Type 2.

Type 1 diabetes

Type 1 diabetes develops when the body's immune system attacks and destroys the cells of the pancreas that produce insulin. As a result, the pancreas is unable to produce insulin and this leads to increased blood glucose levels. It is treated by daily insulin administration through injections or a pump. There are various types of insulin available and your diabetes healthcare team will help to tailor the insulin to your individual needs.

Type 2 diabetes

Type 2 diabetes is more common than Type 1 diabetes and it develops when the pancreas does not produce enough insulin, or when the body is unable to use the insulin effectively (known as insulin resistance). Type 2 diabetes is often associated with being overweight and usually occurs after the age of 40, although in people of South Asian origin it often appears from the age of 25. It is also becoming more common in younger people of all ethnicities, due to the rising levels of obesity.

Usually, Type 2 diabetes is treated primarily with a healthy diet and increased physical activity. However, it is a progressive condition and following a healthy eating plan and being physically active is often not enough to control blood glucose levels. If this is the case, your healthcare team may advise you to take diabetes medication and/or insulin to control your blood glucose levels.

The risk of developing Type 2 diabetes can be reduced. There is strong evidence that lifestyle changes, including a combination of weight loss strategies such as calorie restriction and increased physical activity, can prevent Type 2 diabetes in high-risk individuals. In fact, every 1kg lost has been associated with a 16% reduction in the risk of developing Type 2 diabetes in overweight people.

Carbohydrate Counting

For people with Type 1 diabetes, carbohydrate counting is not a new concept; it has been around for over 50 years. However, in recent years, its popularity has increased and nowadays carbohydrate counting has been incorporated more and more into the education and management of Type 1 diabetes, Type 2 diabetes and diabetes in pregnancy.

Carbohydrate is the main nutrient that affects the rise in blood glucose levels. For people with Type 1 diabetes, there is strong evidence that matching insulin doses to carbohydrate intake improves blood glucose levels. It is important for people with Type 1 diabetes to have an understanding of the amount of carbohydrate in the food and drink they consume, in order to be able to adjust insulin doses accurately. As well as the amount of carbohydrate consumed, other factors such as alcohol consumption and illness can influence how much insulin is needed. Following a healthy diet and regular physical activity are also important in the management of Type 1 diabetes.

In Type 2 diabetes, the evidence about the effect of carbohydrate counting even on those treated with insulin is still inconclusive. Nevertheless, the larger the carbohydrate intake, the greater the rise in blood glucose levels after eating. Using carbohydrate counting as a tool to help people with Type 2 diabetes manage the amount of carbohydrate at each meal may be an effective strategy in controlling blood glucose levels.

People with Type 2 diabetes on a flexible insulin regimen may find that matching their insulin dose to carbohydrate improves their blood glucose levels. Your healthcare team will be able to provide you with the appropriate advice on which treatment is best for you.

If you are starting out with carbohydrate counting, there are three areas that you may wish to familiarise yourself with:

1. Learning about the concept of carbohydrate counting and how to estimate the amount of carbohydrate in food and drink. You can practice carbohydrate counting by using this book, along with other methods, such as weighing your food portions and checking food labels.
2. Understanding the effect of food and drink, diabetes medication, alcohol and physical activity on blood glucose levels and learning how to manage these factors.
3. If you have diabetes and are on multiple daily injections (basal bolus) or using an insulin pump, this book can help you with insulin dose adjustment, i.e. how to match your quick-acting insulin to carbohydrate using your personal insulin-to-carbohydrate ratio.

The carbohydrate content of food and drink can be estimated either in grams or as carbohydrate portions (CPs). One CP usually contains 10g of carbohydrate. For example, 100g of oven chips contain 30g of carbohydrate or 3 CPs. Some people work in grams and some use CPs. It is important to use the method that works best for you. This book shows the carbohydrate content of food and drink in grams. If you are using CPs, all you have to do is find the total carbohydrate content of your meal in grams and divide that figure by 10.

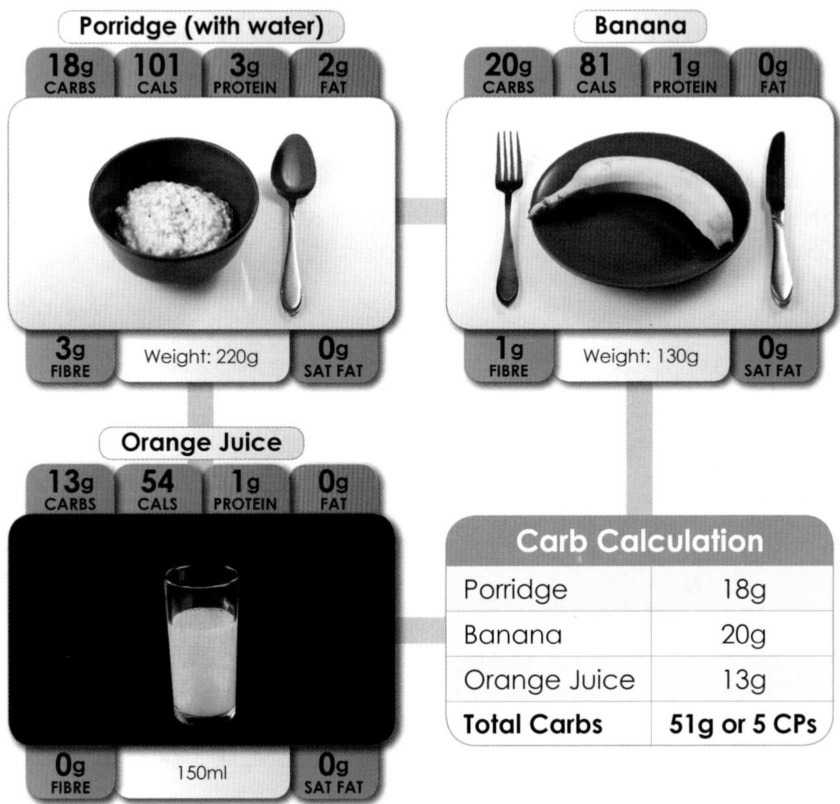

Carb Calculation	
Porridge	18g
Banana	20g
Orange Juice	13g
Total Carbs	**51g or 5 CPs**

Learning to estimate the carbohydrate content of food and drink is a valuable skill that is worth mastering and it becomes easier with practice. You might find it more difficult to estimate the carbohydrate content of your meals when eating out or having a takeaway or dinner with friends, as it is not easy to know which ingredients have been used. For most people with diabetes, however, with time and the right support, carbohydrate counting becomes second nature.

The main disadvantage of carbohydrate counting is that by focusing on carbohydrate only, it is easy to lose sight of the overall nutrient composition of the diet. For example, it is common to overlook the calorie and fat content of food and this may lead to undesirable weight gain and increased risk of complications, such as heart disease. It is important to take into consideration all the nutrients of your food and drink, not just carbohydrate. This book can be of great help with carbohydrate counting as well as for keeping an eye on the overall nutrient composition and calorie content of your diet too!

Examples: A portion of crème brûlée only contains 19g carbohydrate, but it has 27g fat and 333 calories. On the contrary, a portion of basmati rice contains 51g carbohydrate, 233 calories and only 1g fat.

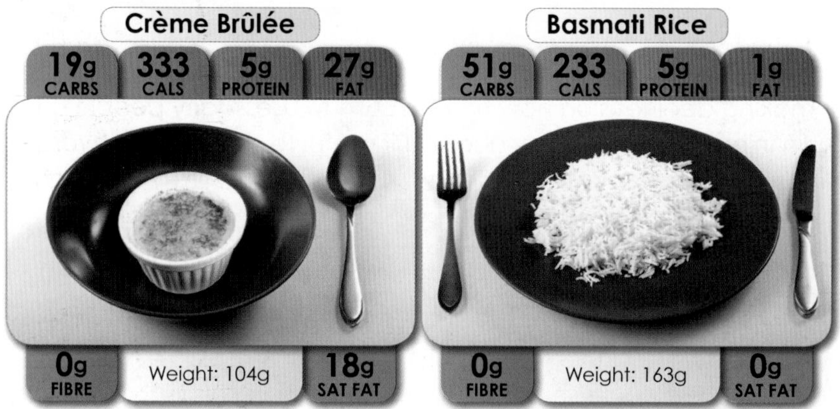

Carbohydrate counting and insulin dose adjustment

The development of insulin has enabled people with diabetes to effectively adjust insulin doses to the carbohydrate content of their meals. This offers more flexible eating, reduces the risk of hypoglycaemia and improves blood glucose control.

As mentioned earlier, the carbohydrate from the food and drink we consume is broken down into glucose when it is digested. This glucose is transferred into the blood and from there it is carried into the cells of the body by the hormone insulin. Long-acting insulin (basal) deals with the glucose produced by the liver and influences the blood glucose levels between meals. Quick-acting insulin (bolus) deals with the glucose produced from the carbohydrate in the food and drink that is consumed.

The amount of quick-acting insulin that is required is directly related to the total amount of carbohydrate consumed. The more carbohydrate you eat or drink, the greater the quick-acting insulin requirements; the less carbohydrate you eat or drink, the lower the quick-acting insulin requirements. If you have a carbohydrate-free meal or negligible amounts of carbohydrate, there is generally no need for quick-acting insulin, as your long-acting insulin will deal with the glucose that is produced by the liver, if the dose is correct for you.

For people on multiple daily injections of insulin (basal-bolus insulin regimen) or on insulin pumps, carbohydrate counting is important for making decisions on how much insulin to use. Many people on 2 insulin injections a day may also find it useful to count carbohydrate in order to maintain consistent amounts of carbohydrate at meals and to reduce the risk of wide fluctuations in blood glucose.

The amount of insulin that is required (known as insulin-to-carbohydrate ratio) varies from person to person and can also vary at different times of the day. Typically, most people start with 1 unit of quick-acting insulin for every 10g carbohydrate or 1CP. Your diabetes team will work with you to help you understand the appropriate insulin-to-carbohydrate ratio for you.

Learning how to adjust insulin doses and how to count carbohydrate can be a complex process. This book is not designed to teach you how to adjust your insulin; it is important that you have the support of appropriately trained healthcare professionals, such as a diabetes specialist nurse and diabetes specialist dietitian. Many areas in the UK now offer structured education programmes, such as BERTIE and DAFNE for Type 1 diabetes, DESMOND for Type 2 diabetes and X-PERT for Type 1 diabetes, Type 2 diabetes and for those at risk of developing diabetes.

Through the X-PERT Programme, for example, people with Type 1 and Type 2 diabetes learn how to self-manage their condition in order to improve their health and wellbeing and reduce the risk of diabetes-related complications and the need for tablets and/or insulin. Those at risk of developing diabetes learn to recognise the importance of making dietary and other lifestyle changes to improve blood pressure, blood glucose and cholesterol levels, all of which can help to prevent the development of diabetes. Visit **www.xperthealth.org.uk** for more information about X-PERT or to find your local centre. You can also ask your diabetes team which diabetes structured education programme is available in your area.

Alcohol and carbohydrate counting

This book includes a variety of alcoholic drinks and displays their carbohydrate values. People who are carbohydrate counting and adjusting their insulin should use these values as a reference guide only, as it is not recommended to take additional insulin for the carbohydrate found in most alcoholic drinks. Extreme caution should be taken when giving additional units of insulin with alcohol, as alcohol is associated with an increased risk of hypoglycaemia. Your diabetes team can advise you on this in greater detail.

Glycaemic Index

The rate at which carbohydrate is broken down depends on the type of carbohydrate consumed; this is known as the Glycaemic Index (GI). Food or drinks with a high GI (such as Lucozade or jelly sweets) are broken down quickly, causing a rapid rise in blood glucose levels. Foods with a low GI (such as porridge oats or pasta) are broken down slowly, giving a more gradual rise in blood glucose levels.

For people with diabetes, having an idea of the GI of food and drink can be helpful in predicting blood glucose fluctuations after eating or drinking. A registered dietitian can help you with more information on this subject.

It is important to bear in mind that GI does not take into account the other nutrients in a meal (protein, fat and fibre), which can slow down the absorption of glucose in the blood, or the amount of carbohydrate in the meal, which is a much better predictor of how high the blood glucose levels will go.

A note of caution: It is important to note that certain foods release glucose at a very slow rate and may not require insulin, or may require a reduced or delayed dose. Examples include foods such as pearl barley, peas, beans and lentils, and some vegetables such as sweetcorn, squash/pumpkin and parsnips. It is advisable to speak to your diabetes team about your insulin requirements for these foods as they may vary from person to person and depend on the portion size consumed.

Diabetes and Weight Management

Weight loss is the primary strategy to control blood glucose levels, especially in overweight or obese people with Type 2 diabetes. People with Type 1 diabetes should also keep to a healthy weight, as being overweight may put them at a higher risk of complications, such as heart disease.

Reducing the total calorie content of the diet and increasing physical activity levels are the best ways of losing weight healthily and keeping it off for good. To date, it is still unclear which is the most effective weight loss plan and which proportion of carbohydrate, protein and fat people with diabetes should consume in order to lose weight. Some people lose weight by following a low fat diet, while others do well on a low carbohydrate diet.

Recent evidence has shown that a very low calorie diet of approximately 450-800 calories per day for two months could reverse the insulin resistance that is common in Type 2 diabetes and slow down the progressive decline of the insulin-producing cells of the pancreas. However, more research is required to show the long-term benefit and it is important to discuss this kind of diet with your healthcare team before considering it as an option for weight loss.

Commercial diet programmes utilise a variety of weight loss methods, such as dietary advice, personalised meal plans, physical activity and group therapy. The evidence about the effect of such programmes on people with diabetes is still unknown. Fad diets, which usually promise quick weight loss by following a restrictive, nutrient-deficient diet of an unusual combination of foods, offer no benefit in the long term and most people put the weight back on.

How to Use This Book

This book has been written with complete practicality in mind. Simply follow the steps outlined below:

1. Decide what you want to eat or drink and find the meal, drink or snack in the book.
2. Look at the tabs above and below the photo for the values you are interested in. These show the carbohydrate, calorie, protein, fat, saturated fat and fibre values.
3. Choose your portion size and assemble your meal.
4. Add up the Carbs, Cals, Protein, Fat, Sat Fat and Fibre values for the different food components to give the totals for your meal.

To help with scale, each food photo displays either a knife and fork, or a dessert spoon. To make it as easy as possible, you can measure your own dinnerware and compare the size of your plates and bowls to the dinnerware in the photos. Alternatively, you may wish to use plates and bowls that are the same size as the ones in the book. The weight of each portion is stated below each photo, just in case you want to double check the weight of your own portion. **This is always the cooked/prepared weight.**

If you are eating a meal with more than one component (e.g. steak, chips and salad), you will need to find each component in the book and add them up separately. For example, your steak, chips and salad meal may comprise of sirloin steak from page 175, oven chips from page 216, Hollandaise sauce from page 261 and mixed lettuce leaves from page 304.

All foods in the book are displayed on one of the following dishes. The type of dish used is displayed at the top of each page as a reminder.

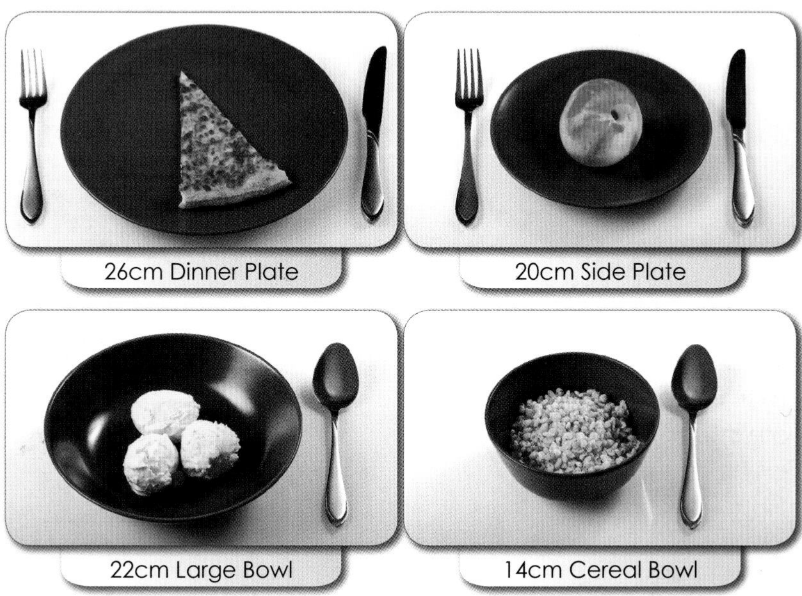

26cm Dinner Plate

20cm Side Plate

22cm Large Bowl

14cm Cereal Bowl

Each food in the book has between 1 and 6 portion photos to help you easily judge the nutrient and calorie content of your particular portion simply by looking at the different photos. For example, a digestive biscuit is always the same size and therefore only 1 photo has been included. However, there are 6 different portion pictures of lasagne included so that you can choose the portion that is closest to the portion on your plate.

Please note that values for carbohydrate, protein, fat, saturated fat and fibre are given to the nearest gram. Therefore, if a food has 0.4g of fat, the fat value will be listed as 0g. If a food has 0.6g of fat, the fat value will be listed as 1g.

Bourbon Cream

8g CARBS	58 CALS	1g PROTEIN	3g FAT
0g FIBRE	Weight: 12g		2g SAT FAT

Chocolate Digestive

9g CARBS	74 CALS	1g PROTEIN	4g FAT
0g FIBRE	Weight: 15g		2g SAT FAT

Chocolate Chip Cookie

6g CARBS	49 CALS	1g PROTEIN	2g FAT
0g FIBRE	Weight: 10g		1g SAT FAT

48g CARBS	366 CALS	4g PROTEIN	17g FAT
2g FIBRE	Weight: 74g		9g SAT FAT

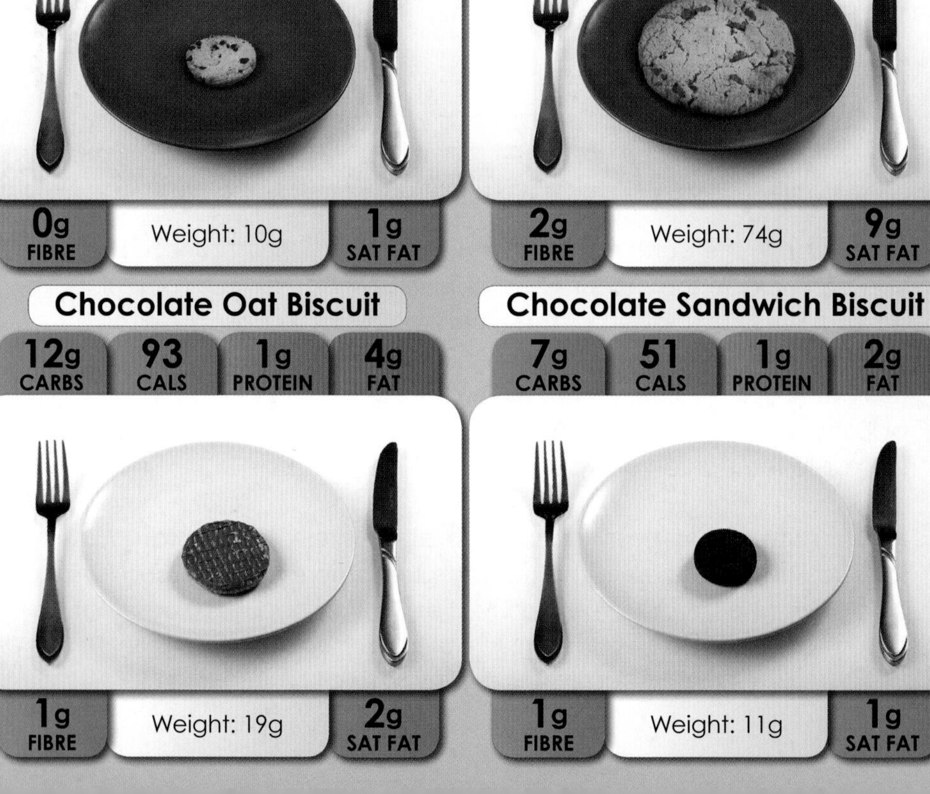

Chocolate Oat Biscuit

12g CARBS	93 CALS	1g PROTEIN	4g FAT
1g FIBRE	Weight: 19g		2g SAT FAT

Chocolate Sandwich Biscuit

7g CARBS	51 CALS	1g PROTEIN	2g FAT
1g FIBRE	Weight: 11g		1g SAT FAT

Custard Cream

CARBS	CALS	PROTEIN	FAT
8g	60	1g	2g

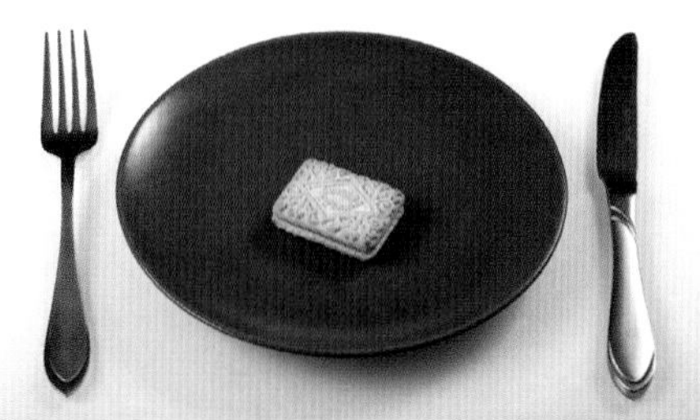

FIBRE	Weight	SAT FAT
0g	Weight: 12g	2g

Digestive

CARBS	CALS	PROTEIN	FAT
11g	69	1g	2g

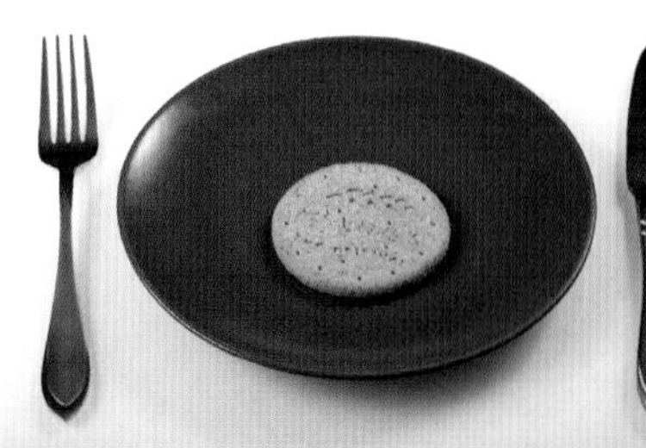

FIBRE	Weight	SAT FAT
0g	Weight: 15g	1g

Fig Roll

CARBS	CALS	PROTEIN	FAT
14g	80	1g	2g

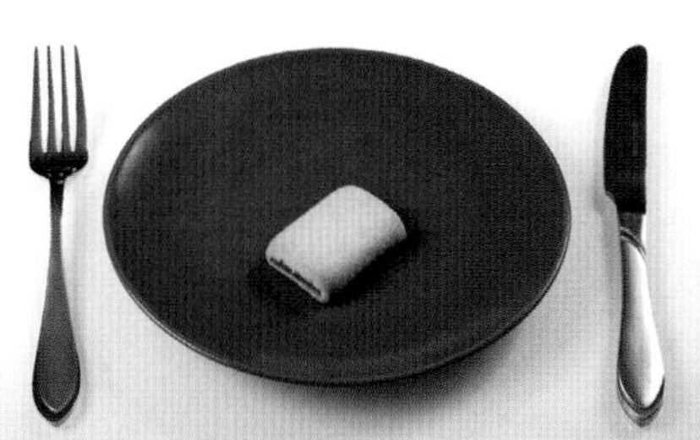

FIBRE	Weight	SAT FAT
1g	Weight: 21g	1g

Ginger Biscuit

CARBS	CALS	PROTEIN	FAT
8g	44	1g	1g

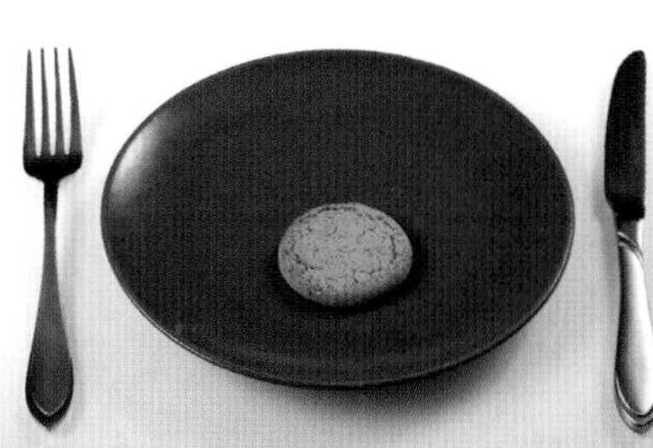

FIBRE	Weight	SAT FAT
0g	Weight: 10g	1g

Gingerbread Man

CARBS	CALS	PROTEIN	FAT
38g	222	3g	8g

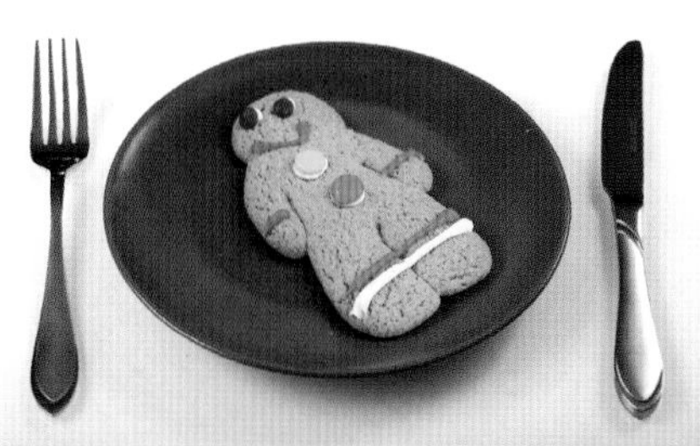

FIBRE	Weight	SAT FAT
1g	Weight: 58g	2g

Iced Ring

CARBS	CALS	PROTEIN	FAT
5g	27	0g	1g

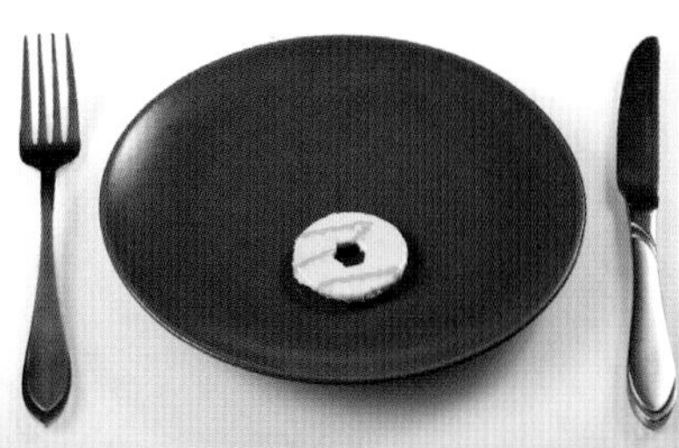

FIBRE	Weight	SAT FAT
0g	Weight: 6g	0g

20cm Side Plate

Jaffa Cake

CARBS	CALS	PROTEIN	FAT	FIBRE	SAT FAT	Weight
10g	49	1g	1g	0g	1g	13g

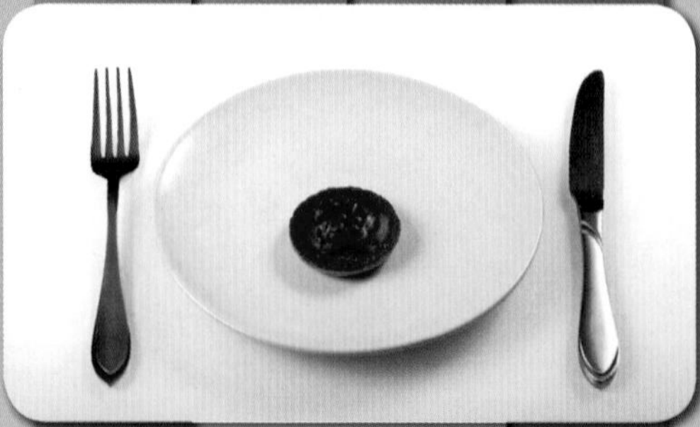

Jam Ring

CARBS	CALS	PROTEIN	FAT	FIBRE	SAT FAT	Weight
13g	79	1g	3g	0g	1g	18g

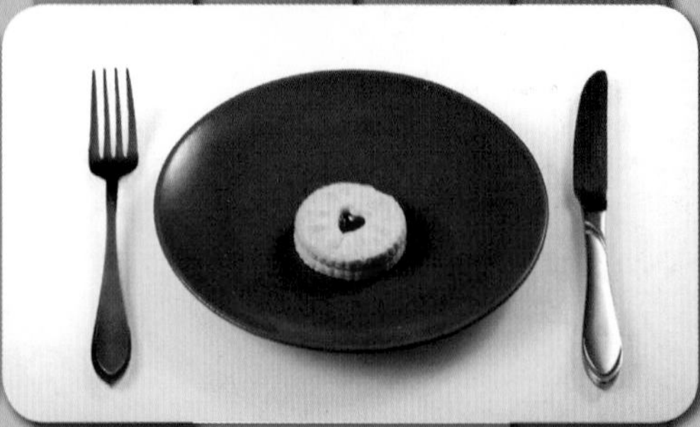

Malted Milk

CARBS	CALS	PROTEIN	FAT	FIBRE	SAT FAT	Weight
5g	40	1g	2g	0g	1g	8g

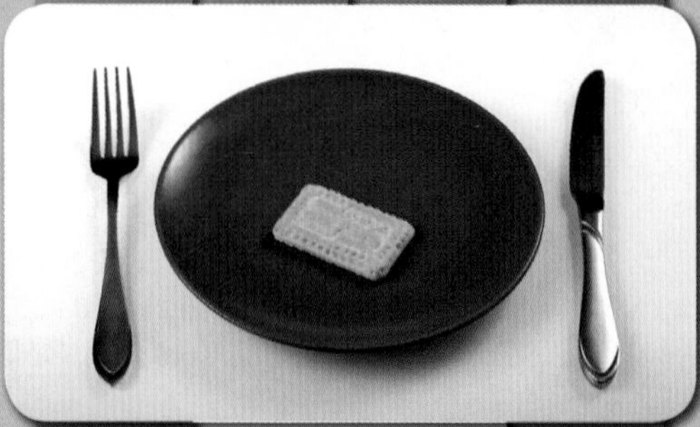

Milk Chocolate Biscuit Bar

CARBS	CALS	PROTEIN	FAT	FIBRE	SAT FAT	Weight
12g	103	1g	5g	1g	3g	20g

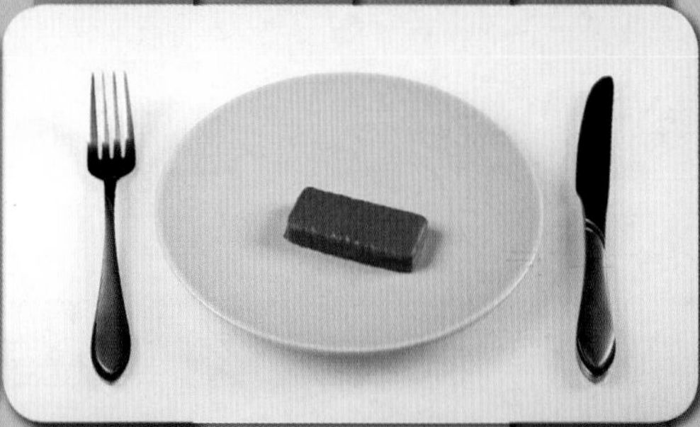

Milk Chocolate Finger

CARBS	CALS	PROTEIN	FAT	FIBRE	SAT FAT	Weight
3g	26	0g	1g	0g	1g	5g

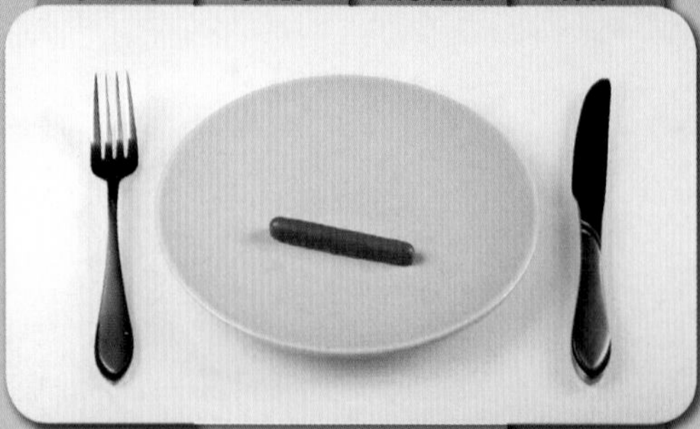

Milk Chocolate Wafer

CARBS	CALS	PROTEIN	FAT	FIBRE	SAT FAT	Weight
13g	107	1g	6g	0g	4g	21g

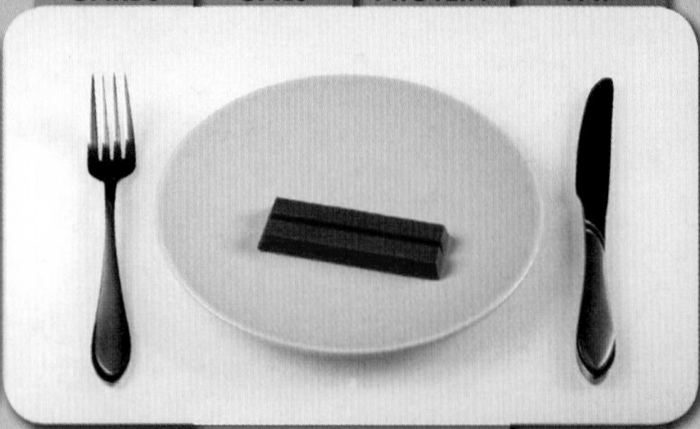

Nice Biscuit

5g CARBS	40 CALS	1g PROTEIN	2g FAT

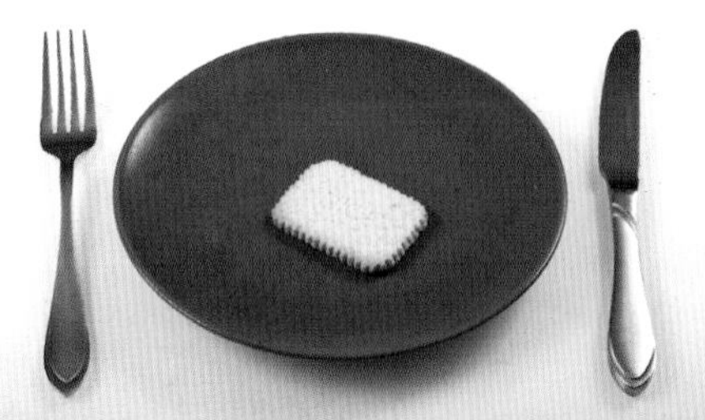

0g FIBRE	Weight: 8g	1g SAT FAT

Oat Biscuit

10g CARBS	76 CALS	1g PROTEIN	3g FAT

1g FIBRE	Weight: 16g	0g SAT FAT

Pink Wafer

6g CARBS	49 CALS	0g PROTEIN	3g FAT

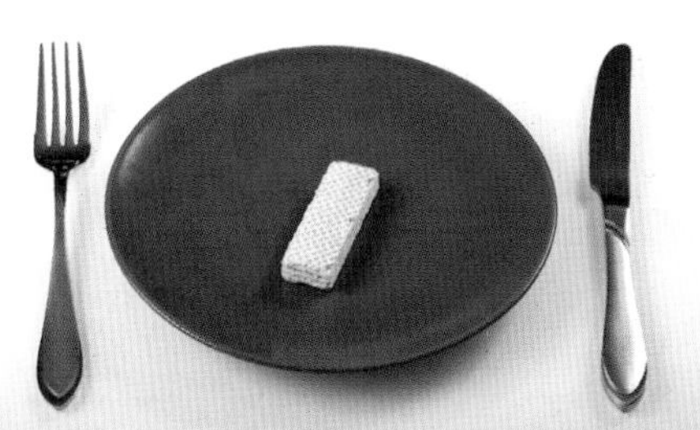

0g FIBRE	Weight: 9g	2g SAT FAT

Rich Tea

5g CARBS	31 CALS	1g PROTEIN	1g FAT

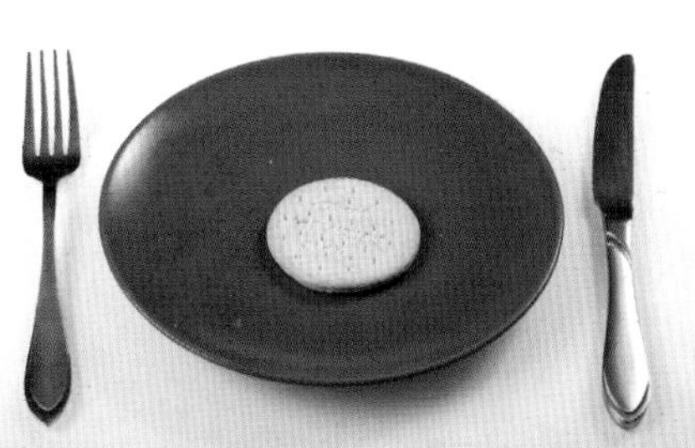

0g FIBRE	Weight: 7g	0g SAT FAT

Shortbread Finger

10g CARBS	81 CALS	1g PROTEIN	4g FAT

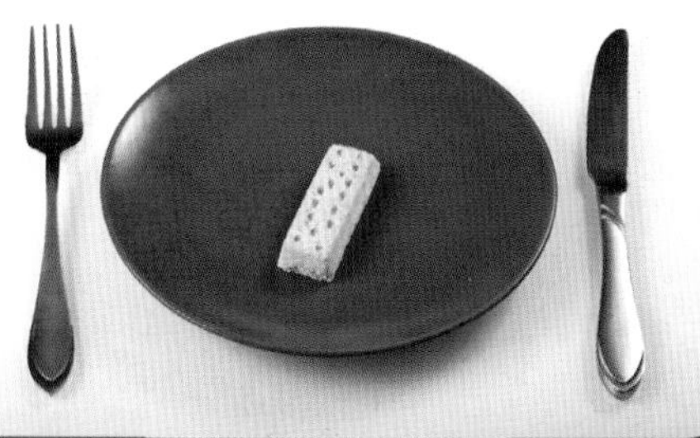

0g FIBRE	Weight: 16g	3g SAT FAT

Shortcake

6g CARBS	50 CALS	1g PROTEIN	3g FAT

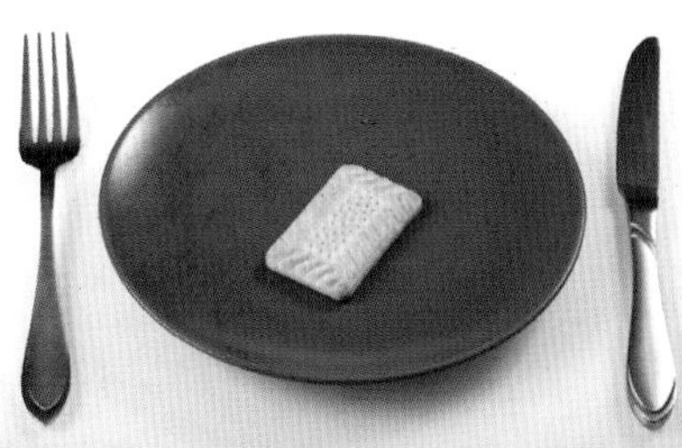

0g FIBRE	Weight: 10g	1g SAT FAT

Breadstick

CARBS	CALS	PROTEIN	FAT	FIBRE	SAT FAT	Weight
4g	20	1g	0g	0g	0g	5g

Cheddar

CARBS	CALS	PROTEIN	FAT	FIBRE	SAT FAT	Weight
3g	26	1g	2g	0g	1g	5g

Cheese Straw

CARBS	CALS	PROTEIN	FAT	FIBRE	SAT FAT	Weight
3g	35	1g	2g	0g	1g	7g

Cream Cracker

CARBS	CALS	PROTEIN	FAT	FIBRE	SAT FAT	Weight
6g	33	1g	1g	0g	0g	8g

Crispbread

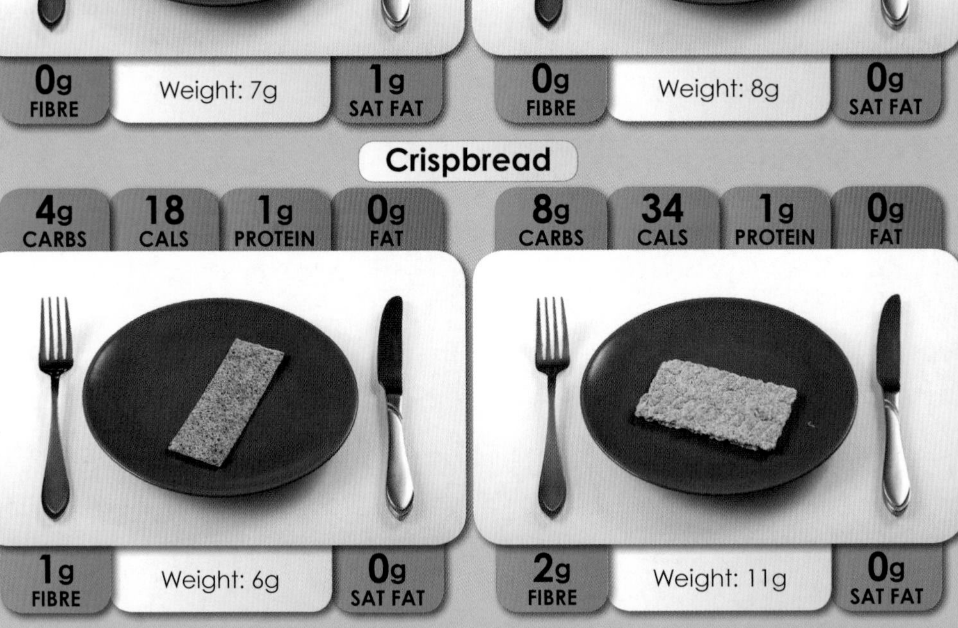

CARBS	CALS	PROTEIN	FAT	FIBRE	SAT FAT	Weight
4g	18	1g	0g	1g	0g	6g

CARBS	CALS	PROTEIN	FAT	FIBRE	SAT FAT	Weight
8g	34	1g	0g	2g	0g	11g

Digestive (savoury)

9g CARBS	61 CALS	1g PROTEIN	3g FAT

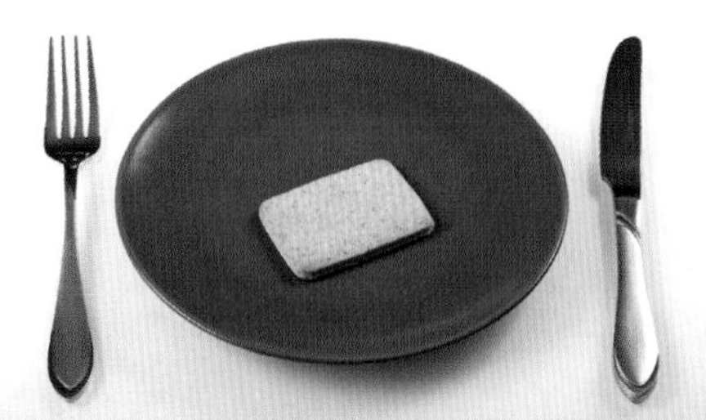

1g FIBRE	Weight: 13g	1g SAT FAT

Oatcake

6g CARBS	45 CALS	1g PROTEIN	2g FAT

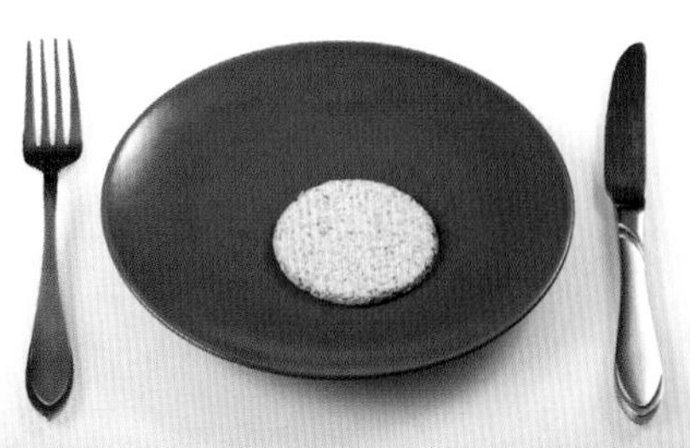

1g FIBRE	Weight: 10g	1g SAT FAT

Puffed Cracker

5g CARBS	47 CALS	1g PROTEIN	3g FAT

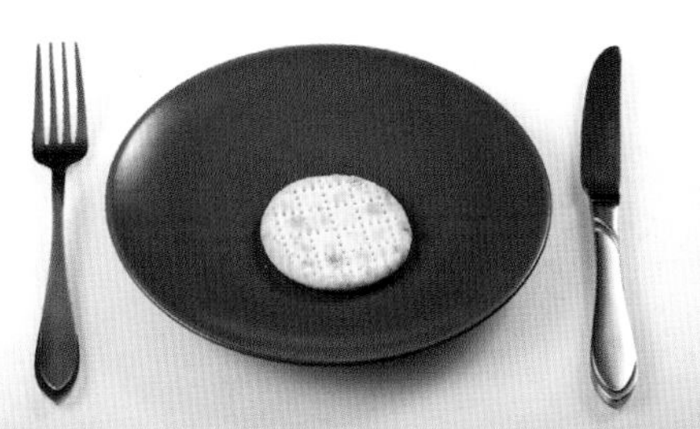

0g FIBRE	Weight: 9g	1g SAT FAT

Rice Cake

7g CARBS	30 CALS	1g PROTEIN	0g FAT

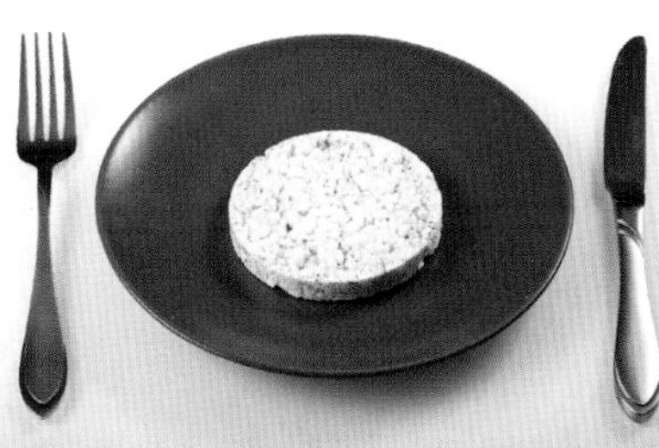

0g FIBRE	Weight: 8g	0g SAT FAT

Water Biscuit

5g CARBS	26 CALS	1g PROTEIN	1g FAT

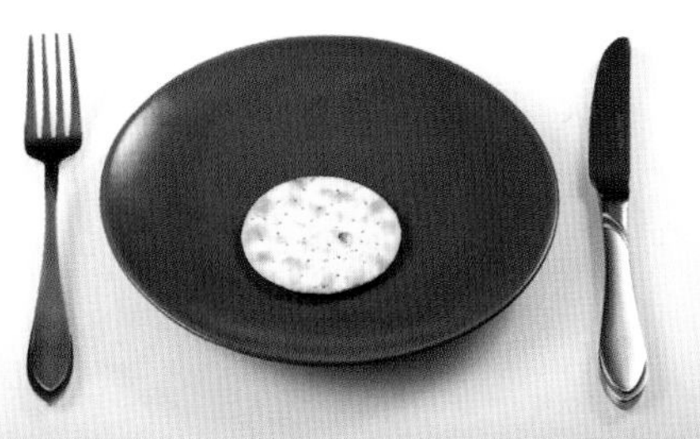

0g FIBRE	Weight: 6g	0g SAT FAT

Wholegrain Cracker

6g CARBS	33 CALS	1g PROTEIN	1g FAT

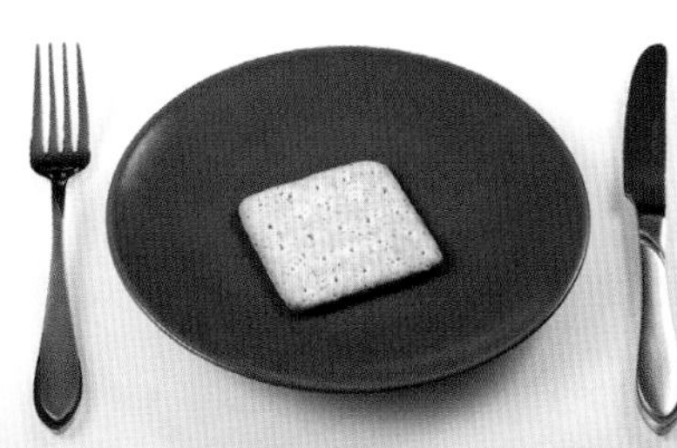

1g FIBRE	Weight: 8g	0g SAT FAT

Granary Bread

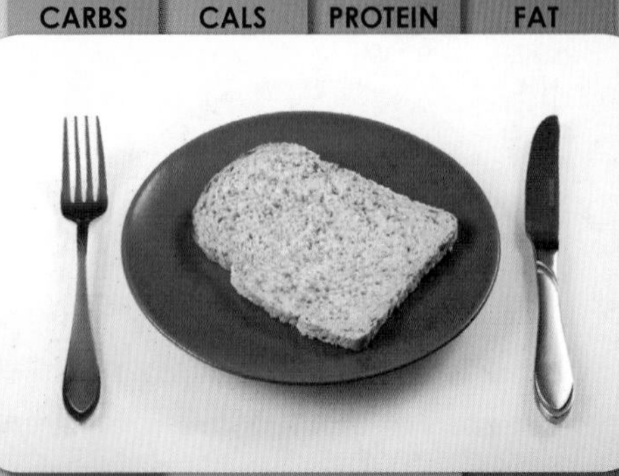

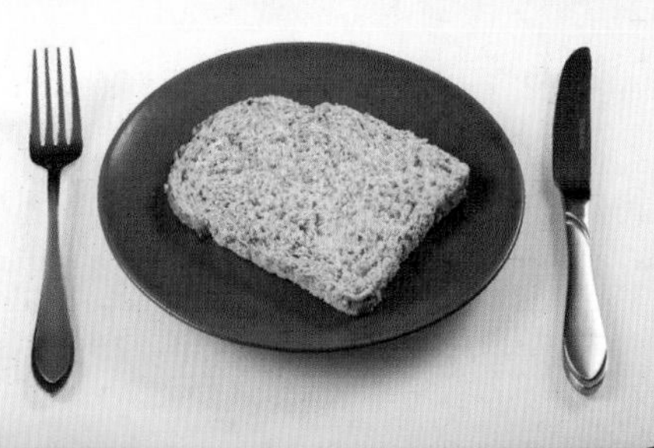

Weight	Carbs	Cals	Protein	Fat	Fibre	Sat Fat
22g (thin slice)	10g	52	2g	1g	1g	0g
33g (medium slice)	16g	78	3g	1g	2g	0g
44g (thick slice)	21g	104	4g	1g	2g	0g

White Bread

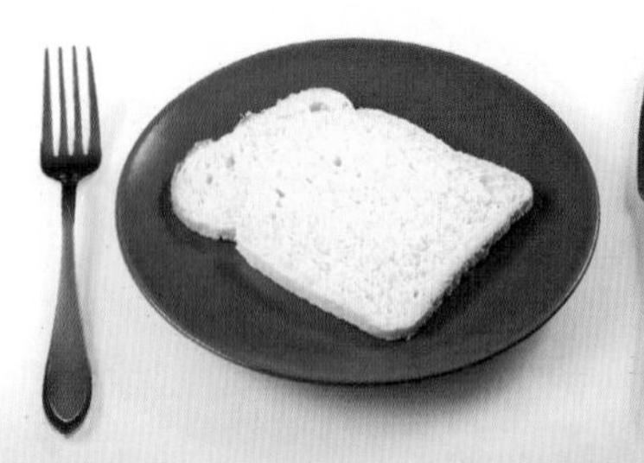

Weight	Carbs	Cals	Protein	Fat	Fibre	Sat Fat
22g (thin slice)	10g	48	2g	0g	1g	0g
33g (medium slice)	15g	72	3g	1g	1g	0g
44g (thick slice)	20g	96	4g	1g	1g	0g

Wholemeal Bread

9g CARBS	48 CALS	2g PROTEIN	1g FAT

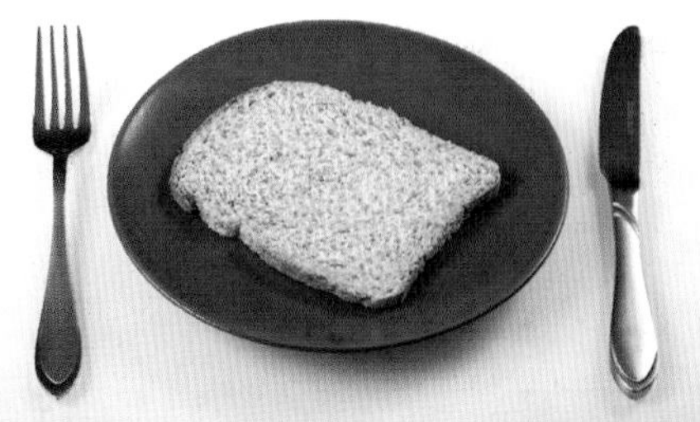

2g FIBRE	Weight: 22g (thin slice)	0g SAT FAT

14g CARBS	72 CALS	3g PROTEIN	1g FAT

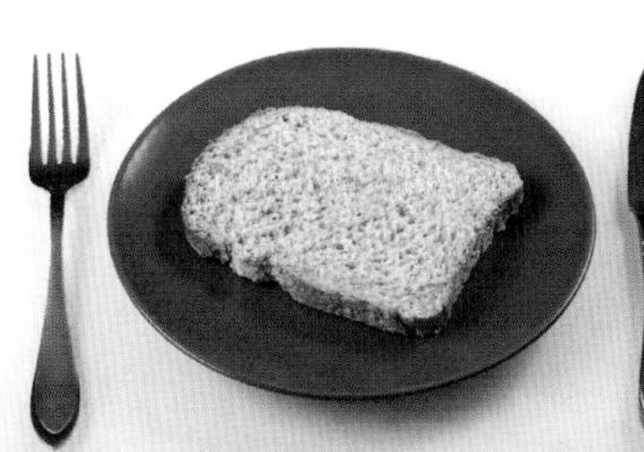

2g FIBRE	Weight: 33g (medium slice)	0g SAT FAT

19g CARBS	96 CALS	4g PROTEIN	1g FAT

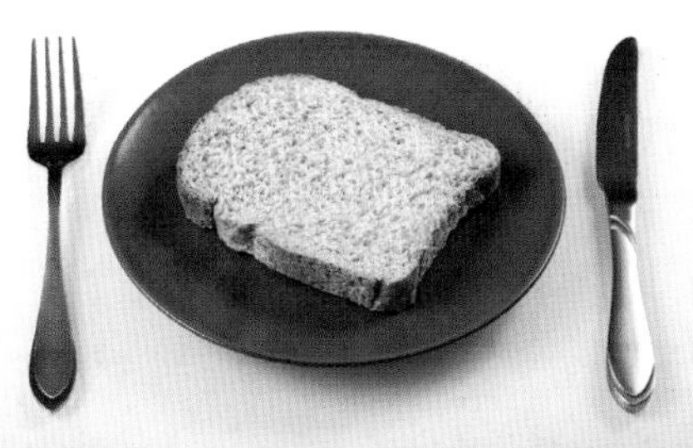

3g FIBRE	Weight: 44g (thick slice)	0g SAT FAT

White Wholemeal Bread

9g CARBS	51 CALS	2g PROTEIN	1g FAT

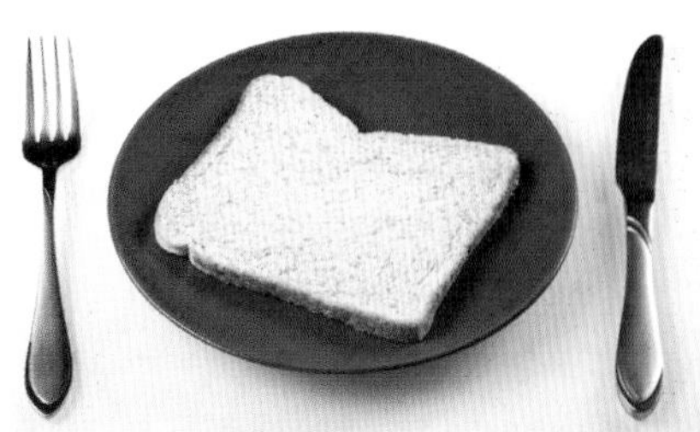

1g FIBRE	Weight: 22g (thin slice)	0g SAT FAT

14g CARBS	76 CALS	3g PROTEIN	1g FAT

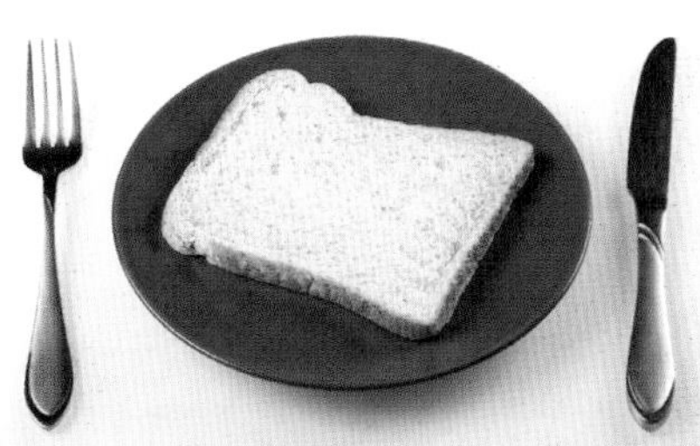

2g FIBRE	Weight: 33g (medium slice)	0g SAT FAT

18g CARBS	102 CALS	4g PROTEIN	1g FAT

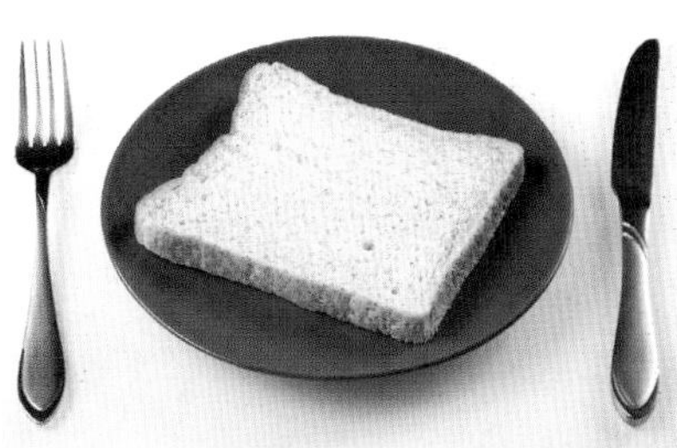

2g FIBRE	Weight: 44g (thick slice)	0g SAT FAT

Bap (white)

CARBS	CALS	PROTEIN	FAT	FIBRE	Weight	SAT FAT
25g	122	5g	1g	1g	Weight: 48g	0g
60g	295	11g	3g	3g	Weight: 116g	1g

Bap (wholemeal)

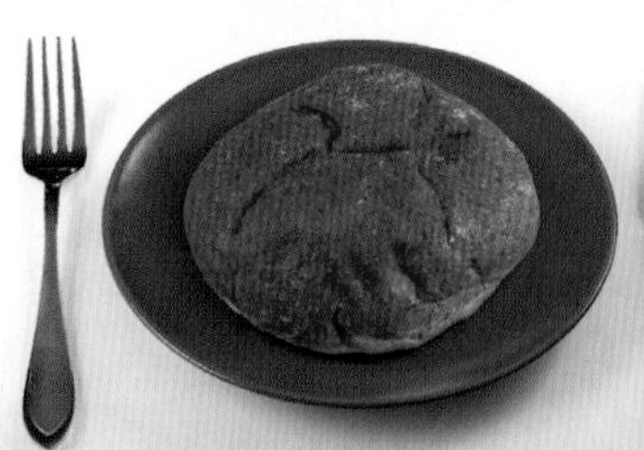

CARBS	CALS	PROTEIN	FAT	FIBRE	Weight	SAT FAT
24g	124	5g	2g	3g	Weight: 51g	0g
53g	278	12g	4g	6g	Weight: 114g	1g

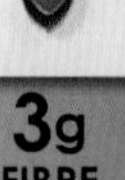

Crusty Roll (white)

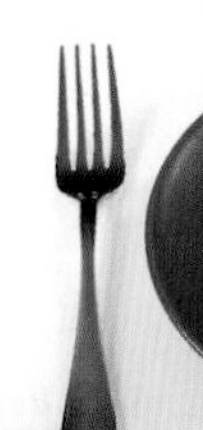

CARBS	CALS	PROTEIN	FAT	FIBRE	Weight	SAT FAT
24g	113	4g	1g	1g	Weight: 43g	0g
47g	225	8g	2g	3g	Weight: 86g	0g

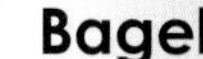

Bagel

CARBS	CALS	PROTEIN	FAT
45g	227	8g	1g

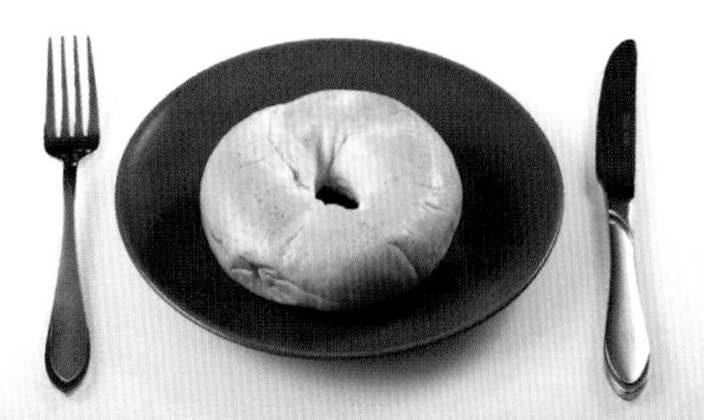

FIBRE	Weight	SAT FAT
3g	Weight: 86g	0g

English Muffin

CARBS	CALS	PROTEIN	FAT
35g	178	8g	2g

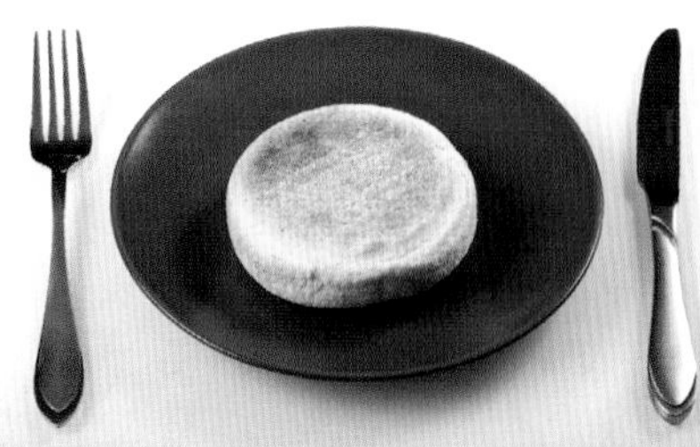

FIBRE	Weight	SAT FAT
2g	Weight: 68g	0g

Crumpet

CARBS	CALS	PROTEIN	FAT
17g	86	3g	0g

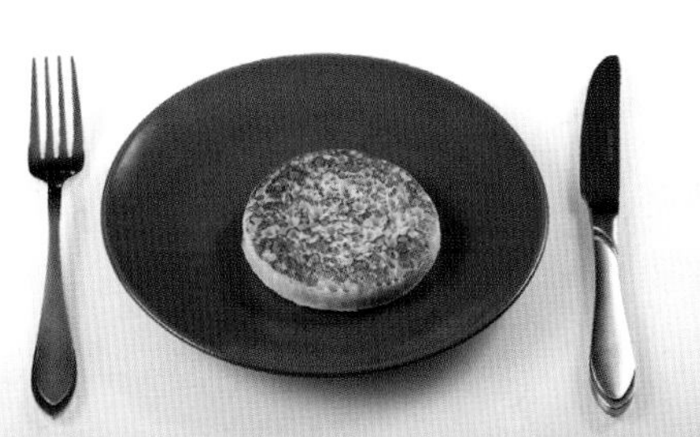

FIBRE	Weight	SAT FAT
1g	Weight: 45g	0g

Crumpet (square)

CARBS	CALS	PROTEIN	FAT
26g	118	4g	1g

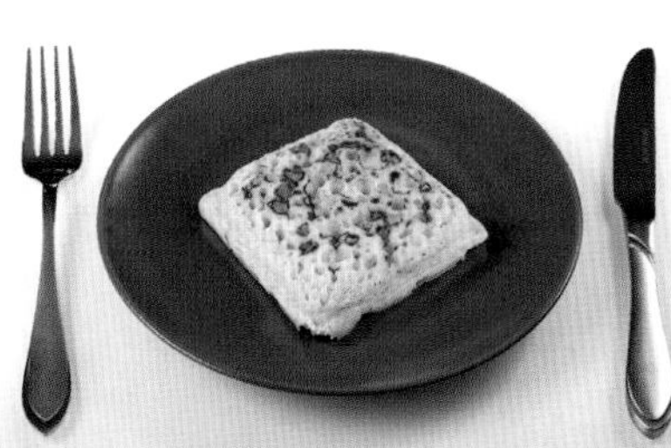

FIBRE	Weight	SAT FAT
1g	Weight: 57g	0g

Poppy Seeded Roll

CARBS	CALS	PROTEIN	FAT
26g	161	6g	4g

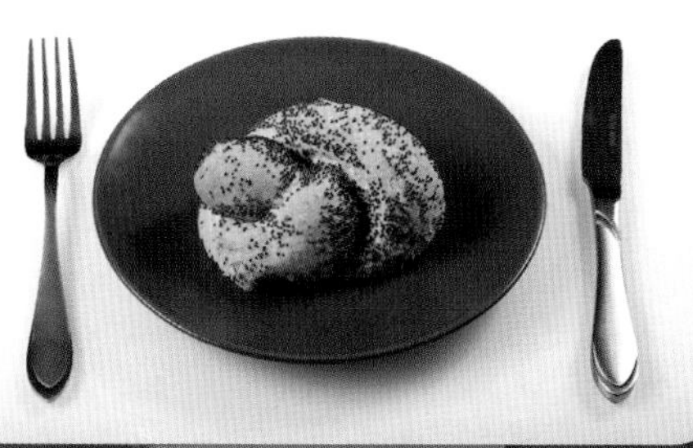

FIBRE	Weight	SAT FAT
2g	Weight: 54g	1g

Tea Cake

CARBS	CALS	PROTEIN	FAT
43g	239	7g	4g

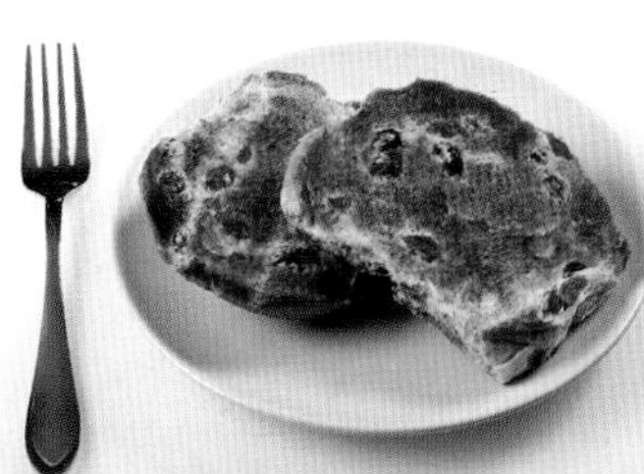

FIBRE	Weight	SAT FAT
3g	Weight: 85g	1g

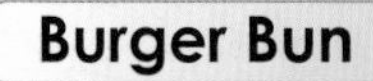

Burger Bun

40g CARBS	217 CALS	8g PROTEIN	4g FAT

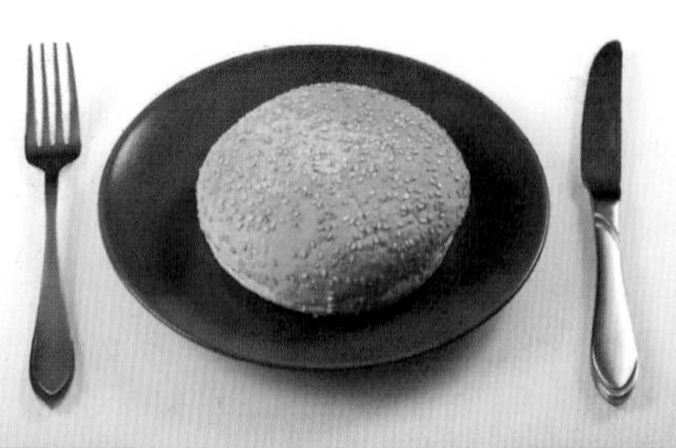

2g FIBRE	Weight: 82g	1g SAT FAT

Finger Roll

21g CARBS	104 CALS	4g PROTEIN	1g FAT

1g FIBRE	Weight: 41g	0g SAT FAT

Ciabatta

50g CARBS	263 CALS	10g PROTEIN	4g FAT

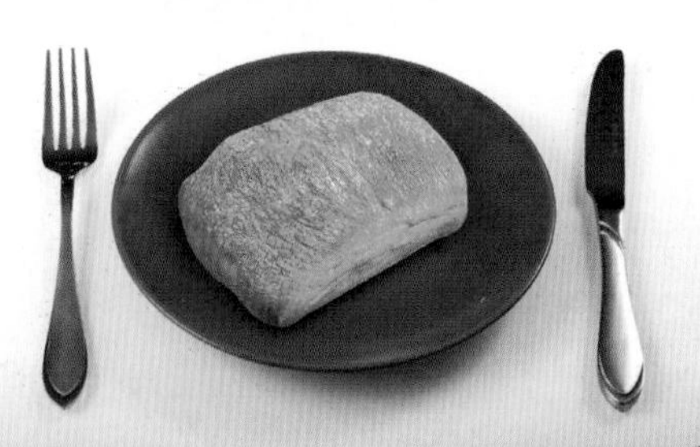

3g FIBRE	Weight: 97g	1g SAT FAT

Panini

47g CARBS	277 CALS	10g PROTEIN	5g FAT

3g FIBRE	Weight: 100g	1g SAT FAT

Focaccia

28g CARBS	192 CALS	6g PROTEIN	7g FAT

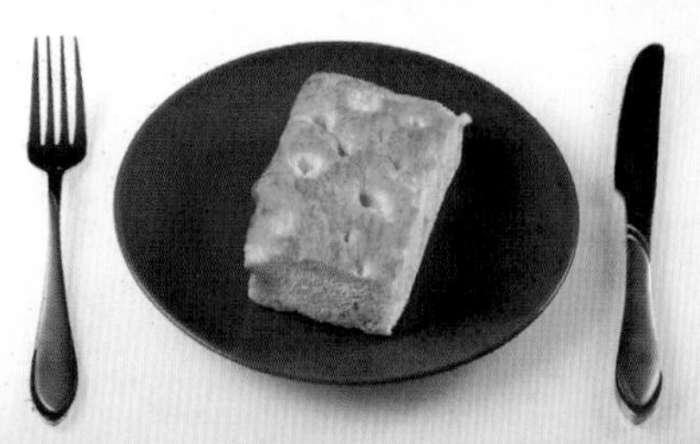

1g FIBRE	Weight: 60g	1g SAT FAT

57g CARBS	384 CALS	12g PROTEIN	13g FAT

3g FIBRE	Weight: 120g	2g SAT FAT

Baguette

CARBS	CALS	PROTEIN	FAT	FIBRE	Weight	SAT FAT
17g	79	3g	1g	1g	Weight: 30g	0g
48g	224	8g	2g	3g	Weight: 85g	0g

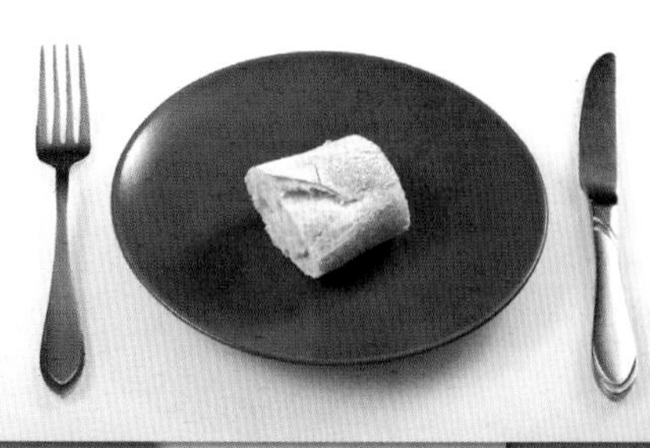

Croutons

CARBS	CALS	PROTEIN	FAT	FIBRE	Weight	SAT FAT
10g	66	2g	2g	1g	Weight: 15g	0g
20g	132	4g	4g	1g	Weight: 30g	0g

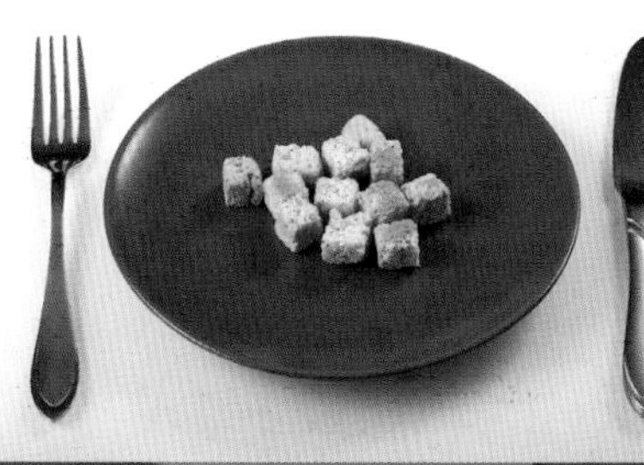

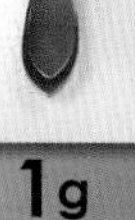

Garlic Bread

CARBS	CALS	PROTEIN	FAT	FIBRE	Weight	SAT FAT
10g	76	2g	3g	1g	Weight: 22g	2g

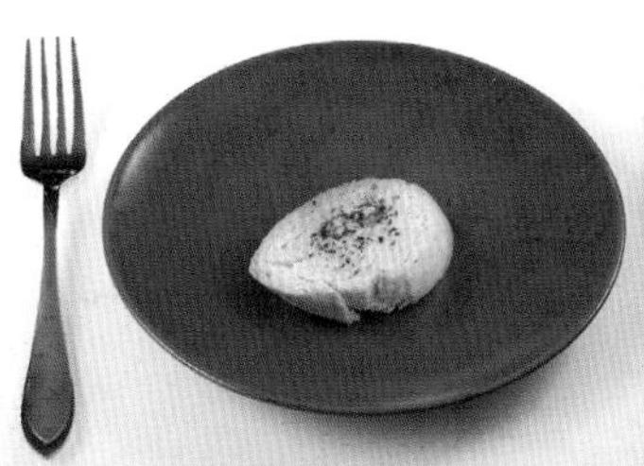

Rye Bread

CARBS	CALS	PROTEIN	FAT	FIBRE	Weight	SAT FAT
33g	158	6g	1g	4g	Weight: 72g	0g

20cm Side Plate / 26cm Dinner Plate

Pitta Bread (white)

CARBS	CALS	PROTEIN	FAT	FIBRE	SAT FAT	Weight
19g	89	3g	1g	1g	0g	35g (mini)
38g	176	6g	1g	2g	0g	69g

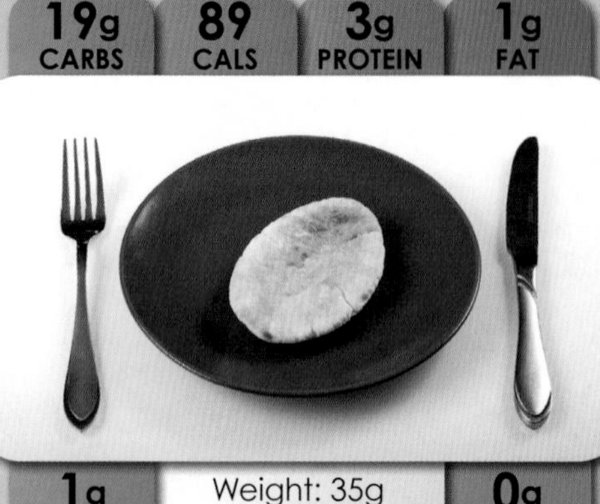

Pitta Bread (wholemeal)

CARBS	CALS	PROTEIN	FAT	FIBRE	SAT FAT	Weight
14g	73	3g	1g	2g	0g	30g (mini)
27g	147	7g	1g	4g	0g	60g

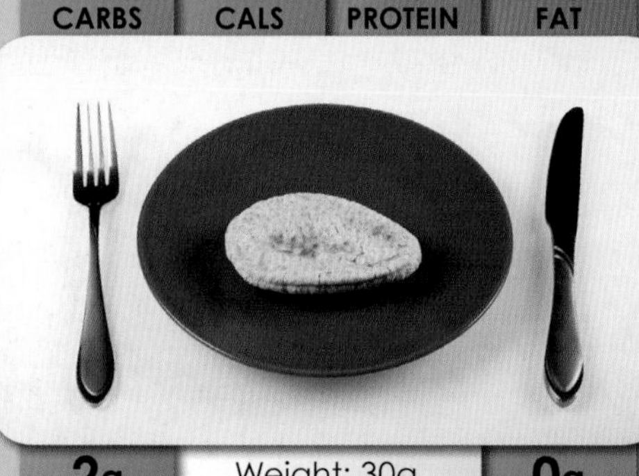

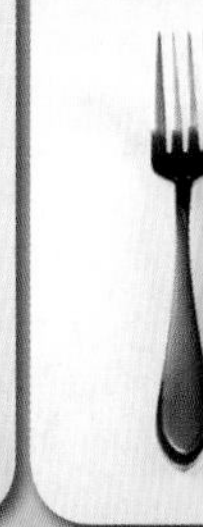

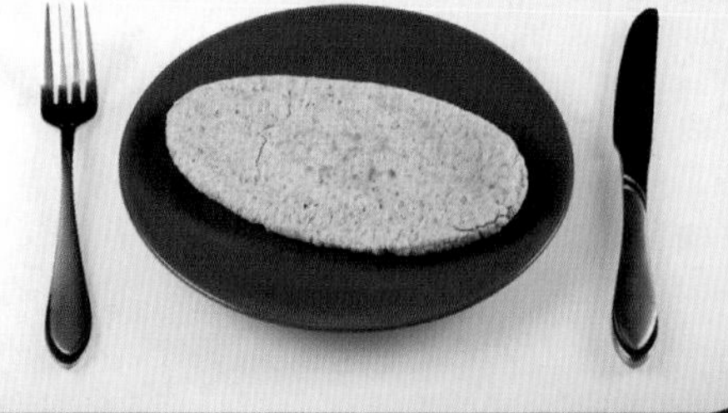

Turkish Flatbread

CARBS	CALS	PROTEIN	FAT	FIBRE	SAT FAT	Weight
35g	169	6g	1g	2g	0g	60g

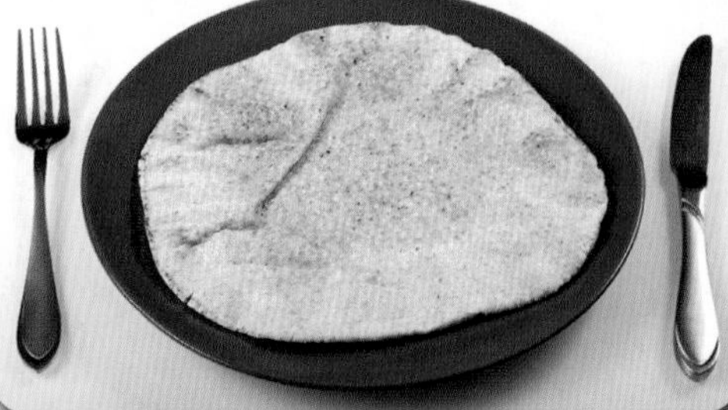

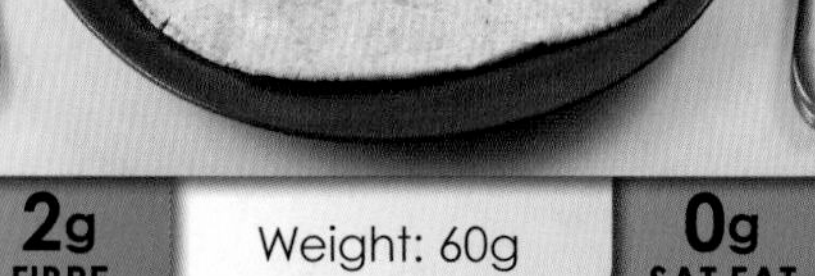

Taco Shell

CARBS	CALS	PROTEIN	FAT	FIBRE	SAT FAT	Weight
9g	77	1g	4g	1g	2g	15g

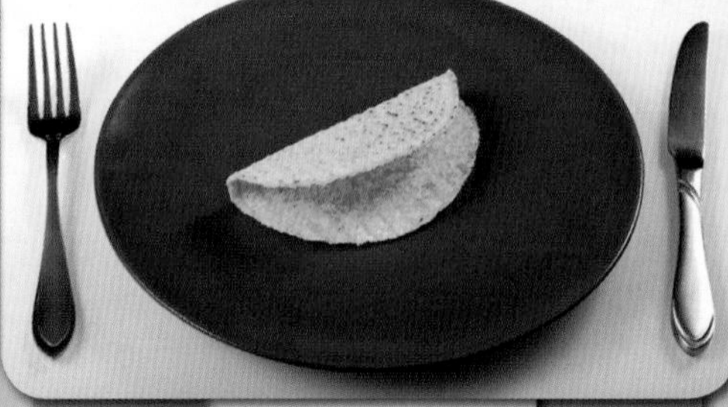

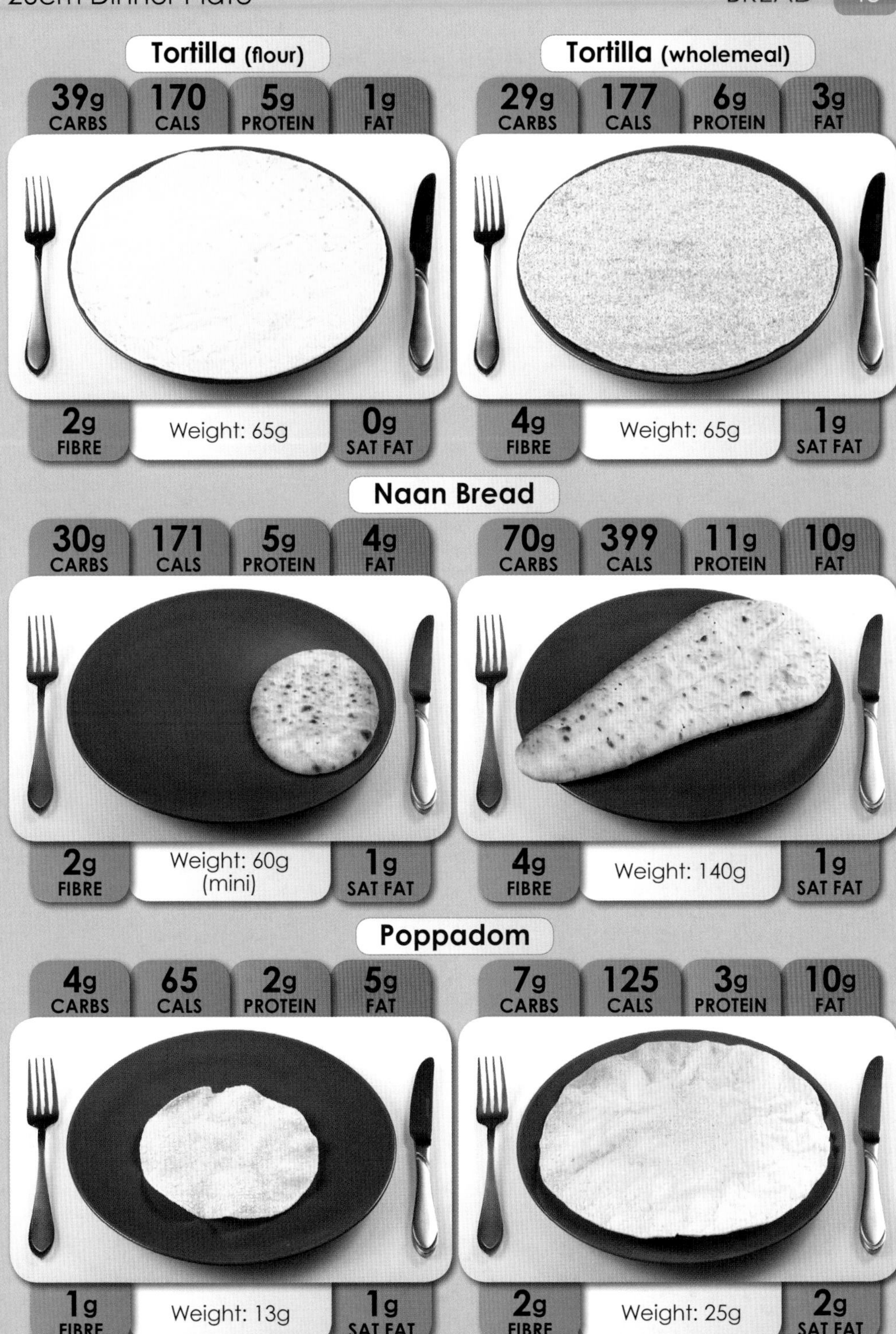

Tortilla (flour)

CARBS	CALS	PROTEIN	FAT	FIBRE	SAT FAT	Weight
39g	170	5g	1g	2g	0g	65g

Tortilla (wholemeal)

CARBS	CALS	PROTEIN	FAT	FIBRE	SAT FAT	Weight
29g	177	6g	3g	4g	1g	65g

Naan Bread

CARBS	CALS	PROTEIN	FAT	FIBRE	SAT FAT	Weight
30g	171	5g	4g	2g	1g	60g (mini)
70g	399	11g	10g	4g	1g	140g

Poppadom

CARBS	CALS	PROTEIN	FAT	FIBRE	SAT FAT	Weight
4g	65	2g	5g	1g	1g	13g
7g	125	3g	10g	2g	2g	25g

Chapati (without fat)

Carbs	Cals	Protein	Fat
39g	182	7g	1g

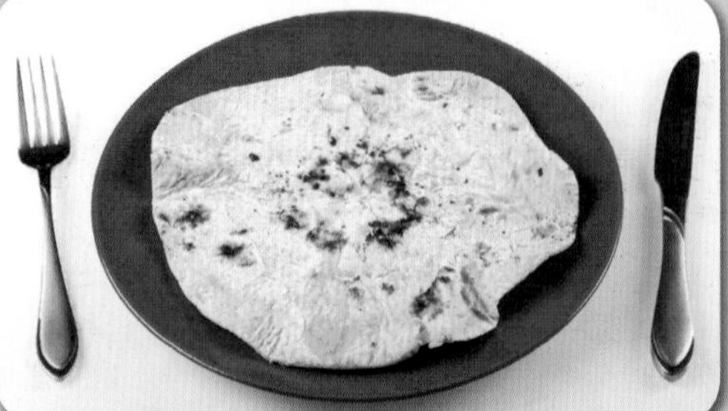

Fibre	Weight	Sat Fat
3g	Weight: 90g	0g

Carbs	Cals	Protein	Fat
52g	242	9g	1g

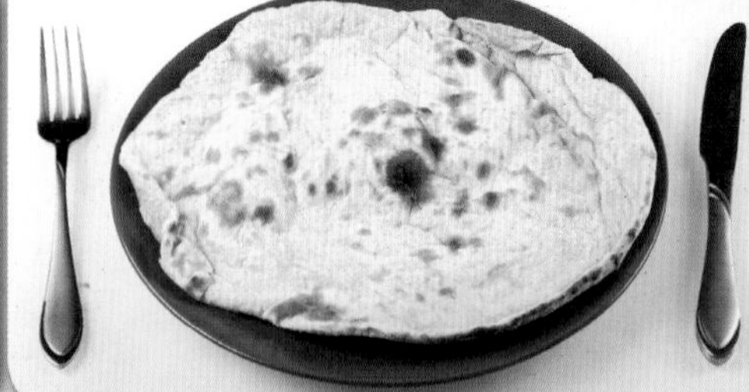

Fibre	Weight	Sat Fat
3g	Weight: 120g	0g

Chapati (with butter)

Carbs	Cals	Protein	Fat
36g	219	6g	7g

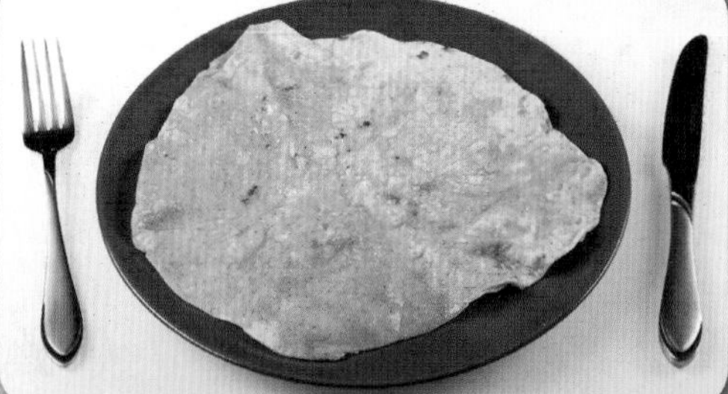

Fibre	Weight	Sat Fat
2g	Weight: 90g	4g

Paratha

Carbs	Cals	Protein	Fat
40g	297	8g	13g

Fibre	Weight	Sat Fat
5g	Weight: 92g	8g

Puri

Carbs	Cals	Protein	Fat
46g	392	8g	21g

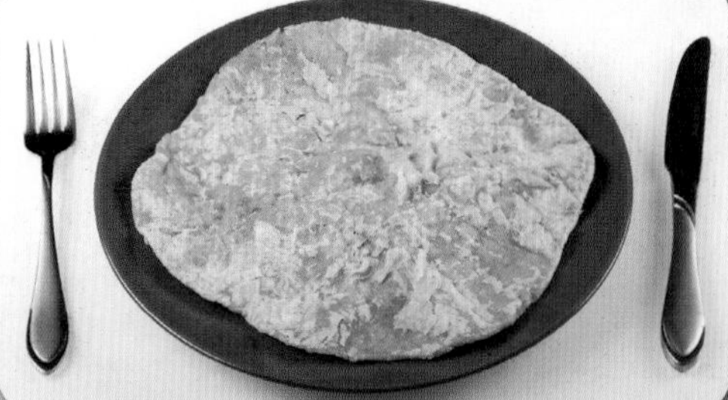

Fibre	Weight	Sat Fat
3g	Weight: 125g	3g

Roti

Carbs	Cals	Protein	Fat
20g	94	4g	1g

Fibre	Weight	Sat Fat
2g	Weight: 43g	0g

Brioche

	Carbs	Cals	Protein	Fat	Fibre	Sat Fat	Weight
Small	9g	64	1g	2g	0g	1g	18g
Large	24g	159	4g	5g	1g	3g	45g

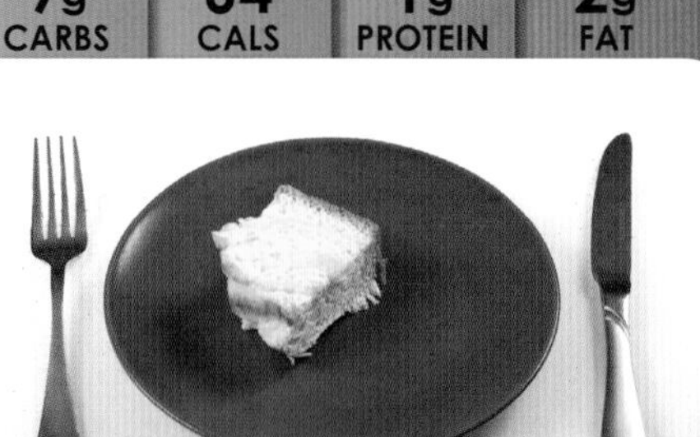
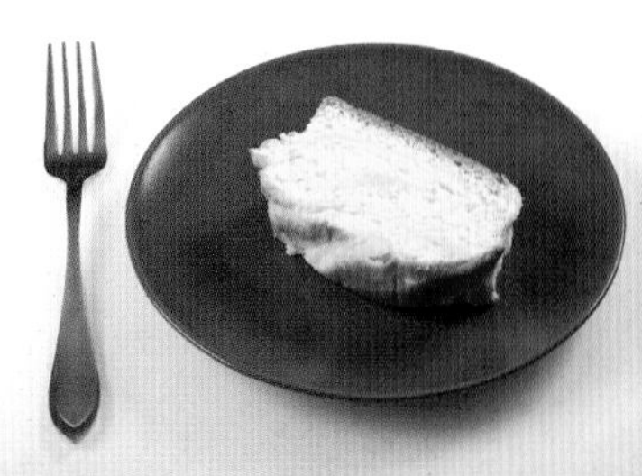

Croissant

	Carbs	Cals	Protein	Fat	Fibre	Sat Fat	Weight
Small	11g	97	2g	5g	1g	3g	26g
Large	22g	190	4g	10g	2g	5g	51g

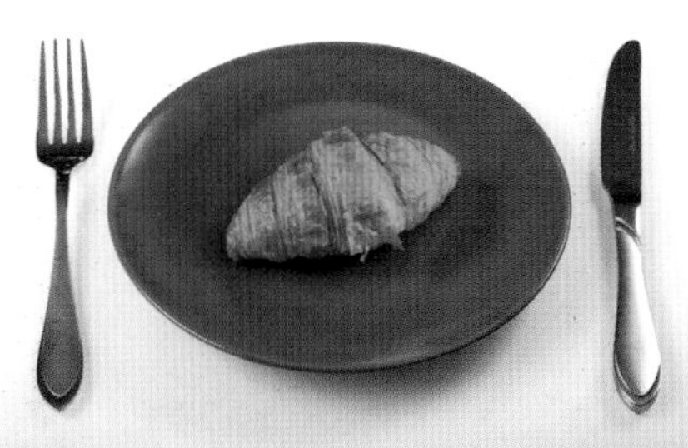

Pain au Chocolat

	Carbs	Cals	Protein	Fat	Fibre	Sat Fat	Weight
Small	15g	142	3g	8g	1g	5g	32g
Large	29g	274	5g	15g	2g	9g	64g

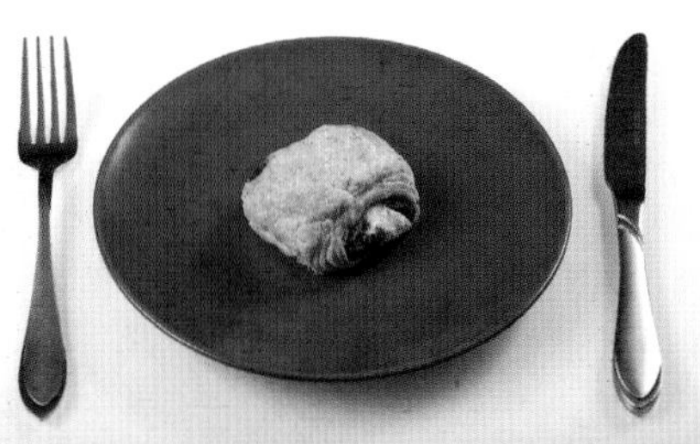
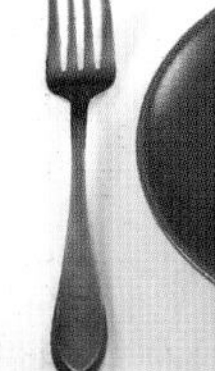

All Bran

9g CARBS	54 CALS	3g PROTEIN	1g FAT
6g FIBRE	Weight: 20g	0g SAT FAT	

18g CARBS	108 CALS	5g PROTEIN	2g FAT
12g FIBRE	Weight: 40g	0g SAT FAT	

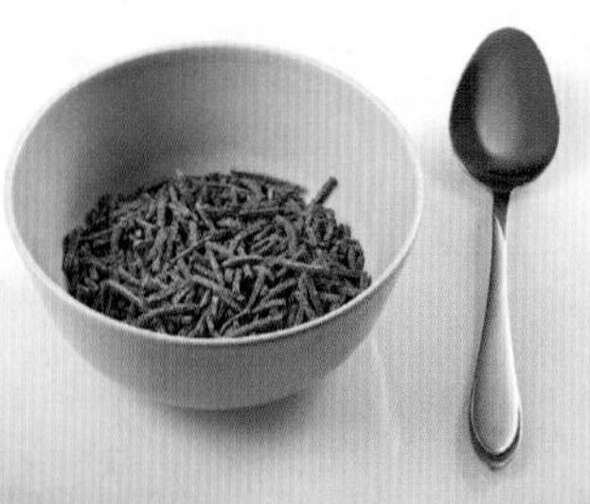

37g CARBS	216 CALS	10g PROTEIN	3g FAT
23g FIBRE	Weight: 80g	1g SAT FAT	

Bran Flakes

11g CARBS	50 CALS	2g PROTEIN	0g FAT
2g FIBRE	Weight: 15g	0g SAT FAT	

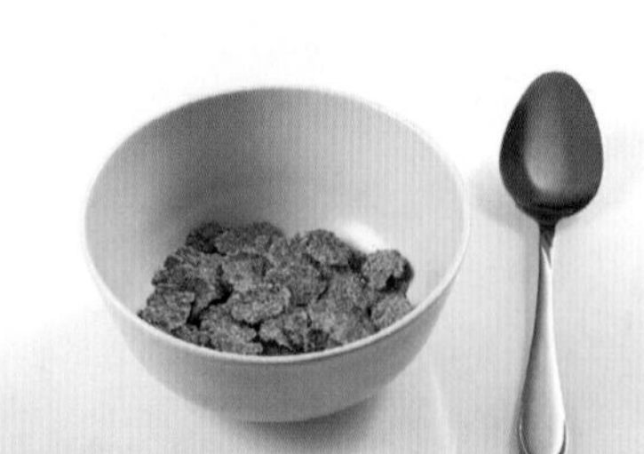

21g CARBS	99 CALS	3g PROTEIN	1g FAT
5g FIBRE	Weight: 30g	0g SAT FAT	

43g CARBS	198 CALS	6g PROTEIN	2g FAT
9g FIBRE	Weight: 60g	0g SAT FAT	

Chocolate Snaps

CARBS	CALS	PROTEIN	FAT
14g	58	1g	0g

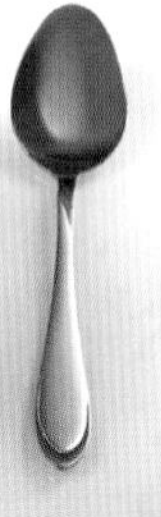

FIBRE	Weight	SAT FAT
0g	Weight: 15g	0g

CARBS	CALS	PROTEIN	FAT
28g	115	1g	1g

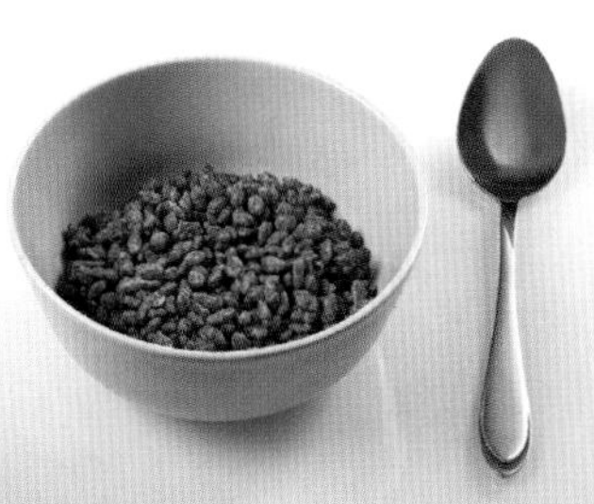

FIBRE	Weight	SAT FAT
1g	Weight: 30g	0g

CARBS	CALS	PROTEIN	FAT
55g	230	3g	2g

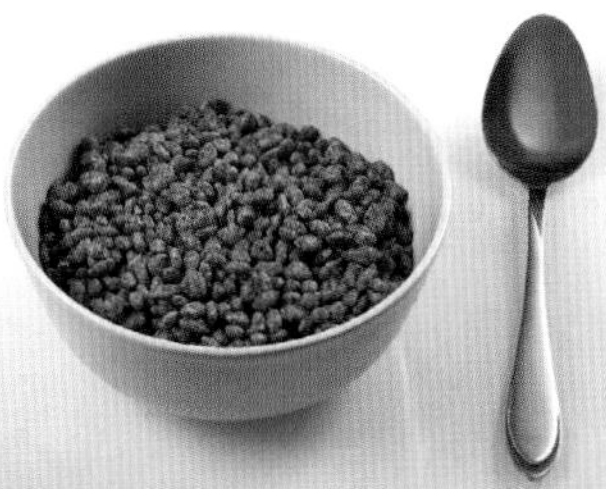

FIBRE	Weight	SAT FAT
2g	Weight: 60g	1g

Corn Flakes

CARBS	CALS	PROTEIN	FAT
13g	56	1g	0g

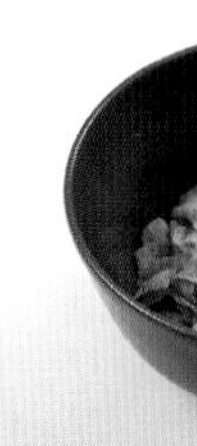

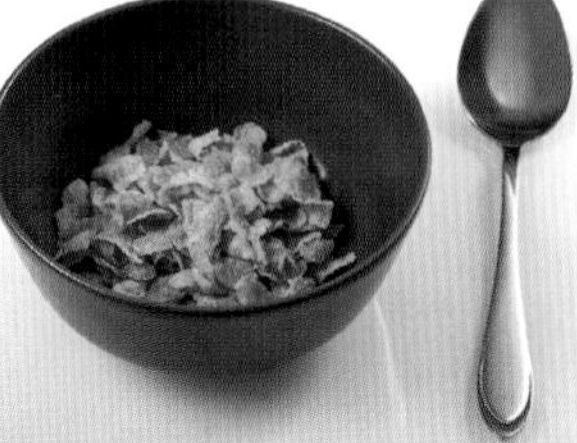

FIBRE	Weight	SAT FAT
1g	Weight: 15g	0g

CARBS	CALS	PROTEIN	FAT
27g	113	2g	0g

FIBRE	Weight	SAT FAT
1g	Weight: 30g	0g

CARBS	CALS	PROTEIN	FAT
54g	226	5g	1g

FIBRE	Weight	SAT FAT
2g	Weight: 60g	0g

Frosted Flakes

14g CARBS	57 CALS	1g PROTEIN	0g FAT

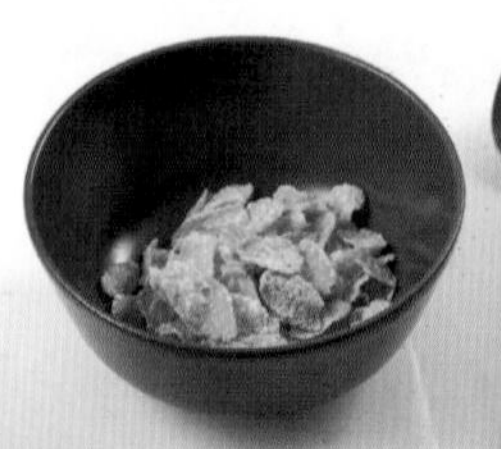

0g FIBRE	Weight: 15g	0g SAT FAT

28g CARBS	114 CALS	2g PROTEIN	0g FAT

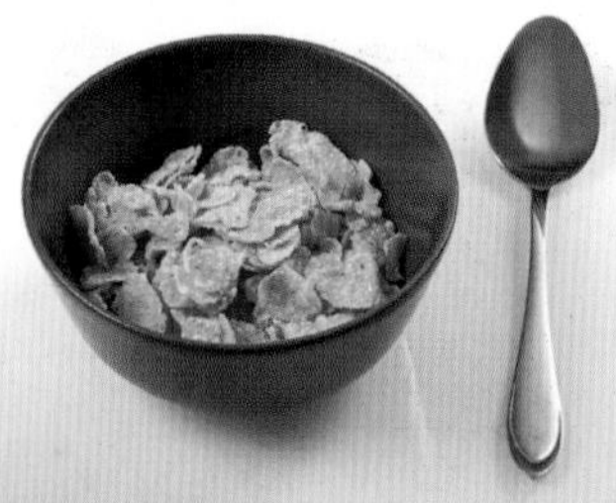

0g FIBRE	Weight: 30g	0g SAT FAT

57g CARBS	229 CALS	3g PROTEIN	0g FAT

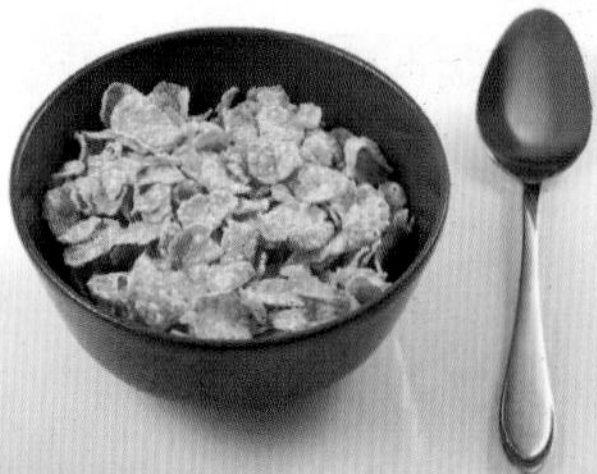

0g FIBRE	Weight: 60g	0g SAT FAT

Fruit & Fibre

15g CARBS	71 CALS	2g PROTEIN	1g FAT

2g FIBRE	Weight: 20g	1g SAT FAT

29g CARBS	141 CALS	4g PROTEIN	2g FAT

4g FIBRE	Weight: 40g	1g SAT FAT

58g CARBS	282 CALS	7g PROTEIN	4g FAT

7g FIBRE	Weight: 80g	2g SAT FAT

Granola

CARBS	CALS	PROTEIN	FAT	FIBRE	SAT FAT	Weight
22g	157	3g	6g	2g	1g	35g
44g	313	7g	12g	4g	2g	70g
66g	470	10g	18g	6g	3g	105g

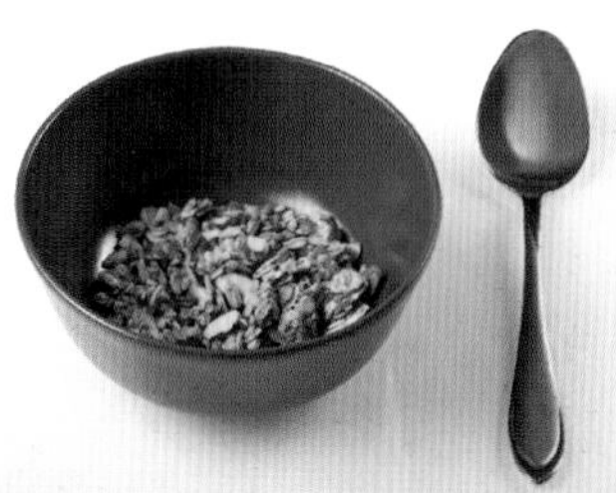

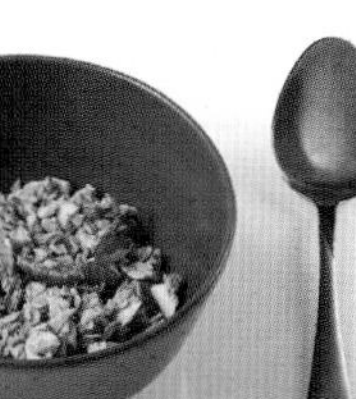

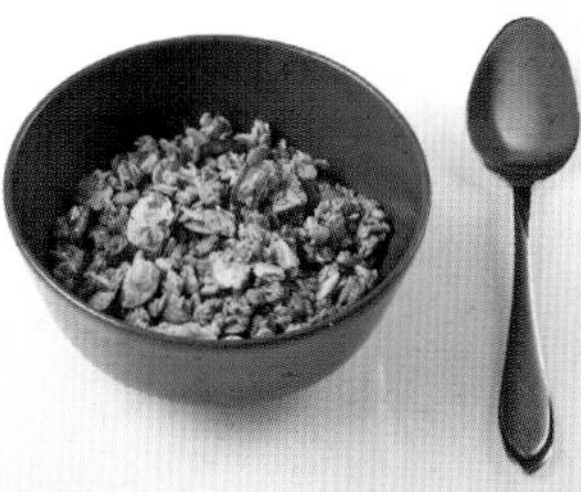

Honey Nut Flakes

CARBS	CALS	PROTEIN	FAT	FIBRE	SAT FAT	Weight
14g	61	1g	1g	0g	0g	15g
27g	122	2g	1g	1g	0g	30g
55g	243	4g	2g	2g	0g	60g

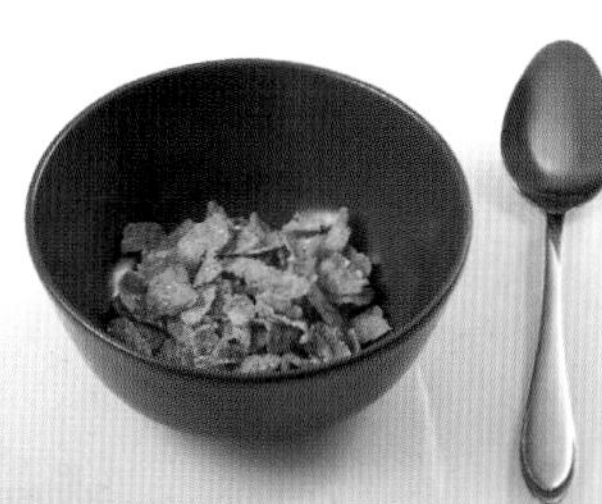

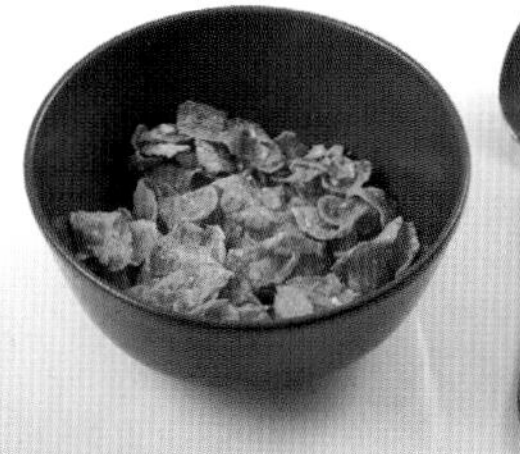

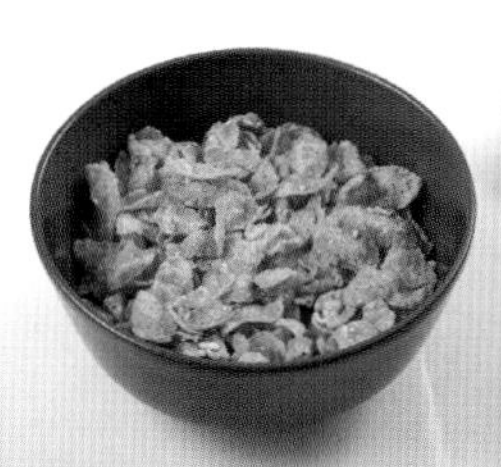

Honey Puffed Wheat

11g	46	1g	0g
CARBS	CALS	PROTEIN	FAT

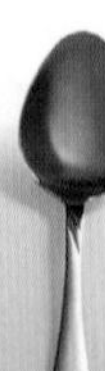

0g FIBRE	Weight: 12g	0g SAT FAT

32g	133	2g	0g
CARBS	CALS	PROTEIN	FAT

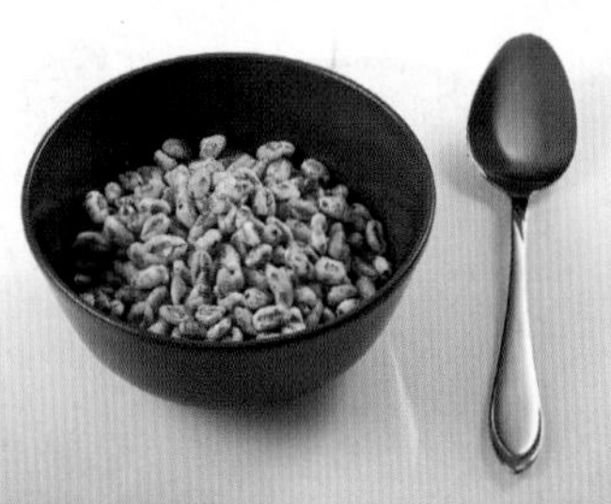

1g FIBRE	Weight: 35g	0g SAT FAT

54g	221	4g	1g
CARBS	CALS	PROTEIN	FAT

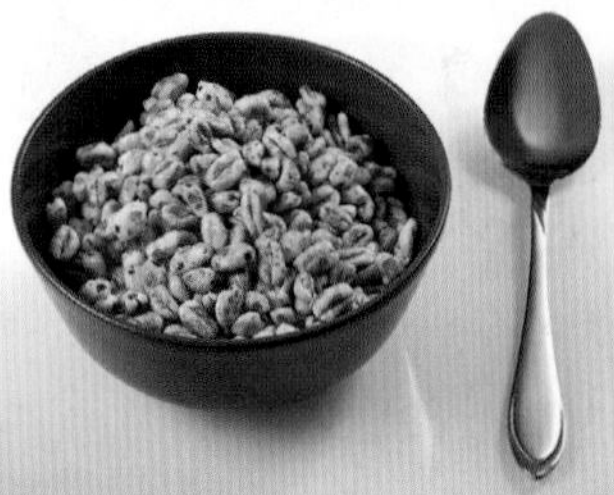

2g FIBRE	Weight: 58g	0g SAT FAT

Malted Wheats

11g	48	1g	0g
CARBS	CALS	PROTEIN	FAT

2g FIBRE	Weight: 14g	0g SAT FAT

33g	145	4g	1g
CARBS	CALS	PROTEIN	FAT

5g FIBRE	Weight: 42g	0g SAT FAT

54g	242	7g	1g
CARBS	CALS	PROTEIN	FAT

8g FIBRE	Weight: 70g	0g SAT FAT

Muesli

CARBS	CALS	PROTEIN	FAT
22g	109	3g	2g

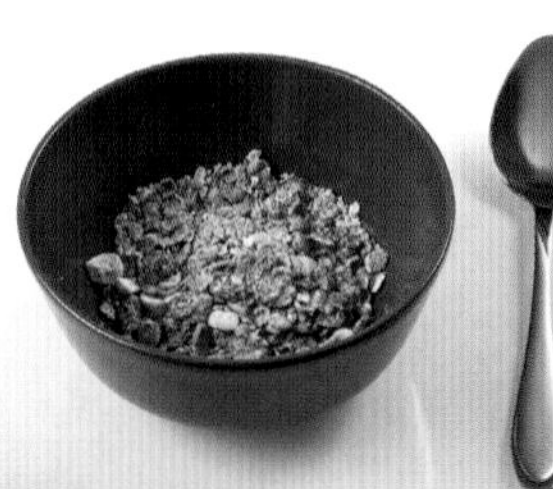

FIBRE	Weight	SAT FAT
3g	Weight: 30g	0g

CARBS	CALS	PROTEIN	FAT
43g	218	6g	4g

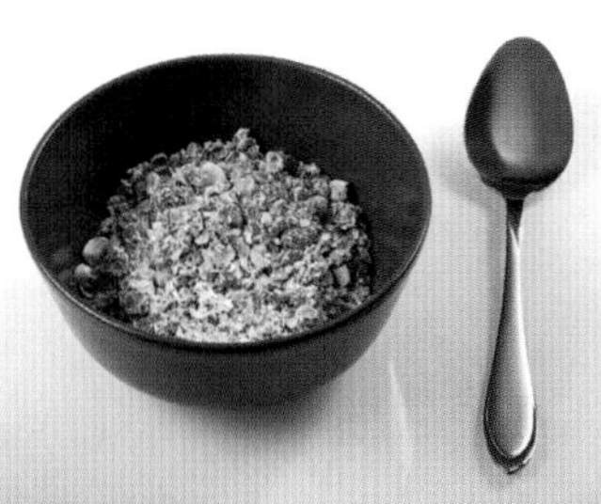

FIBRE	Weight	SAT FAT
5g	Weight: 60g	1g

CARBS	CALS	PROTEIN	FAT
86g	432	12g	7g

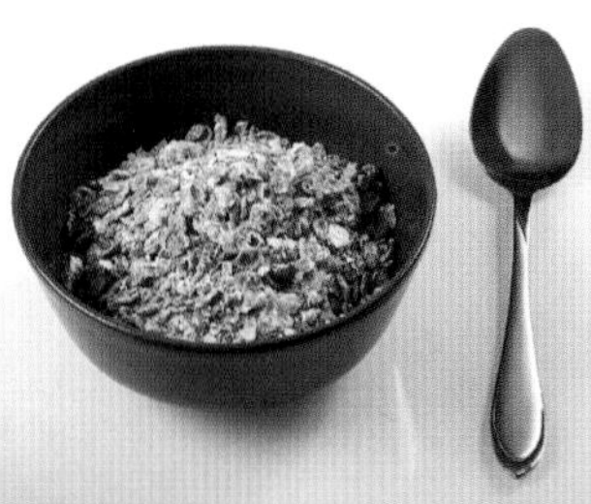

FIBRE	Weight	SAT FAT
10g	Weight: 119g	1g

Muesli (no added sugar)

CARBS	CALS	PROTEIN	FAT
20g	110	3g	2g

FIBRE	Weight	SAT FAT
3g	Weight: 30g	0g

CARBS	CALS	PROTEIN	FAT
40g	220	6g	5g

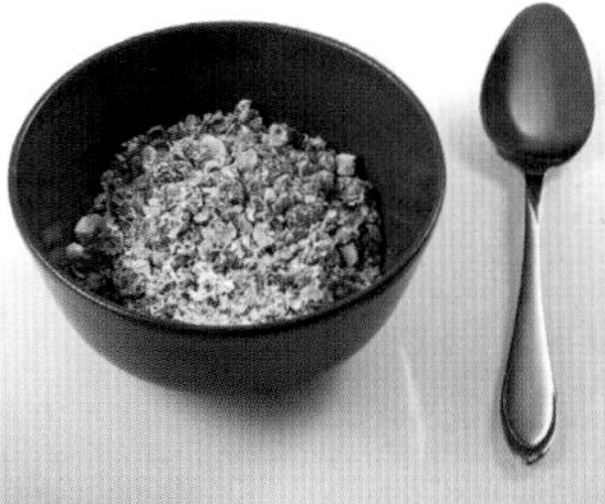

FIBRE	Weight	SAT FAT
6g	Weight: 60g	1g

CARBS	CALS	PROTEIN	FAT
80g	436	12g	9g

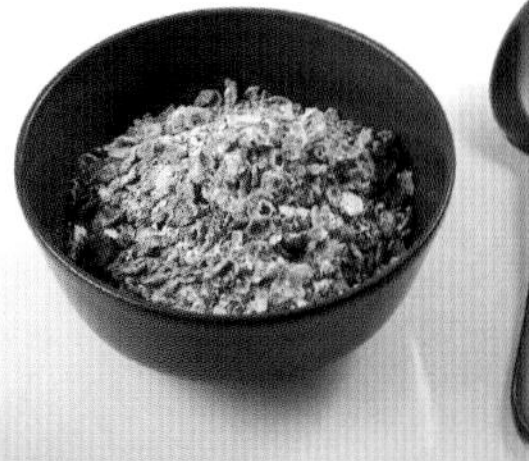

FIBRE	Weight	SAT FAT
12g	Weight: 119g	2g

Multigrain Hoops

Carbs	Cals	Protein	Fat
12g	55	1g	1g

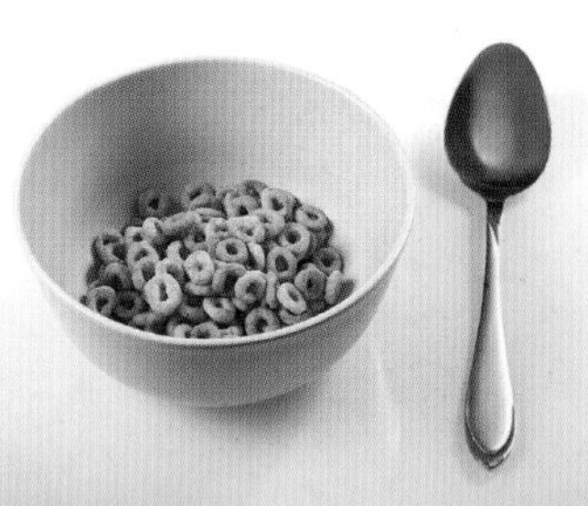

Fibre	Weight	Sat Fat
1g	Weight: 15g	0g

Carbs	Cals	Protein	Fat
24g	110	2g	1g

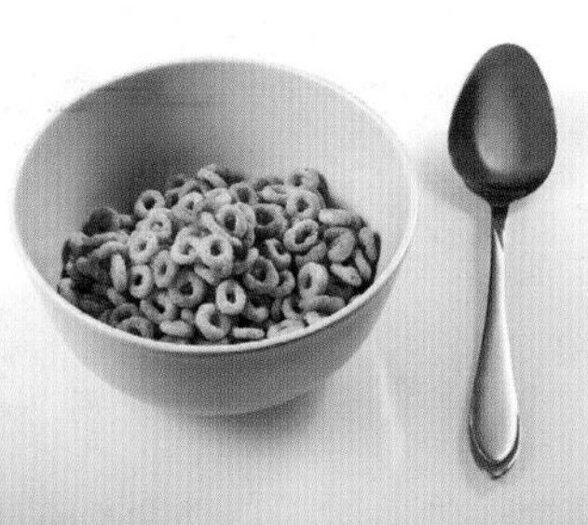
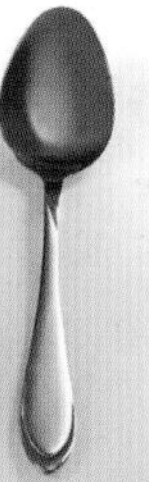

Fibre	Weight	Sat Fat
2g	Weight: 30g	1g

Carbs	Cals	Protein	Fat
48g	221	5g	2g

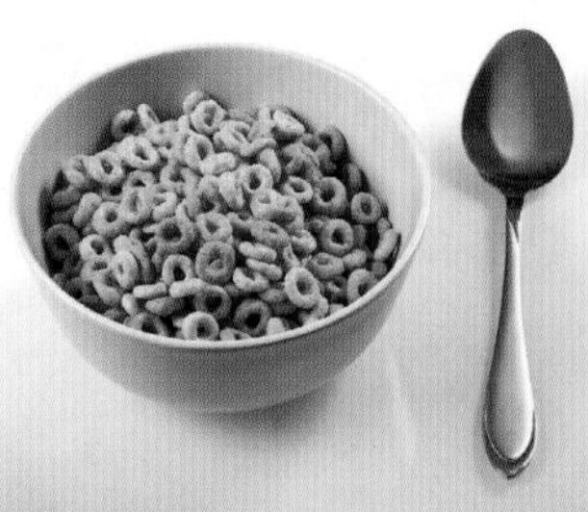
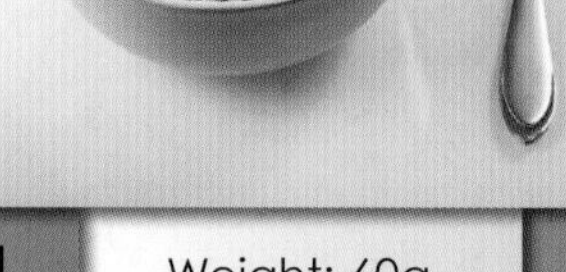

Fibre	Weight	Sat Fat
4g	Weight: 60g	1g

Raisin Bites

Carbs	Cals	Protein	Fat
17g	74	2g	0g

Fibre	Weight	Sat Fat
2g	Weight: 22g	0g

Carbs	Cals	Protein	Fat
34g	152	4g	1g

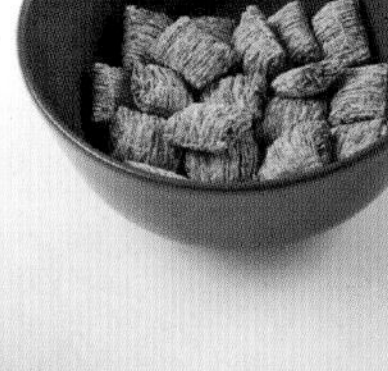
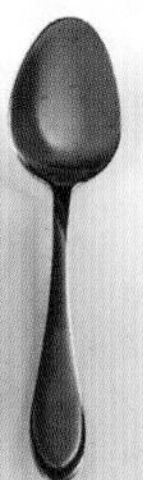

Fibre	Weight	Sat Fat
5g	Weight: 45g	0g

Carbs	Cals	Protein	Fat
75g	337	9g	2g

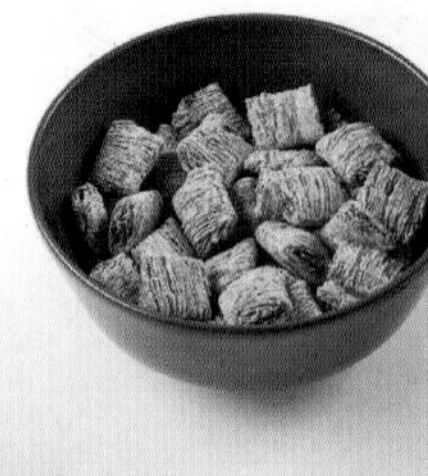

Fibre	Weight	Sat Fat
11g	Weight: 100g	0g

Rice Snaps

9g	38	1g	0g
CARBS	CALS	PROTEIN	FAT

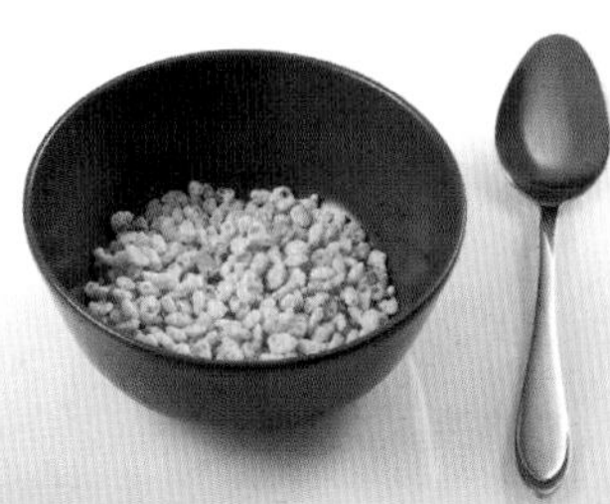

0g	Weight: 10g	0g
FIBRE		SAT FAT

19g	76	1g	0g
CARBS	CALS	PROTEIN	FAT

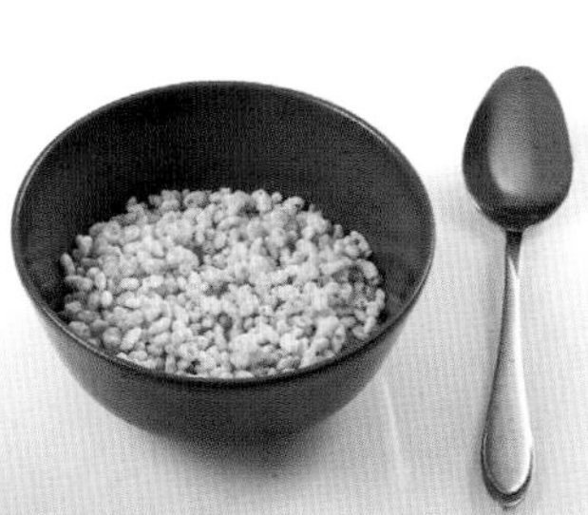

0g	Weight: 20g	0g
FIBRE		SAT FAT

37g	153	2g	0g
CARBS	CALS	PROTEIN	FAT

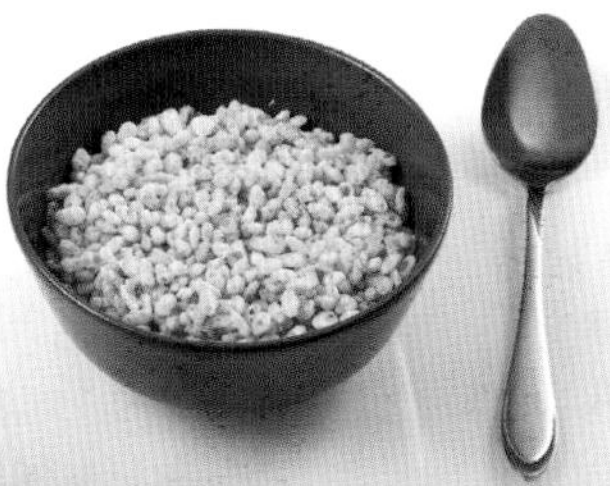
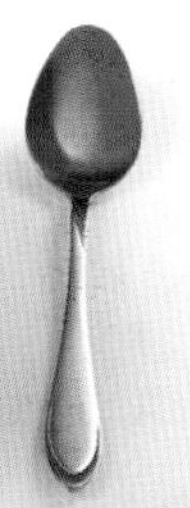

1g	Weight: 40g	0g
FIBRE		SAT FAT

Special Flakes with Berries

12g	57	2g	0g
CARBS	CALS	PROTEIN	FAT

1g	Weight: 15g	0g
FIBRE		SAT FAT

23g	114	4g	1g
CARBS	CALS	PROTEIN	FAT

1g	Weight: 30g	0g
FIBRE		SAT FAT

46g	228	8g	1g
CARBS	CALS	PROTEIN	FAT

2g	Weight: 60g	0g
FIBRE		SAT FAT

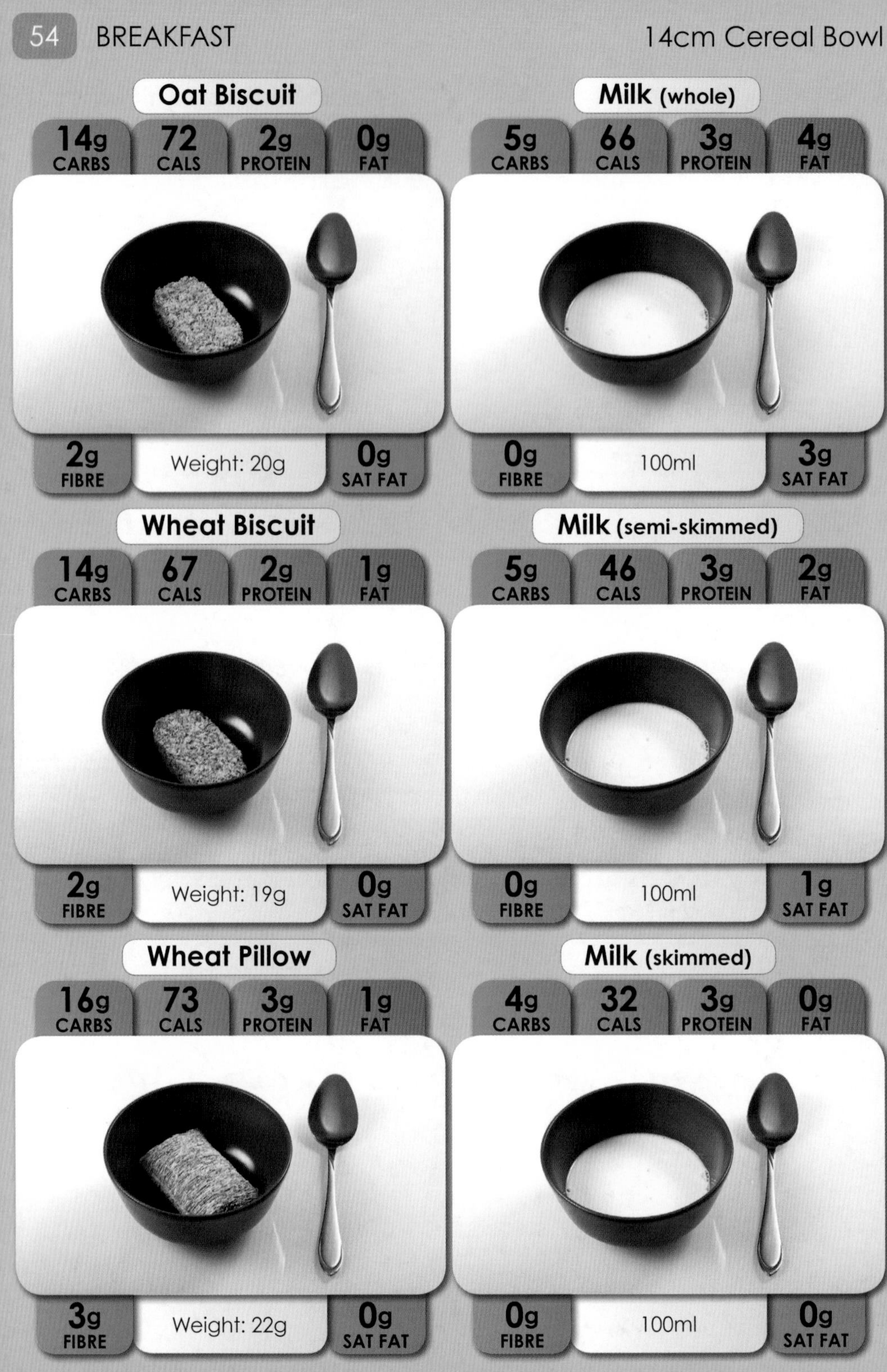

Oat Biscuit

CARBS	CALS	PROTEIN	FAT	FIBRE	SAT FAT
14g	72	2g	0g	2g	0g

Weight: 20g

Milk (whole)

CARBS	CALS	PROTEIN	FAT	FIBRE	SAT FAT
5g	66	3g	4g	0g	3g

100ml

Wheat Biscuit

CARBS	CALS	PROTEIN	FAT	FIBRE	SAT FAT
14g	67	2g	1g	2g	0g

Weight: 19g

Milk (semi-skimmed)

CARBS	CALS	PROTEIN	FAT	FIBRE	SAT FAT
5g	46	3g	2g	0g	1g

100ml

Wheat Pillow

CARBS	CALS	PROTEIN	FAT	FIBRE	SAT FAT
16g	73	3g	1g	3g	0g

Weight: 22g

Milk (skimmed)

CARBS	CALS	PROTEIN	FAT	FIBRE	SAT FAT
4g	32	3g	0g	0g	0g

100ml

Cornmeal Porridge (condensed milk)

CARBS	CALS	PROTEIN	FAT
19g	104	3g	2g

FIBRE	Weight	SAT FAT
0g	Weight: 100g	1g

CARBS	CALS	PROTEIN	FAT
56g	311	9g	7g

FIBRE	Weight	SAT FAT
0g	Weight: 300g	4g

CARBS	CALS	PROTEIN	FAT
94g	518	14g	11g

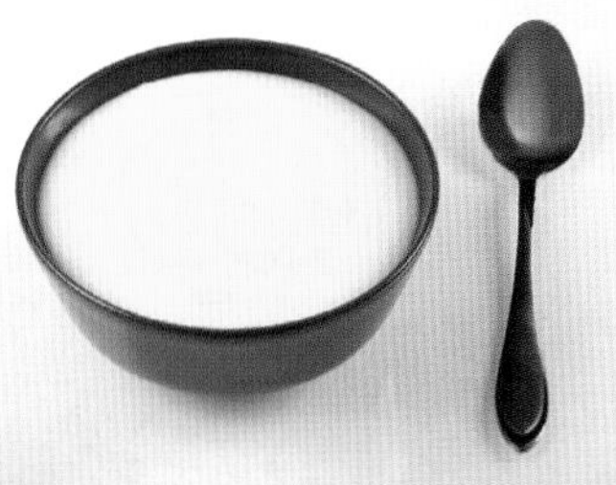

FIBRE	Weight	SAT FAT
0g	Weight: 500g	7g

Cornmeal Porridge (water)

CARBS	CALS	PROTEIN	FAT
12g	53	1g	0g

FIBRE	Weight	SAT FAT
0g	Weight: 100g	0g

CARBS	CALS	PROTEIN	FAT
35g	158	3g	1g

FIBRE	Weight	SAT FAT
0g	Weight: 300g	0g

CARBS	CALS	PROTEIN	FAT
59g	262	4g	1g

FIBRE	Weight	SAT FAT
0g	Weight: 500g	0g

Porridge (with semi-skimmed milk)

CARBS	CALS	PROTEIN	FAT
11g	84	4g	2g

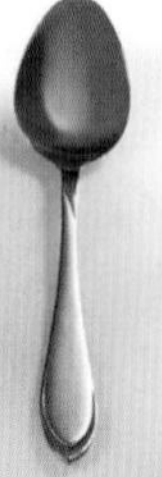

FIBRE	Weight	SAT FAT
1g	Weight: 75g	1g

CARBS	CALS	PROTEIN	FAT
33g	246	13g	7g

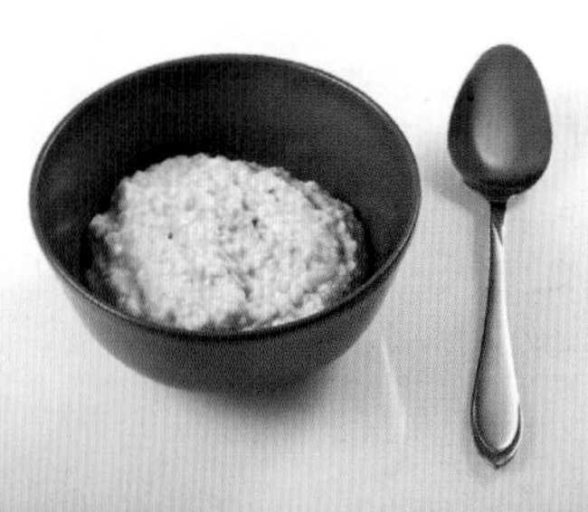

FIBRE	Weight	SAT FAT
3g	Weight: 220g	3g

CARBS	CALS	PROTEIN	FAT
54g	407	21g	12g

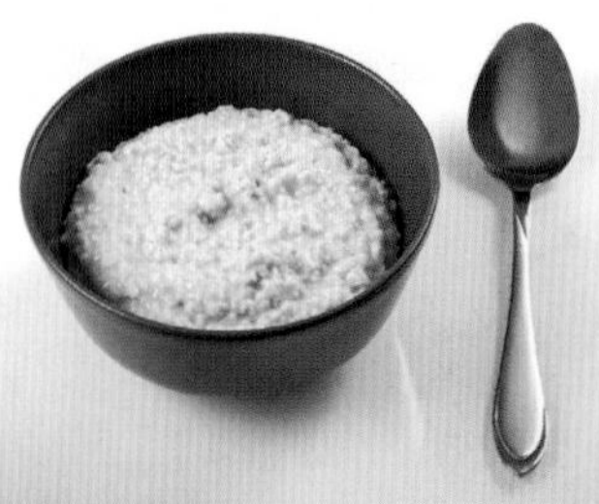

FIBRE	Weight	SAT FAT
5g	Weight: 365g	6g

Porridge (with water)

CARBS	CALS	PROTEIN	FAT
6g	35	1g	1g

FIBRE	Weight	SAT FAT
1g	Weight: 75g	0g

CARBS	CALS	PROTEIN	FAT
18g	101	3g	2g

FIBRE	Weight	SAT FAT
3g	Weight: 220g	0g

CARBS	CALS	PROTEIN	FAT
30g	168	5g	4g

FIBRE	Weight	SAT FAT
4g	Weight: 365g	1g

Toast with Choc Spread & Margarine

18g CARBS	136 CALS	3g PROTEIN	7g FAT

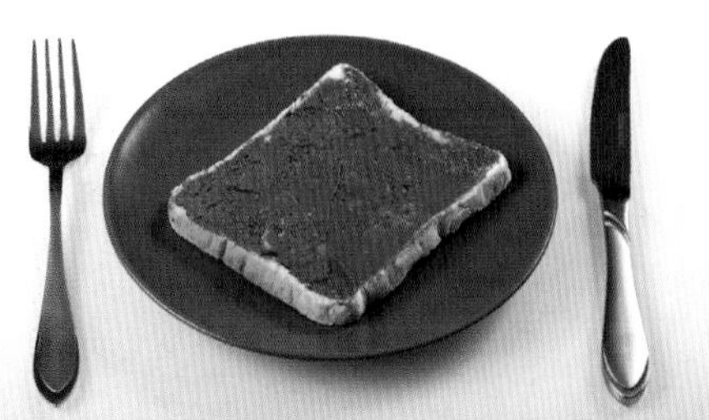

1g FIBRE	26g toast, 5g marg, 5g choc	1g SAT FAT

Toast with Honey & Margarine

19g CARBS	124 CALS	3g PROTEIN	5g FAT

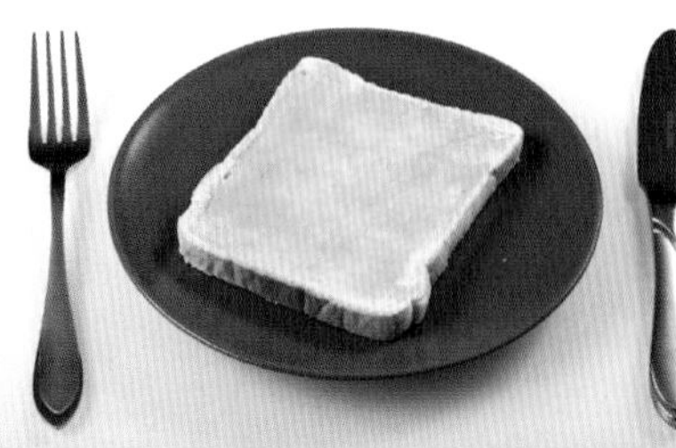

1g FIBRE	26g toast, 5g marg, 5g honey	1g SAT FAT

Toast with Jam & Margarine

18g CARBS	122 CALS	3g PROTEIN	5g FAT

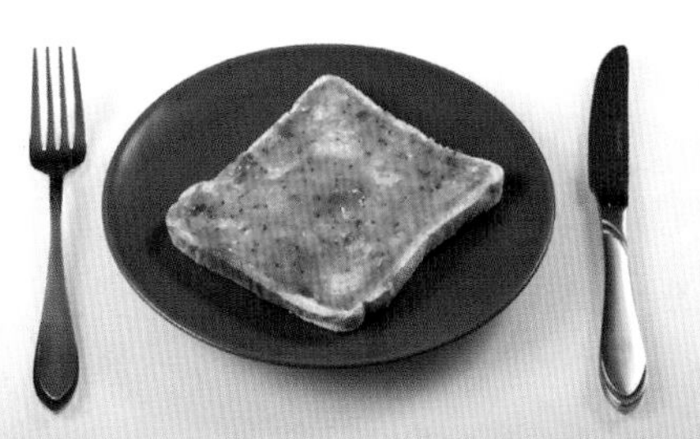

1g FIBRE	26g toast, 5g marg, 5g jam	1g SAT FAT

Toast with Lemon Curd & Margarine

18g CARBS	124 CALS	3g PROTEIN	5g FAT

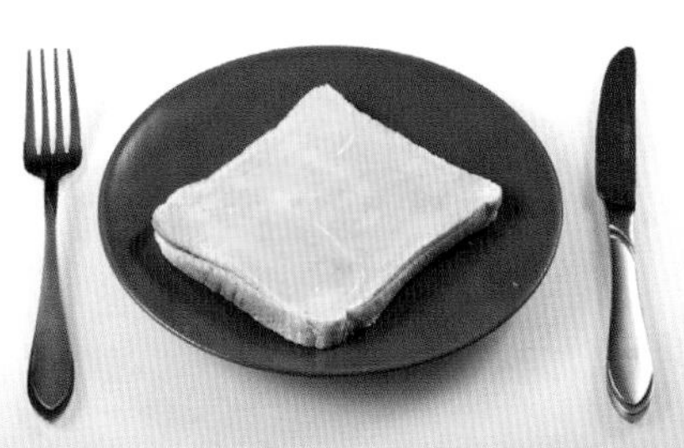

1g FIBRE	26g toast, 5g marg, 5g lemon	1g SAT FAT

Toast with Marmalade & Margarine

19g CARBS	123 CALS	3g PROTEIN	5g FAT

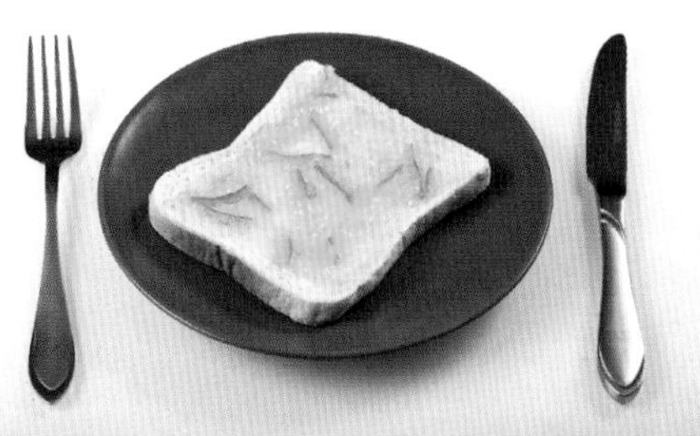

1g FIBRE	26g toast, 5g marg, 5g marm	1g SAT FAT

Toast with Peanut Butter & Margarine

16g CARBS	140 CALS	4g PROTEIN	7g FAT

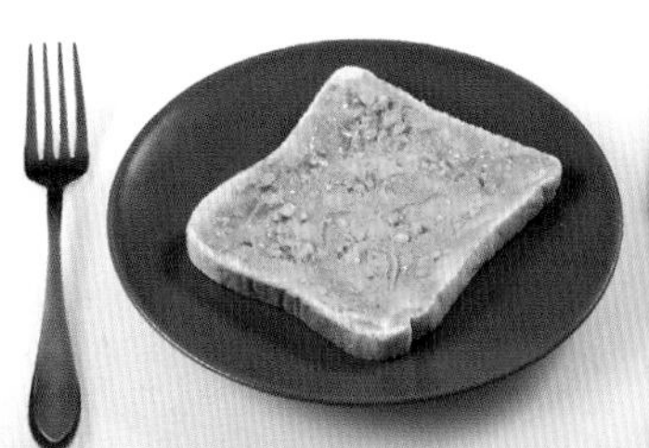

1g FIBRE	26g toast, 5g marg, 5g peanut	1g SAT FAT

Pancake (plain)

5g CARBS	56 CALS	1g PROTEIN	3g FAT

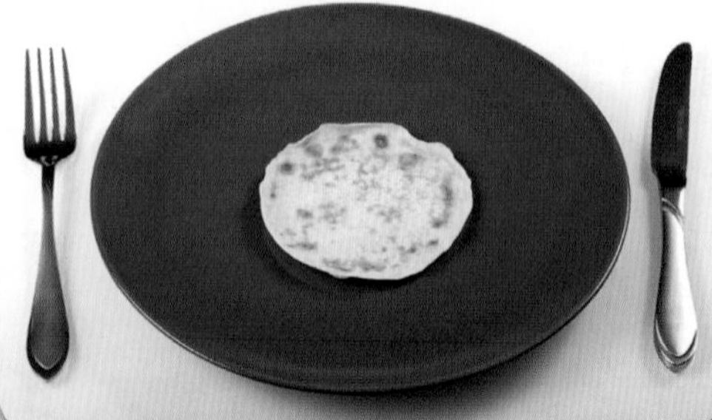

0g FIBRE	Weight: 22g	1g SAT FAT

10g CARBS	110 CALS	3g PROTEIN	7g FAT

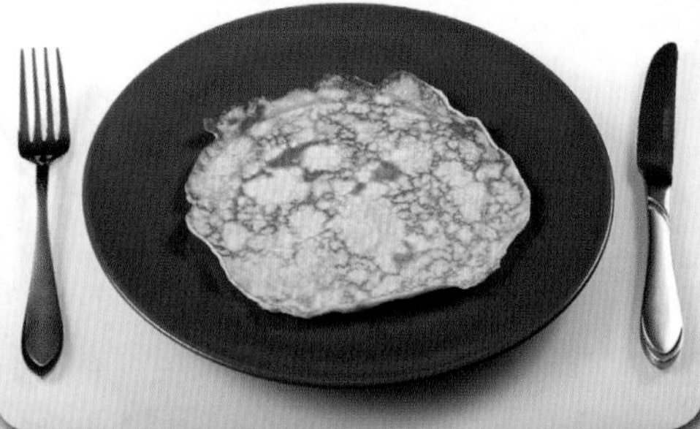

1g FIBRE	Weight: 43g	2g SAT FAT

20g CARBS	217 CALS	5g PROTEIN	13g FAT

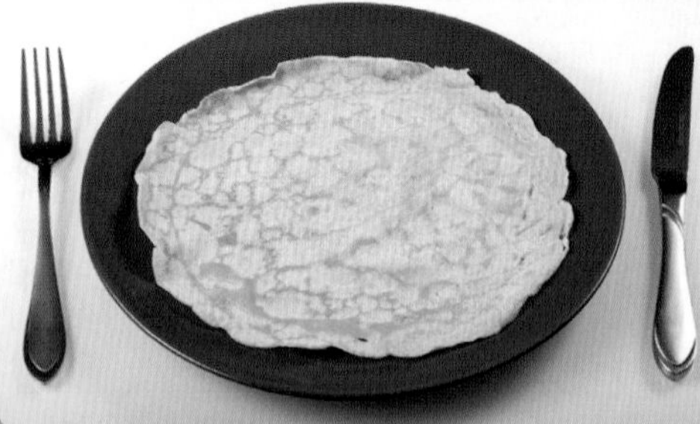

1g FIBRE	Weight: 85g	4g SAT FAT

Pancake with Choc Spread

14g CARBS	106 CALS	2g PROTEIN	5g FAT

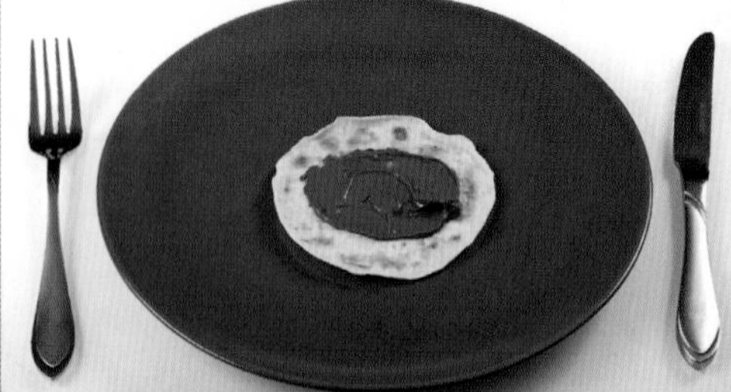

1g FIBRE	22g pancake, 8g choc spread	1g SAT FAT

22g CARBS	166 CALS	3g PROTEIN	8g FAT

1g FIBRE	43g pancake, 8g choc spread	2g SAT FAT

43g CARBS	329 CALS	7g PROTEIN	15g FAT

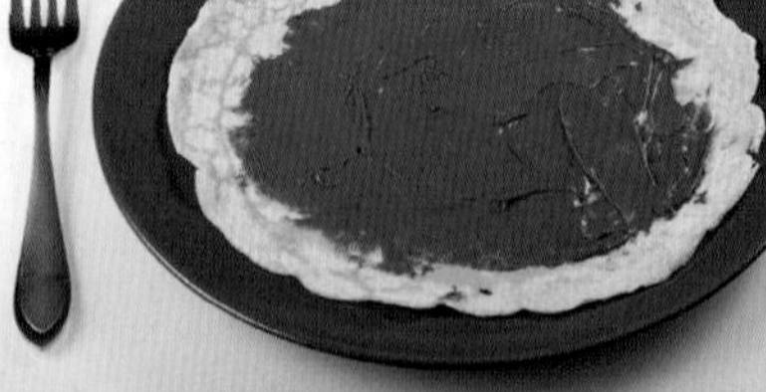

2g FIBRE	85g pancake, 16g choc spread	4g SAT FAT

Pancake with Maple Syrup

14g CARBS	83 CALS	2g PROTEIN	3g FAT

0g FIBRE	22g pancake, 8g maple syrup	1g SAT FAT

22g CARBS	143 CALS	3g PROTEIN	5g FAT

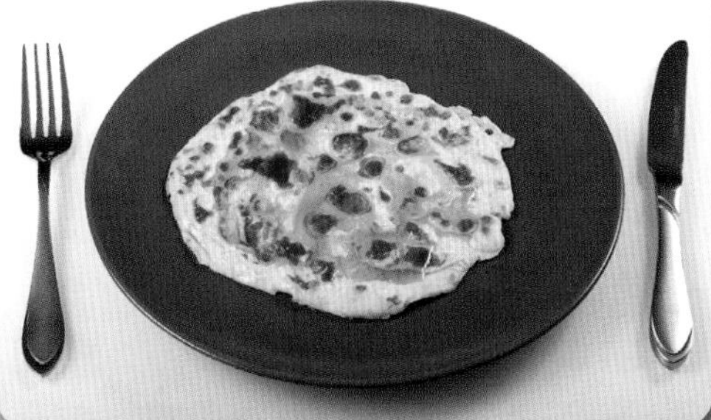

1g FIBRE	43g pancake, 8g maple syrup	1g SAT FAT

44g CARBS	283 CALS	6g PROTEIN	10g FAT

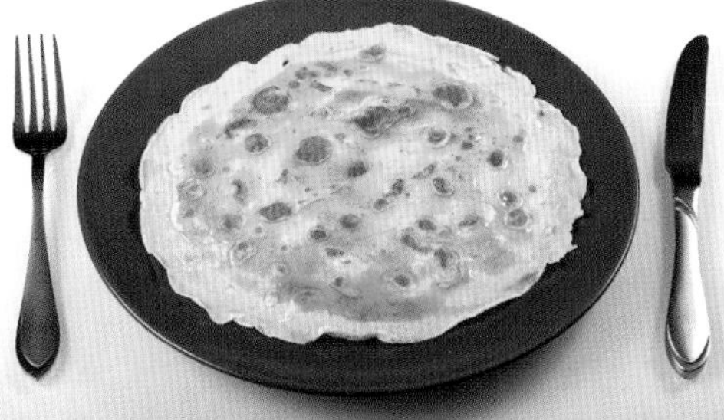

1g FIBRE	85g pancake, 16g maple syrup	3g SAT FAT

Pancake with Sugar & Lemon

14g CARBS	82 CALS	2g PROTEIN	3g FAT

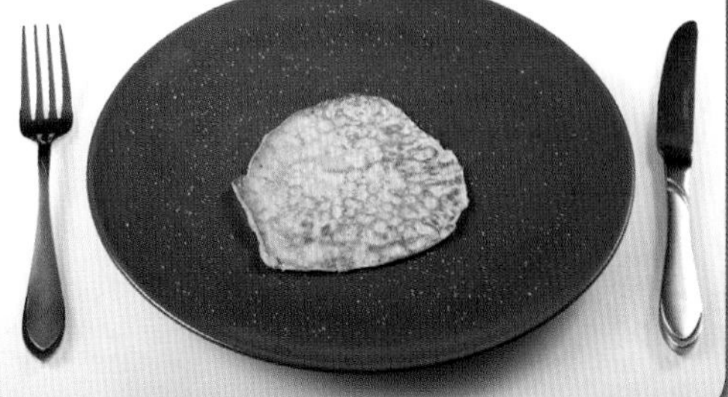

0g FIBRE	22g pancake, 5g sugar	1g SAT FAT

22g CARBS	142 CALS	3g PROTEIN	5g FAT

1g FIBRE	43g pancake, 5g sugar	1g SAT FAT

44g CARBS	281 CALS	6g PROTEIN	10g FAT

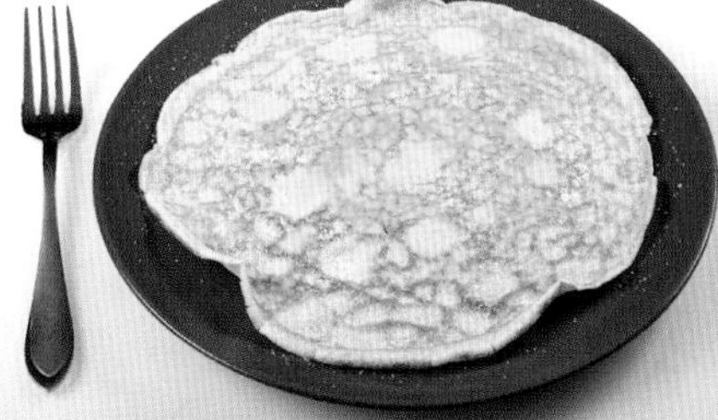

1g FIBRE	85g pancake, 10g sugar	3g SAT FAT

20cm Side Plate / 26cm Dinner Plate

Breakfast Tart

CARBS	CALS	PROTEIN	FAT
36g	207	2g	6g

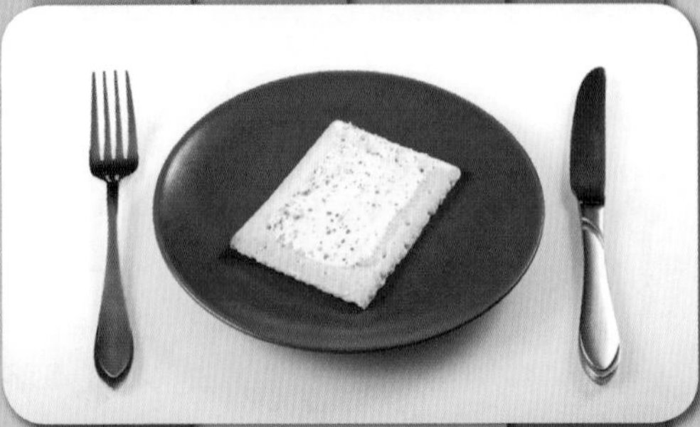

FIBRE	Weight	SAT FAT
1g	Weight: 52g	3g

Scotch Pancake

CARBS	CALS	PROTEIN	FAT
12g	88	2g	4g

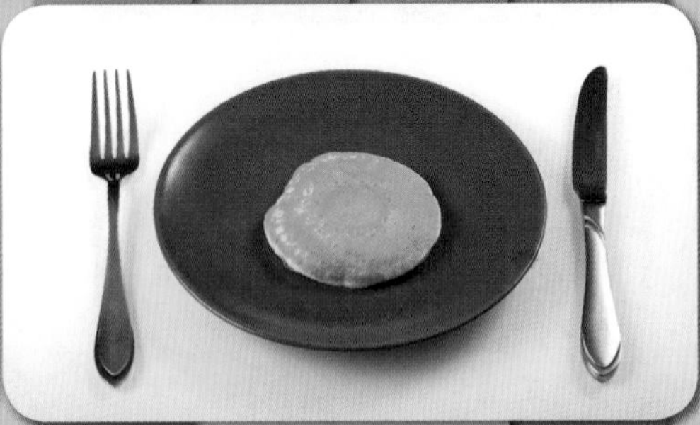

FIBRE	Weight	SAT FAT
1g	Weight: 31g	1g

Eggy Bread

CARBS	CALS	PROTEIN	FAT
10g	194	8g	14g

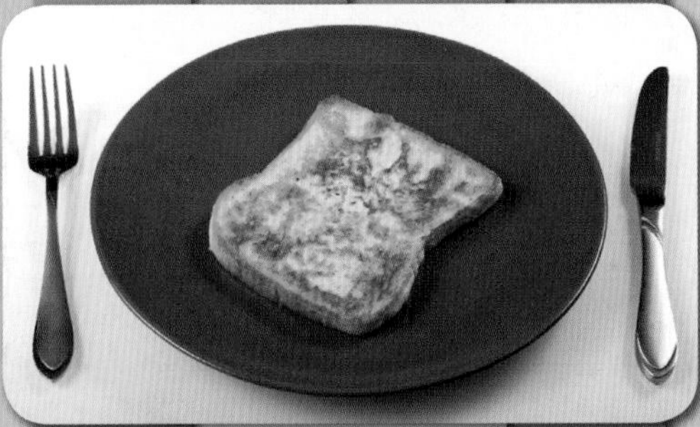

FIBRE	Weight	SAT FAT
1g	Weight: 50g	7g

Fried Bread

CARBS	CALS	PROTEIN	FAT
10g	160	2g	13g

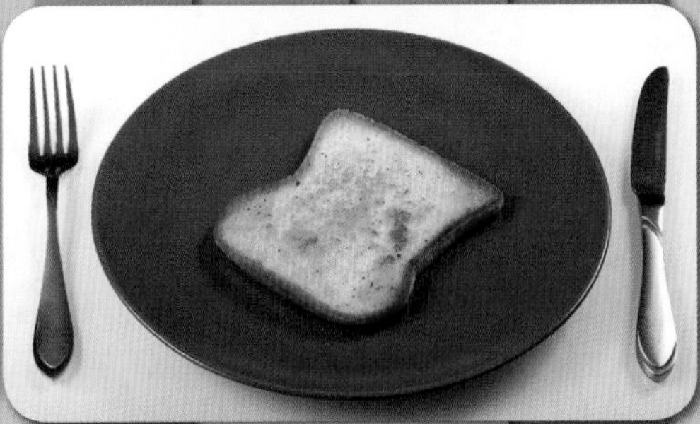

FIBRE	Weight	SAT FAT
1g	Weight: 30g	8g

Waffle (sweet)

CARBS	CALS	PROTEIN	FAT
15g	129	3g	7g

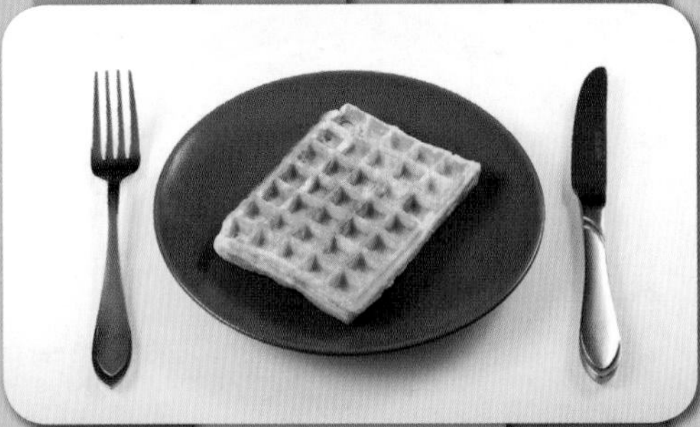

CARBS	CALS	PROTEIN	FAT
24g	201	5g	10g

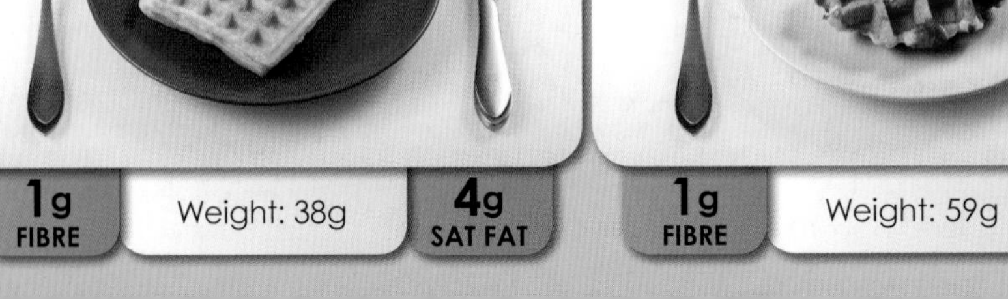

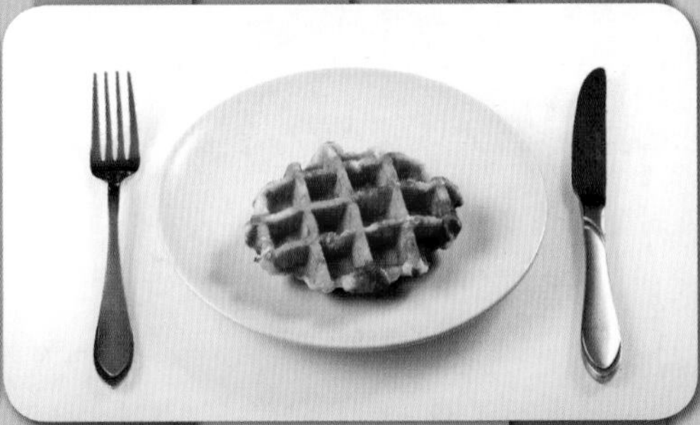

FIBRE	Weight	SAT FAT
1g	Weight: 38g	4g

FIBRE	Weight	SAT FAT
1g	Weight: 59g	6g

Bakewell Tart

15g CARBS	155 CALS	2g PROTEIN	10g FAT

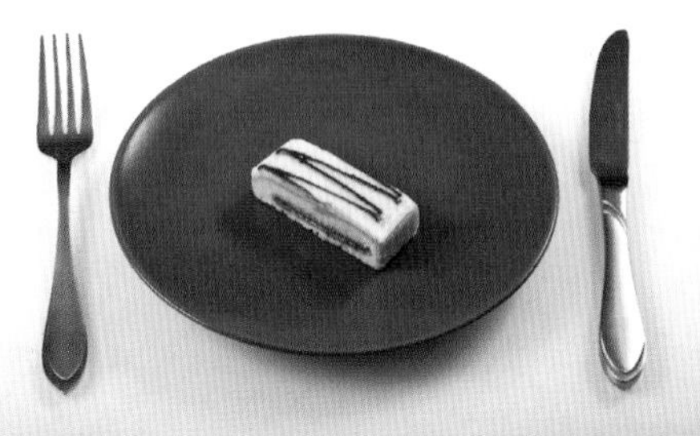

1g FIBRE	Weight: 34g	3g SAT FAT

20g CARBS	205 CALS	3g PROTEIN	13g FAT

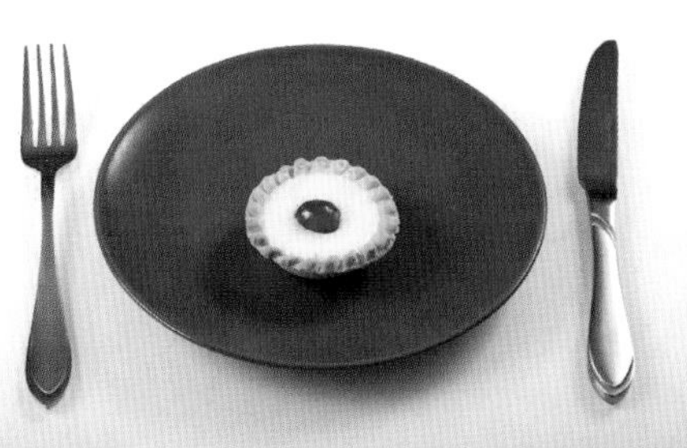

1g FIBRE	Weight: 45g	5g SAT FAT

41g CARBS	424 CALS	6g PROTEIN	28g FAT

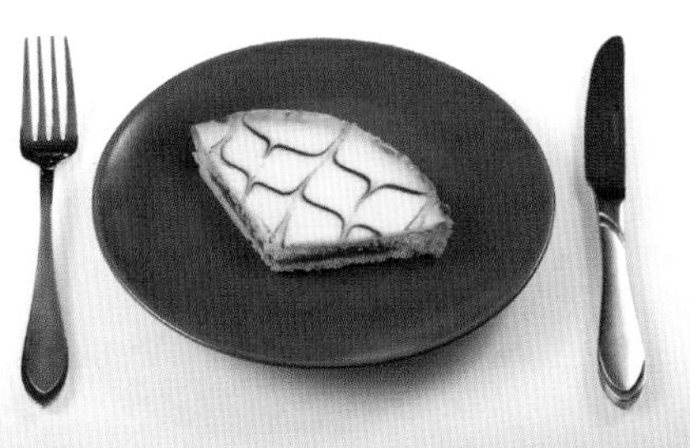

2g FIBRE	Weight: 93g	9g SAT FAT

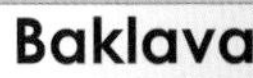

Baklava

7g CARBS	71 CALS	1g PROTEIN	4g FAT

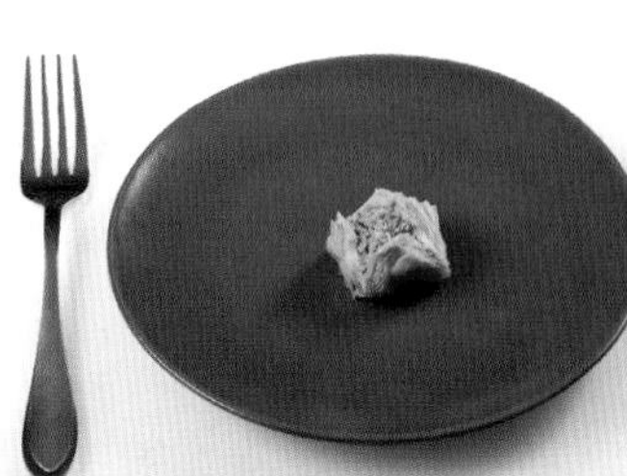

1g FIBRE	Weight: 14g	2g SAT FAT

10g CARBS	102 CALS	2g PROTEIN	6g FAT

1g FIBRE	Weight: 20g	2g SAT FAT

14g CARBS	142 CALS	2g PROTEIN	9g FAT

1g FIBRE	Weight: 28g	3g SAT FAT

20cm Side Plate

Carrot Cake

CARBS	CALS	PROTEIN	FAT
19g	180	2g	11g

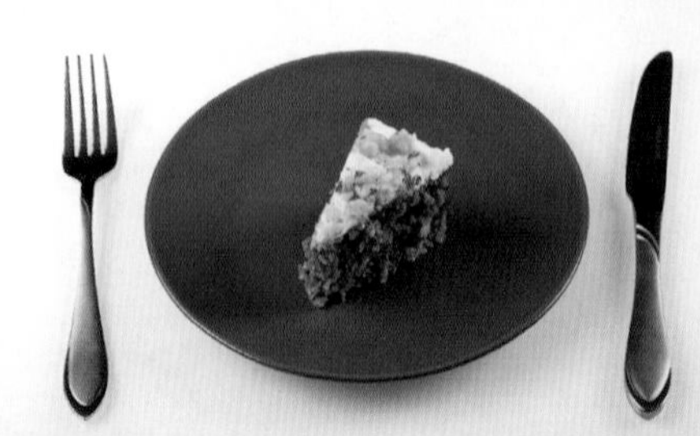
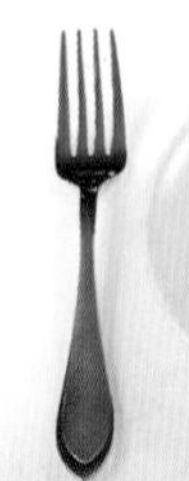

FIBRE	Weight	SAT FAT
1g	Weight: 50g	3g

CARBS	CALS	PROTEIN	FAT
37g	359	4g	23g

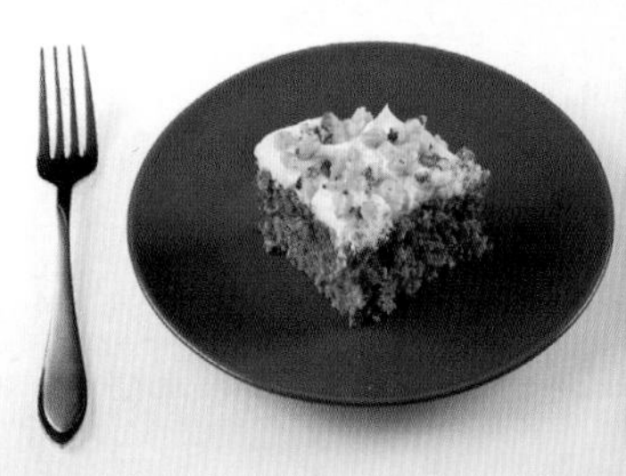

FIBRE	Weight	SAT FAT
2g	Weight: 100g	6g

CARBS	CALS	PROTEIN	FAT
74g	718	9g	45g

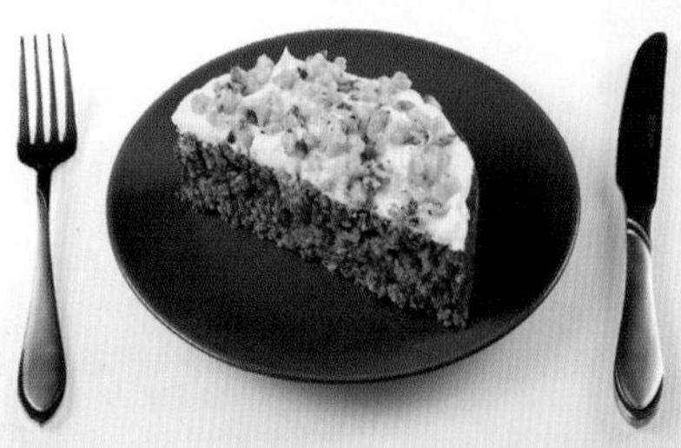
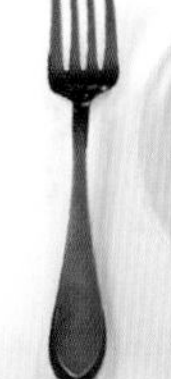

FIBRE	Weight	SAT FAT
3g	Weight: 200g	11g

Chocolate Cake

CARBS	CALS	PROTEIN	FAT
20g	186	3g	11g

FIBRE	Weight	SAT FAT
1g	Weight: 40g	3g

CARBS	CALS	PROTEIN	FAT
35g	325	5g	19g

FIBRE	Weight	SAT FAT
2g	Weight: 70g	5g

CARBS	CALS	PROTEIN	FAT
70g	640	10g	38g

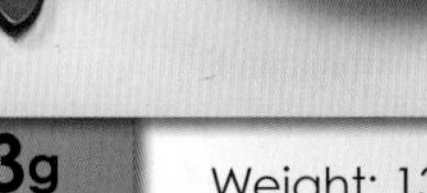

FIBRE	Weight	SAT FAT
3g	Weight: 138g	9g

Coffee & Walnut Cake

CARBS	CALS	PROTEIN	FAT
27g	216	2g	11g

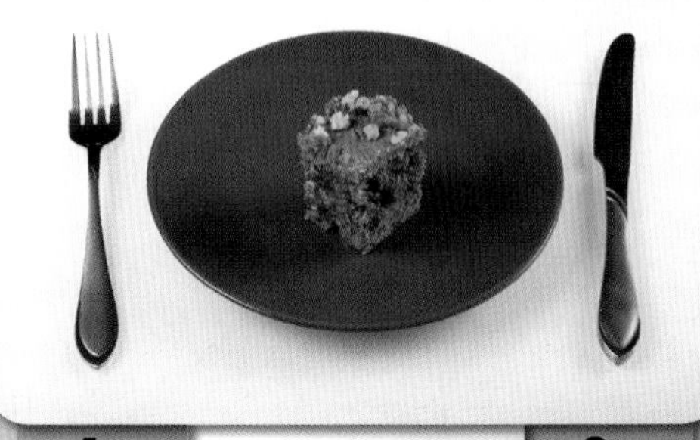

FIBRE	Weight	SAT FAT
1g	Weight: 50g	3g

CARBS	CALS	PROTEIN	FAT
53g	431	4g	22g

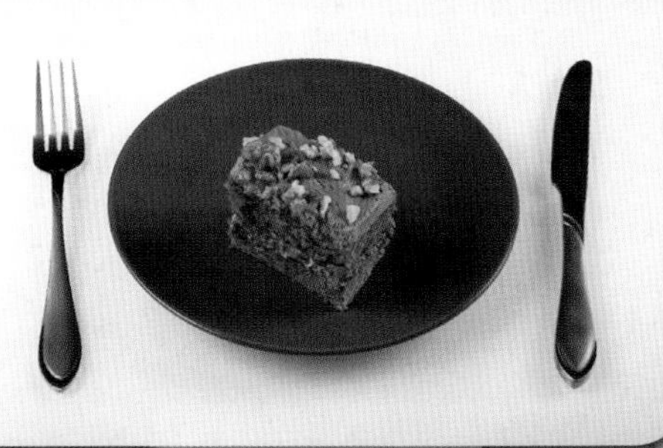

FIBRE	Weight	SAT FAT
2g	Weight: 100g	7g

CARBS	CALS	PROTEIN	FAT
106g	863	9g	44g

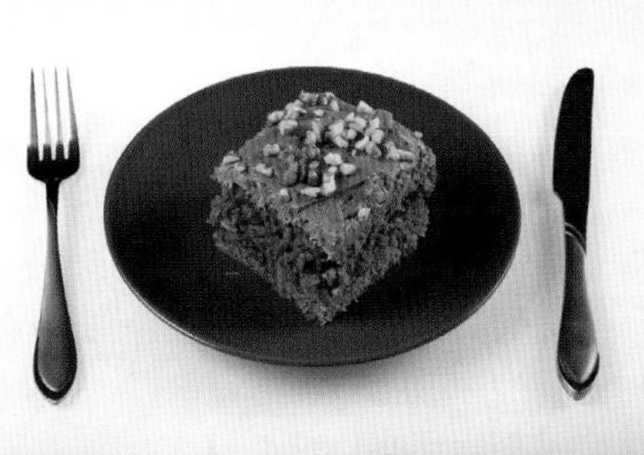

FIBRE	Weight	SAT FAT
4g	Weight: 200g	13g

Fruit Cake

CARBS	CALS	PROTEIN	FAT
16g	89	1g	3g

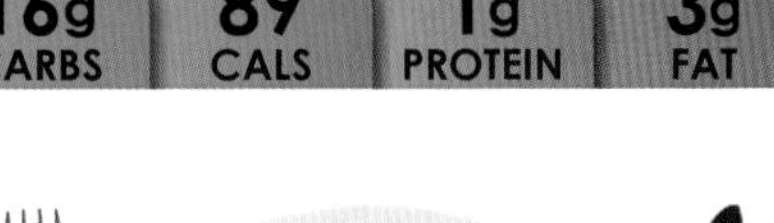

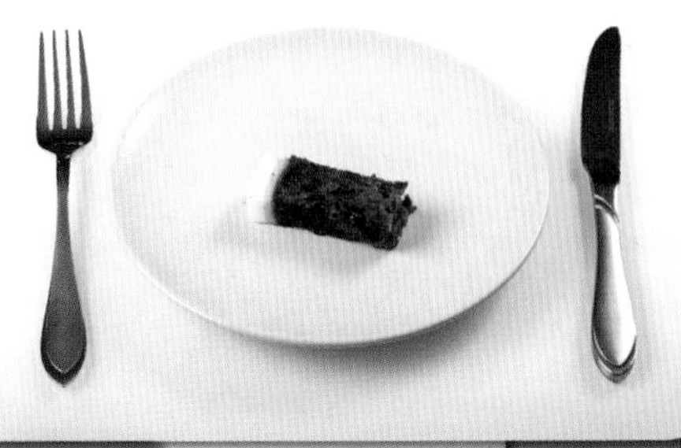

FIBRE	Weight	SAT FAT
1g	Weight: 26g	1g

CARBS	CALS	PROTEIN	FAT
36g	206	2g	7g

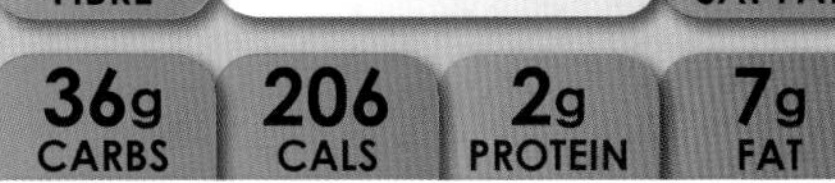

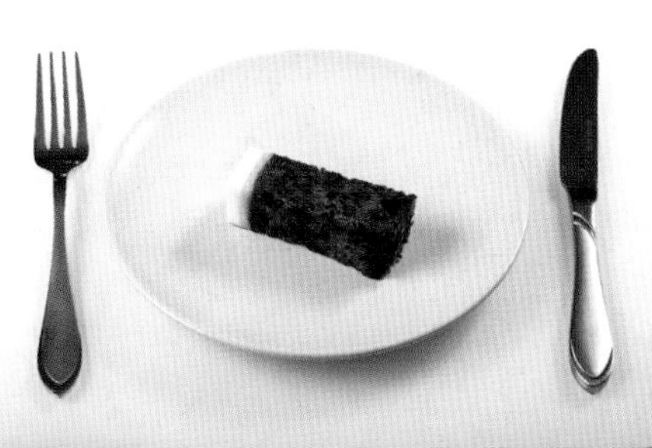

FIBRE	Weight	SAT FAT
1g	Weight: 60g	1g

CARBS	CALS	PROTEIN	FAT
73g	415	5g	14g

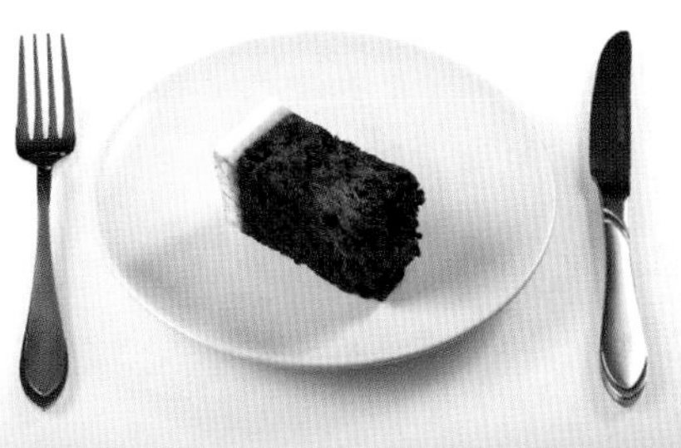

FIBRE	Weight	SAT FAT
2g	Weight: 121g	3g

Ginger Cake

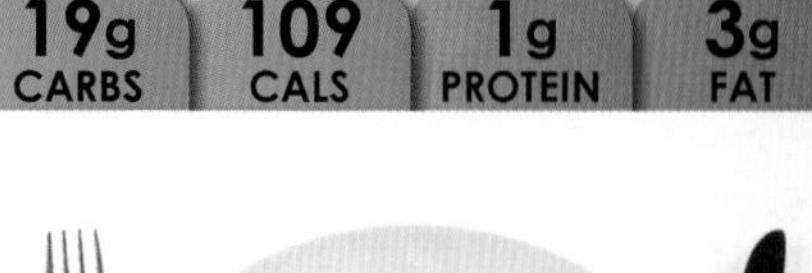

CARBS	CALS	PROTEIN	FAT	FIBRE	SAT FAT	Weight
19g	109	1g	3g	1g	1g	30g

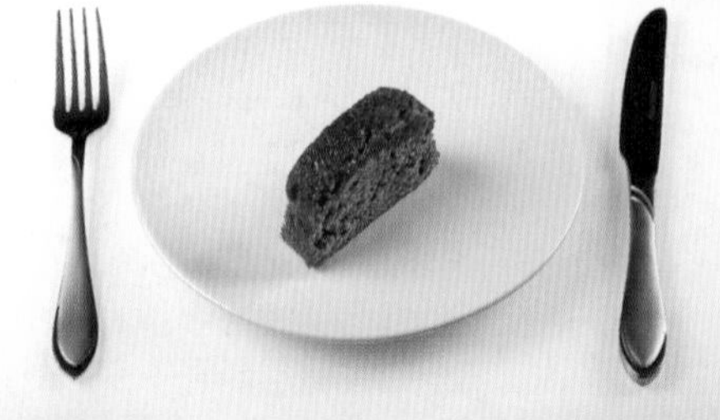

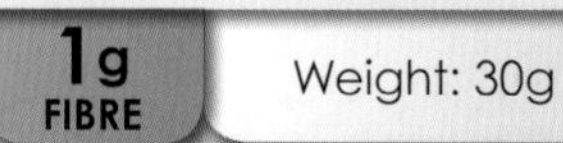

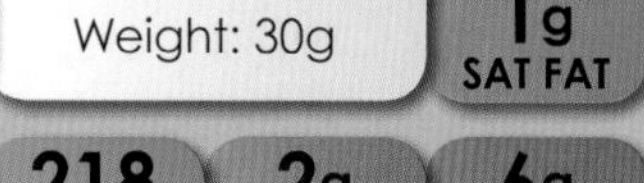

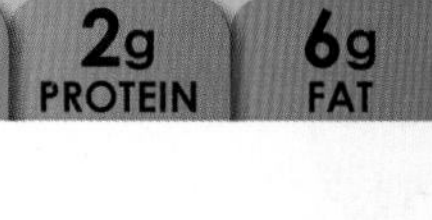

CARBS	CALS	PROTEIN	FAT	FIBRE	SAT FAT	Weight
38g	218	2g	6g	1g	2g	60g

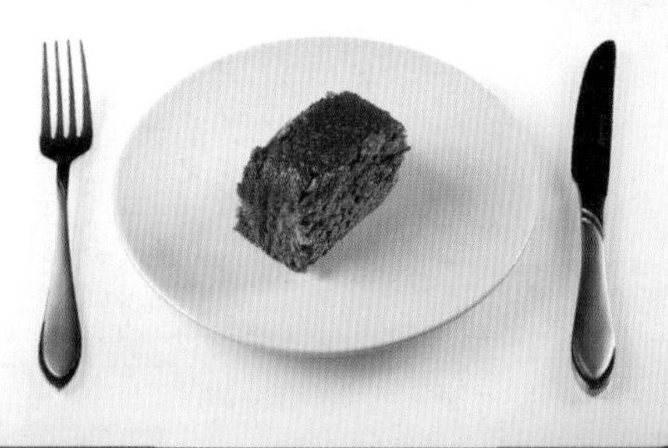

CARBS	CALS	PROTEIN	FAT	FIBRE	SAT FAT	Weight
76g	437	4g	13g	2g	4g	120g

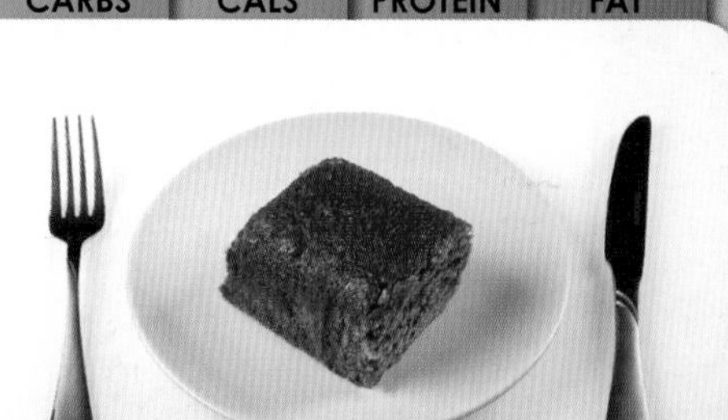

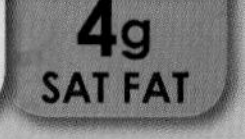

Malt Loaf

CARBS	CALS	PROTEIN	FAT	FIBRE	SAT FAT	Weight
20g	89	2g	1g	1g	0g	30g

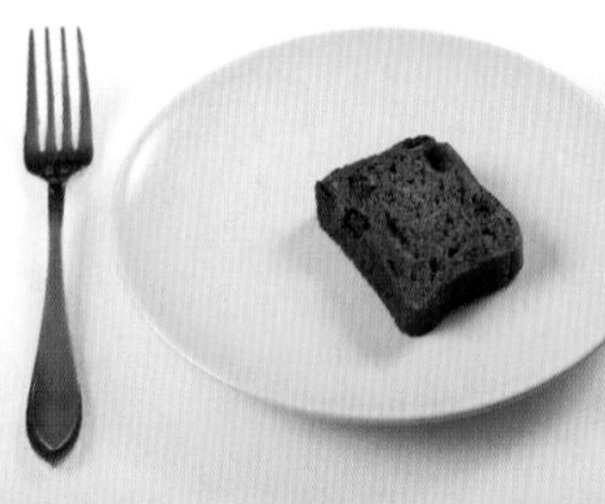

CARBS	CALS	PROTEIN	FAT	FIBRE	SAT FAT	Weight
40g	180	5g	1g	2g	0g	61g

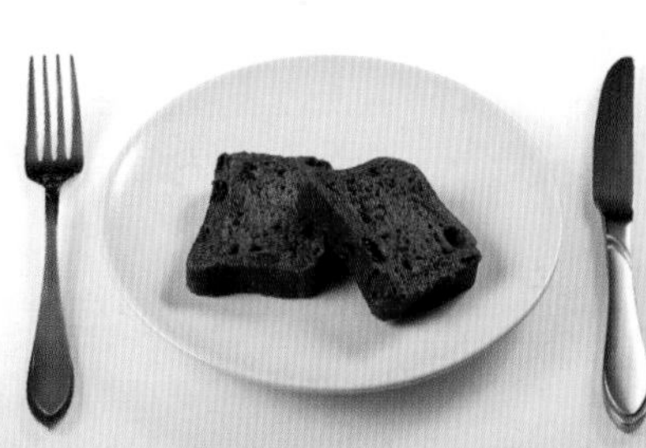

CARBS	CALS	PROTEIN	FAT	FIBRE	SAT FAT	Weight
59g	269	7g	2g	3g	1g	91g

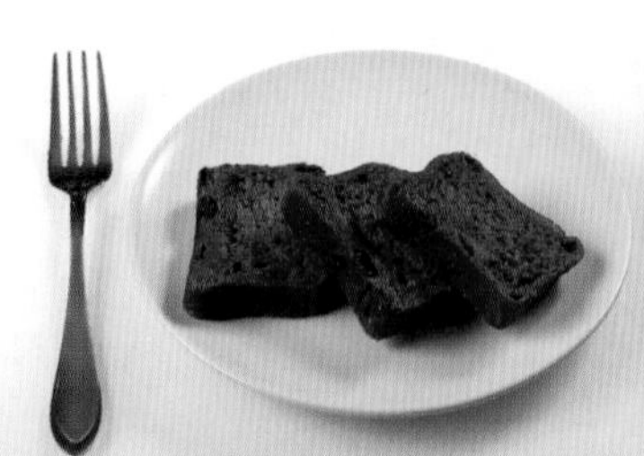

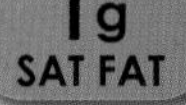

Swiss Roll

20g CARBS	138 CALS	2g PROTEIN	6g FAT

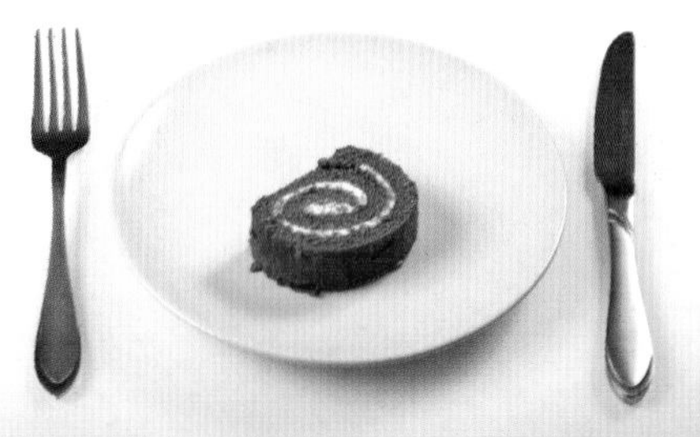

1g FIBRE	Weight: 35g	2g SAT FAT

40g CARBS	264 CALS	3g PROTEIN	11g FAT

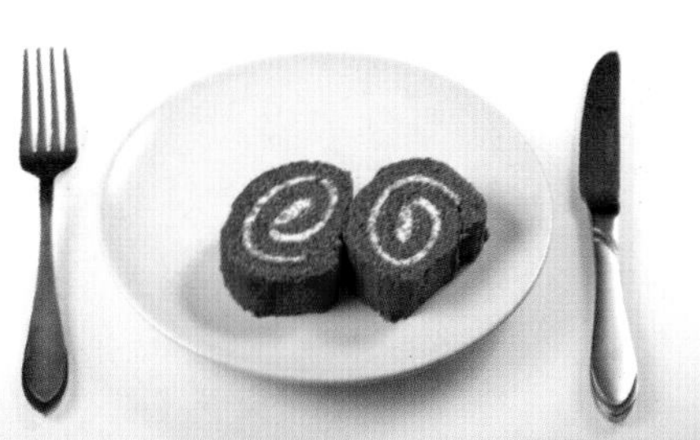

2g FIBRE	Weight: 69g	4g SAT FAT

59g CARBS	395 CALS	5g PROTEIN	16g FAT

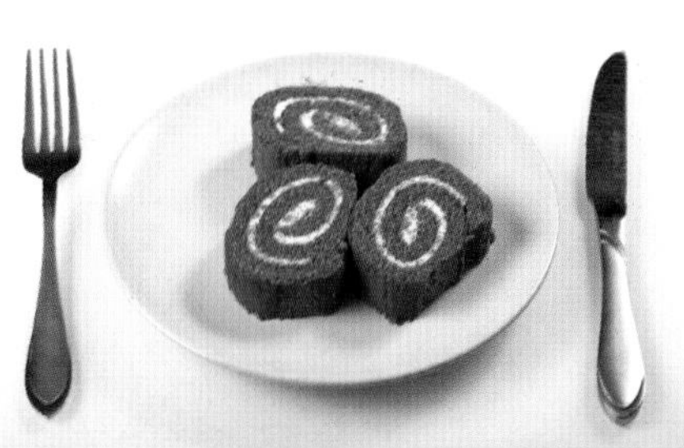

2g FIBRE	Weight: 103g	6g SAT FAT

Victoria Sponge

23g CARBS	184 CALS	2g PROTEIN	8g FAT

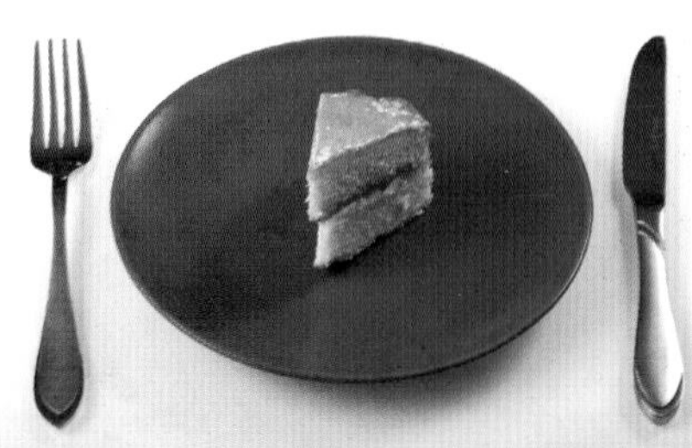

1g FIBRE	Weight: 44g	5g SAT FAT

39g CARBS	323 CALS	4g PROTEIN	15g FAT

2g FIBRE	Weight: 77g	9g SAT FAT

79g CARBS	650 CALS	8g PROTEIN	30g FAT

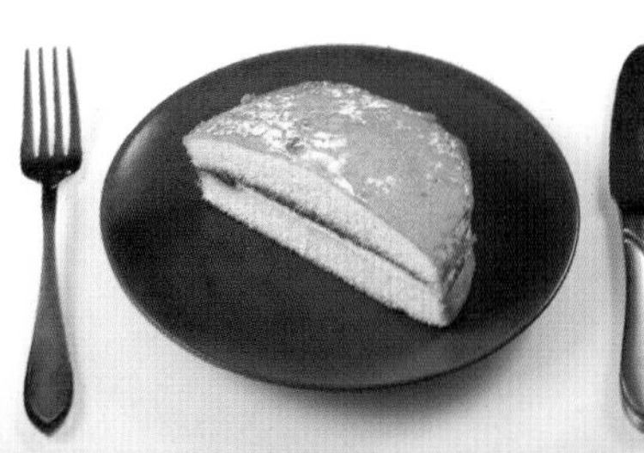

3g FIBRE	Weight: 155g	17g SAT FAT

Apple Danish

39g CARBS	308 CALS	6g PROTEIN	14g FAT

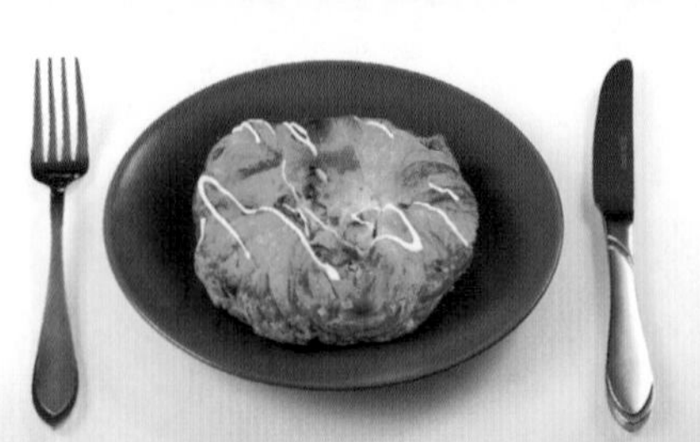

3g FIBRE	Weight: 87g	6g SAT FAT

Chocolate Chip Twist

32g CARBS	340 CALS	4g PROTEIN	22g FAT

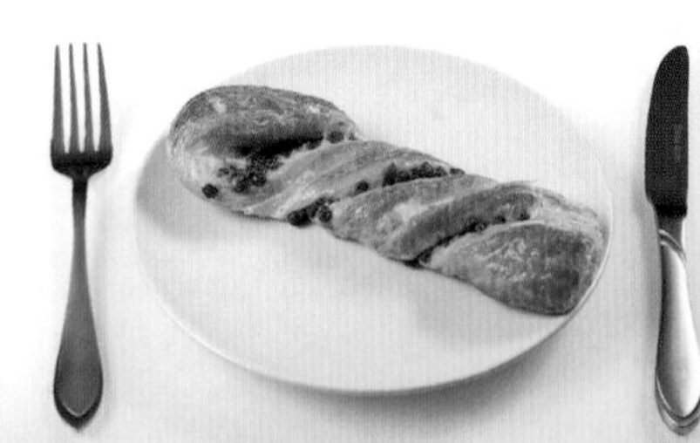

2g FIBRE	Weight: 85g	8g SAT FAT

Cinnamon Swirl

36g CARBS	357 CALS	4g PROTEIN	22g FAT

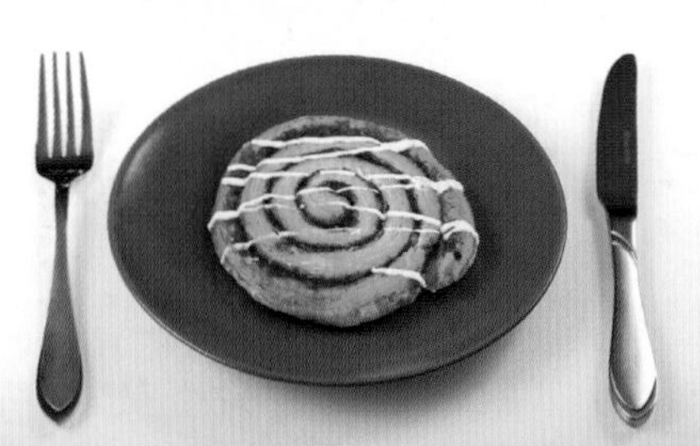

2g FIBRE	Weight: 79g	9g SAT FAT

Fruit Trellis

27g CARBS	238 CALS	3g PROTEIN	13g FAT

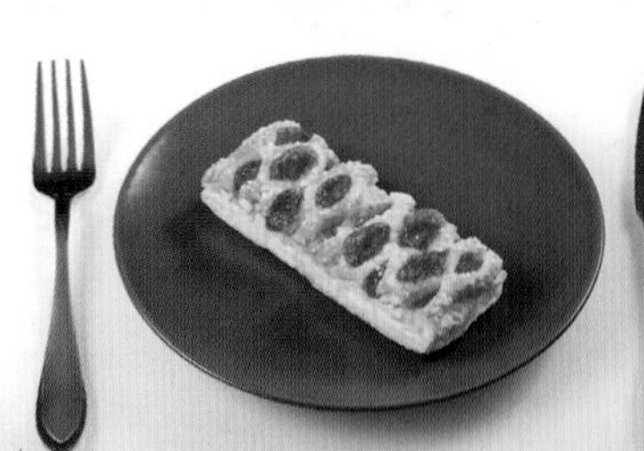

1g FIBRE	Weight: 58g	6g SAT FAT

Pain au Raisin

37g CARBS	318 CALS	7g PROTEIN	16g FAT

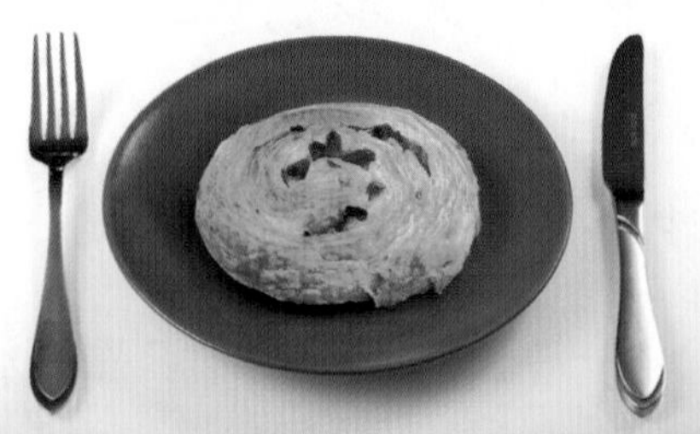

2g FIBRE	Weight: 95g	11g SAT FAT

Pecan Plait

36g CARBS	340 CALS	5g PROTEIN	19g FAT

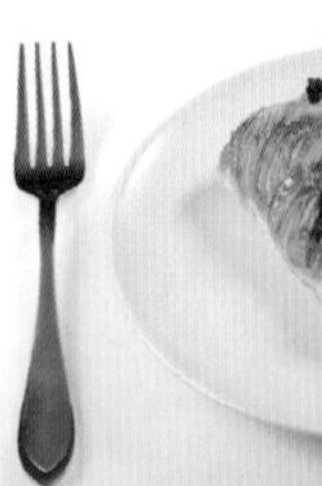

1g FIBRE	Weight: 81g	8g SAT FAT

Chocolate Éclair

21g CARBS	217 CALS	2g PROTEIN	14g FAT

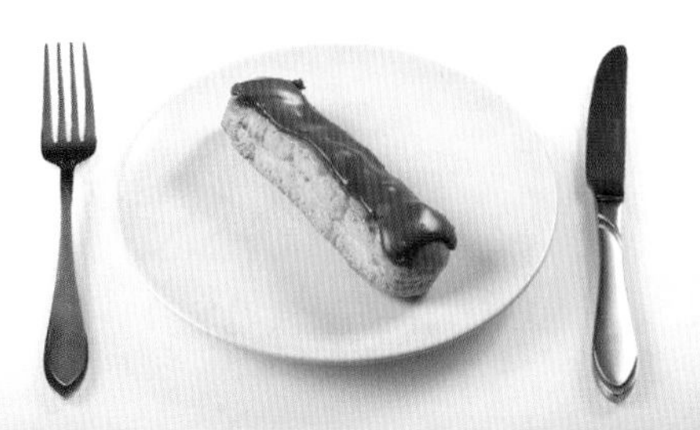

0g FIBRE	Weight: 56g	7g SAT FAT

Corn Flake Cake

40g CARBS	249 CALS	3g PROTEIN	10g FAT

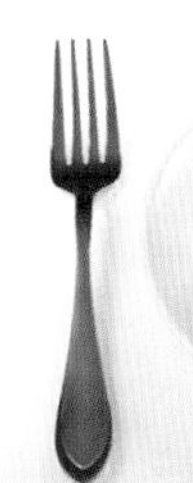
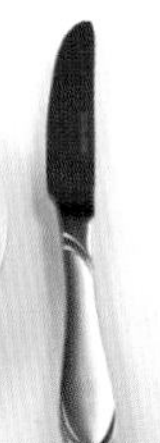

0g FIBRE	Weight: 54g	6g SAT FAT

Cup Cake

34g CARBS	272 CALS	2g PROTEIN	14g FAT

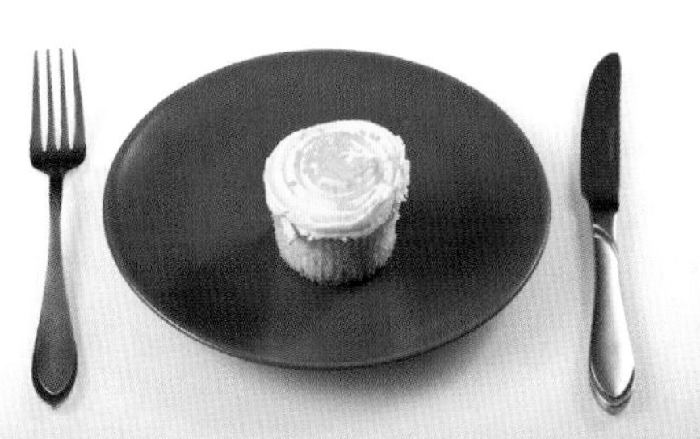

0g FIBRE	Weight: 56g	5g SAT FAT

Custard Slice

40g CARBS	286 CALS	2g PROTEIN	13g FAT

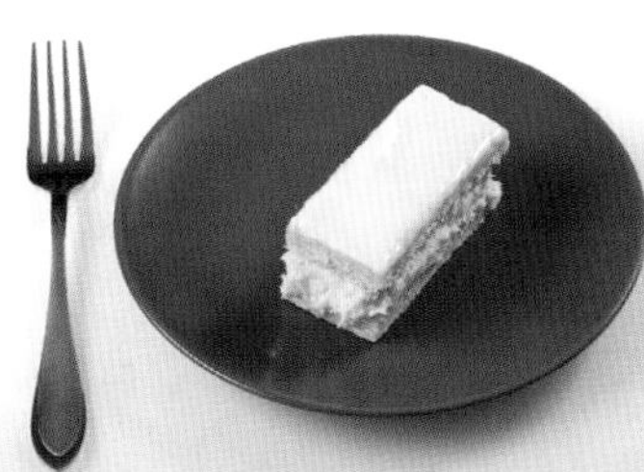

2g FIBRE	Weight: 106g	7g SAT FAT

Custard Tart

27g CARBS	263 CALS	5g PROTEIN	16g FAT

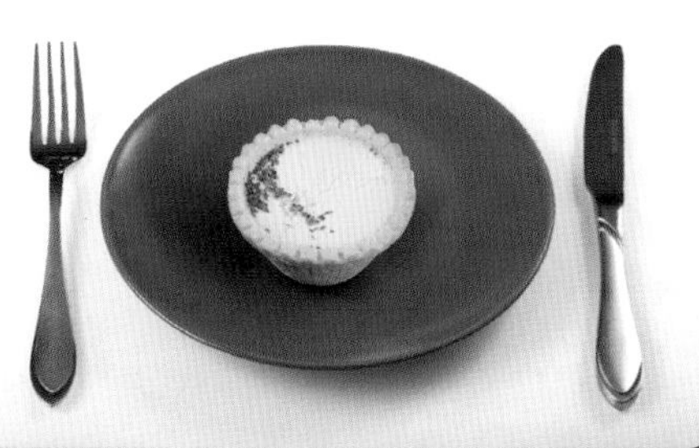

1g FIBRE	Weight: 92g	5g SAT FAT

Mini Battenburg

21g CARBS	120 CALS	1g PROTEIN	3g FAT

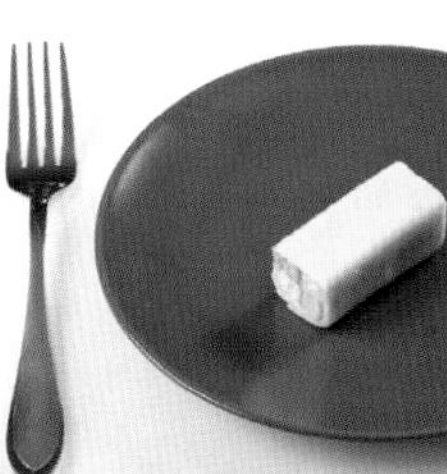

0g FIBRE	Weight: 30g	1g SAT FAT

Choc Ring Doughnut

CARBS	CALS	PROTEIN	FAT
36g	279	3g	13g

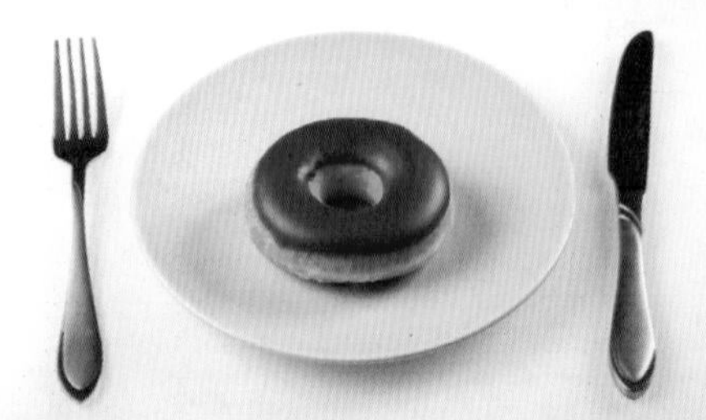

FIBRE	Weight	SAT FAT
1g	Weight: 66g	7g

Glazed Ring Doughnut

CARBS	CALS	PROTEIN	FAT
25g	223	3g	12g

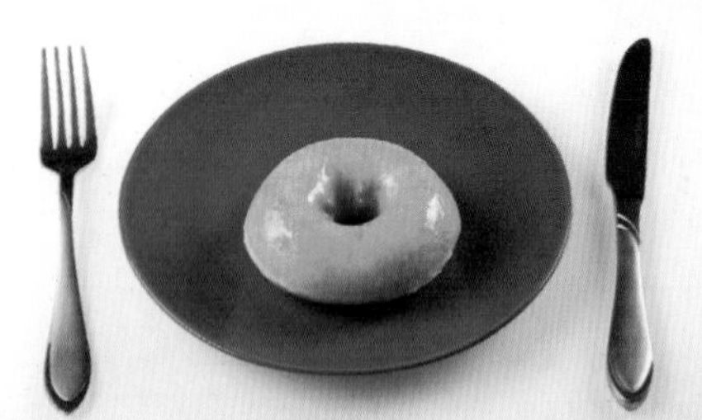

FIBRE	Weight	SAT FAT
1g	Weight: 52g	6g

Jam Doughnut

CARBS	CALS	PROTEIN	FAT
35g	238	4g	9g

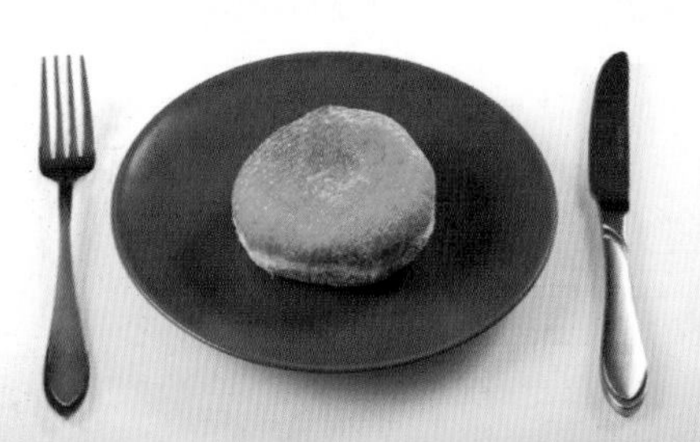

FIBRE	Weight	SAT FAT
2g	Weight: 71g	4g

Mini Doughnut

CARBS	CALS	PROTEIN	FAT
6g	45	1g	2g

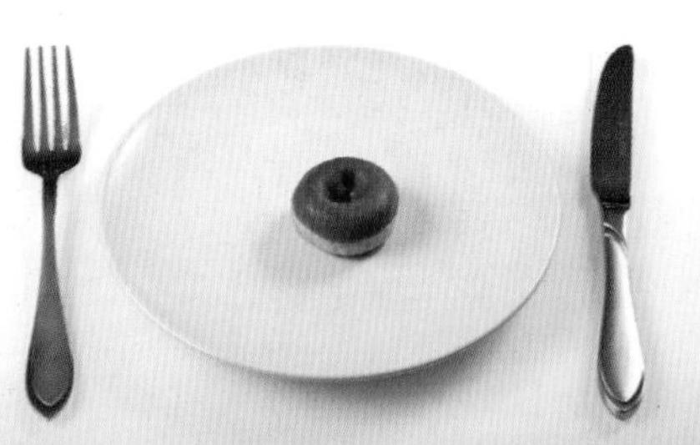

FIBRE	Weight	SAT FAT
0g	Weight: 11g	1g

Sprinkle Ring Doughnut

CARBS	CALS	PROTEIN	FAT
39g	299	4g	13g

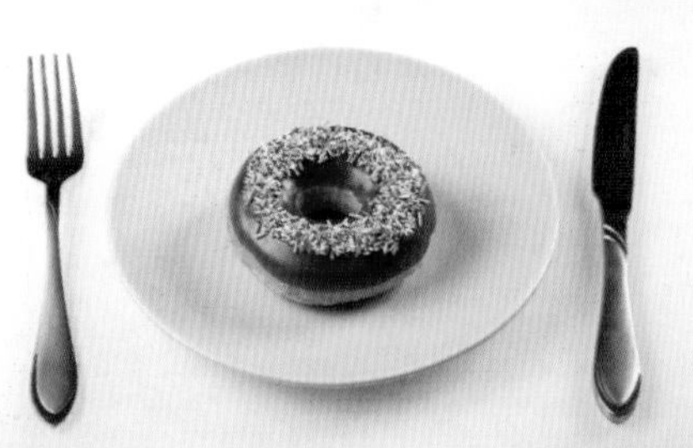

FIBRE	Weight	SAT FAT
1g	Weight: 71g	6g

Sugar Ring Doughnut

CARBS	CALS	PROTEIN	FAT
32g	274	3g	14g

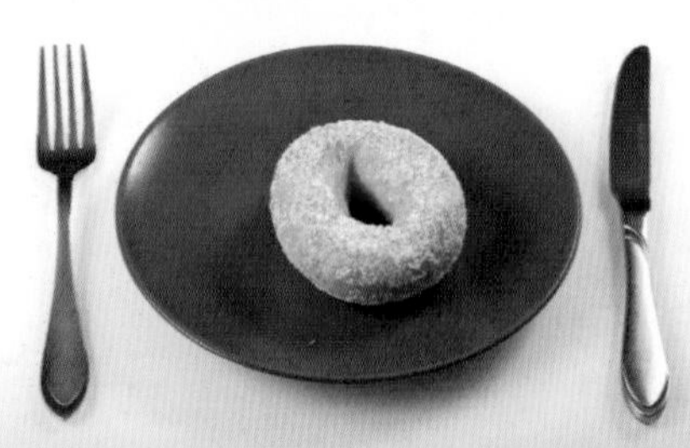

FIBRE	Weight	SAT FAT
1g	Weight: 66g	7g

Fresh Cream Doughnut

CARBS	CALS	PROTEIN	FAT
30g	276	4g	15g

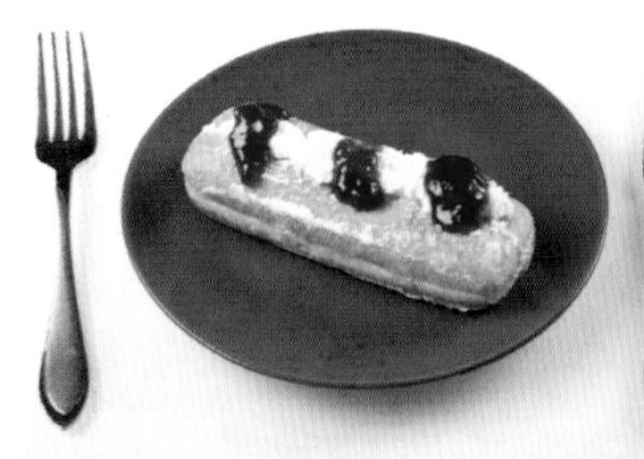

FIBRE	Weight	SAT FAT
1g	Weight: 80g	7g

Yum Yum

CARBS	CALS	PROTEIN	FAT
29g	287	3g	17g

FIBRE	Weight	SAT FAT
1g	Weight: 70g	8g

Blueberry Muffin

CARBS	CALS	PROTEIN	FAT
11g	96	1g	5g

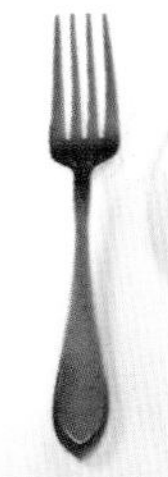

FIBRE	Weight	SAT FAT
1g	Weight: 25g (mini)	1g

CARBS	CALS	PROTEIN	FAT
46g	393	5g	21g

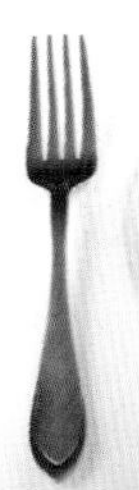

FIBRE	Weight	SAT FAT
2g	Weight: 102g	2g

Chocolate Muffin

CARBS	CALS	PROTEIN	FAT
15g	108	2g	5g

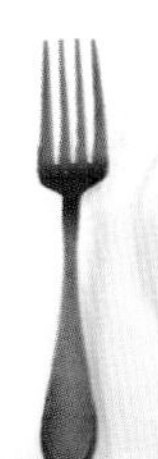

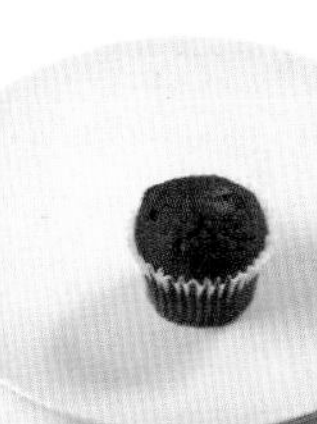

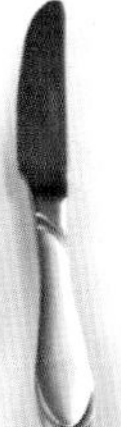

FIBRE	Weight	SAT FAT
1g	Weight: 28g (mini)	3g

CARBS	CALS	PROTEIN	FAT
55g	404	7g	19g

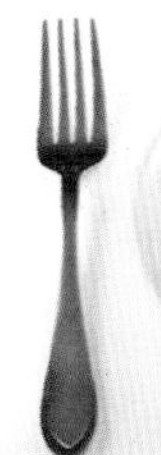

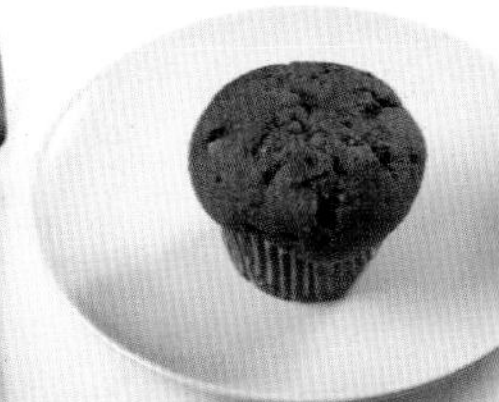

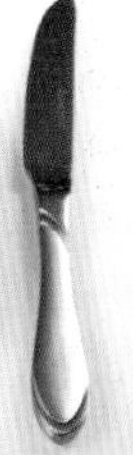

FIBRE	Weight	SAT FAT
2g	Weight: 105g	11g

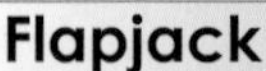

Flapjack

31g CARBS	247 CALS	2g PROTEIN	14g FAT

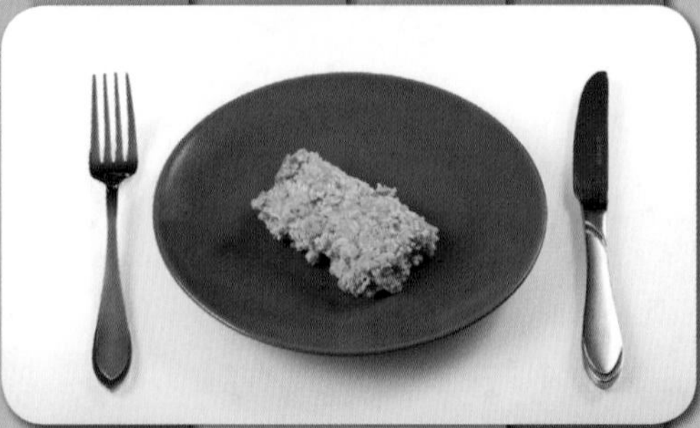

2g FIBRE	Weight: 50g	3g SAT FAT

51g CARBS	404 CALS	4g PROTEIN	22g FAT

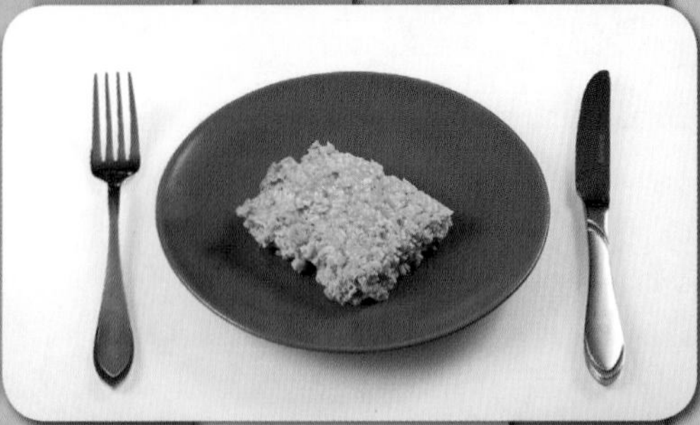

3g FIBRE	Weight: 82g	4g SAT FAT

Meringue Nest

5g CARBS	20 CALS	0g PROTEIN	0g FAT

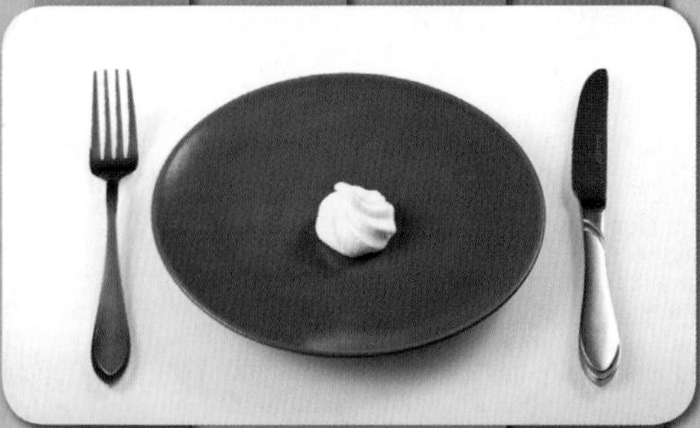

0g FIBRE	Weight: 5g (mini)	0g SAT FAT

15g CARBS	63 CALS	1g PROTEIN	0g FAT

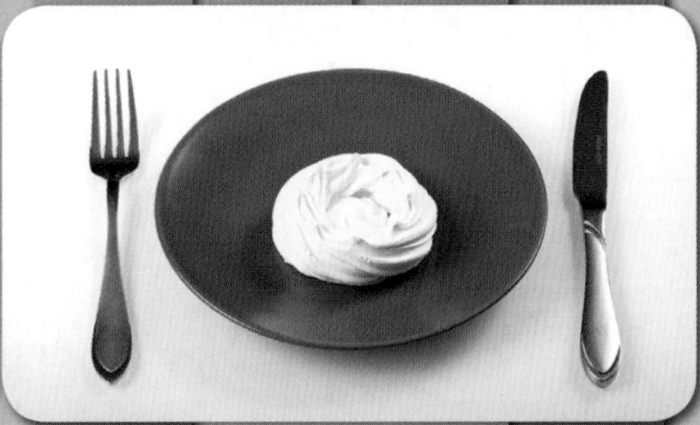

0g FIBRE	Weight: 16g	0g SAT FAT

Mince Pie

26g CARBS	167 CALS	2g PROTEIN	6g FAT

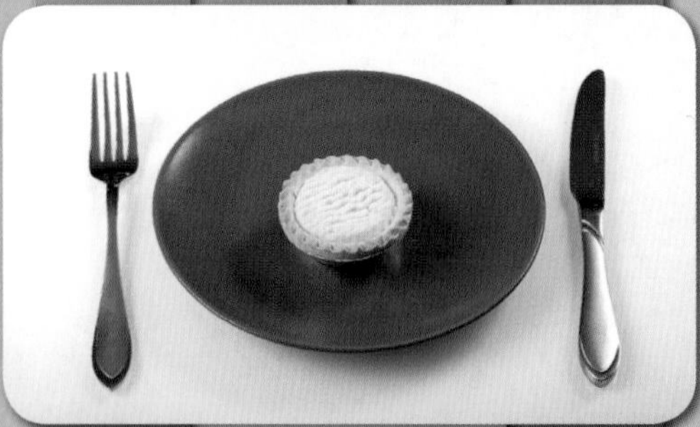

1g FIBRE	Weight: 42g	1g SAT FAT

37g CARBS	239 CALS	2g PROTEIN	9g FAT

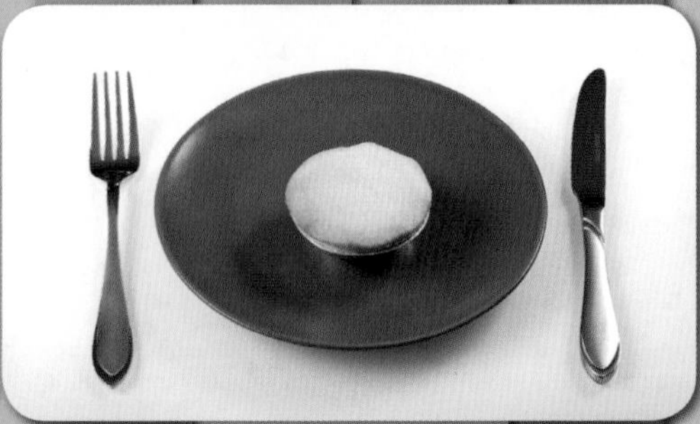

2g FIBRE	Weight: 60g	2g SAT FAT

Belgian Bun

71g CARBS	416 CALS	6g PROTEIN	12g FAT

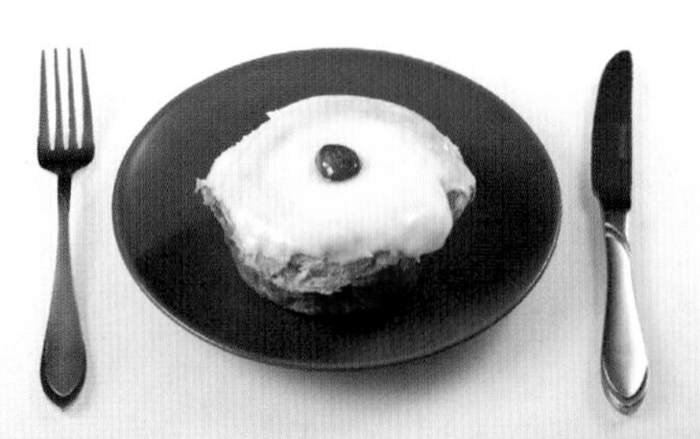

3g FIBRE	Weight: 116g	6g SAT FAT

Iced Bun

21g CARBS	123 CALS	2g PROTEIN	3g FAT

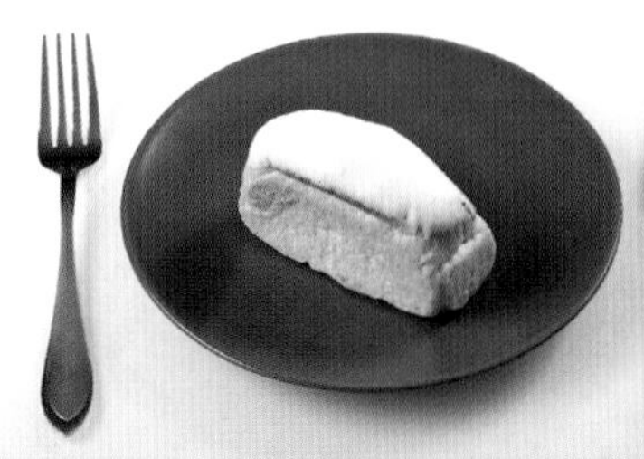

1g FIBRE	Weight: 37g	1g SAT FAT

Hot Cross Bun

30g CARBS	159 CALS	4g PROTEIN	4g FAT

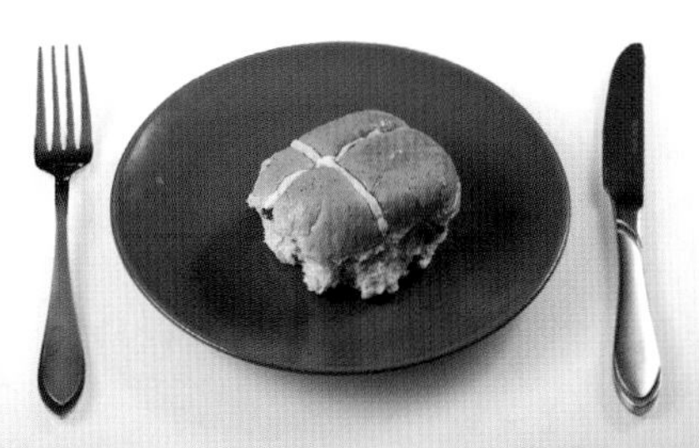

1g FIBRE	Weight: 51g	1g SAT FAT

Cheese Scone

30g CARBS	251 CALS	7g PROTEIN	12g FAT

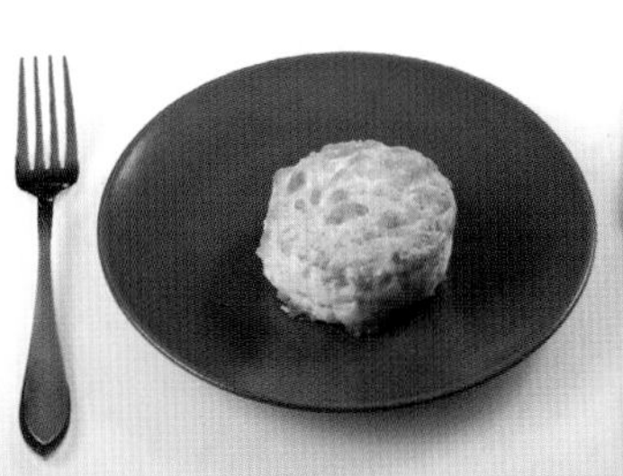

1g FIBRE	Weight: 68g	4g SAT FAT

Fruit Scone

21g CARBS	120 CALS	3g PROTEIN	3g FAT

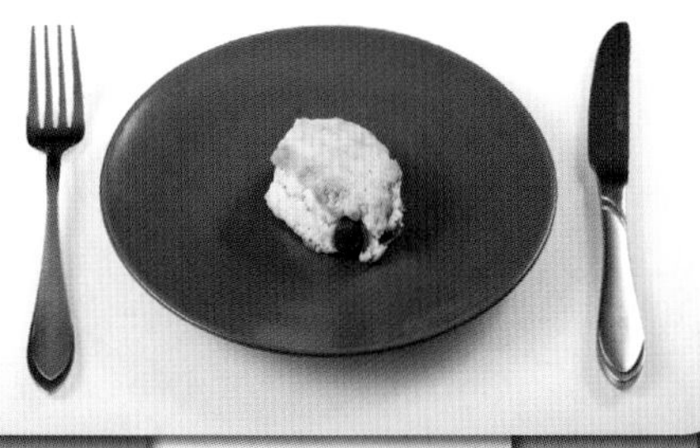

1g FIBRE	Weight: 38g	1g SAT FAT

37g CARBS	208 CALS	4g PROTEIN	6g FAT

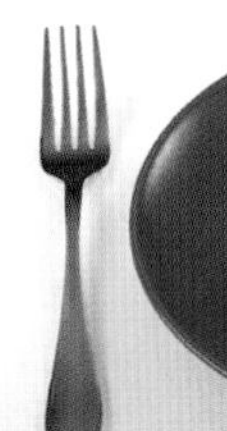

2g FIBRE	Weight: 66g	2g SAT FAT

Blue Stilton

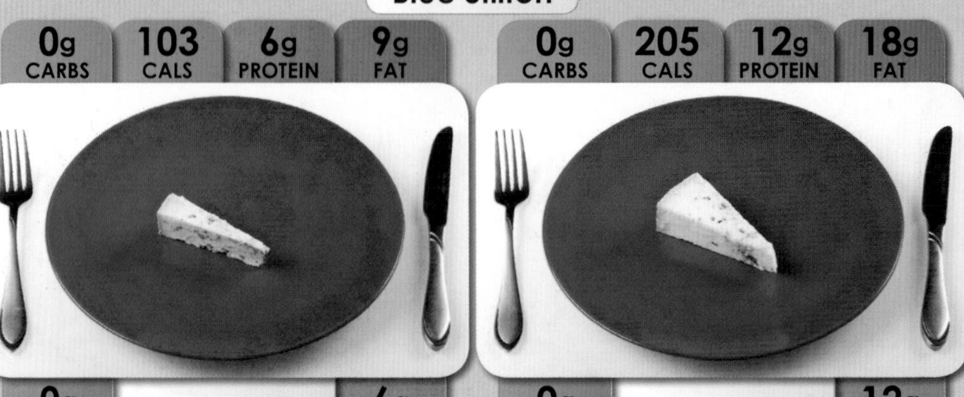

Weight	Carbs	Cals	Protein	Fat	Fibre	Sat Fat
25g	0g	103	6g	9g	0g	6g
50g	0g	205	12g	18g	0g	12g

Brie

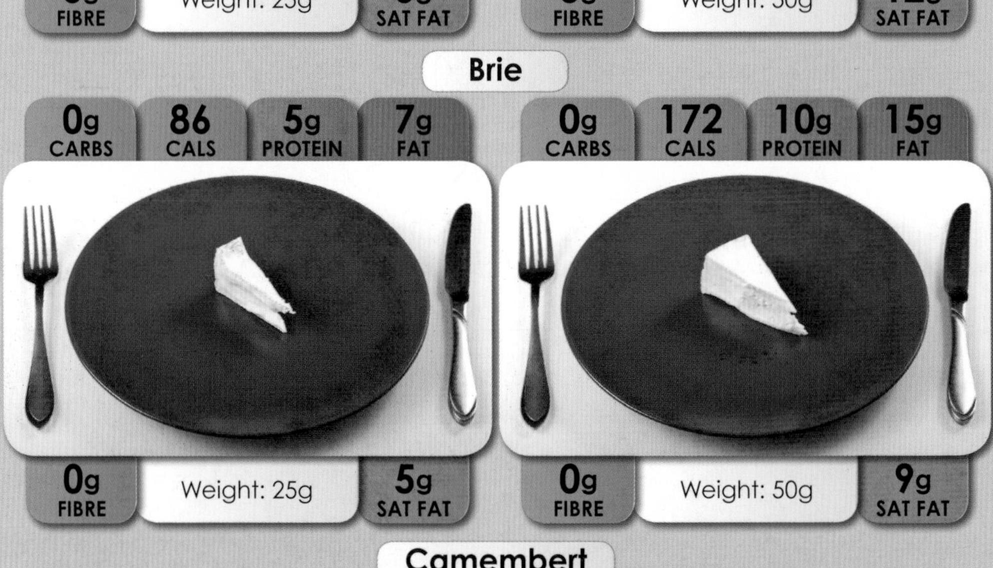

Weight	Carbs	Cals	Protein	Fat	Fibre	Sat Fat
25g	0g	86	5g	7g	0g	5g
50g	0g	172	10g	15g	0g	9g

Camembert

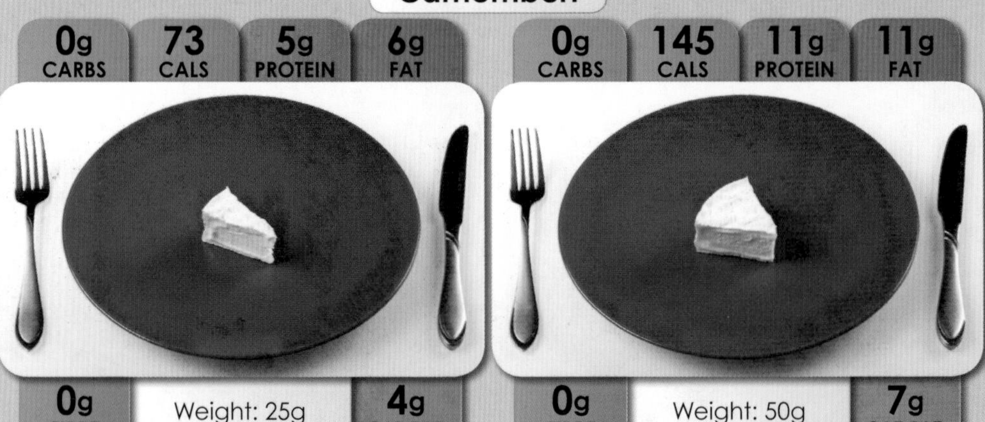

Weight	Carbs	Cals	Protein	Fat	Fibre	Sat Fat
25g	0g	73	5g	6g	0g	4g
50g	0g	145	11g	11g	0g	7g

Cheddar

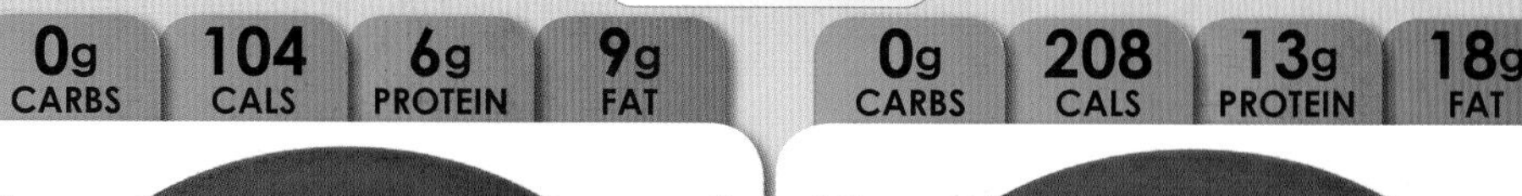

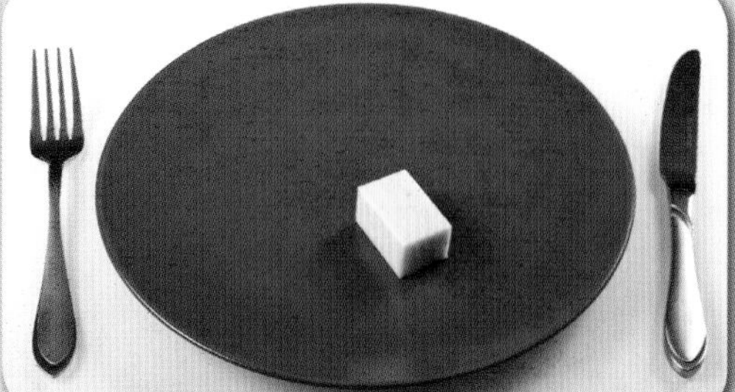

	Weight: 25g	Weight: 50g
CARBS	0g	0g
CALS	104	208
PROTEIN	6g	13g
FAT	9g	18g
FIBRE	0g	0g
SAT FAT	5g	11g

Cheddar (grated)

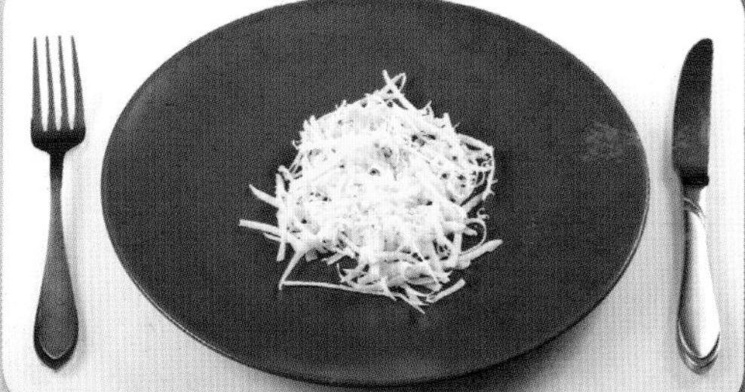

	Weight: 25g	Weight: 50g
CARBS	0g	0g
CALS	104	208
PROTEIN	6g	13g
FAT	9g	18g
FIBRE	0g	0g
SAT FAT	5g	11g

Cheddar (sliced)

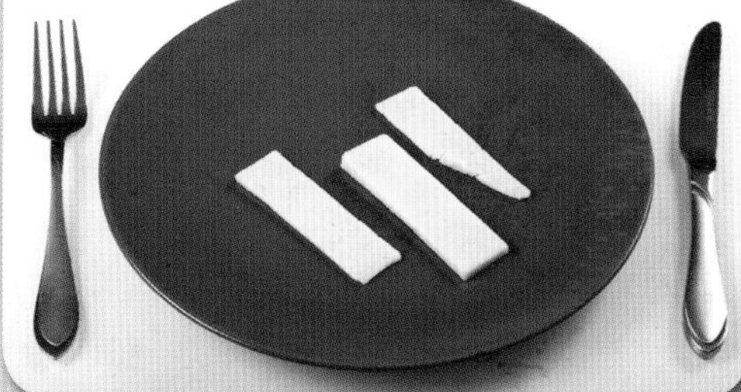

	Weight: 25g	Weight: 50g
CARBS	0g	0g
CALS	104	208
PROTEIN	6g	13g
FAT	9g	18g
FIBRE	0g	0g
SAT FAT	5g	11g

Cheddar (reduced fat)

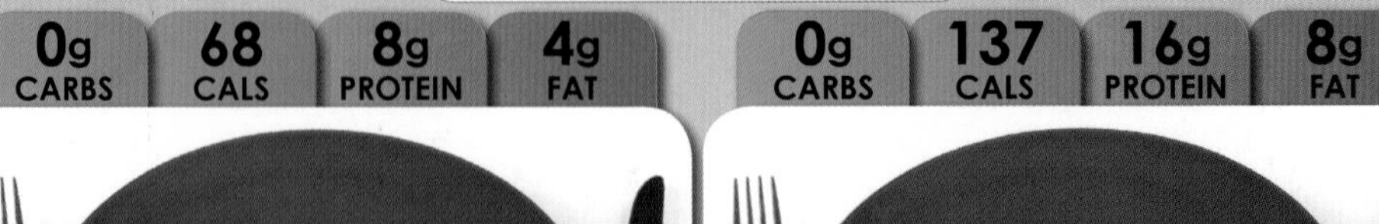

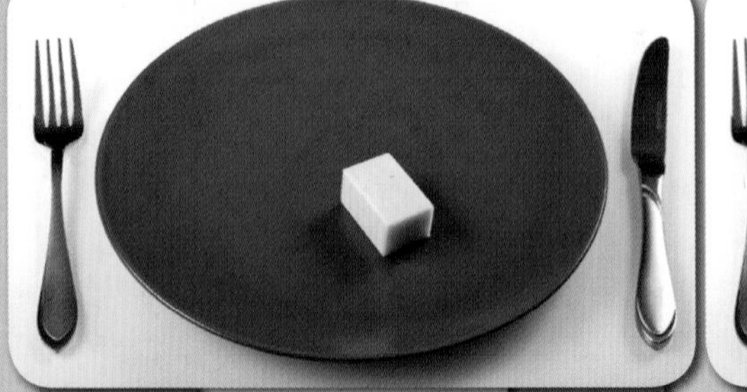

Weight	Carbs	Cals	Protein	Fat	Fibre	Sat Fat
25g	0g	68	8g	4g	0g	3g
50g	0g	137	16g	8g	0g	5g

Cottage Cheese

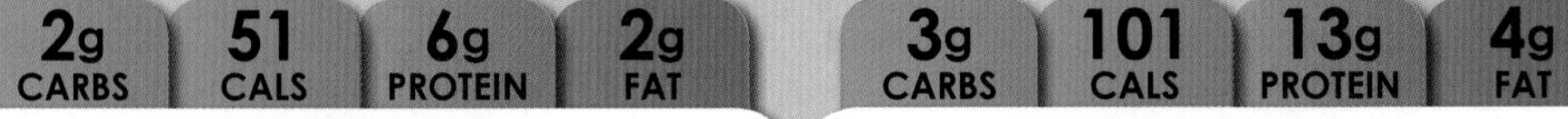

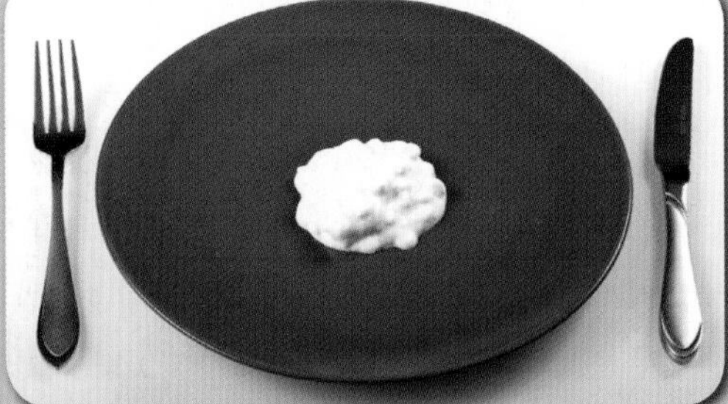

Weight	Carbs	Cals	Protein	Fat	Fibre	Sat Fat
50g	2g	51	6g	2g	0g	1g
100g	3g	101	13g	4g	0g	2g

Cream Cheese

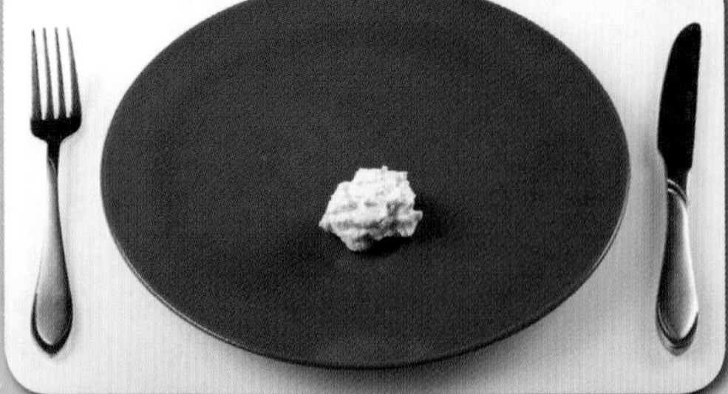

Weight	Carbs	Cals	Protein	Fat	Fibre	Sat Fat
25g	1g	62	1g	6g	0g	4g
50g	2g	125	3g	12g	0g	7g

Edam

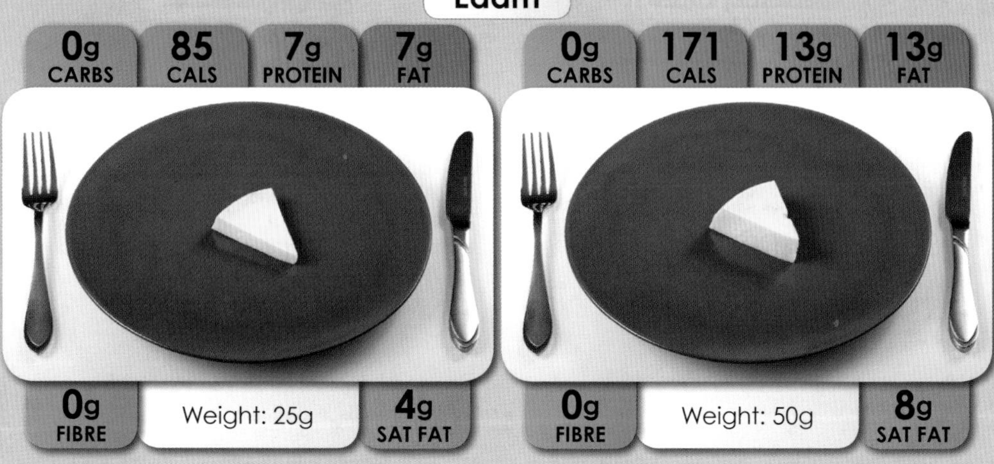

	Weight: 25g	Weight: 50g
CARBS	0g	0g
CALS	85	171
PROTEIN	7g	13g
FAT	7g	13g
FIBRE	0g	0g
SAT FAT	4g	8g

Feta

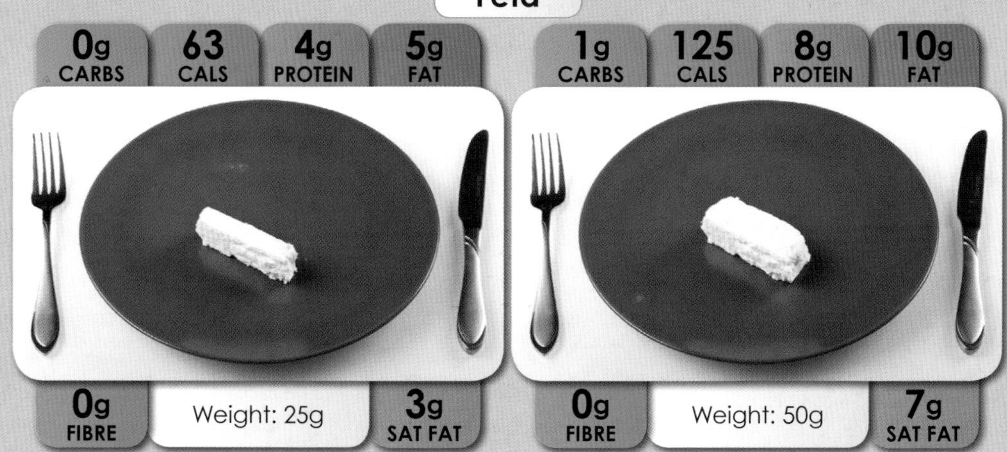

	Weight: 25g	Weight: 50g
CARBS	0g	1g
CALS	63	125
PROTEIN	4g	8g
FAT	5g	10g
FIBRE	0g	0g
SAT FAT	3g	7g

Goat's Cheese

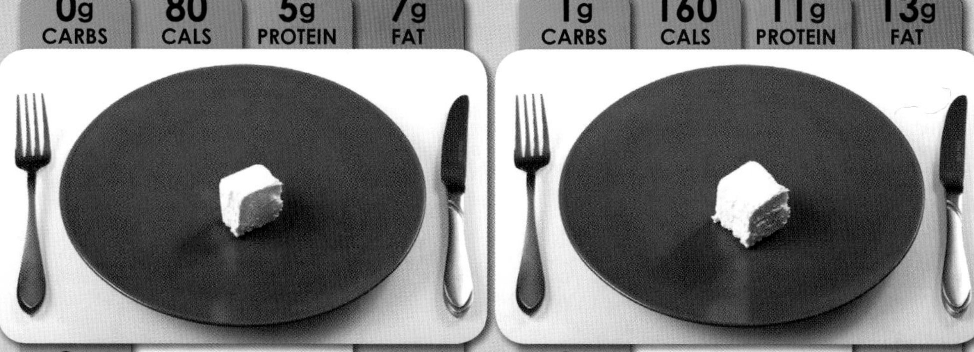

	Weight: 25g	Weight: 50g
CARBS	0g	1g
CALS	80	160
PROTEIN	5g	11g
FAT	7g	13g
FIBRE	0g	0g
SAT FAT	5g	9g

Halloumi

CARBS	CALS	PROTEIN	FAT	FIBRE	Weight	SAT FAT
1g	80	5g	6g	0g	25g	4g
1g	160	10g	13g	0g	50g	8g

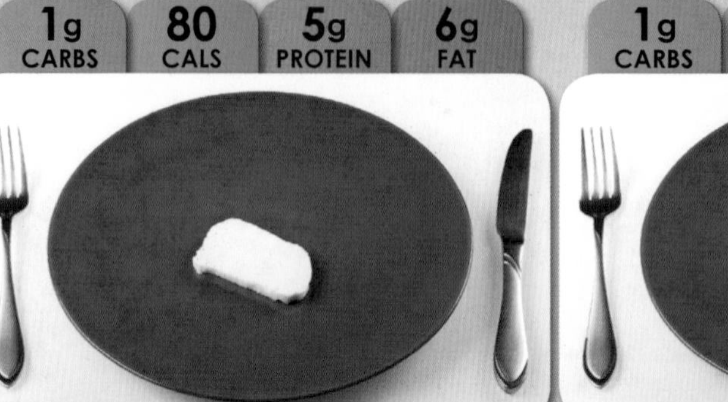

Mozzarella

CARBS	CALS	PROTEIN	FAT	FIBRE	Weight	SAT FAT
0g	64	5g	5g	0g	25g	4g
0g	129	9g	10g	0g	50g	7g

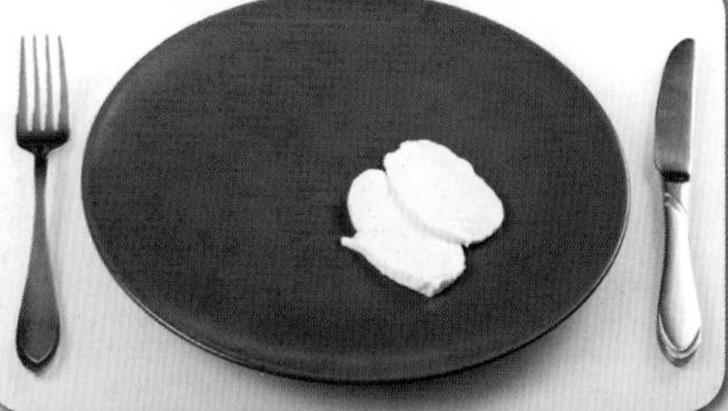

Processed Cheese Slice

CARBS	CALS	PROTEIN	FAT	FIBRE	Weight	SAT FAT
1g	59	4g	5g	0g	20g	3g

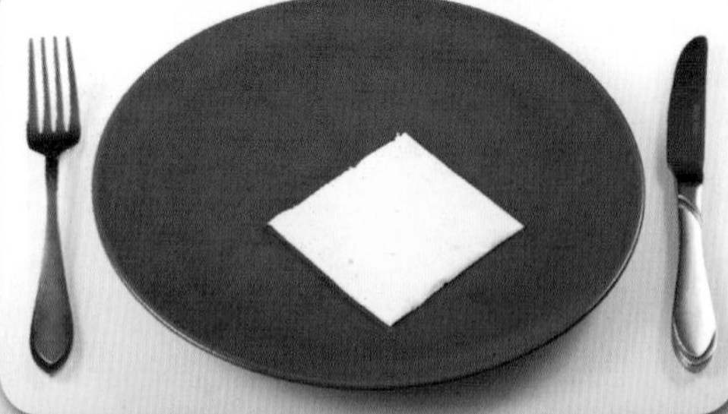

Spreadable Cheese

CARBS	CALS	PROTEIN	FAT	FIBRE	Weight	SAT FAT
1g	48	2g	4g	0g	18g	3g

Parmesan

	Carbs	Cals	Protein	Fat	Fibre	Weight	Sat Fat
	0g	104	9g	7g	0g	Weight: 25g	5g
	1g	208	18g	15g	0g	Weight: 50g	10g

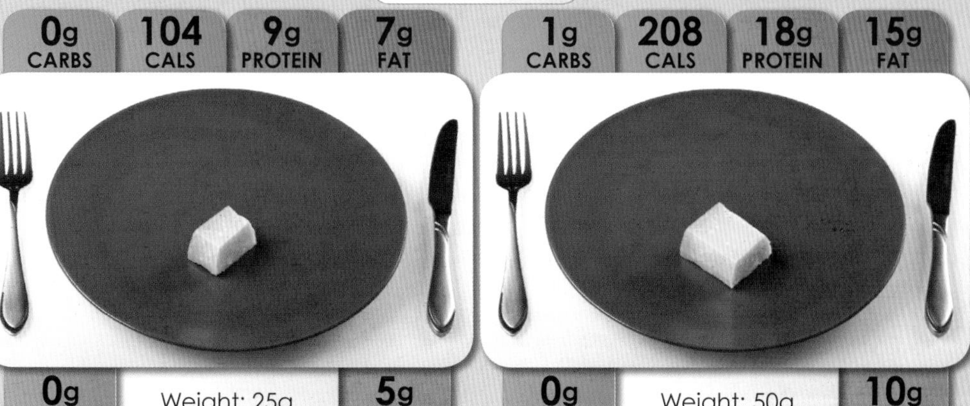

Parmesan (grated)

	Carbs	Cals	Protein	Fat	Fibre	Weight	Sat Fat
	0g	42	4g	3g	0g	Weight: 10g	2g
	0g	83	7g	6g	0g	Weight: 20g	4g

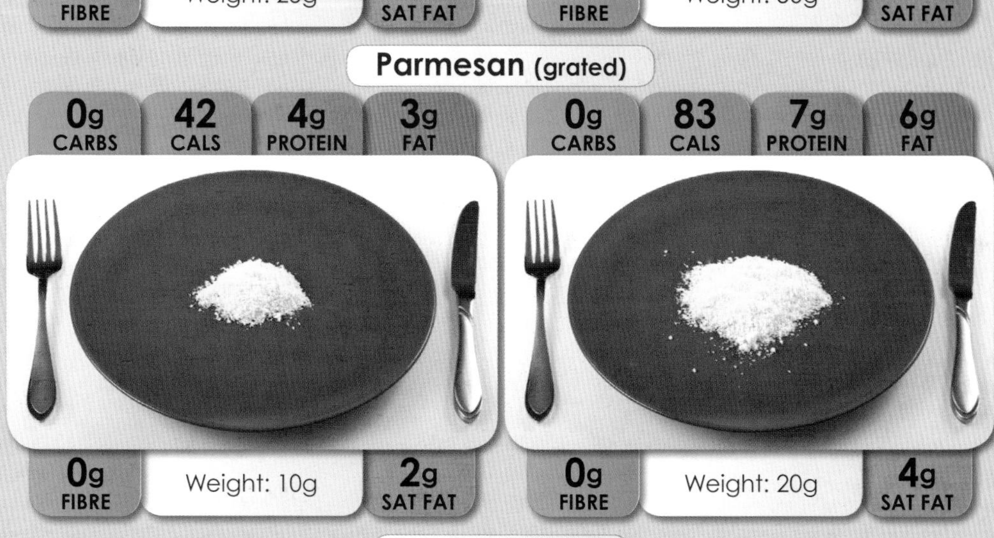

Red Leicester

	Carbs	Cals	Protein	Fat	Fibre	Weight	Sat Fat
	0g	100	6g	8g	0g	Weight: 25g	5g
	0g	201	12g	17g	0g	Weight: 50g	11g

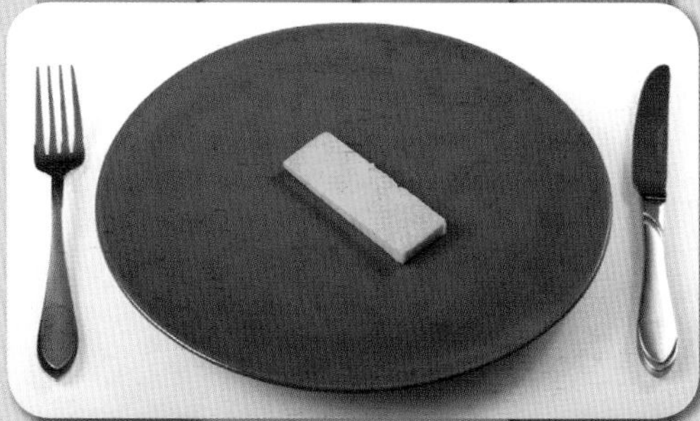

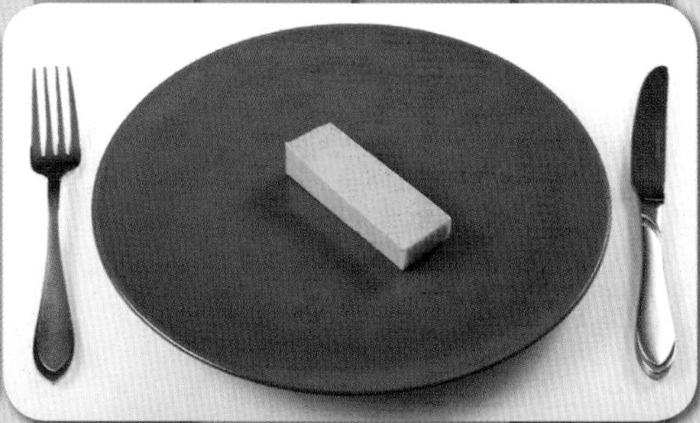

Ricotta

CARBS	CALS	PROTEIN	FAT
1g	36	2g	3g

FIBRE	Weight	SAT FAT
0g	Weight: 25g	2g

CARBS	CALS	PROTEIN	FAT
1g	72	5g	6g

FIBRE	Weight	SAT FAT
0g	Weight: 50g	4g

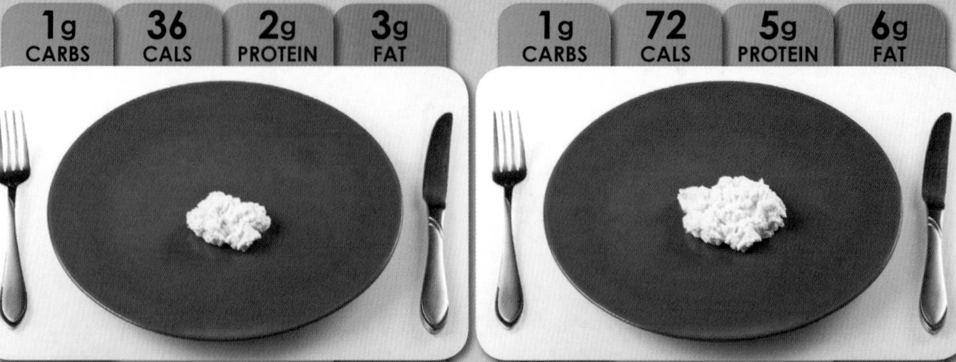

Squirty Cheese

CARBS	CALS	PROTEIN	FAT
0g	24	2g	2g

FIBRE	Weight	SAT FAT
1g	Weight: 12g	1g

CARBS	CALS	PROTEIN	FAT
1g	48	3g	4g

FIBRE	Weight	SAT FAT
1g	Weight: 24g	3g

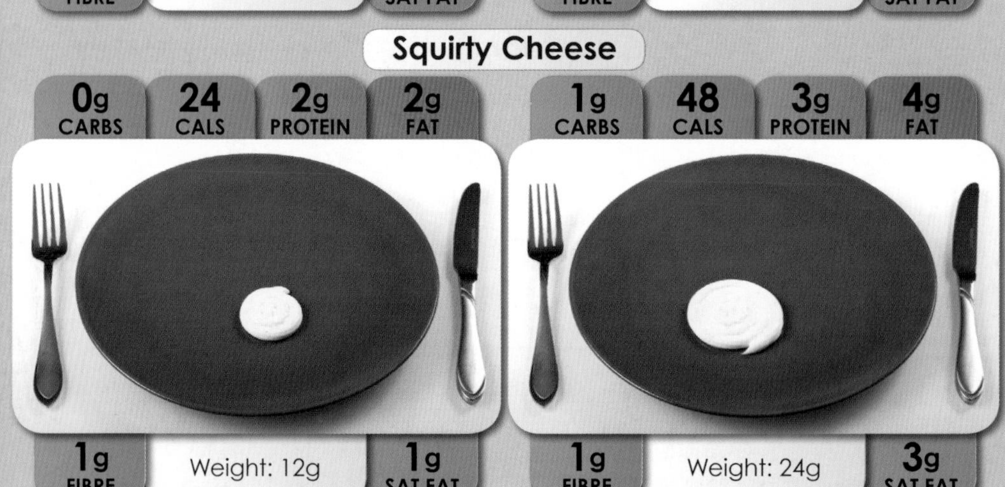

Wensleydale with Cranberries

CARBS	CALS	PROTEIN	FAT
3g	94	5g	7g

FIBRE	Weight	SAT FAT
0g	Weight: 25g	5g

CARBS	CALS	PROTEIN	FAT
6g	188	10g	13g

FIBRE	Weight	SAT FAT
1g	Weight: 50g	9g

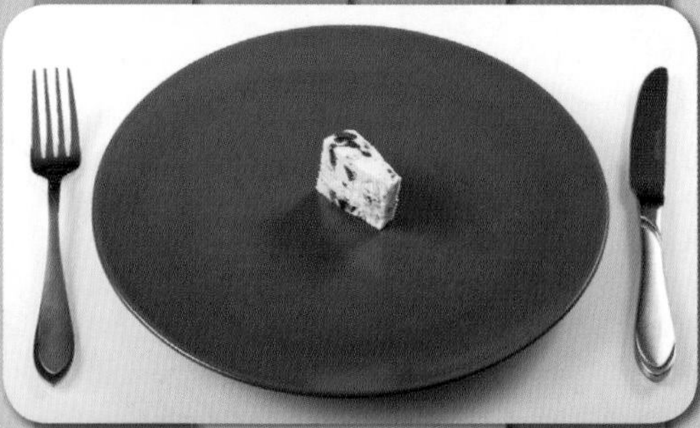

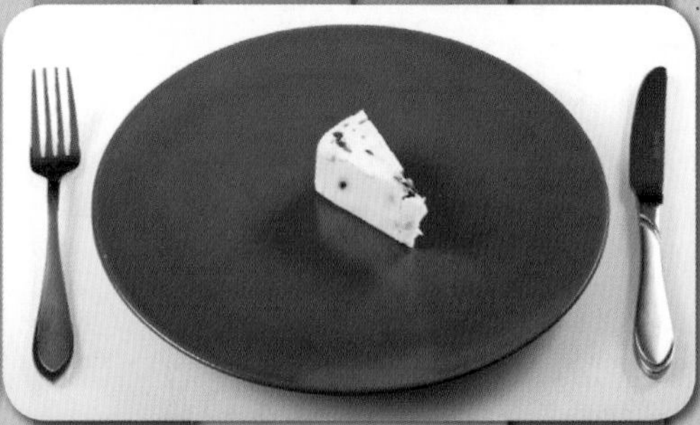

Apple Pie

CARBS	CALS	PROTEIN	FAT
29g	214	2g	11g

FIBRE	Weight	SAT FAT
2g	Weight: 80g	3g

CARBS	CALS	PROTEIN	FAT
57g	427	5g	22g

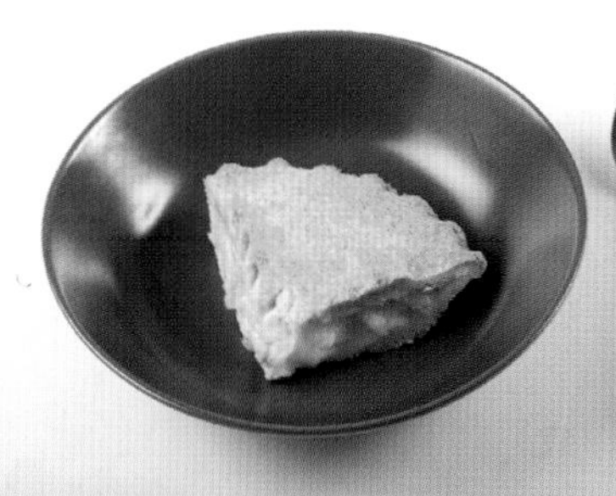
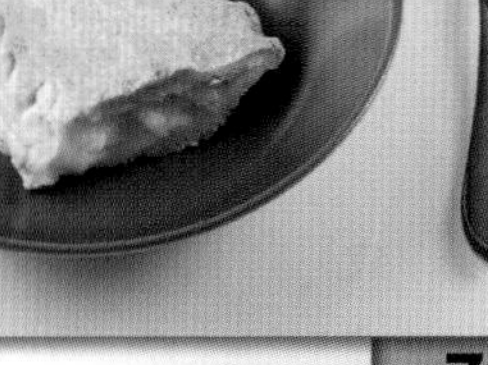

FIBRE	Weight	SAT FAT
4g	Weight: 160g	7g

CARBS	CALS	PROTEIN	FAT
114g	854	9g	43g

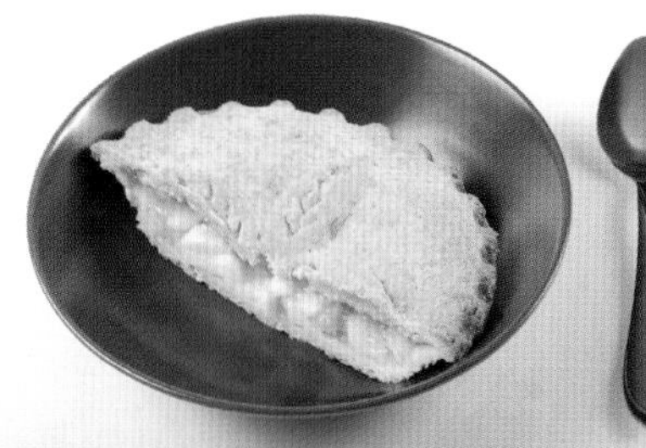

FIBRE	Weight	SAT FAT
7g	Weight: 320g	13g

Apple & Rhubarb Crumble

CARBS	CALS	PROTEIN	FAT
20g	120	1g	4g

FIBRE	Weight	SAT FAT
1g	Weight: 60g	1g

CARBS	CALS	PROTEIN	FAT
40g	234	2g	8g

FIBRE	Weight	SAT FAT
3g	Weight: 117g	2g

CARBS	CALS	PROTEIN	FAT
80g	470	5g	17g

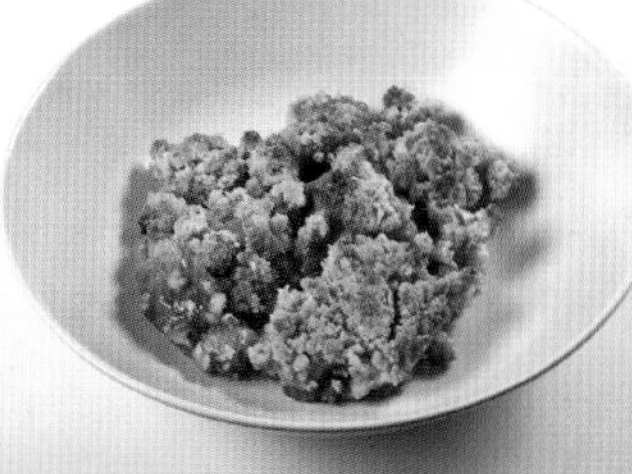

FIBRE	Weight	SAT FAT
5g	Weight: 235g	3g

Apple Strudel

CARBS	CALS	PROTEIN	FAT	FIBRE	Weight	SAT FAT
15g	109	1g	5g	0g	45g	2g
45g	328	4g	15g	1g	135g	7g
76g	554	6g	25g	2g	228g	11g

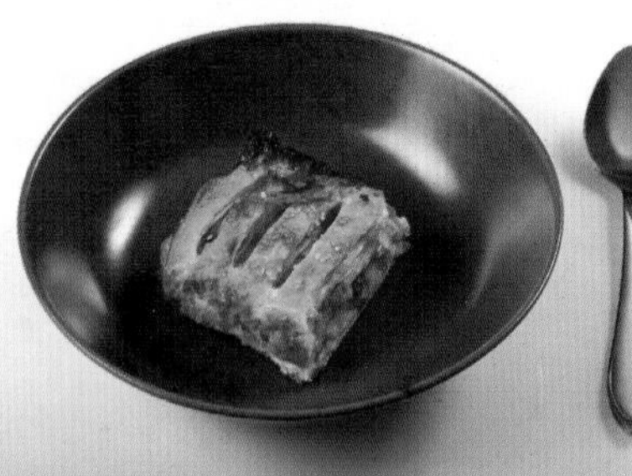

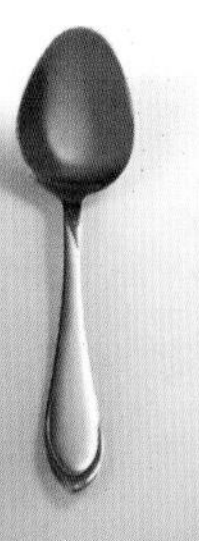

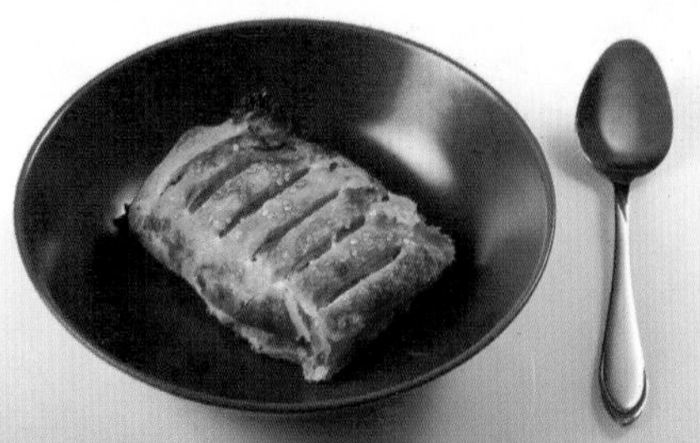

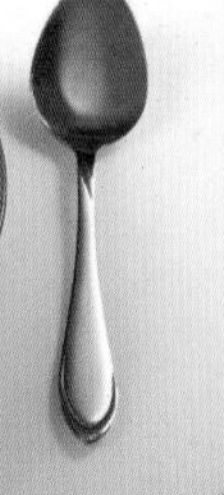

Banoffee Pie

CARBS	CALS	PROTEIN	FAT	FIBRE	Weight	SAT FAT
16g	148	1g	9g	0g	43g	5g
48g	456	4g	27g	1g	133g	15g
80g	755	7g	44g	2g	220g	25g

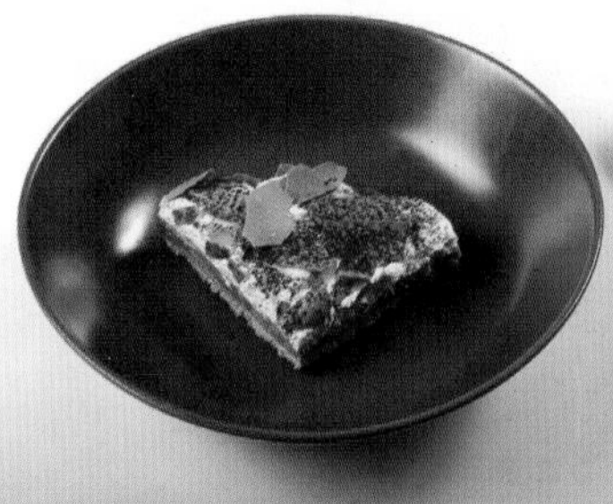

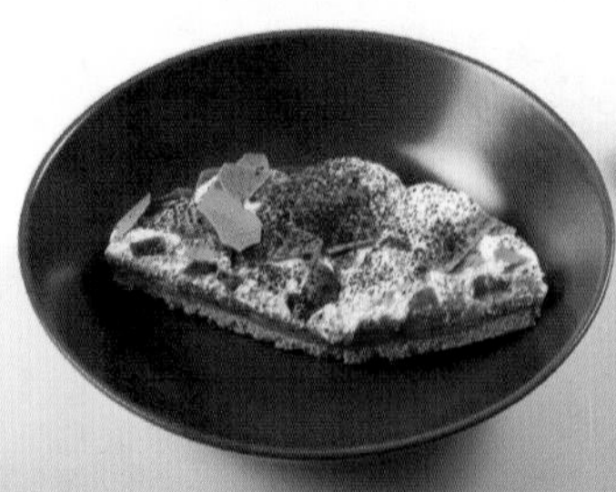

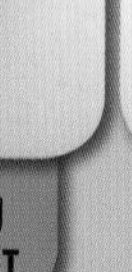

Black Forest Gateau

CARBS	CALS	PROTEIN	FAT
22g	177	2g	9g

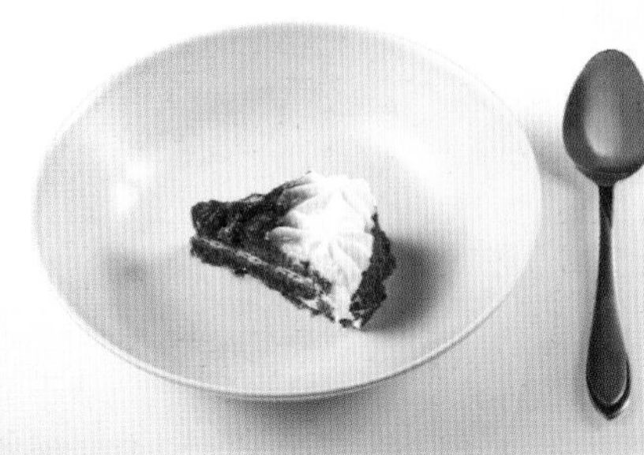

FIBRE	Weight	SAT FAT
1g	Weight: 60g	6g

CARBS	CALS	PROTEIN	FAT
45g	354	4g	19g

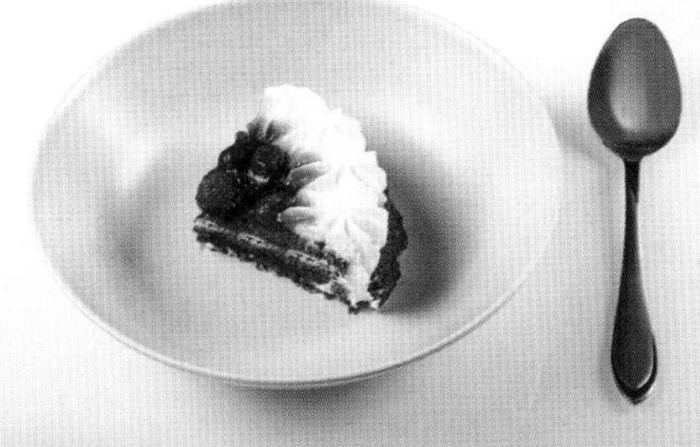

FIBRE	Weight	SAT FAT
2g	Weight: 120g	12g

CARBS	CALS	PROTEIN	FAT
89g	708	8g	38g

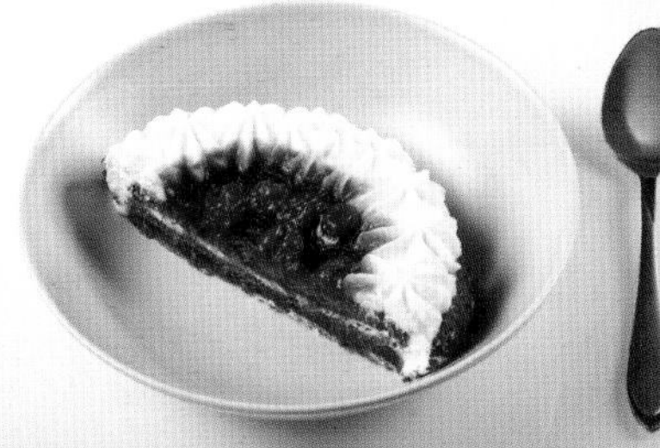

FIBRE	Weight	SAT FAT
5g	Weight: 240g	25g

Bread & Butter Pudding

CARBS	CALS	PROTEIN	FAT
19g	201	4g	11g

FIBRE	Weight	SAT FAT
1g	Weight: 81g	6g

CARBS	CALS	PROTEIN	FAT
39g	407	9g	22g

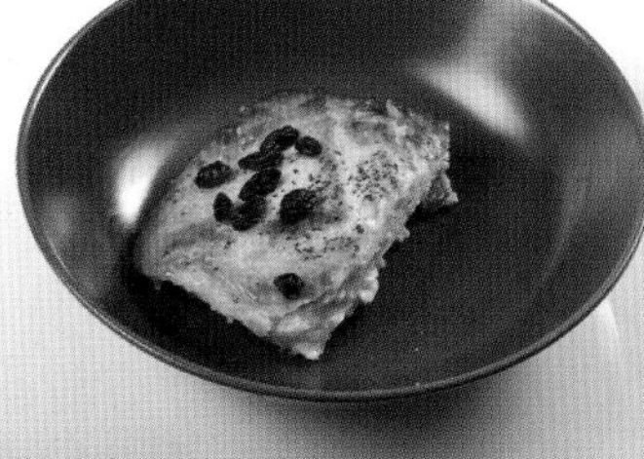

FIBRE	Weight	SAT FAT
1g	Weight: 164g	13g

CARBS	CALS	PROTEIN	FAT
59g	610	14g	33g

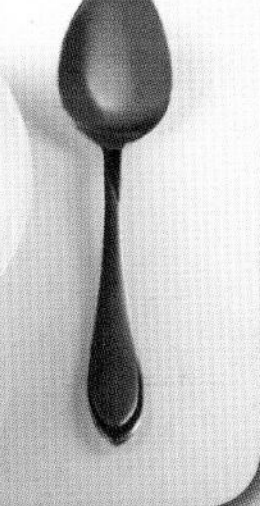

FIBRE	Weight	SAT FAT
2g	Weight: 246g	19g

Brownie

CARBS	CALS	PROTEIN	FAT
24g	199	2g	11g

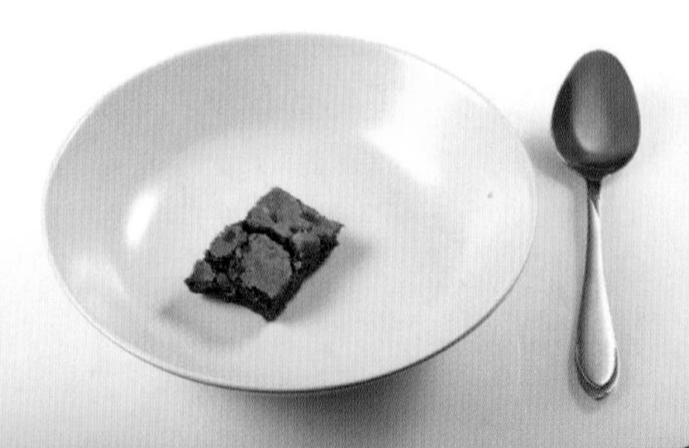

FIBRE	Weight	SAT FAT
1g	Weight: 45g	7g

CARBS	CALS	PROTEIN	FAT
67g	561	6g	31g

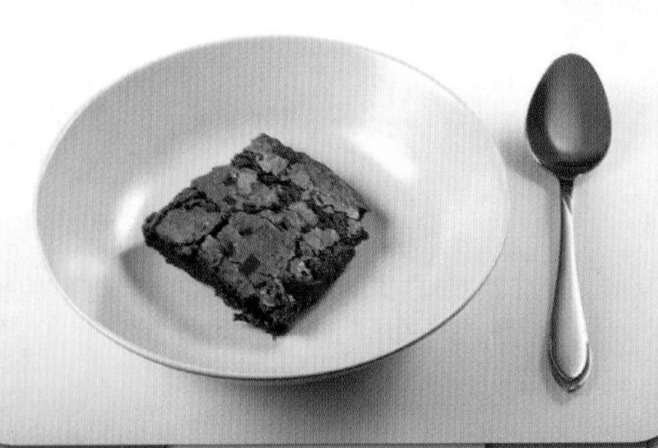

FIBRE	Weight	SAT FAT
3g	Weight: 127g	19g

CARBS	CALS	PROTEIN	FAT
111g	924	10g	51g

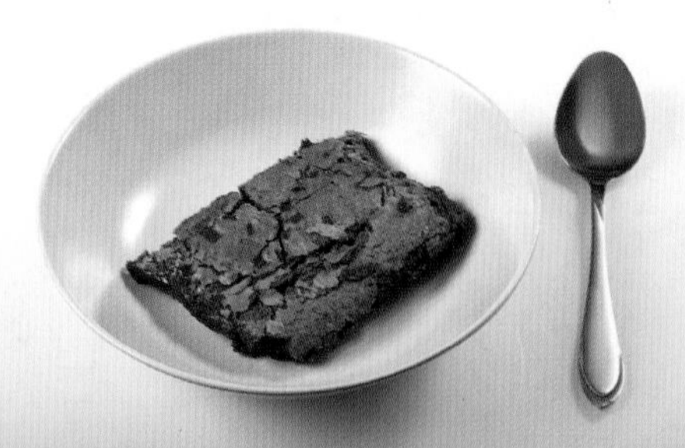

FIBRE	Weight	SAT FAT
4g	Weight: 209g	31g

Chocolate Torte

CARBS	CALS	PROTEIN	FAT
10g	141	2g	10g

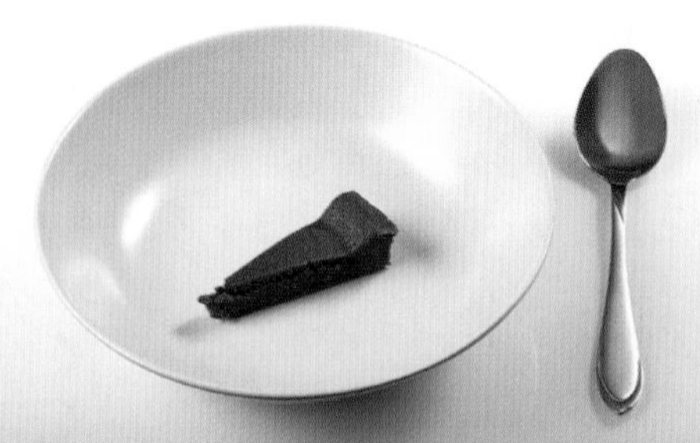

FIBRE	Weight	SAT FAT
1g	Weight: 33g	6g

CARBS	CALS	PROTEIN	FAT
31g	427	6g	31g

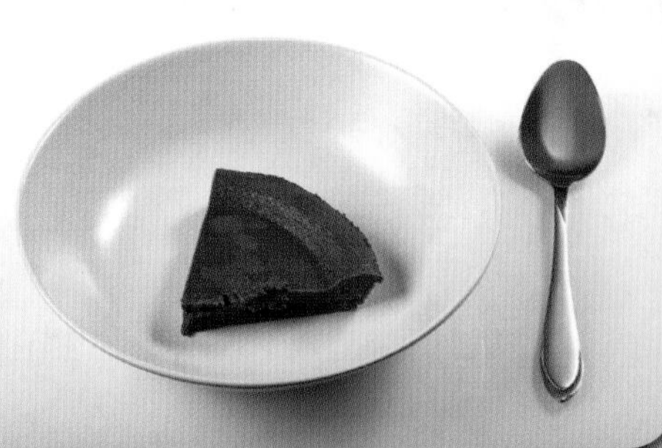

FIBRE	Weight	SAT FAT
2g	Weight: 100g	19g

CARBS	CALS	PROTEIN	FAT
52g	709	10g	52g

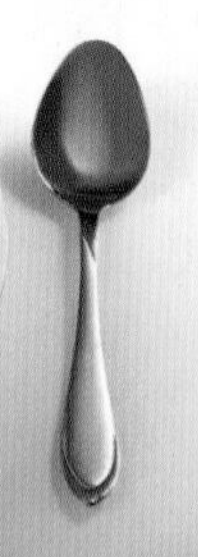

FIBRE	Weight	SAT FAT
3g	Weight: 166g	31g

Cheesecake

18g	147	2g	8g
CARBS	CALS	PROTEIN	FAT

1g FIBRE	Weight: 50g	5g SAT FAT

35g	294	4g	16g
CARBS	CALS	PROTEIN	FAT

1g FIBRE	Weight: 100g	9g SAT FAT

53g	441	6g	24g
CARBS	CALS	PROTEIN	FAT

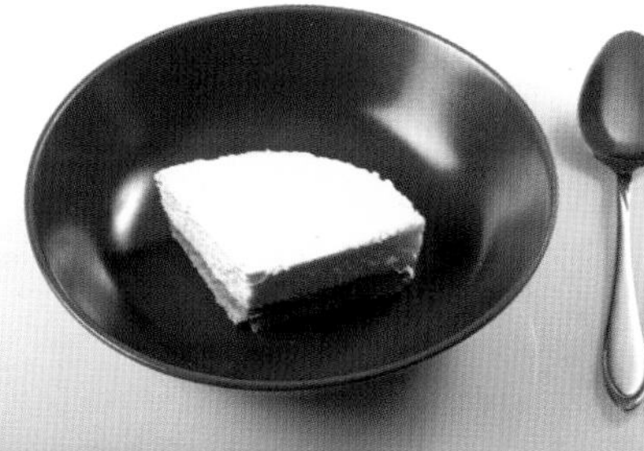

2g FIBRE	Weight: 150g	14g SAT FAT

70g	588	8g	32g
CARBS	CALS	PROTEIN	FAT

2g FIBRE	Weight: 200g	19g SAT FAT

88g	735	10g	41g
CARBS	CALS	PROTEIN	FAT

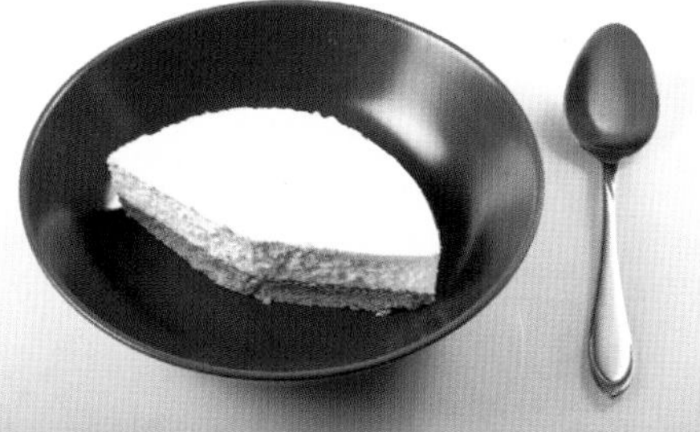

3g FIBRE	Weight: 250g	24g SAT FAT

106g	882	12g	49g
CARBS	CALS	PROTEIN	FAT

3g FIBRE	Weight: 300g	28g SAT FAT

Christmas Pudding

20g CARBS	115 CALS	1g PROTEIN	4g FAT

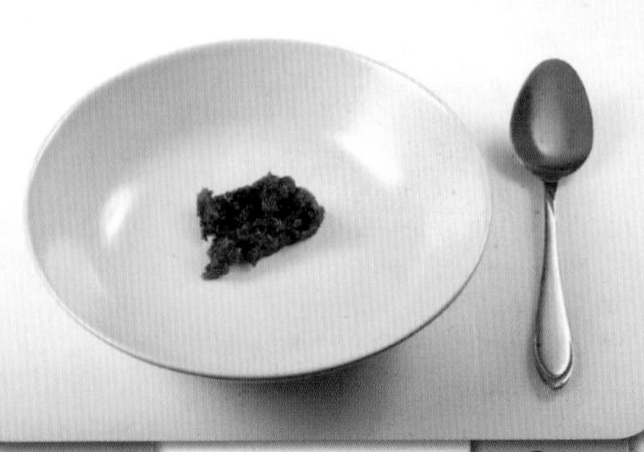

1g FIBRE	Weight: 35g	2g SAT FAT

60g CARBS	349 CALS	3g PROTEIN	13g FAT

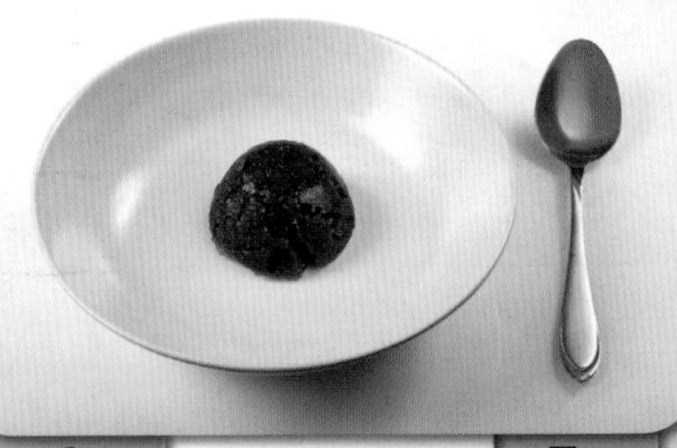

2g FIBRE	Weight: 106g	7g SAT FAT

100g CARBS	582 CALS	5g PROTEIN	21g FAT

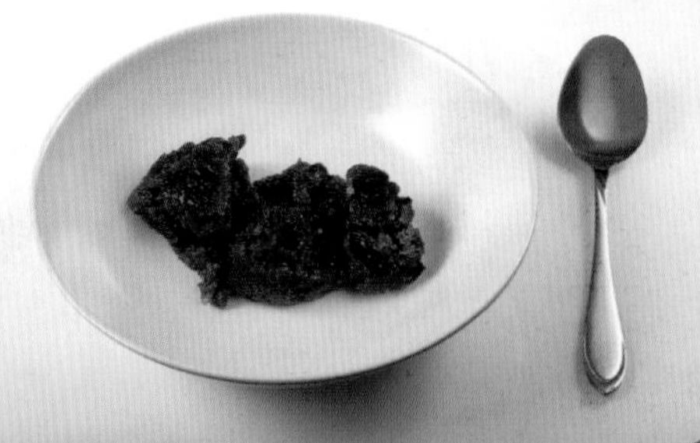

4g FIBRE	Weight: 177g	11g SAT FAT

Custard (with semi-skimmed milk)

10g CARBS	57 CALS	2g PROTEIN	1g FAT

0g FIBRE	Weight: 60g	1g SAT FAT

30g CARBS	171 CALS	7g PROTEIN	4g FAT

0g FIBRE	Weight: 180g	2g SAT FAT

49g CARBS	285 CALS	12g PROTEIN	6g FAT

0g FIBRE	Weight: 300g	4g SAT FAT

Ice Cream (chocolate)

Carbs	Cals	Protein	Fat	Fibre	Sat Fat	Weight
9g	69	1g	3g	0g	2g	40g
18g	137	2g	6g	1g	4g	80g
27g	206	4g	9g	1g	6g	120g

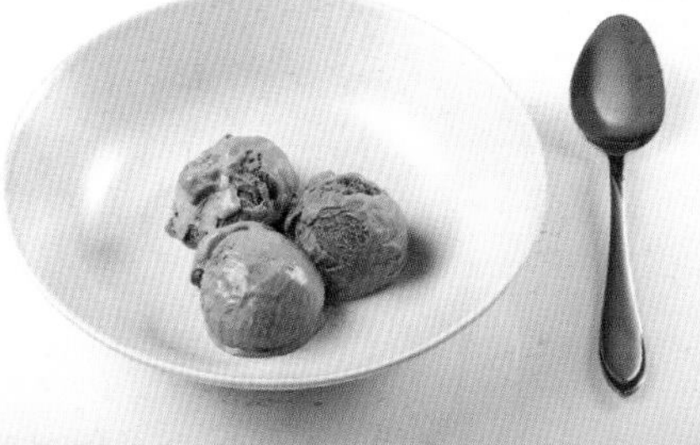

Ice Cream (vanilla)

Carbs	Cals	Protein	Fat	Fibre	Sat Fat	Weight
8g	71	1g	4g	0g	2g	40g
16g	142	3g	8g	0g	5g	80g
24g	214	4g	12g	0g	7g	121g

22cm Large Bowl

Sorbet (lemon)

Weight	Carbs	Cals	Protein	Fat	Fibre	Sat Fat
45g	11g	44	0g	0g	0g	0g
88g	22g	85	0g	0g	1g	0g
132g	33g	128	0g	0g	1g	0g

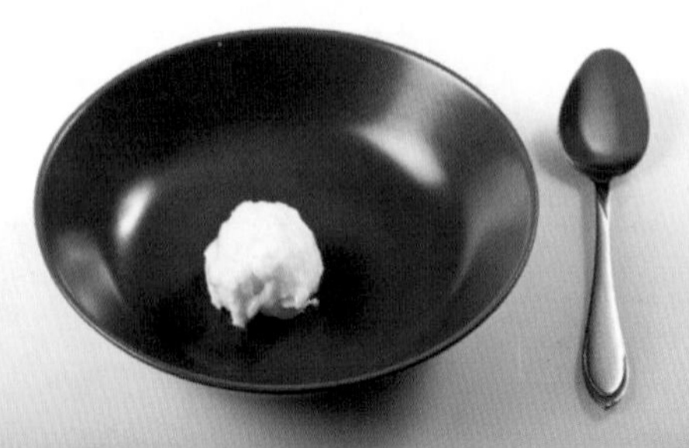

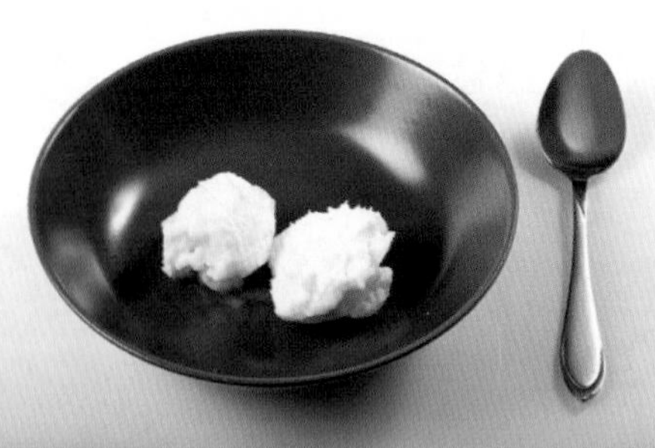

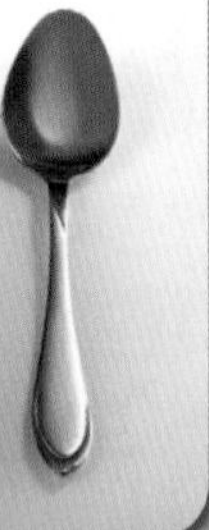

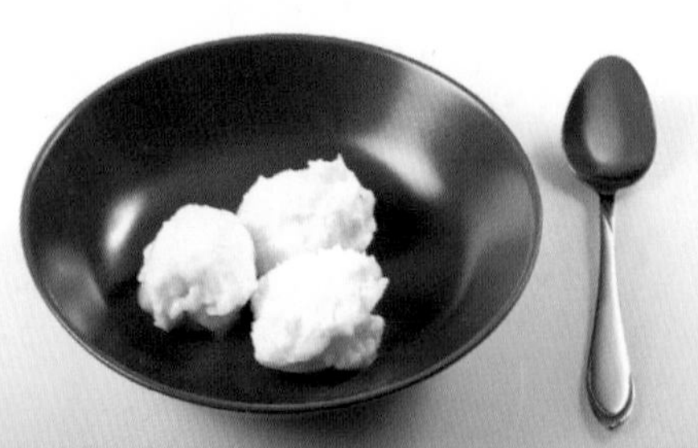

Sorbet (raspberry)

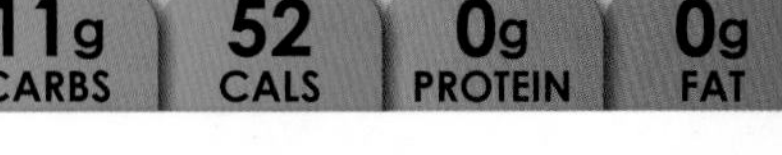

Weight	Carbs	Cals	Protein	Fat	Fibre	Sat Fat
45g	11g	52	0g	0g	0g	0g
88g	22g	101	0g	0g	0g	0g
132g	34g	152	1g	0g	1g	0g

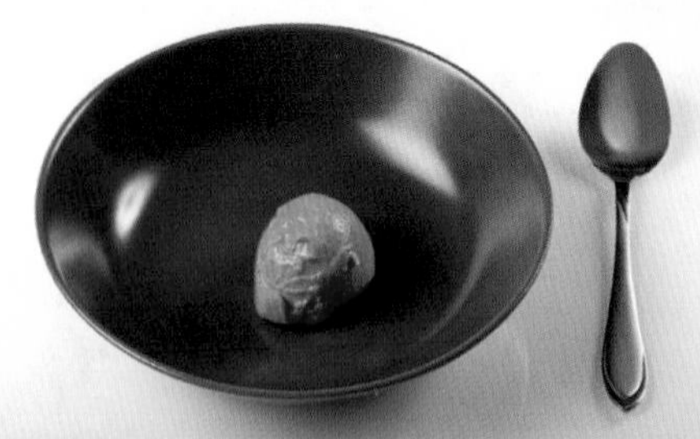

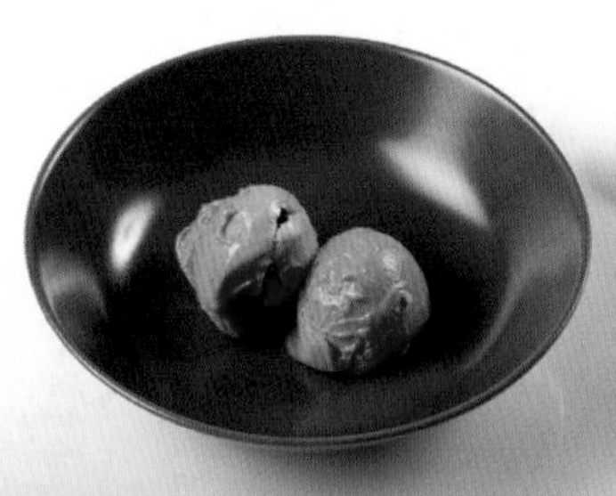

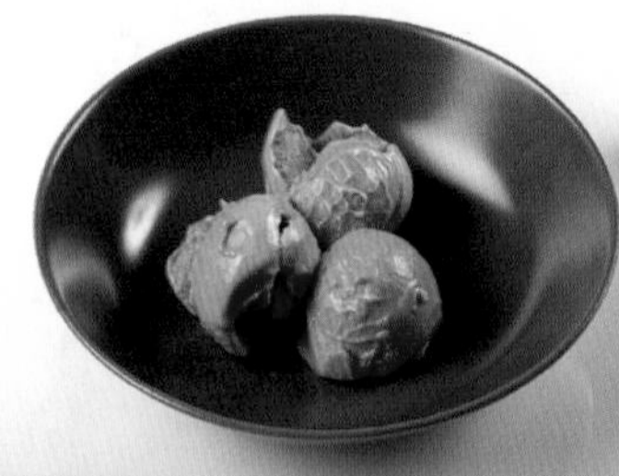

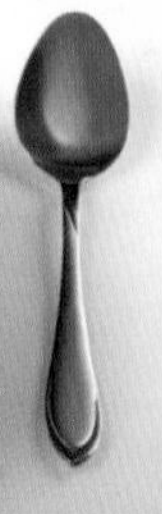

Choc Ice

12g CARBS	153 CALS	2g PROTEIN	11g FAT
0g FIBRE	Weight: 52g		10g SAT FAT

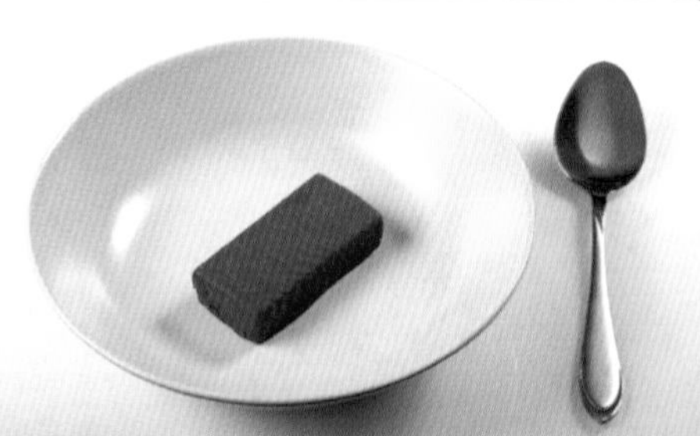

Crème Brûlée

19g CARBS	333 CALS	5g PROTEIN	27g FAT
0g FIBRE	Weight: 104g		18g SAT FAT

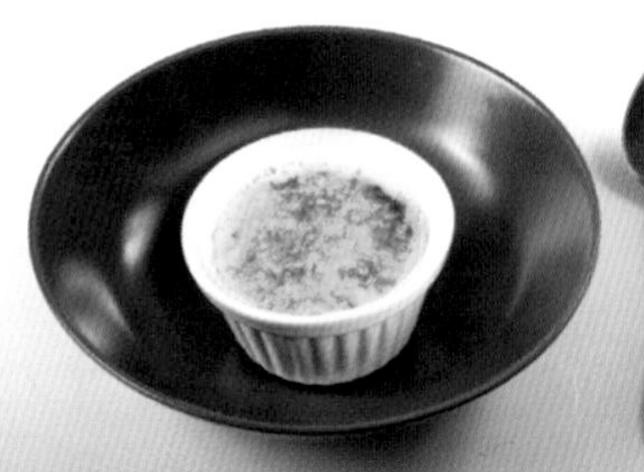

Chocolate & Nut Cone

21g CARBS	207 CALS	3g PROTEIN	13g FAT
0g FIBRE	Weight: 73g		10g SAT FAT

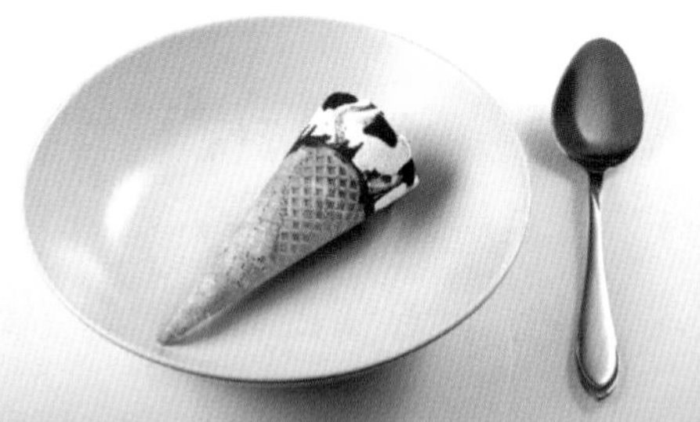

Panna Cotta

35g CARBS	384 CALS	4g PROTEIN	25g FAT
1g FIBRE	Weight: 145g		15g SAT FAT

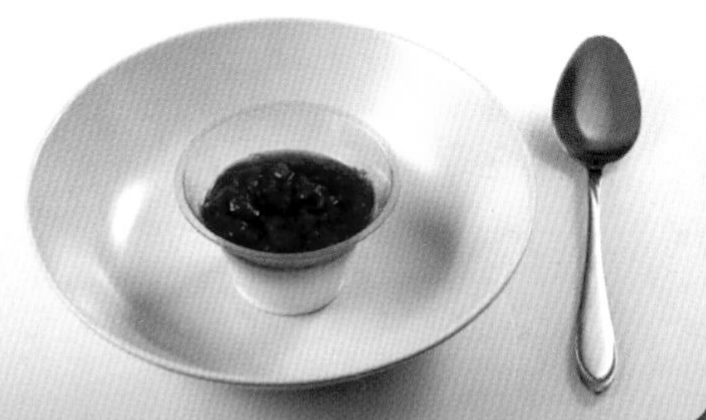

Ice Cream Lolly

26g CARBS	267 CALS	3g PROTEIN	17g FAT
1g FIBRE	Weight: 89g		13g SAT FAT

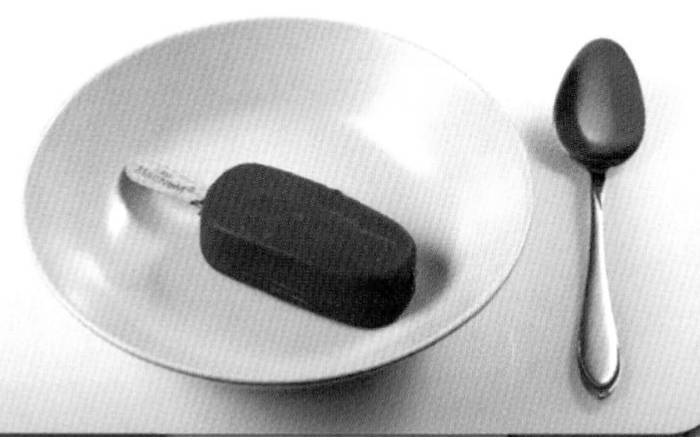

Strawberry Tartlet

35g CARBS	272 CALS	3g PROTEIN	14g FAT
2g FIBRE	Weight: 132g		5g SAT FAT

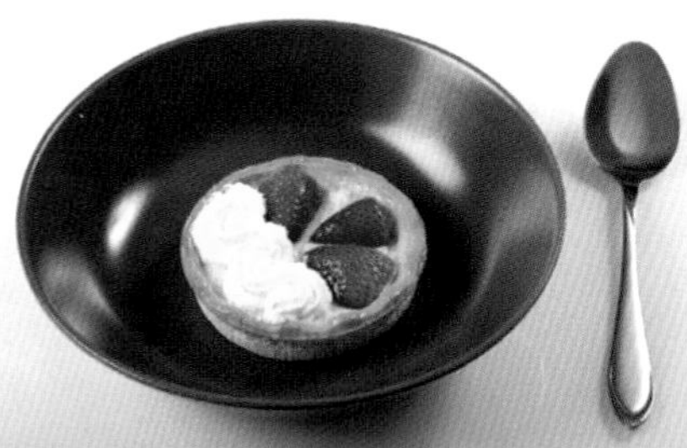

Jelly

13g CARBS	52 CALS	1g PROTEIN	0g FAT
0g FIBRE	Weight: 85g		0g SAT FAT

26g CARBS	104 CALS	2g PROTEIN	0g FAT
0g FIBRE	Weight: 170g		0g SAT FAT

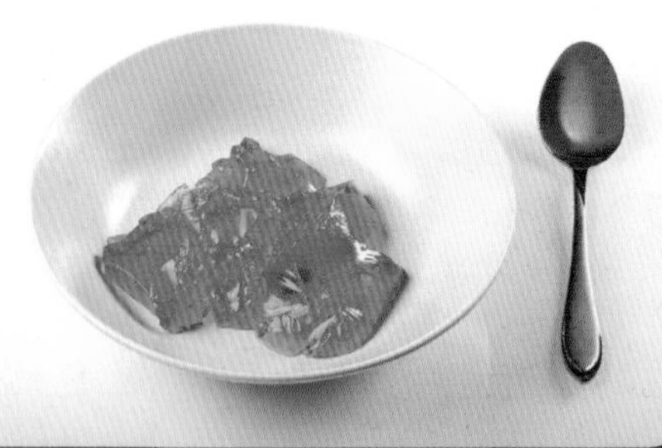

51g CARBS	207 CALS	4g PROTEIN	0g FAT
0g FIBRE	Weight: 340g		0g SAT FAT

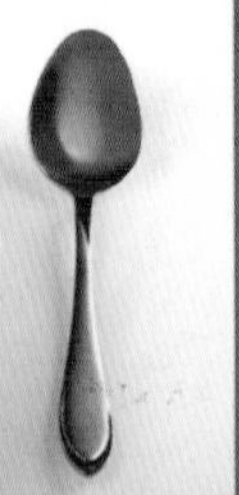

Lemon Meringue Pie

19g CARBS	110 CALS	1g PROTEIN	4g FAT
0g FIBRE	Weight: 44g		1g SAT FAT

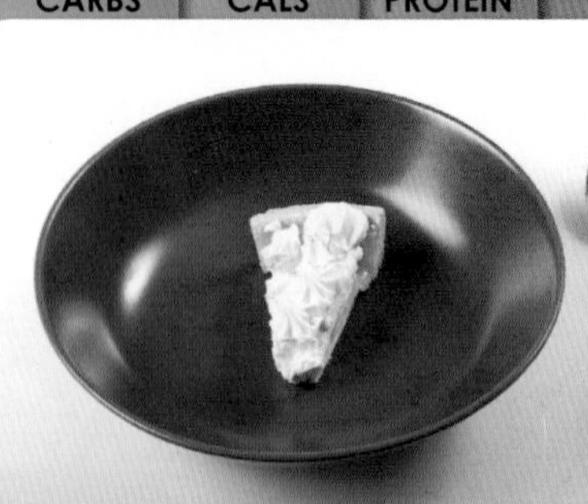

57g CARBS	326 CALS	4g PROTEIN	11g FAT
1g FIBRE	Weight: 130g		4g SAT FAT

95g CARBS	547 CALS	6g PROTEIN	19g FAT
2g FIBRE	Weight: 218g		7g SAT FAT

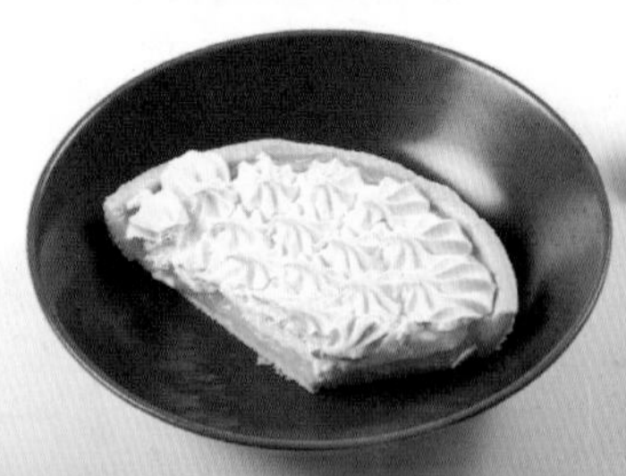

Mousse (chocolate)

CARBS	CALS	PROTEIN	FAT
10g	75	2g	3g

FIBRE	Weight	SAT FAT
0g	Weight: 50g	2g

CARBS	CALS	PROTEIN	FAT
20g	149	4g	7g

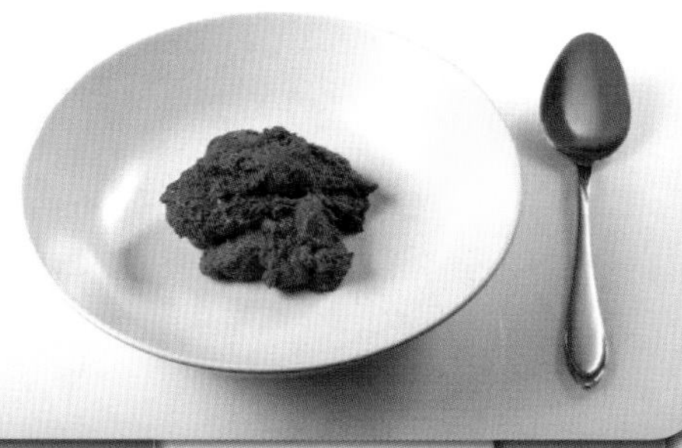

FIBRE	Weight	SAT FAT
1g	Weight: 100g	3g

CARBS	CALS	PROTEIN	FAT
40g	298	8g	13g

FIBRE	Weight	SAT FAT
1g	Weight: 200g	7g

Profiteroles

CARBS	CALS	PROTEIN	FAT
10g	138	2g	10g

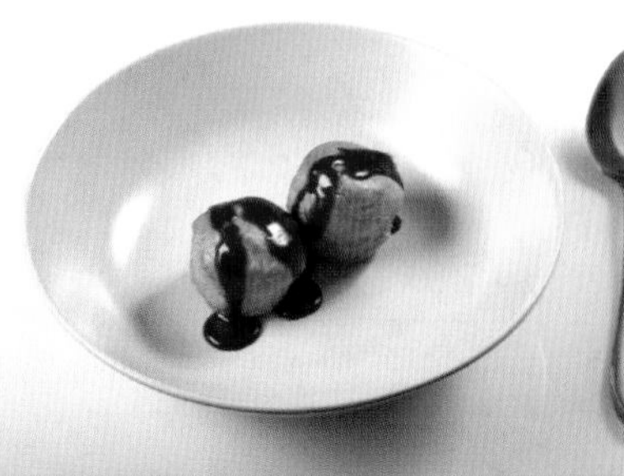

FIBRE	Weight	SAT FAT
1g	Weight: 40g	6g

CARBS	CALS	PROTEIN	FAT
20g	277	4g	21g

FIBRE	Weight	SAT FAT
1g	Weight: 80g	11g

CARBS	CALS	PROTEIN	FAT
30g	415	7g	31g

FIBRE	Weight	SAT FAT
2g	Weight: 120g	17g

14cm Cereal Bowl / 22cm Large Bowl

Rice Pudding

23g CARBS	119 CALS	5g PROTEIN	2g FAT

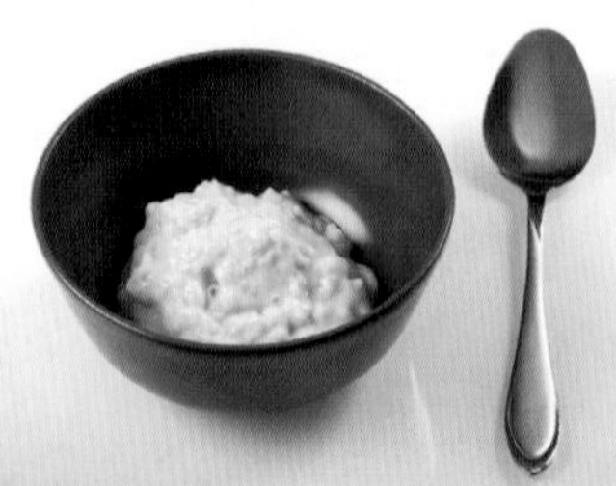

0g FIBRE	Weight: 140g	1g SAT FAT

46g CARBS	242 CALS	9g PROTEIN	4g FAT

1g FIBRE	Weight: 285g	2g SAT FAT

68g CARBS	361 CALS	14g PROTEIN	6g FAT

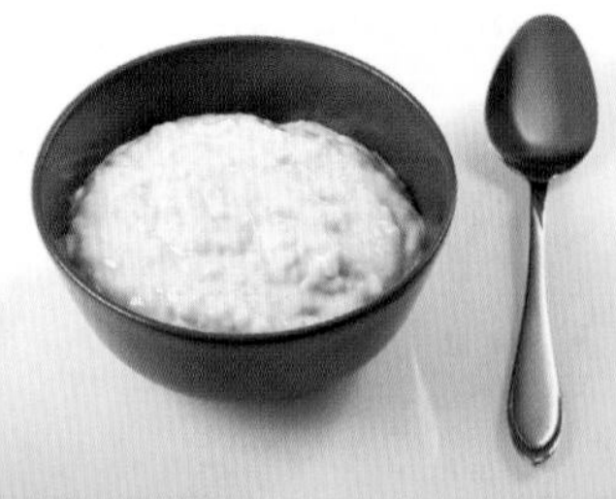

1g FIBRE	Weight: 425g	3g SAT FAT

Roulade

36g CARBS	308 CALS	3g PROTEIN	17g FAT

0g FIBRE	Weight: 76g	10g SAT FAT

54g CARBS	462 CALS	4g PROTEIN	26g FAT

1g FIBRE	Weight: 114g	15g SAT FAT

90g CARBS	778 CALS	7g PROTEIN	43g FAT

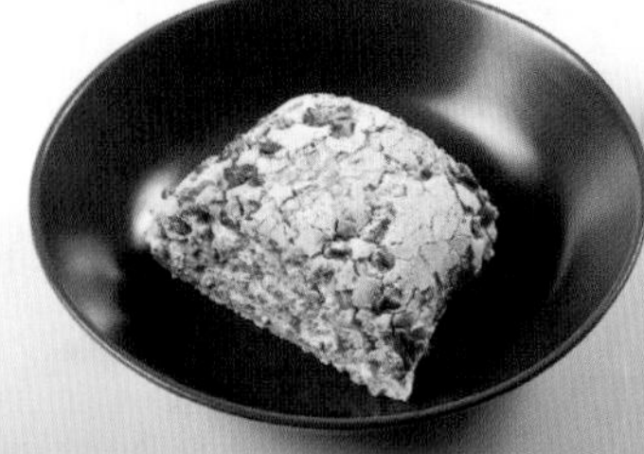

1g FIBRE	Weight: 192g	26g SAT FAT

Spotted Dick

Weight	Carbs	Cals	Protein	Fat	Fibre	Sat Fat
50g	26g	175	2g	7g	1g	3g
100g	51g	350	4g	14g	3g	7g
200g	102g	701	7g	28g	5g	13g

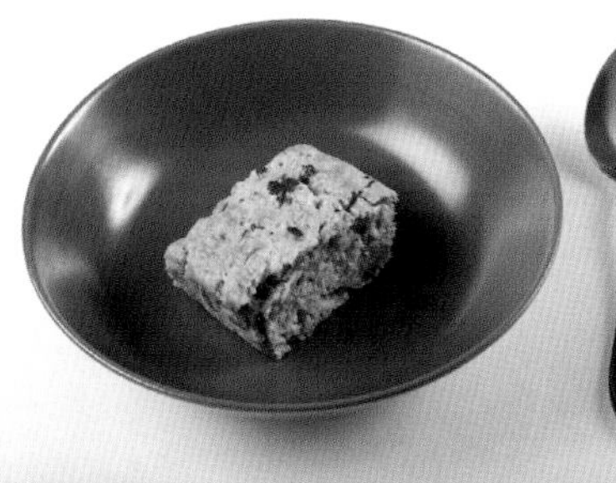
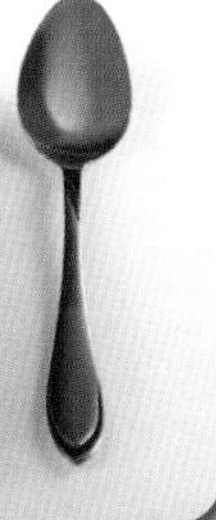
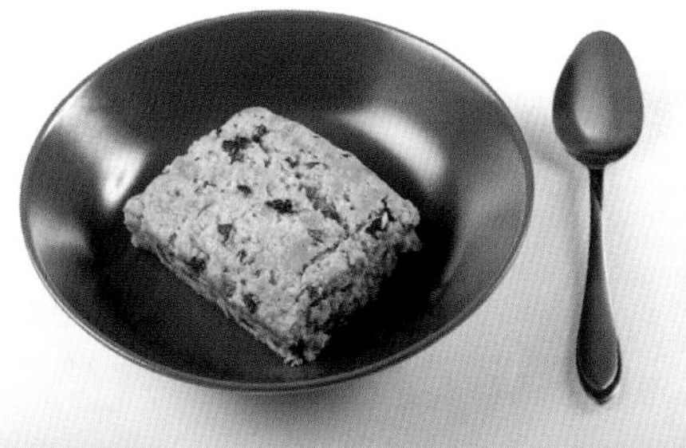
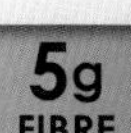

Sticky Toffee Pudding

Weight	Carbs	Cals	Protein	Fat	Fibre	Sat Fat
50g	24g	173	1g	8g	1g	4g
100g	48g	345	2g	16g	2g	9g
200g	95g	690	5g	32g	3g	17g

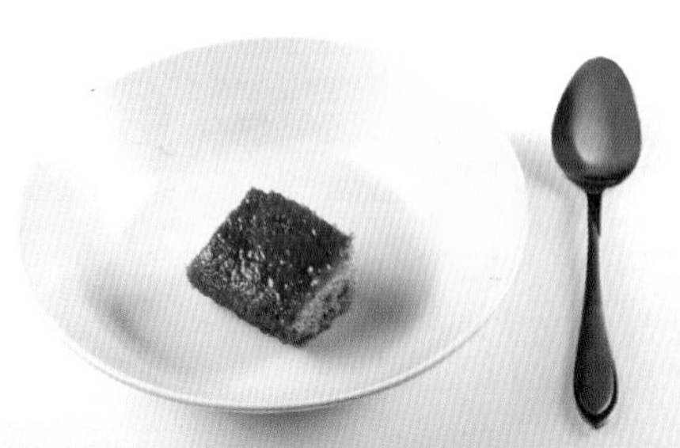
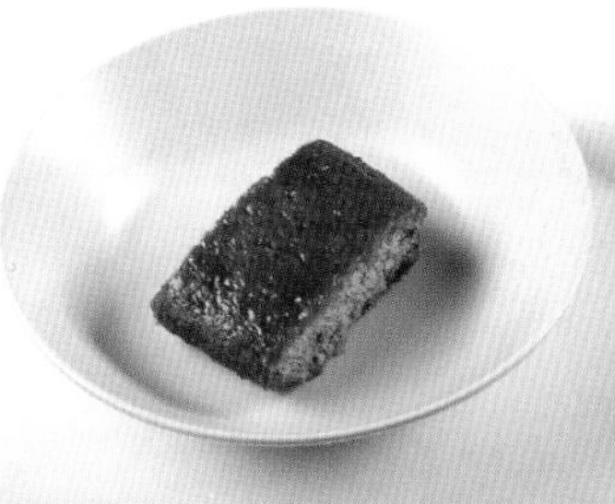
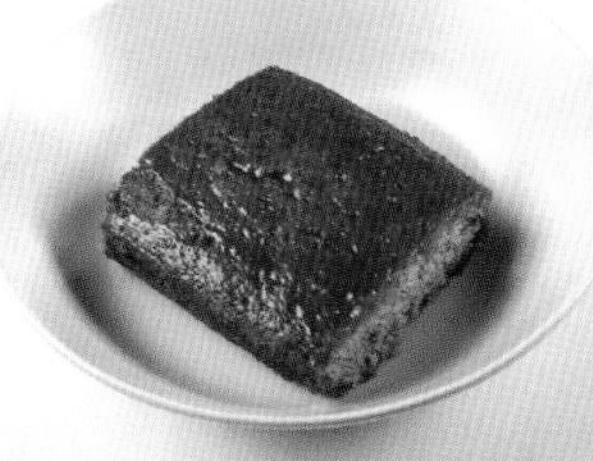
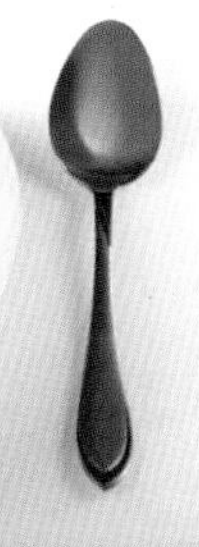

Strawberry Delight

CARBS	CALS	PROTEIN	FAT	FIBRE	SAT FAT	Weight
8g	58	2g	2g	0g	2g	Weight: 50g
15g	116	3g	5g	0g	4g	Weight: 100g
30g	232	7g	10g	1g	7g	Weight: 200g

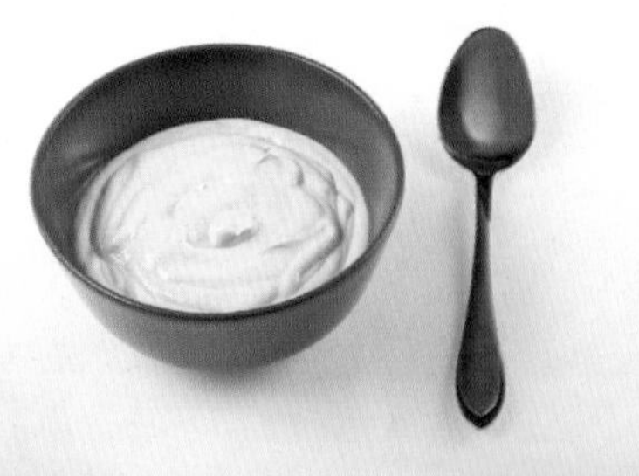

Summer Pudding

CARBS	CALS	PROTEIN	FAT	FIBRE	SAT FAT	Weight
10g	43	1g	0g	1g	0g	Weight: 45g
30g	133	4g	1g	5g	0g	Weight: 140g
49g	221	6g	1g	8g	0g	Weight: 233g

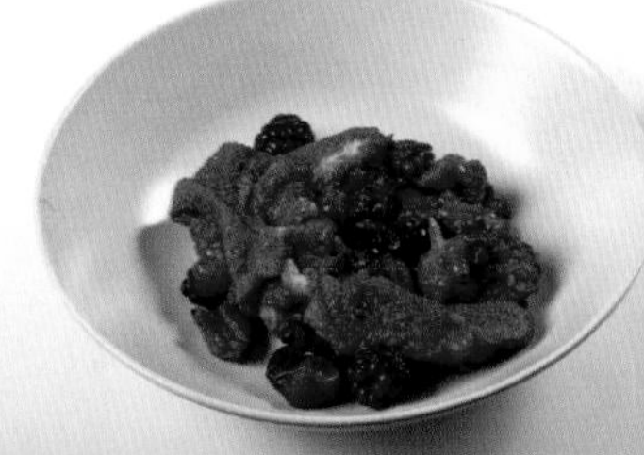

Tiramisu

15g CARBS	115 CALS	2g PROTEIN	5g FAT

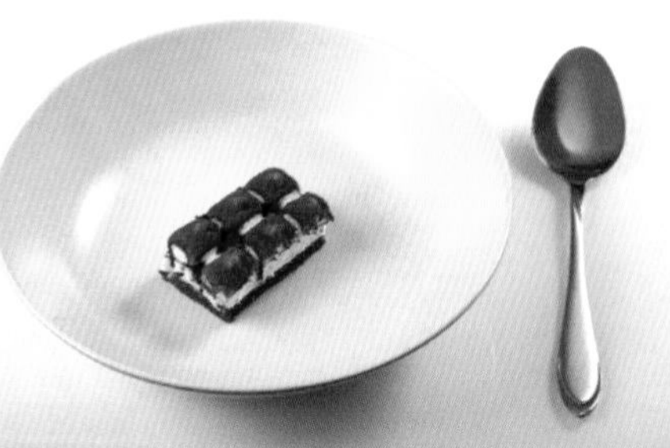

1g FIBRE	Weight: 45g	4g SAT FAT

29g CARBS	230 CALS	4g PROTEIN	10g FAT

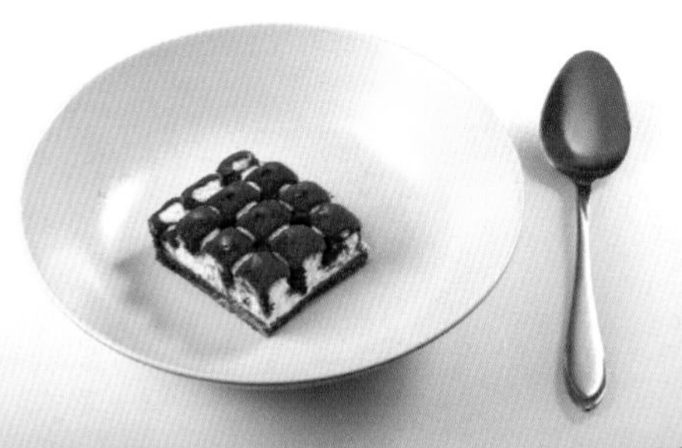
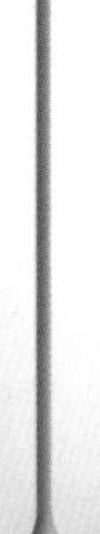

1g FIBRE	Weight: 90g	8g SAT FAT

58g CARBS	456 CALS	7g PROTEIN	21g FAT

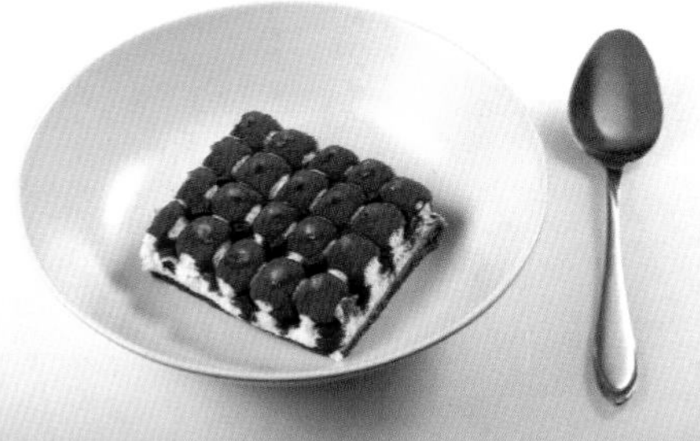
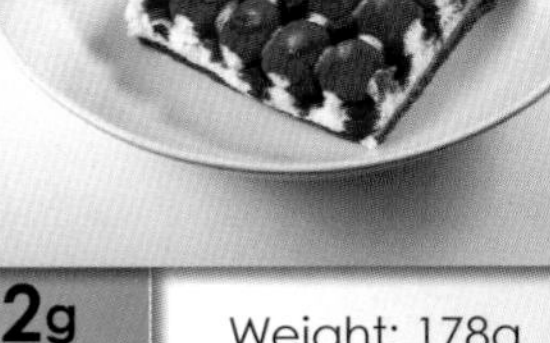
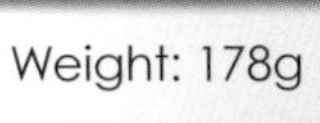

2g FIBRE	Weight: 178g	16g SAT FAT

Trifle

11g CARBS	87 CALS	1g PROTEIN	4g FAT

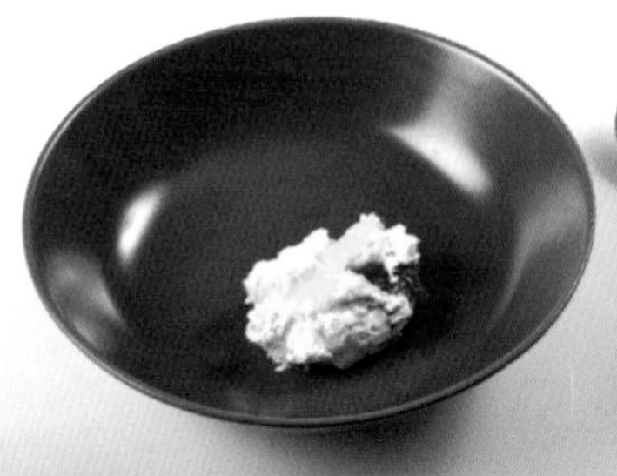

1g FIBRE	Weight: 55g	3g SAT FAT

32g CARBS	256 CALS	3g PROTEIN	13g FAT

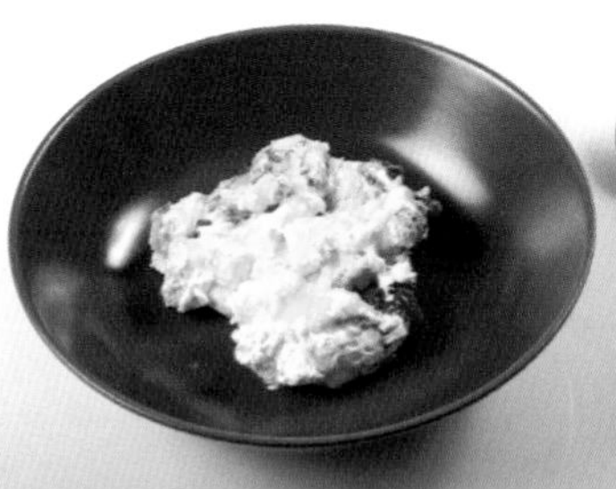
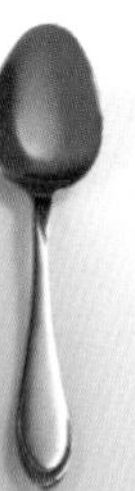

2g FIBRE	Weight: 162g	8g SAT FAT

53g CARBS	426 CALS	5g PROTEIN	21g FAT

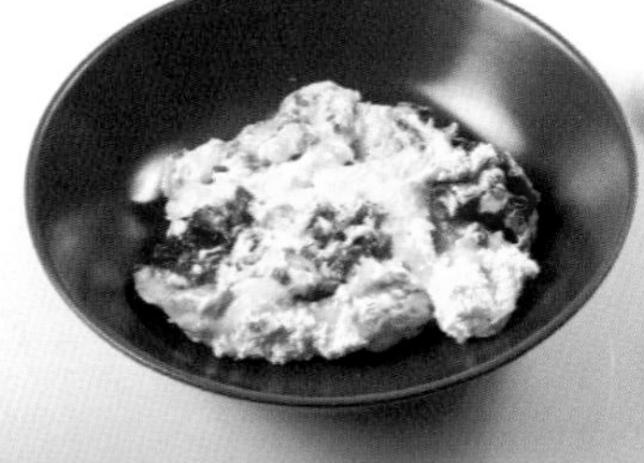

4g FIBRE	Weight: 270g	13g SAT FAT

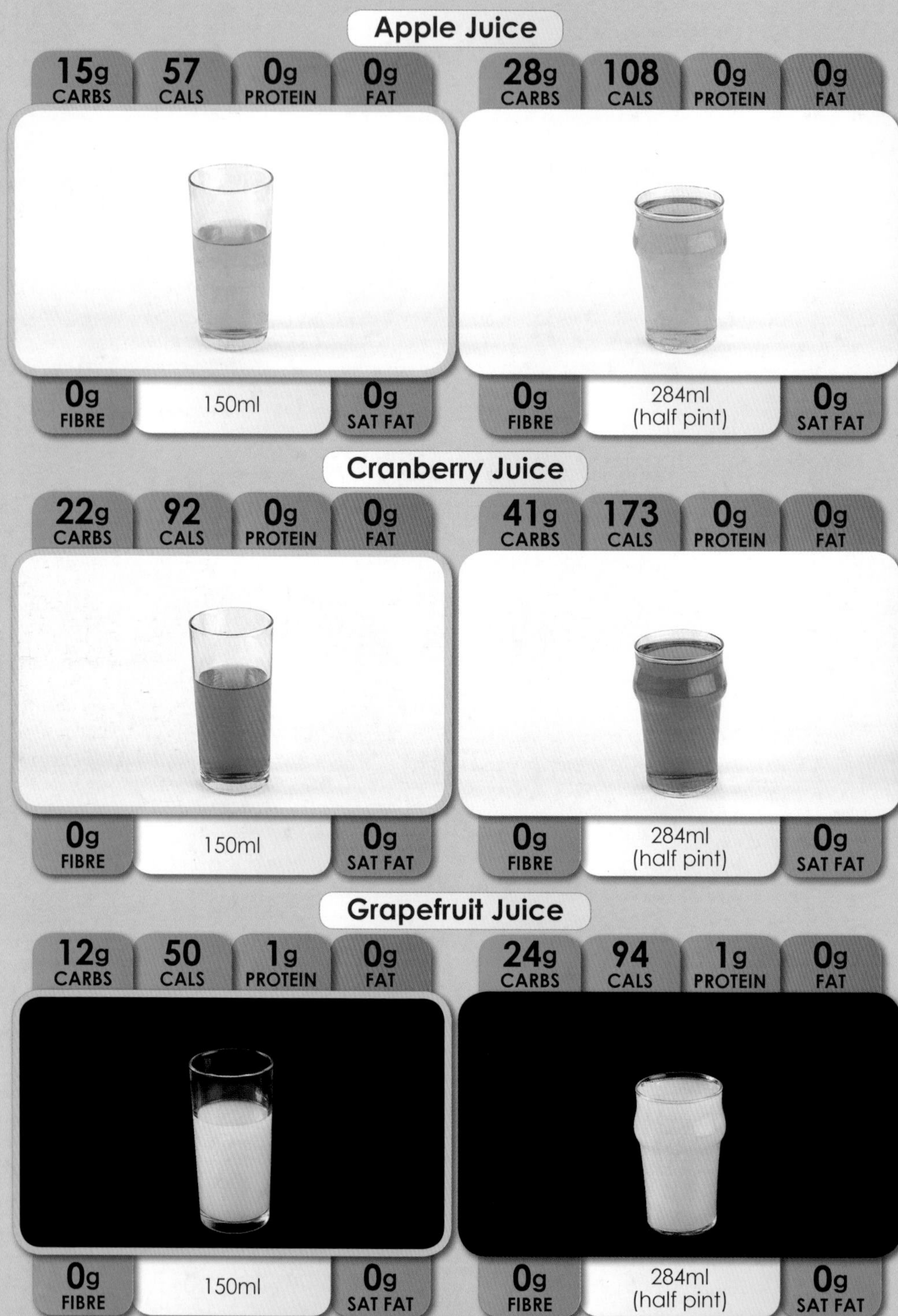

Apple Juice

	150ml	284ml (half pint)
CARBS	15g	28g
CALS	57	108
PROTEIN	0g	0g
FAT	0g	0g
FIBRE	0g	0g
SAT FAT	0g	0g

Cranberry Juice

	150ml	284ml (half pint)
CARBS	22g	41g
CALS	92	173
PROTEIN	0g	0g
FAT	0g	0g
FIBRE	0g	0g
SAT FAT	0g	0g

Grapefruit Juice

	150ml	284ml (half pint)
CARBS	12g	24g
CALS	50	94
PROTEIN	1g	1g
FAT	0g	0g
FIBRE	0g	0g
SAT FAT	0g	0g

Orange Juice

CARBS	CALS	PROTEIN	FAT
13g	54	1g	0g

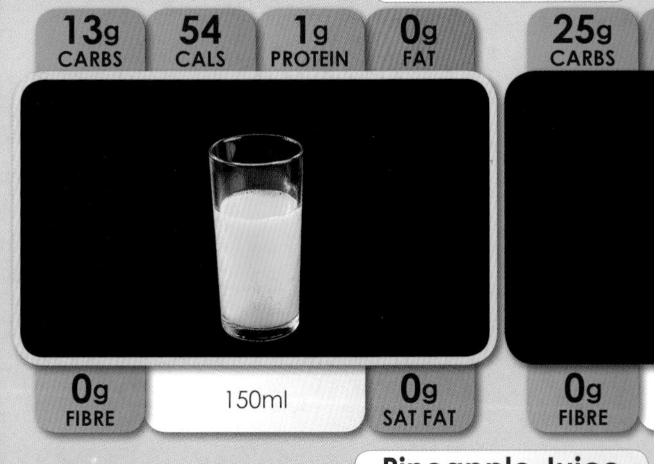

FIBRE	Serving	SAT FAT
0g	150ml	0g

CARBS	CALS	PROTEIN	FAT
25g	102	1g	0g

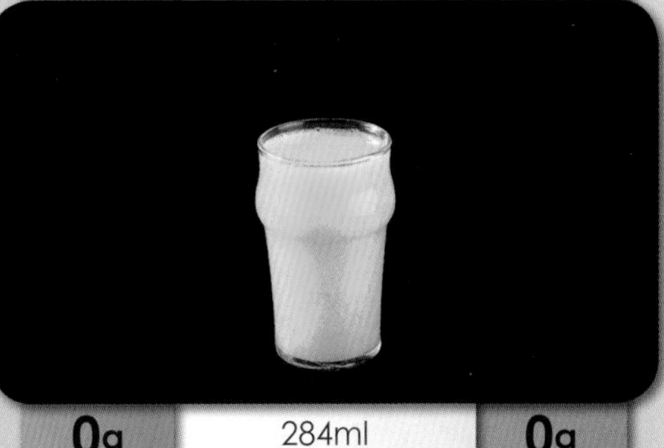

FIBRE	Serving	SAT FAT
0g	284ml (half pint)	0g

Pineapple Juice

CARBS	CALS	PROTEIN	FAT
16g	62	0g	0g

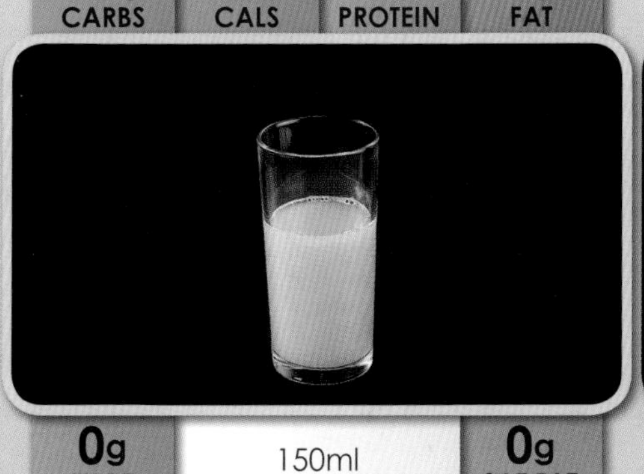

FIBRE	Serving	SAT FAT
0g	150ml	0g

CARBS	CALS	PROTEIN	FAT
30g	116	1g	0g

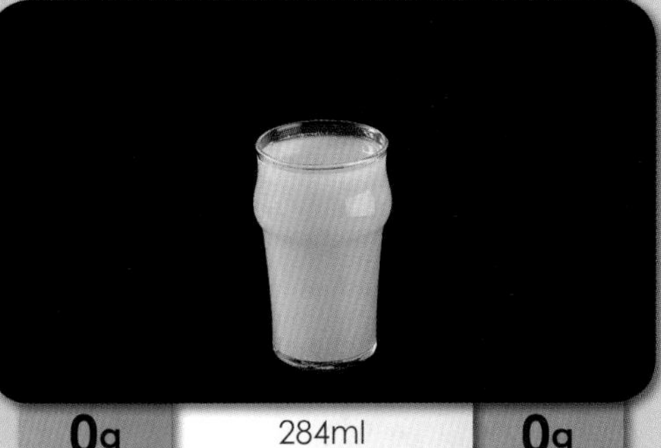

FIBRE	Serving	SAT FAT
0g	284ml (half pint)	0g

Tomato Juice

CARBS	CALS	PROTEIN	FAT
5g	21	1g	0g

FIBRE	Serving	SAT FAT
1g	150ml	0g

CARBS	CALS	PROTEIN	FAT
9g	40	2g	0g

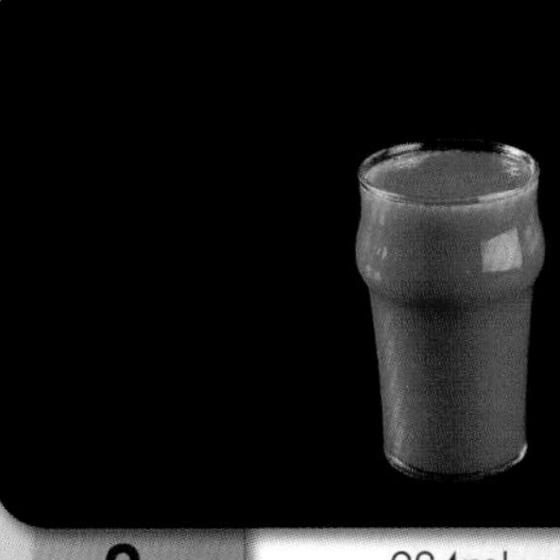

FIBRE	Serving	SAT FAT
2g	284ml (half pint)	0g

Smoothie (strawberry & banana)

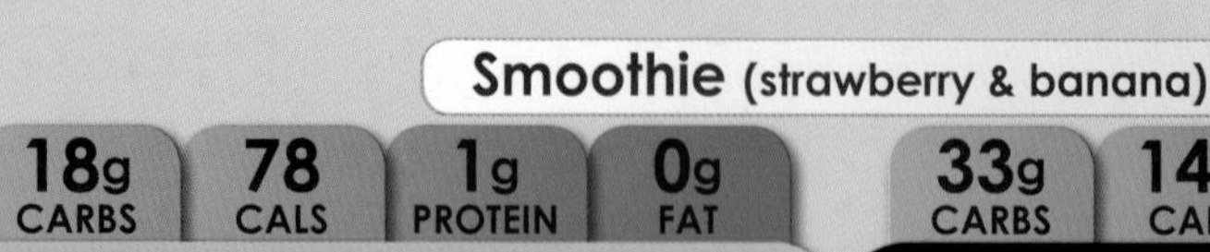

Serving	Carbs	Cals	Protein	Fat	Fibre	Sat Fat
150ml	18g	78	1g	0g	2g	0g
284ml (half pint)	33g	148	2g	0g	3g	0g

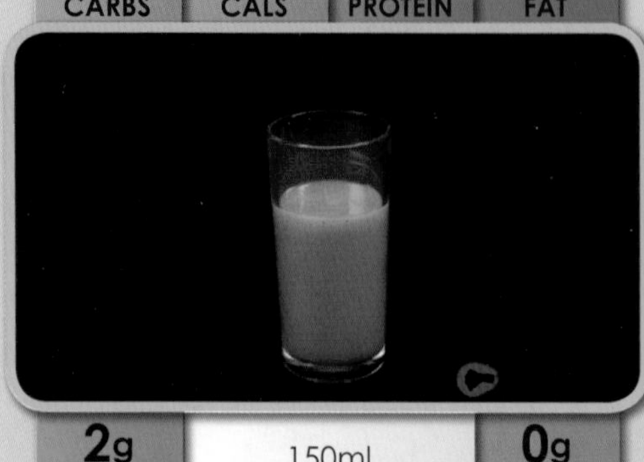

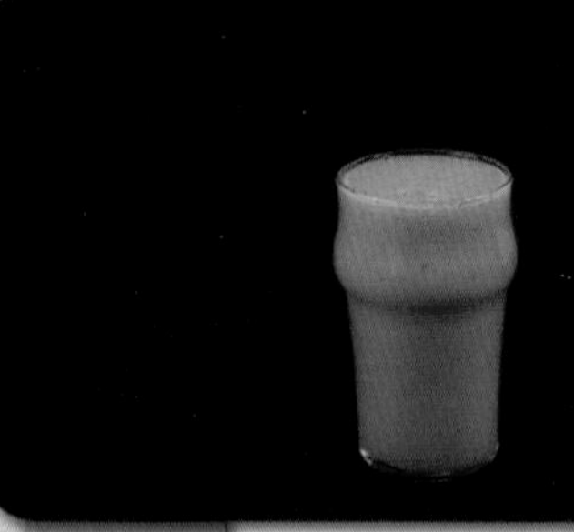

Squash

Serving	Carbs	Cals	Protein	Fat	Fibre	Sat Fat
150ml (120ml water, 30ml squash)	18g	68	0g	0g	0g	0g
284ml (229ml water, 55ml squash)	35g	130	0g	0g	0g	0g

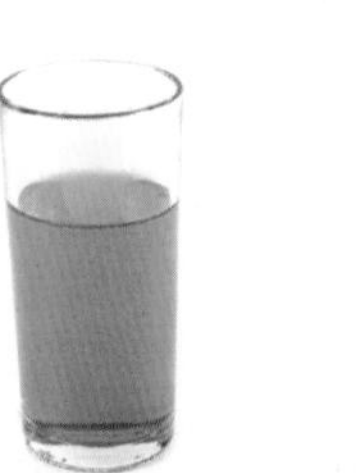

Squash (no added sugar)

Serving	Carbs	Cals	Protein	Fat	Fibre	Sat Fat
150ml (120ml water, 30ml squash)	1g	6	0g	0g	0g	0g
284ml (229ml water, 55ml squash)	2g	12	0g	0g	0g	0g

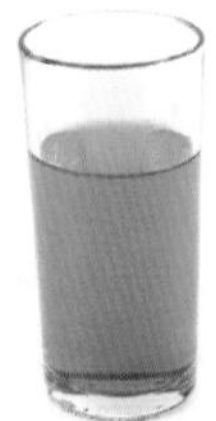

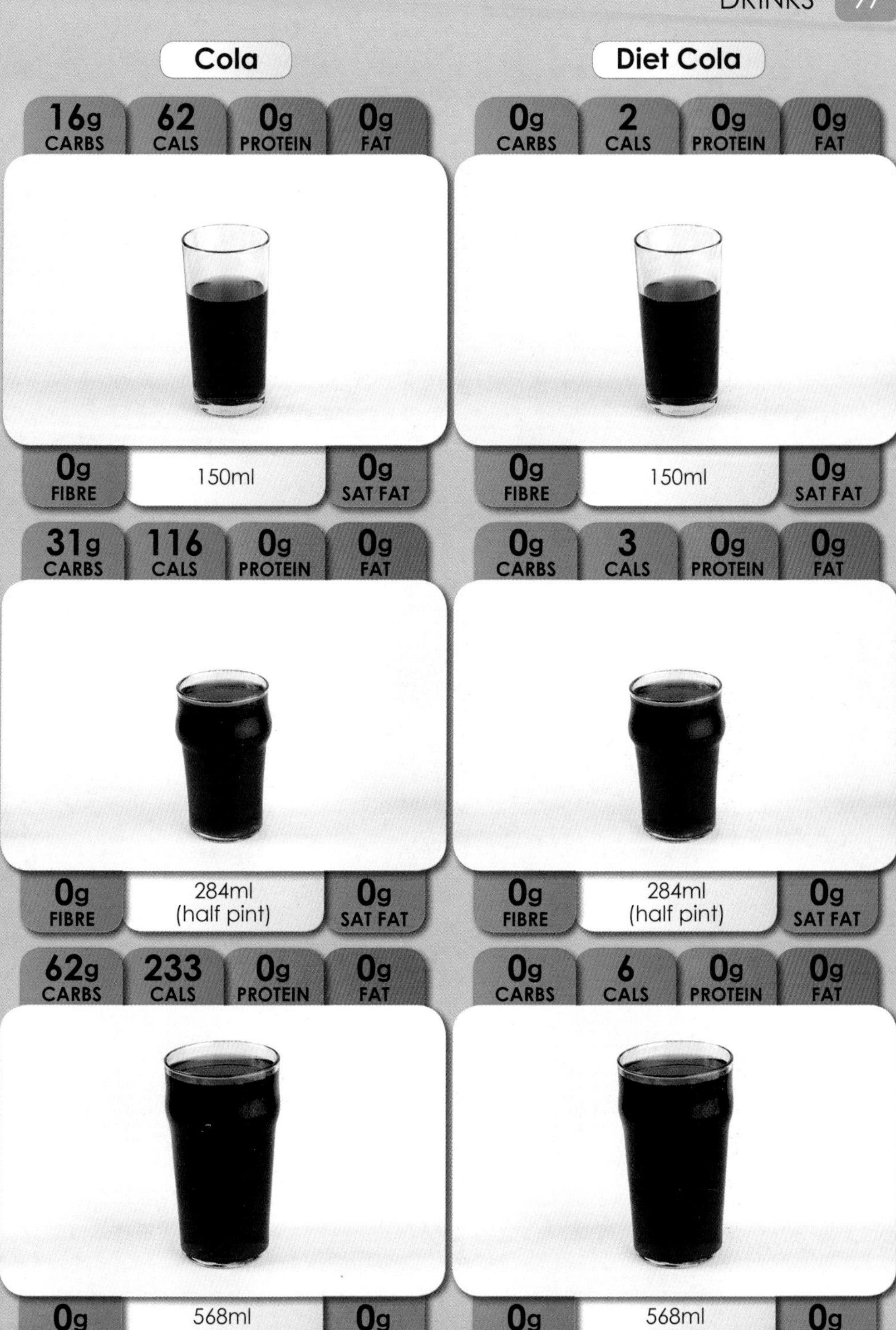
Cola
16g CARBS
62 CALS
0g PROTEIN
0g FAT
0g FIBRE
150ml
0g SAT FAT
31g CARBS
116 CALS
0g PROTEIN
0g FAT
0g FIBRE
284ml (half pint)
0g SAT FAT
62g CARBS
233 CALS
0g PROTEIN
0g FAT
0g FIBRE
568ml (pint)
0g SAT FAT
Diet Cola
0g CARBS
2 CALS
0g PROTEIN
0g FAT
0g FIBRE
150ml
0g SAT FAT
0g CARBS
3 CALS
0g PROTEIN
0g FAT
0g FIBRE
284ml (half pint)
0g SAT FAT
0g CARBS
6 CALS
0g PROTEIN
0g FAT
0g FIBRE
568ml (pint)
0g SAT FAT

Lemonade (sparkling)

9g CARBS	33 CALS	0g PROTEIN	0g FAT

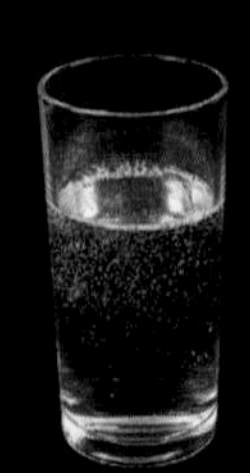

0g FIBRE	150ml	0g SAT FAT

17g CARBS	63 CALS	0g PROTEIN	0g FAT

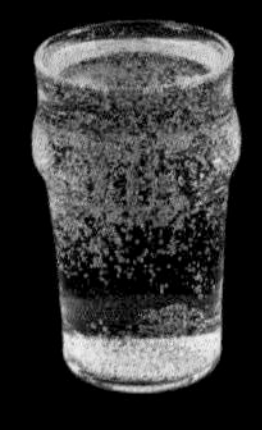

0g FIBRE	284ml (half pint)	0g SAT FAT

33g CARBS	125 CALS	0g PROTEIN	0g FAT

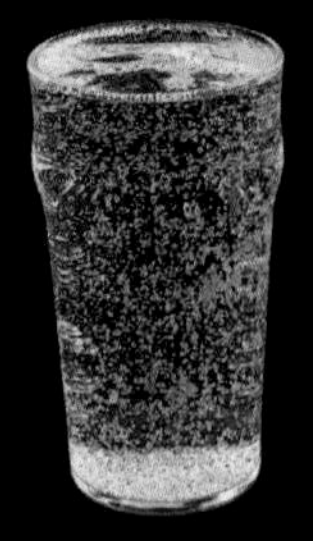

0g FIBRE	568ml (pint)	0g SAT FAT

Lucozade Energy

10g CARBS	39 CALS	0g PROTEIN	0g FAT

0g FIBRE	56ml	0g SAT FAT

20g CARBS	80 CALS	0g PROTEIN	0g FAT

0g FIBRE	114ml	0g SAT FAT

30g CARBS	119 CALS	0g PROTEIN	0g FAT

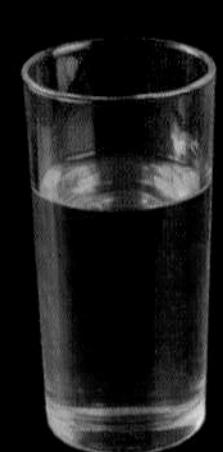

0g FIBRE	170ml	0g SAT FAT

Iced Tea

	150ml	284ml (half pint)
CARBS	10g	18g
CALS	39	74
PROTEIN	0g	0g
FAT	0g	0g
FIBRE	0g	0g
SAT FAT	0g	0g

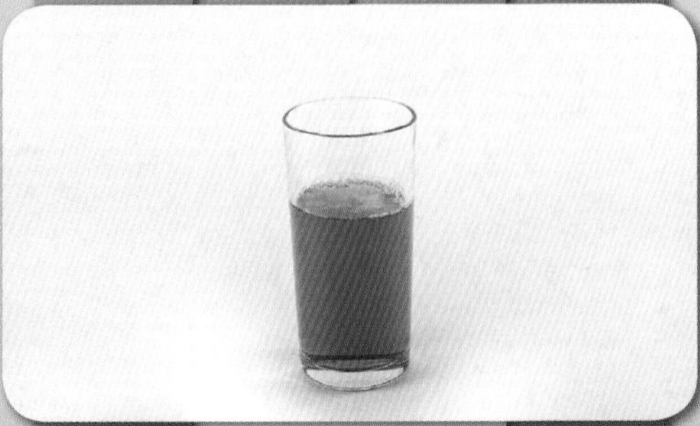

Lemonade (fresh)

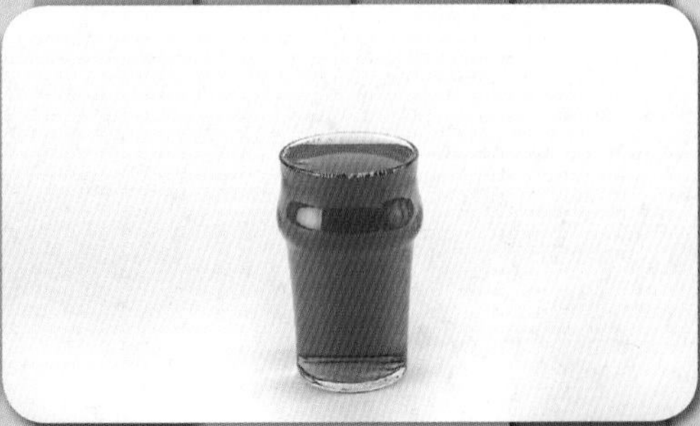

	150ml	284ml (half pint)
CARBS	18g	35g
CALS	79	150
PROTEIN	0g	0g
FAT	0g	0g
FIBRE	0g	1g
SAT FAT	0g	0g

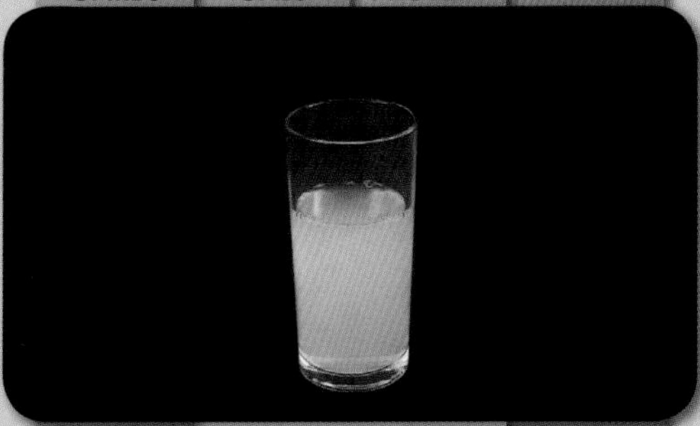

Malt Drink

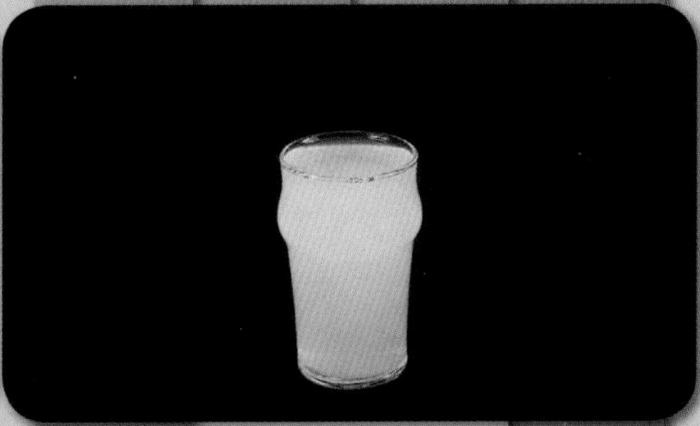

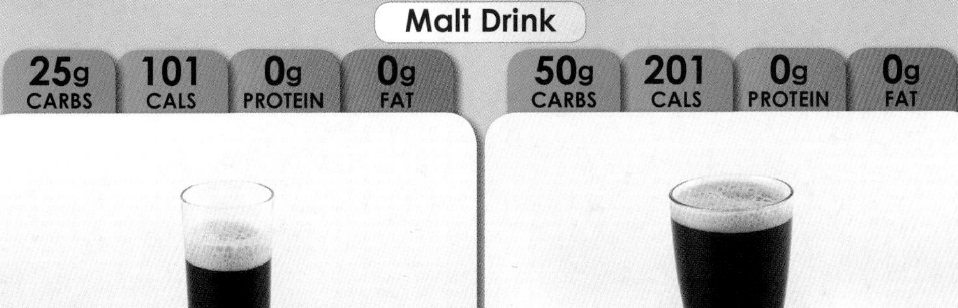

	165ml (half bottle)	330ml (bottle)
CARBS	25g	50g
CALS	101	201
PROTEIN	0g	0g
FAT	0g	0g
FIBRE	0g	0g
SAT FAT	0g	0g

Cappuccino (whole milk)

CARBS	CALS	PROTEIN	FAT	FIBRE	SIZE	SAT FAT
8g	92	5g	5g	0g	235ml (8 fl oz)	3g
10g	116	6g	6g	0g	355ml (12 fl oz)	3g
11g	136	7g	7g	0g	475ml (16 fl oz)	4g

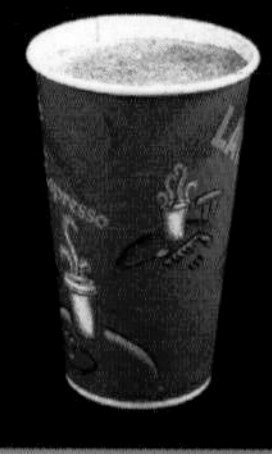

Cappuccino (skimmed milk)

CARBS	CALS	PROTEIN	FAT	FIBRE	SIZE	SAT FAT
8g	55	5g	0g	0g	235ml (8 fl oz)	0g
11g	70	7g	0g	0g	355ml (12 fl oz)	0g
12g	82	8g	0g	0g	475ml (16 fl oz)	0g

Hot Chocolate (whole milk)

CARBS	CALS	PROTEIN	FAT
25g	212	8g	9g

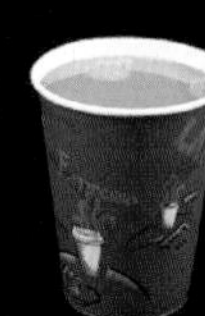

FIBRE	Serving	SAT FAT
2g	235ml (8 fl oz)	6g

CARBS	CALS	PROTEIN	FAT
38g	320	12g	14g

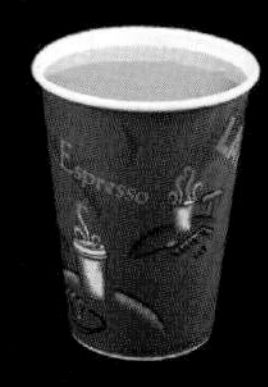

FIBRE	Serving	SAT FAT
4g	355ml (12 fl oz)	9g

CARBS	CALS	PROTEIN	FAT
51g	428	17g	19g

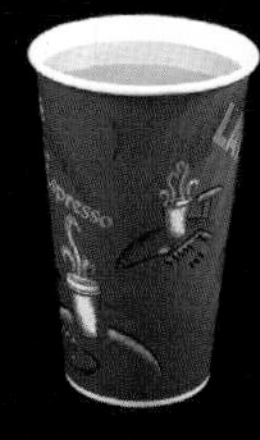

FIBRE	Serving	SAT FAT
5g	475ml (16 fl oz)	12g

Hot Chocolate (skimmed milk)

CARBS	CALS	PROTEIN	FAT
25g	141	8g	2g

FIBRE	Serving	SAT FAT
0g	235ml (8 fl oz)	1g

CARBS	CALS	PROTEIN	FAT
38g	213	13g	2g

FIBRE	Serving	SAT FAT
0g	355ml (12 fl oz)	1g

CARBS	CALS	PROTEIN	FAT
50g	285	17g	3g

FIBRE	Serving	SAT FAT
0g	475ml (16 fl oz)	2g

Latte (whole milk)

Serving	Carbs	Cals	Protein	Fat	Fibre	Sat Fat
235ml (8 fl oz)	9g	113	6g	6g	0g	3g
355ml (12 fl oz)	15g	172	9g	8g	0g	5g
475ml (16 fl oz)	18g	223	12g	12g	0g	7g

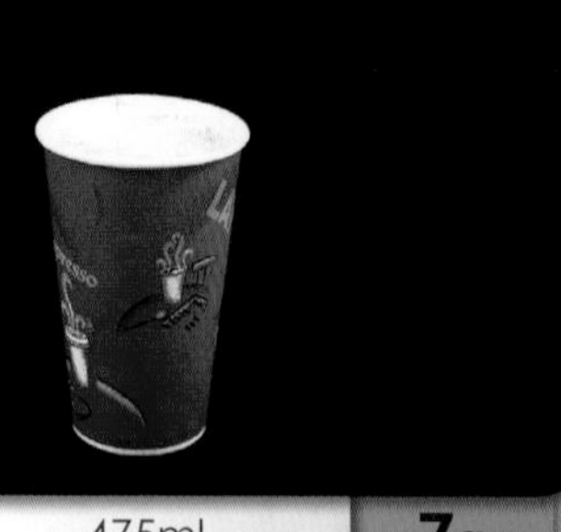

Latte (skimmed milk)

Serving	Carbs	Cals	Protein	Fat	Fibre	Sat Fat
235ml (8 fl oz)	10g	67	6g	0g	0g	0g
355ml (12 fl oz)	15g	102	10g	0g	0g	0g
475ml (16 fl oz)	20g	131	13g	0g	0g	0g

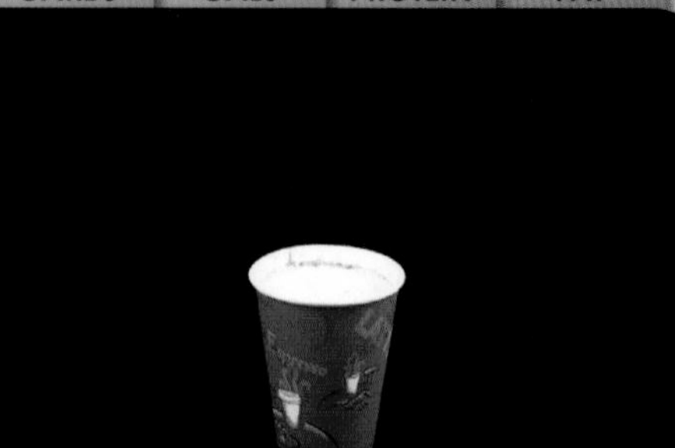

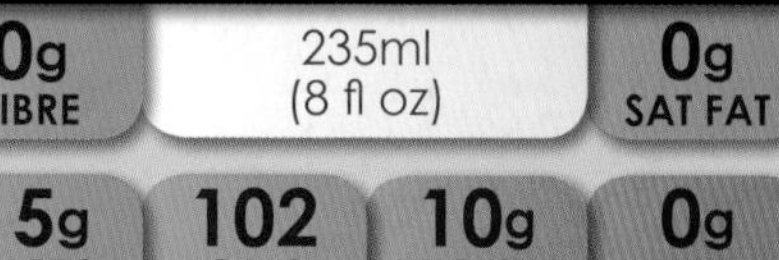

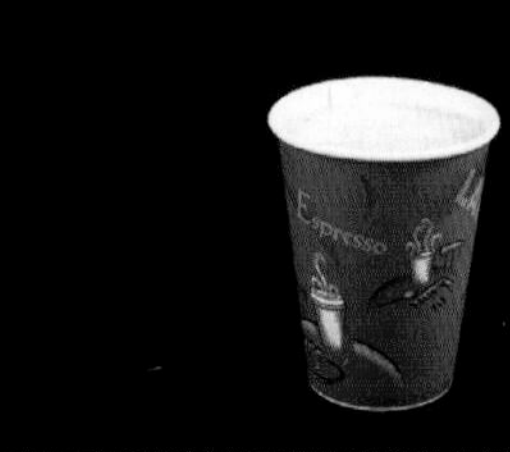

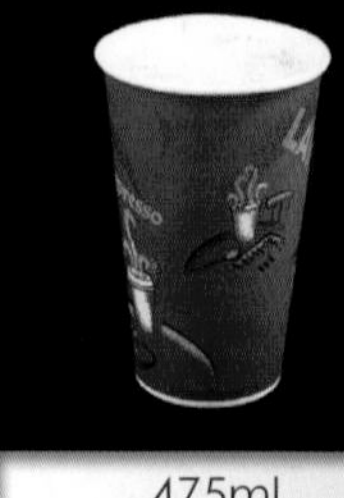

Cup of Coffee (black)

1g CARBS	5 CALS	1g PROTEIN	0g FAT

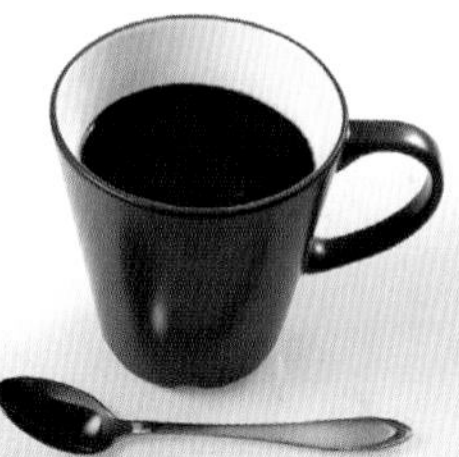

0g FIBRE	260ml	0g SAT FAT

Cup of Coffee (with milk)

2g CARBS	18 CALS	2g PROTEIN	1g FAT

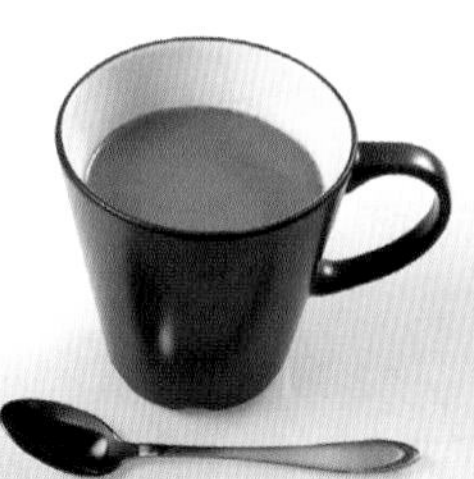

0g FIBRE	260ml	0g SAT FAT

Cup of Tea (with milk)

2g CARBS	18 CALS	1g PROTEIN	1g FAT

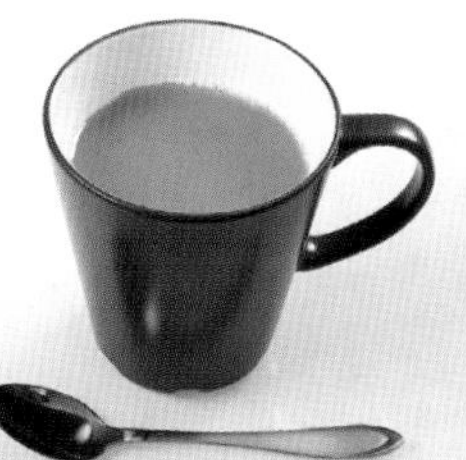

0g FIBRE	260ml	0g SAT FAT

Espresso

0g CARBS	1 CALS	0g PROTEIN	0g FAT

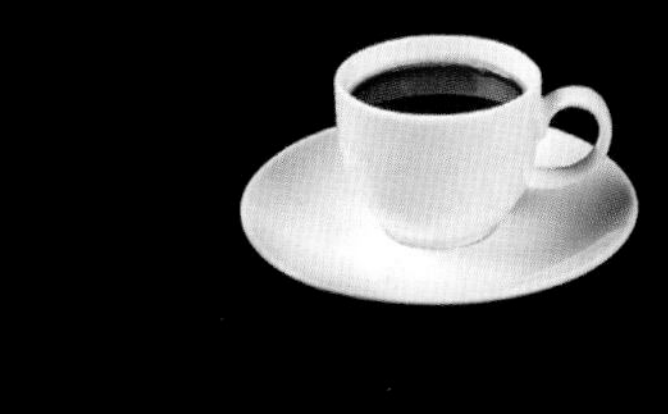

0g FIBRE	60ml	0g SAT FAT

Hot Malt Drink

32g CARBS	218 CALS	11g PROTEIN	5g FAT

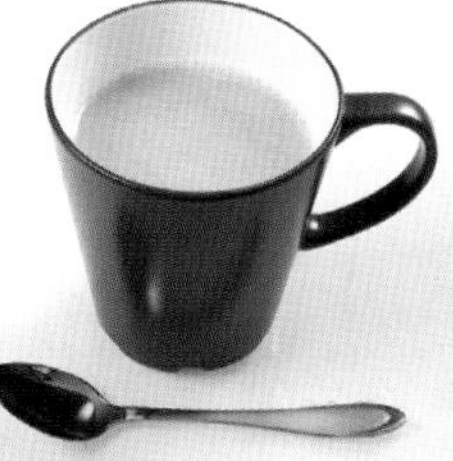

1g FIBRE	260ml	3g SAT FAT

Teaspoon of Sugar

5g CARBS	20 CALS	0g PROTEIN	0g FAT

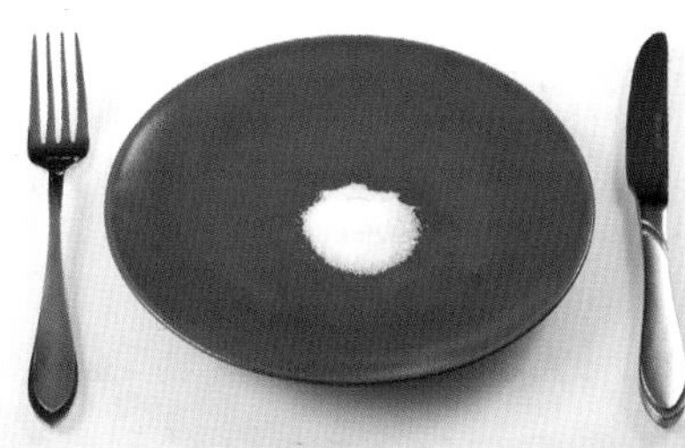

0g FIBRE	Weight: 5g	0g SAT FAT

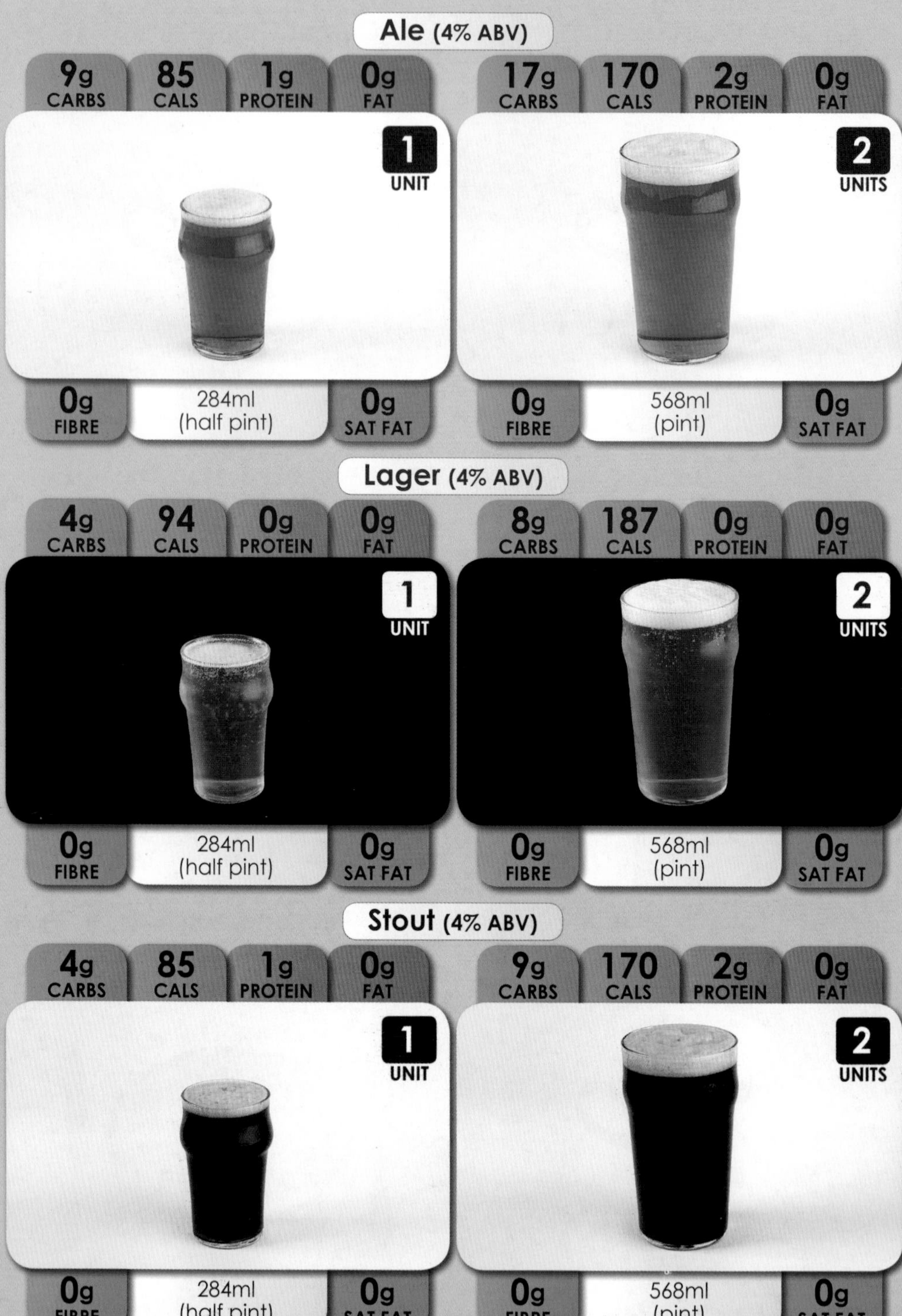
Ale (4% ABV)
9g CARBS
85 CALS
1g PROTEIN
0g FAT
1 UNIT
0g FIBRE
284ml (half pint)
0g SAT FAT
17g CARBS
170 CALS
2g PROTEIN
0g FAT
2 UNITS
0g FIBRE
568ml (pint)
0g SAT FAT
Lager (4% ABV)
4g CARBS
94 CALS
0g PROTEIN
0g FAT
1 UNIT
0g FIBRE
284ml (half pint)
0g SAT FAT
8g CARBS
187 CALS
0g PROTEIN
0g FAT
2 UNITS
0g FIBRE
568ml (pint)
0g SAT FAT
Stout (4% ABV)
4g CARBS
85 CALS
1g PROTEIN
0g FAT
1 UNIT
0g FIBRE
284ml (half pint)
0g SAT FAT
9g CARBS
170 CALS
2g PROTEIN
0g FAT
2 UNITS
0g FIBRE
568ml (pint)
0g SAT FAT

Cider (dry, 5% ABV)

Serving	Carbs	Cals	Protein	Fat	Fibre	Sat Fat	Units
284ml (half pint)	7g	102	0g	0g	0g	0g	1½
568ml (pint)	15g	205	0g	0g	0g	0g	3

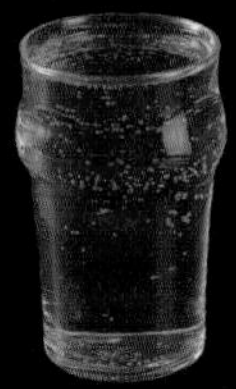

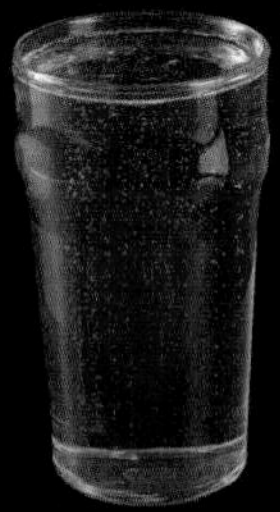

Cider (sweet, 5% ABV)

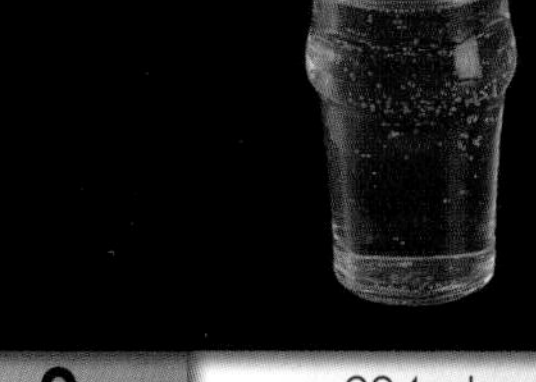

Serving	Carbs	Cals	Protein	Fat	Fibre	Sat Fat	Units
284ml (half pint)	12g	119	0g	0g	0g	0g	1½
568ml (pint)	24g	239	0g	0g	0g	0g	3

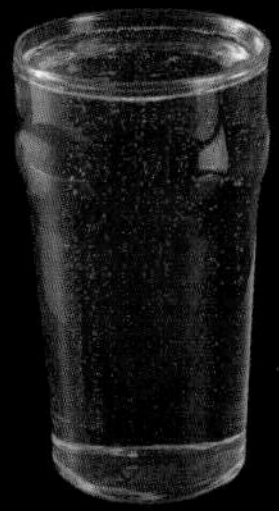

WKD Vodka Blue

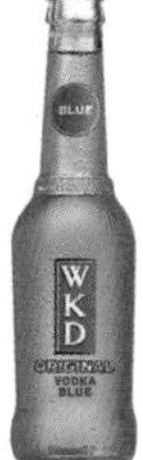

Serving	Carbs	Cals	Protein	Fat	Fibre	Sat Fat	Units
275ml (bottle)	36g	216	0g	0g	0g	0g	1

WKD Iron Brew

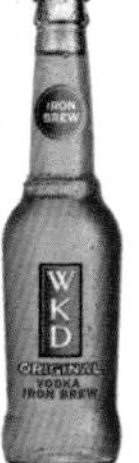

Serving	Carbs	Cals	Protein	Fat	Fibre	Sat Fat	Units
275ml (bottle)	22g	161	0g	0g	0g	0g	1

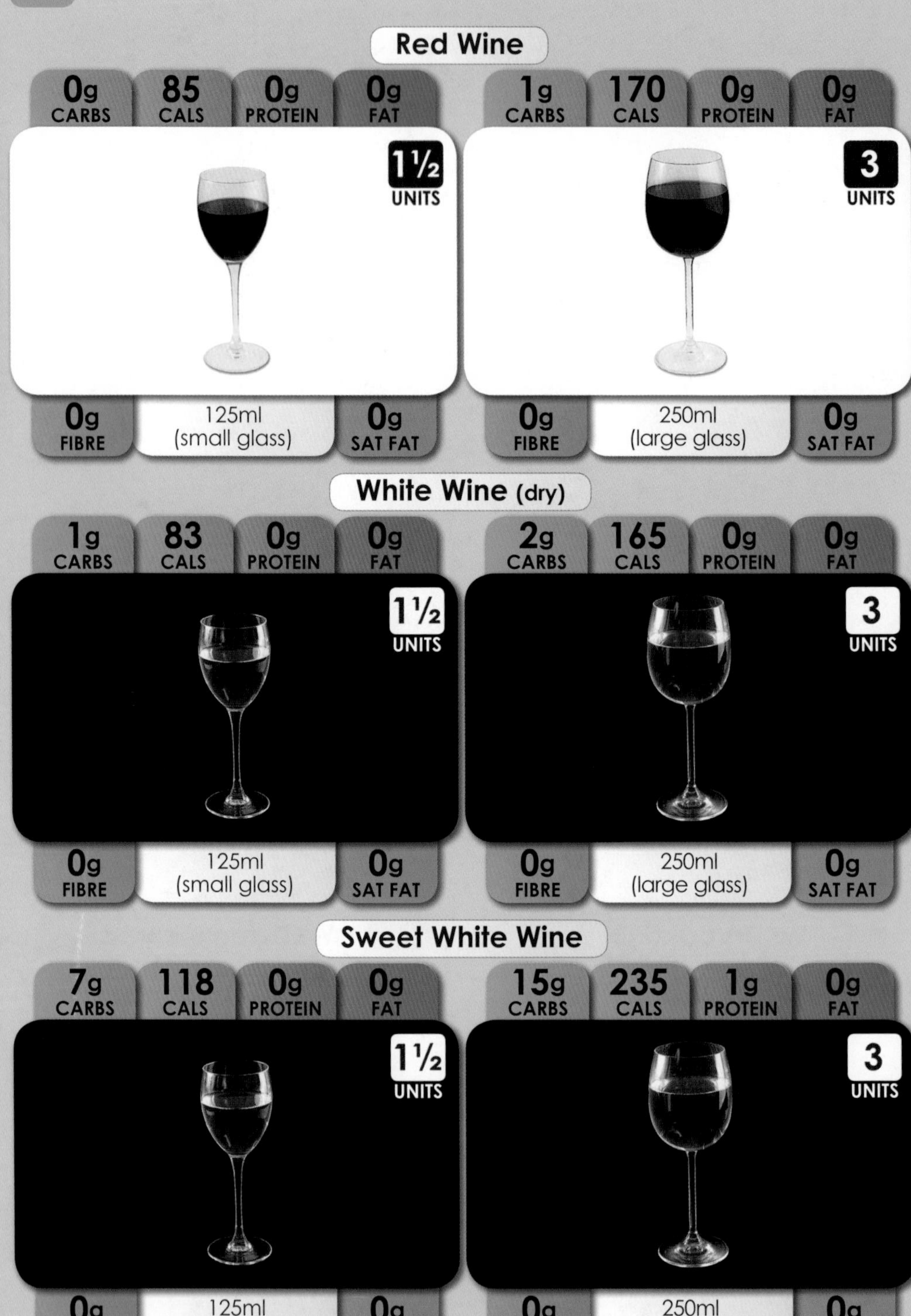

Red Wine

Serving	Units	Carbs	Cals	Protein	Fat	Fibre	Sat Fat
125ml (small glass)	1½	0g	85	0g	0g	0g	0g
250ml (large glass)	3	1g	170	0g	0g	0g	0g

White Wine (dry)

Serving	Units	Carbs	Cals	Protein	Fat	Fibre	Sat Fat
125ml (small glass)	1½	1g	83	0g	0g	0g	0g
250ml (large glass)	3	2g	165	0g	0g	0g	0g

Sweet White Wine

Serving	Units	Carbs	Cals	Protein	Fat	Fibre	Sat Fat
125ml (small glass)	1½	7g	118	0g	0g	0g	0g
250ml (large glass)	3	15g	235	1g	0g	0g	0g

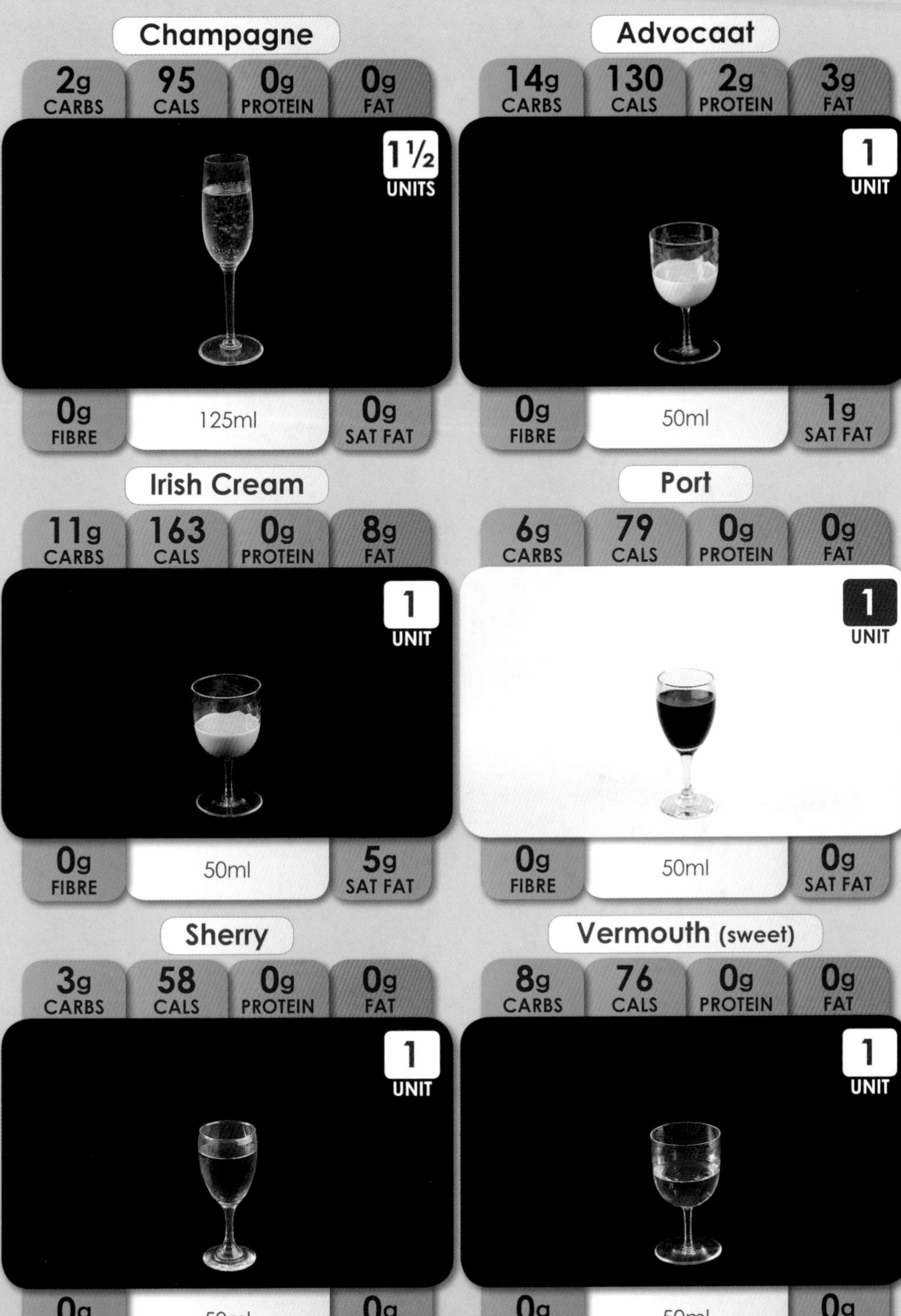

Champagne

CARBS	CALS	PROTEIN	FAT	FIBRE	SAT FAT	Portion	Units
2g	95	0g	0g	0g	0g	125ml	1½ UNITS

Advocaat

CARBS	CALS	PROTEIN	FAT	FIBRE	SAT FAT	Portion	Units
14g	130	2g	3g	0g	1g	50ml	1 UNIT

Irish Cream

CARBS	CALS	PROTEIN	FAT	FIBRE	SAT FAT	Portion	Units
11g	163	0g	8g	0g	5g	50ml	1 UNIT

Port

CARBS	CALS	PROTEIN	FAT	FIBRE	SAT FAT	Portion	Units
6g	79	0g	0g	0g	0g	50ml	1 UNIT

Sherry

CARBS	CALS	PROTEIN	FAT	FIBRE	SAT FAT	Portion	Units
3g	58	0g	0g	0g	0g	50ml	1 UNIT

Vermouth (sweet)

CARBS	CALS	PROTEIN	FAT	FIBRE	SAT FAT	Portion	Units
8g	76	0g	0g	0g	0g	50ml	1 UNIT

Brandy

0g CARBS	56 CALS	0g PROTEIN	0g FAT

1 UNIT

0g FIBRE	25ml	0g SAT FAT

Gin

0g CARBS	56 CALS	0g PROTEIN	0g FAT

1 UNIT

0g FIBRE	25ml	0g SAT FAT

Rum

0g CARBS	56 CALS	0g PROTEIN	0g FAT

1 UNIT

0g FIBRE	25ml	0g SAT FAT

Sweet Liqueur

8g CARBS	64 CALS	0g PROTEIN	0g FAT

1 UNIT

0g FIBRE	25ml	0g SAT FAT

Vodka

0g CARBS	56 CALS	0g PROTEIN	0g FAT

1 UNIT

0g FIBRE	25ml	0g SAT FAT

Whisky

0g CARBS	56 CALS	0g PROTEIN	0g FAT

1 UNIT

0g FIBRE	25ml	0g SAT FAT

Boiled Egg

CARBS	CALS	PROTEIN	FAT
0g	88	8g	6g

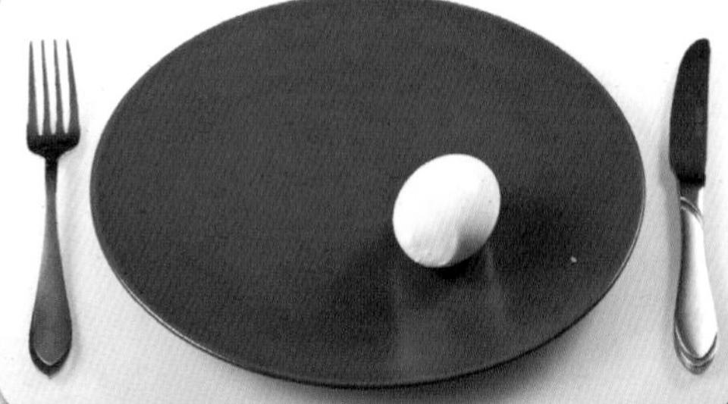

FIBRE		SAT FAT
0g	Weight: 60g	2g

Fried Egg

CARBS	CALS	PROTEIN	FAT
0g	90	7g	7g

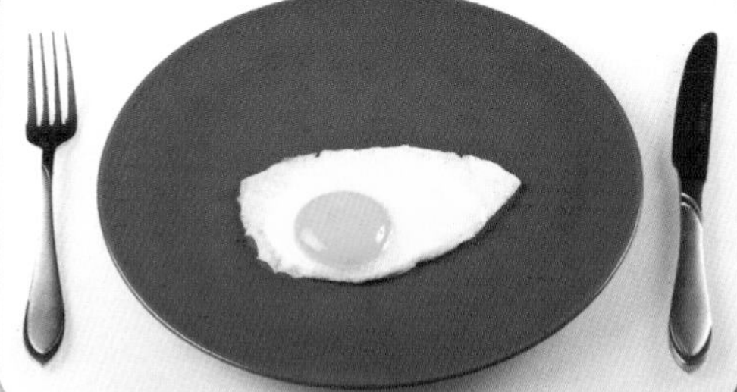

FIBRE		SAT FAT
0g	Weight: 50g	2g

Poached Egg

CARBS	CALS	PROTEIN	FAT
0g	74	6g	5g

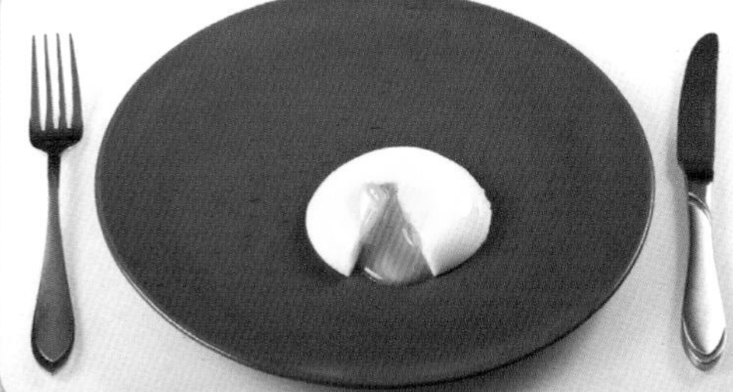

FIBRE		SAT FAT
0g	Weight: 50g	2g

Scrambled Egg (with milk)

CARBS	CALS	PROTEIN	FAT
1g	109	9g	8g

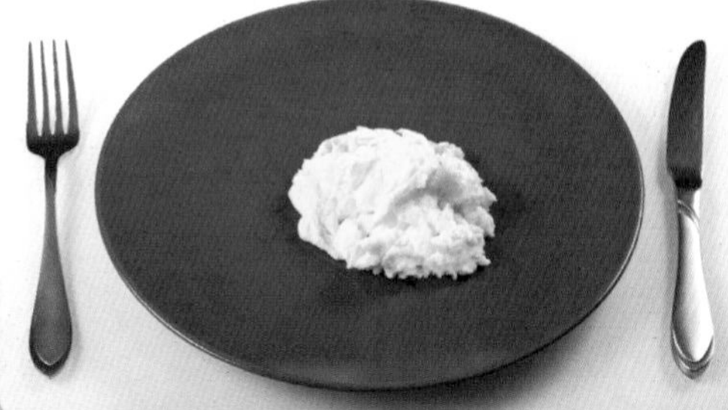

FIBRE		SAT FAT
0g	Weight: 70g (1 egg)	2g

CARBS	CALS	PROTEIN	FAT
2g	187	16g	14g

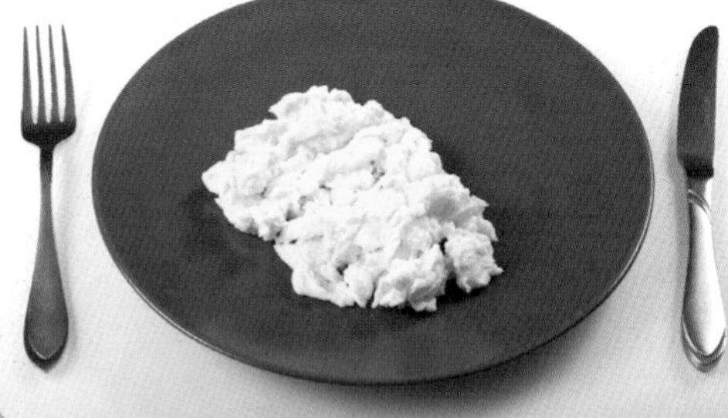

FIBRE		SAT FAT
0g	Weight: 120g (2 eggs)	4g

CARBS	CALS	PROTEIN	FAT
2g	281	24g	20g

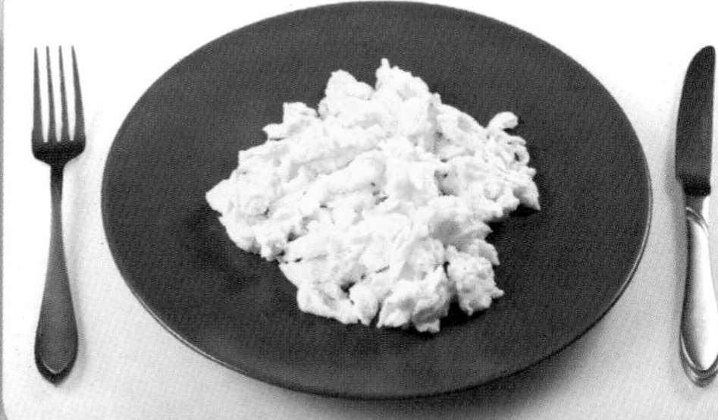

FIBRE		SAT FAT
0g	Weight: 180g (3 eggs)	6g

Omelette (plain)

0g CARBS	98 CALS	6g PROTEIN	8g FAT

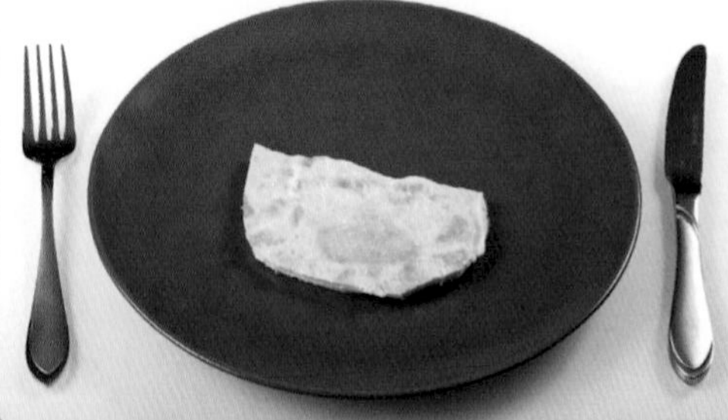

0g FIBRE	Weight: 50g (1 egg)	4g SAT FAT

0g CARBS	195 CALS	11g PROTEIN	17g FAT

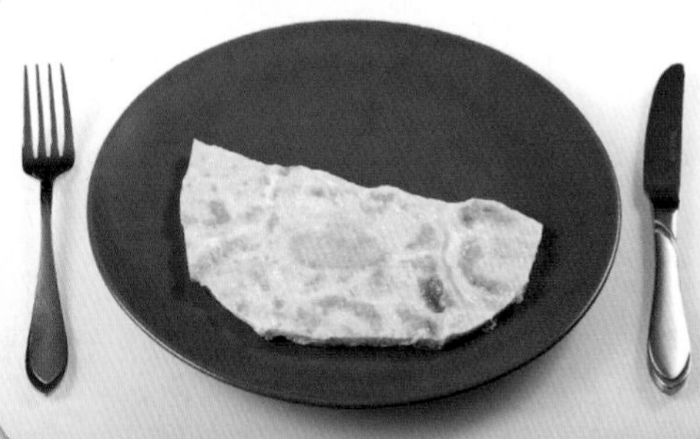

0g FIBRE	Weight: 100g (2 eggs)	7g SAT FAT

0g CARBS	293 CALS	16g PROTEIN	25g FAT

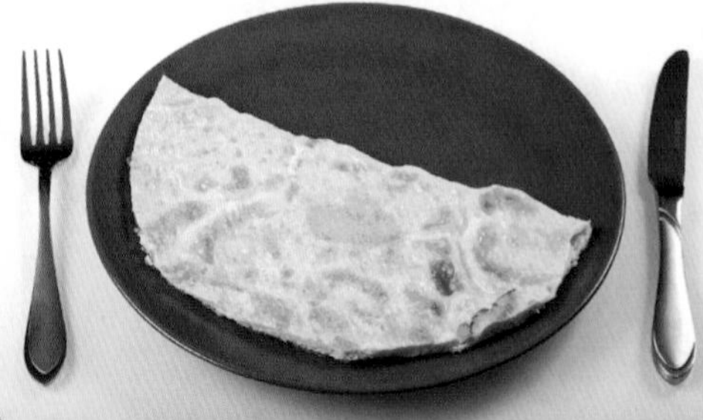

0g FIBRE	Weight: 150g (3 eggs)	11g SAT FAT

Omelette (cheese)

0g CARBS	163 CALS	10g PROTEIN	14g FAT

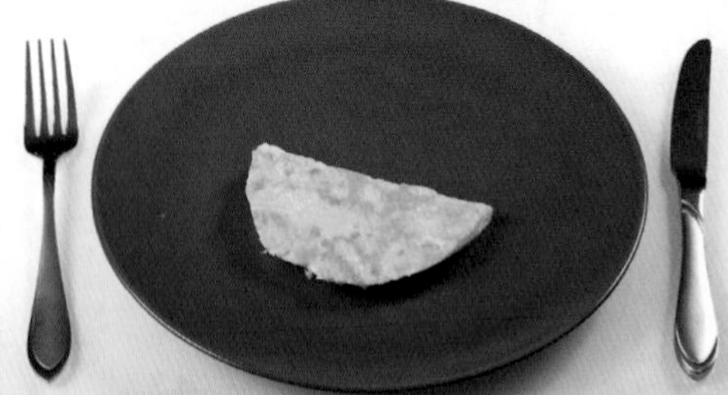

0g FIBRE	60g (1 egg, 10g cheese)	7g SAT FAT

0g CARBS	325 CALS	19g PROTEIN	28g FAT

0g FIBRE	120g (2 eggs, 20g cheese)	15g SAT FAT

0g CARBS	488 CALS	29g PROTEIN	41g FAT

0g FIBRE	180g (3 eggs, 30g cheese)	22g SAT FAT

Eggs Benedict

CARBS	CALS	PROTEIN	FAT
16g	311	17g	21g

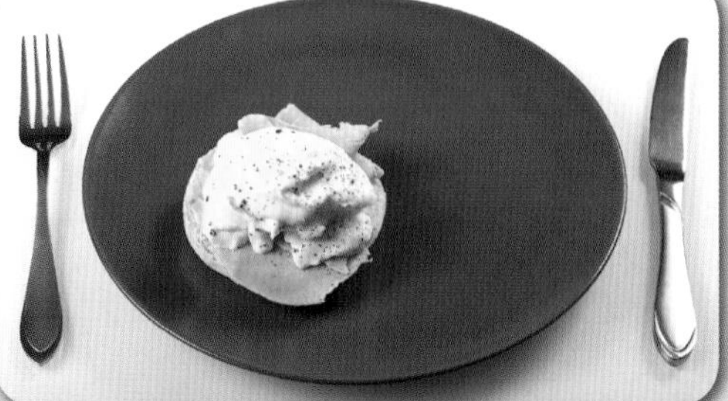

FIBRE		SAT FAT
1g	Weight: 170g	9g

CARBS	CALS	PROTEIN	FAT
31g	623	34g	41g

FIBRE		SAT FAT
2g	Weight: 340g	19g

Eggs Florentine

CARBS	CALS	PROTEIN	FAT
19g	294	16g	17g

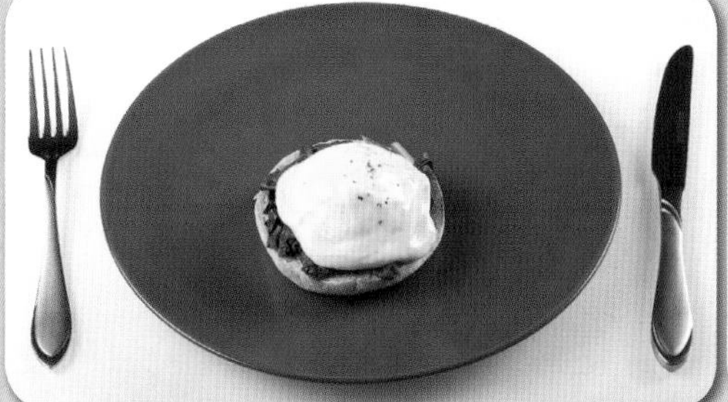

FIBRE		SAT FAT
1g	Weight: 155g	7g

CARBS	CALS	PROTEIN	FAT
38g	588	33g	35g

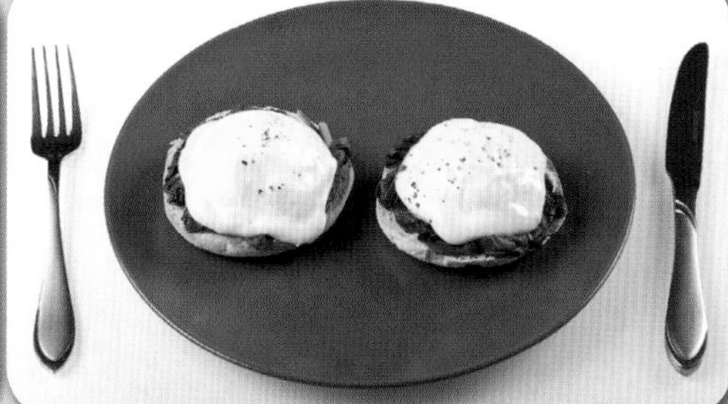

FIBRE		SAT FAT
3g	Weight: 310g	14g

Scotch Egg

CARBS	CALS	PROTEIN	FAT
9g	140	6g	8g

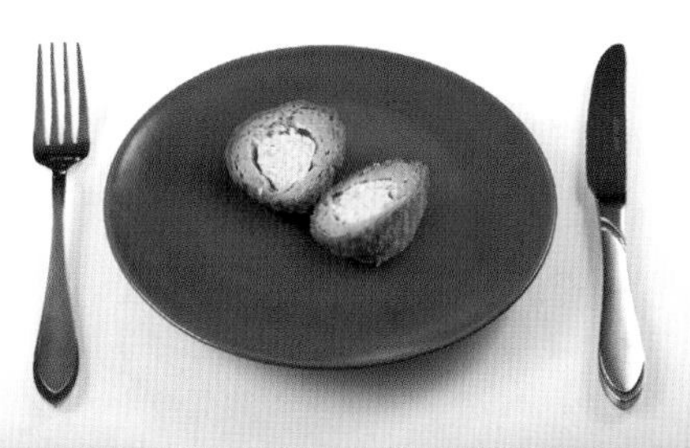

FIBRE		SAT FAT
1g	Weight: 60g (mini)	2g

CARBS	CALS	PROTEIN	FAT
19g	280	13g	17g

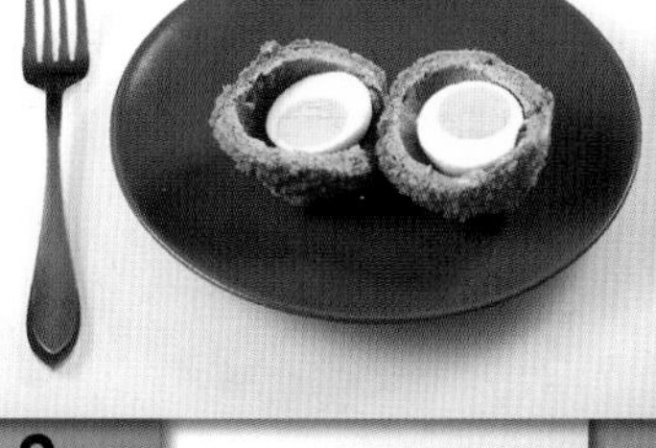

FIBRE		SAT FAT
2g	Weight: 120g	5g

Apricots

4g CARBS	17 CALS	1g PROTEIN	0g FAT

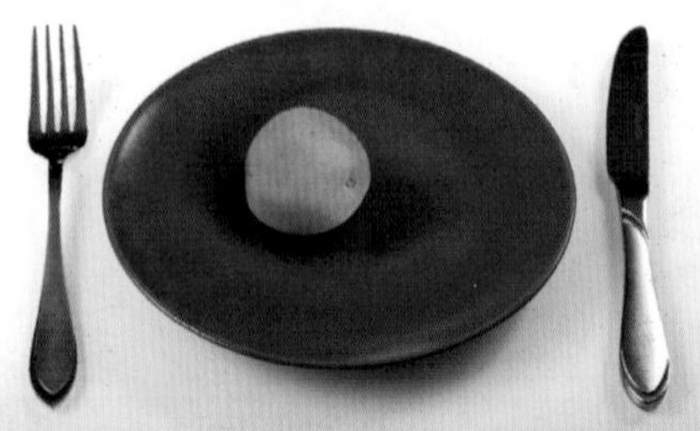

1g FIBRE	Weight: 55g	0g SAT FAT

8g CARBS	34 CALS	1g PROTEIN	0g FAT

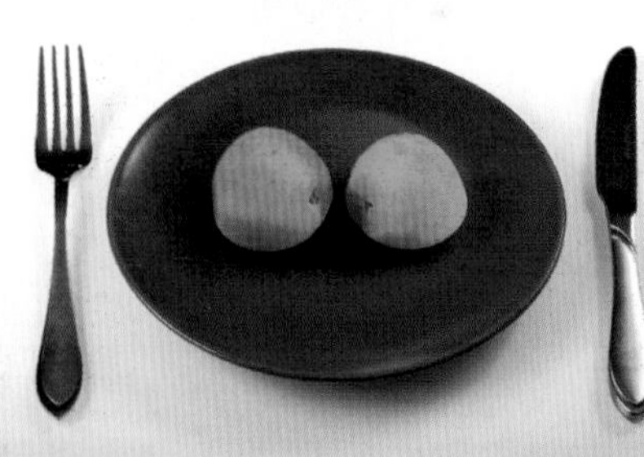

3g FIBRE	Weight: 110g	0g SAT FAT

12g CARBS	51 CALS	2g PROTEIN	0g FAT

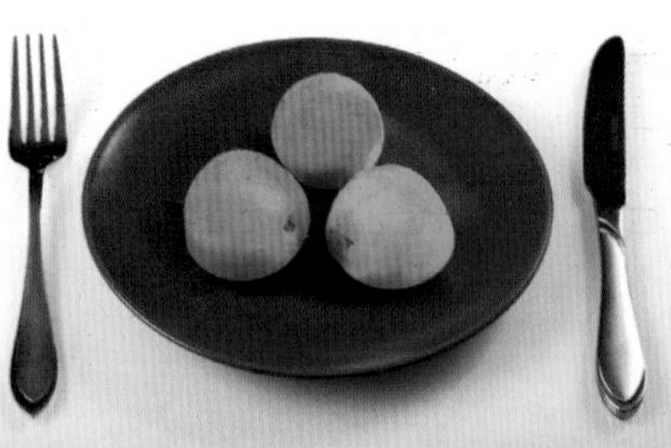

4g FIBRE	Weight: 165g	0g SAT FAT

Apricots (tinned in juice)

7g CARBS	27 CALS	0g PROTEIN	0g FAT

1g FIBRE	Weight: 80g	0g SAT FAT

13g CARBS	54 CALS	1g PROTEIN	0g FAT

1g FIBRE	Weight: 160g	0g SAT FAT

34g CARBS	136 CALS	2g PROTEIN	0g FAT

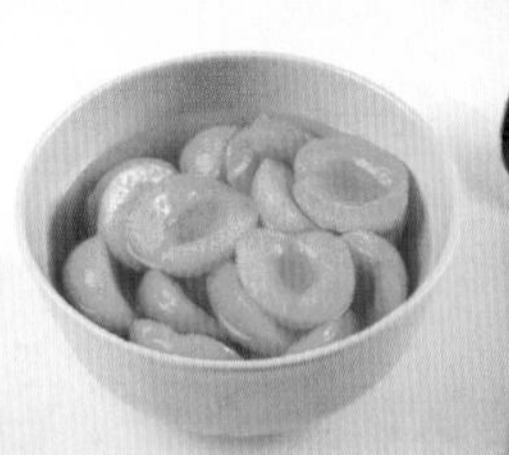

4g FIBRE	Weight: 400g	0g SAT FAT

Apple

CARBS	CALS	PROTEIN	FAT
10g	40	0g	0g

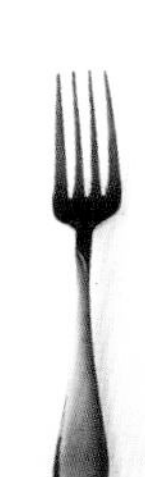
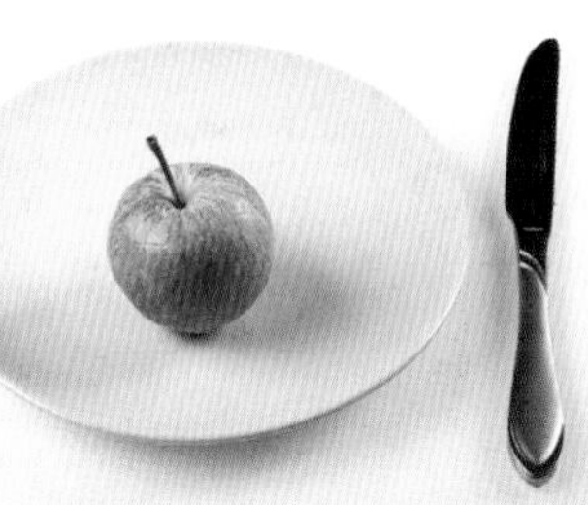

FIBRE	Weight	SAT FAT
2g	Weight: 85g	0g

CARBS	CALS	PROTEIN	FAT
16g	62	1g	0g

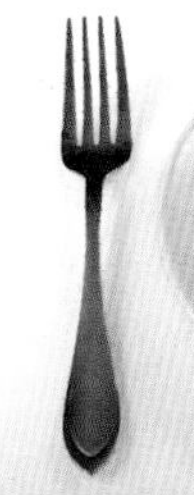
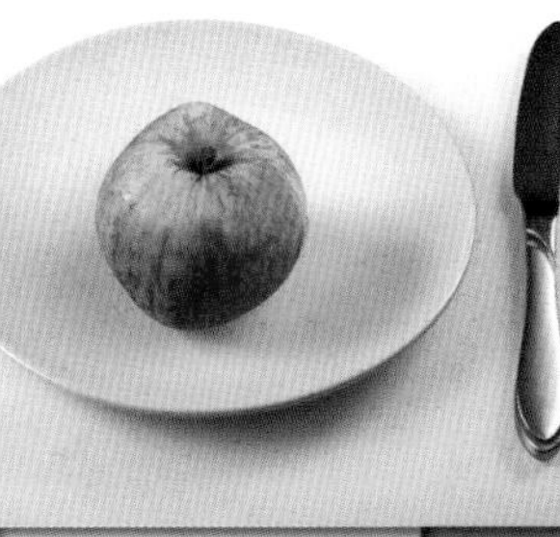
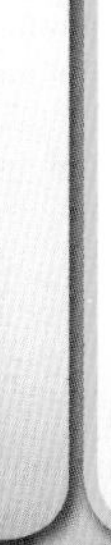

FIBRE	Weight	SAT FAT
3g	Weight: 131g	0g

CARBS	CALS	PROTEIN	FAT
20g	80	1g	0g

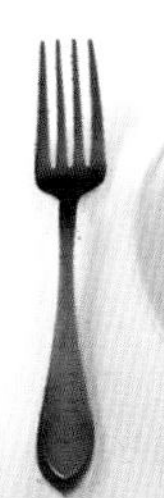
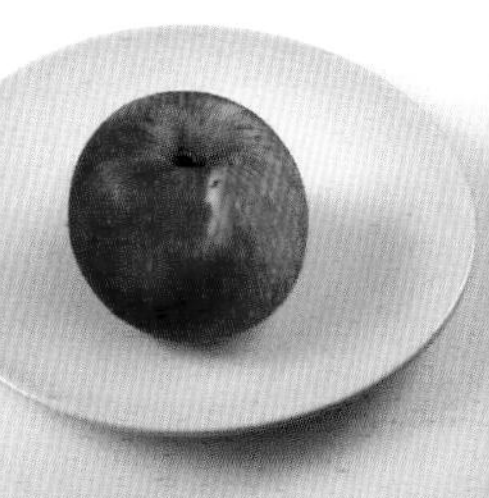
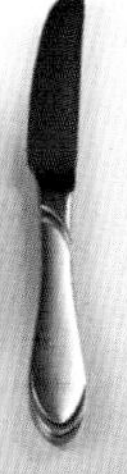

FIBRE	Weight	SAT FAT
4g	Weight: 170g	0g

Blackberries

CARBS	CALS	PROTEIN	FAT
2g	10	0g	0g

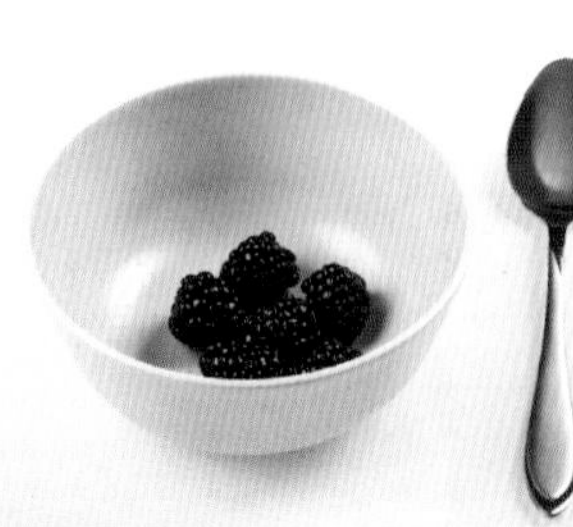

FIBRE	Weight	SAT FAT
2g	Weight: 40g	0g

CARBS	CALS	PROTEIN	FAT
4g	20	1g	0g

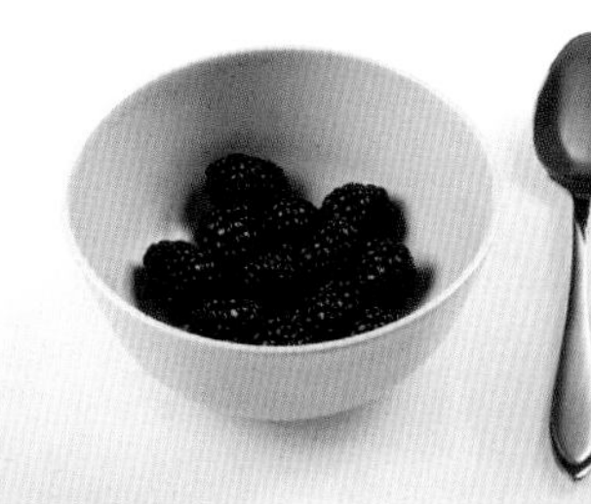

FIBRE	Weight	SAT FAT
3g	Weight: 80g	0g

CARBS	CALS	PROTEIN	FAT
8g	40	1g	0g

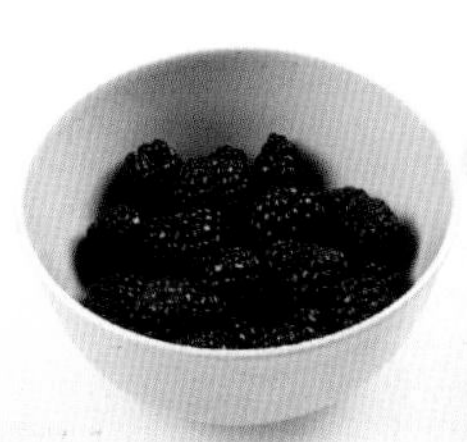
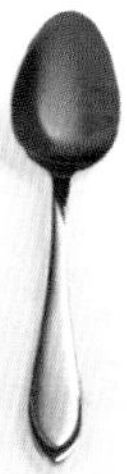

FIBRE	Weight	SAT FAT
7g	Weight: 160g	0g

Banana (with skin)

CARBS	CALS	PROTEIN	FAT
15g	60	1g	0g

FIBRE	Weight	SAT FAT
1g	Weight: 97g	0g

CARBS	CALS	PROTEIN	FAT
20g	81	1g	0g

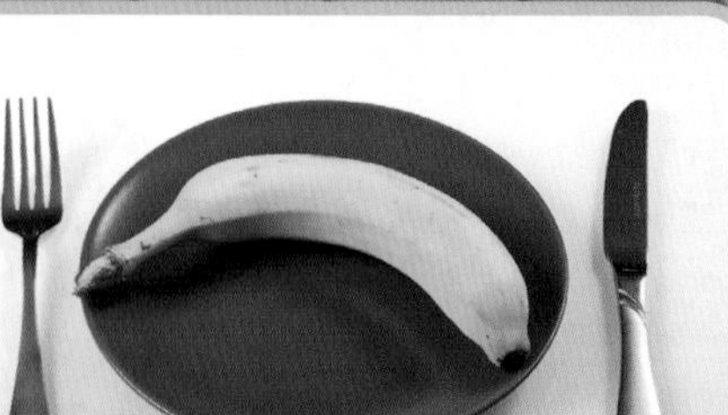

FIBRE	Weight	SAT FAT
1g	Weight: 130g	0g

CARBS	CALS	PROTEIN	FAT
30g	122	2g	0g

FIBRE	Weight	SAT FAT
2g	Weight: 190g	0g

Banana (without skin)

CARBS	CALS	PROTEIN	FAT
15g	60	1g	0g

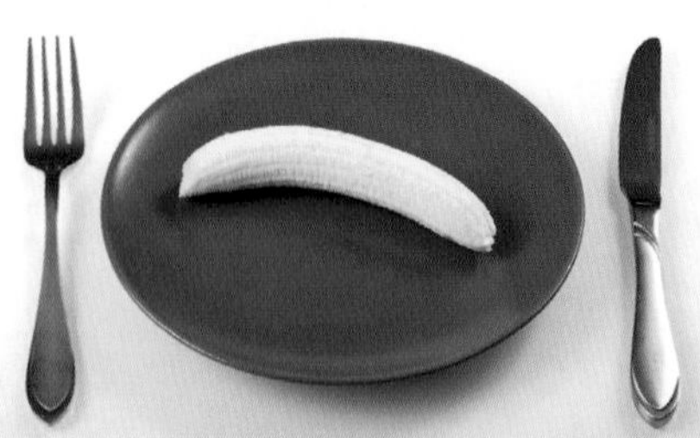

FIBRE	Weight	SAT FAT
1g	Weight: 63g	0g

CARBS	CALS	PROTEIN	FAT
20g	81	1g	0g

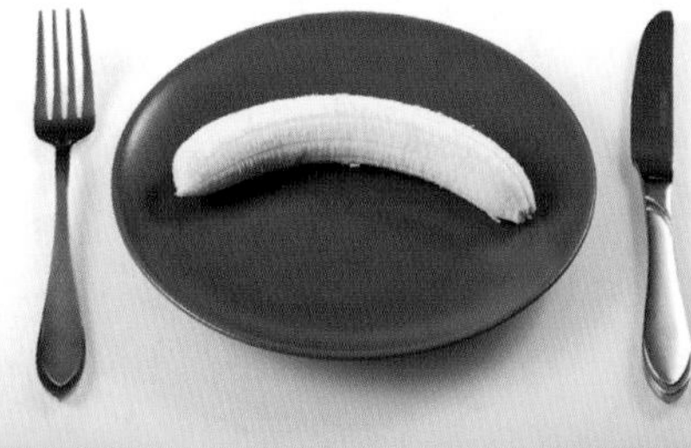

FIBRE	Weight	SAT FAT
1g	Weight: 85g	0g

CARBS	CALS	PROTEIN	FAT
30g	122	2g	0g

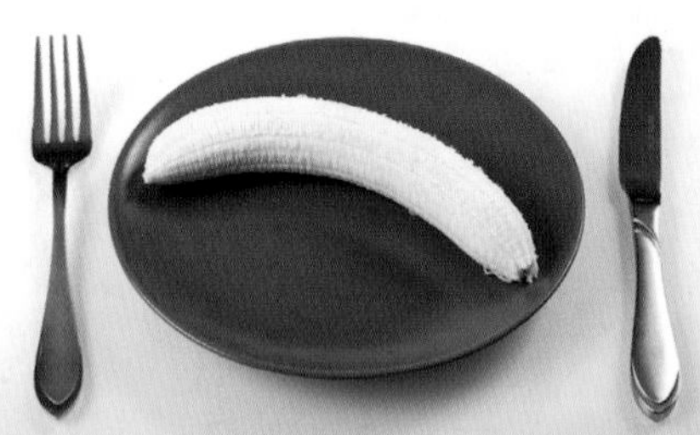

FIBRE	Weight	SAT FAT
2g	Weight: 128g	0g

Blueberries

Weight	Carbs	Cals	Protein	Fat	Fibre	Sat Fat
40g	6g	26	0g	0g	1g	0g
80g	11g	53	1g	0g	2g	0g
160g	23g	106	1g	1g	3g	0g

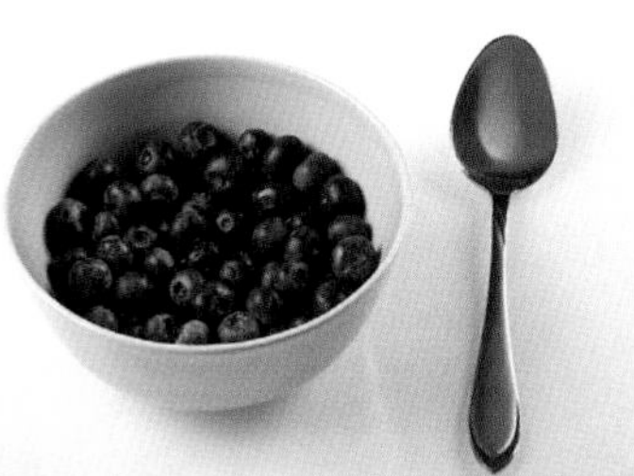

Cherries

Weight	Carbs	Cals	Protein	Fat	Fibre	Sat Fat
50g	6g	24	1g	0g	1g	0g
100g	12g	48	1g	0g	1g	0g
160g	18g	77	1g	0g	2g	0g

20cm Side Plate / 14cm Cereal Bowl

Clementine

5g CARBS	22 CALS	1g PROTEIN	0g FAT

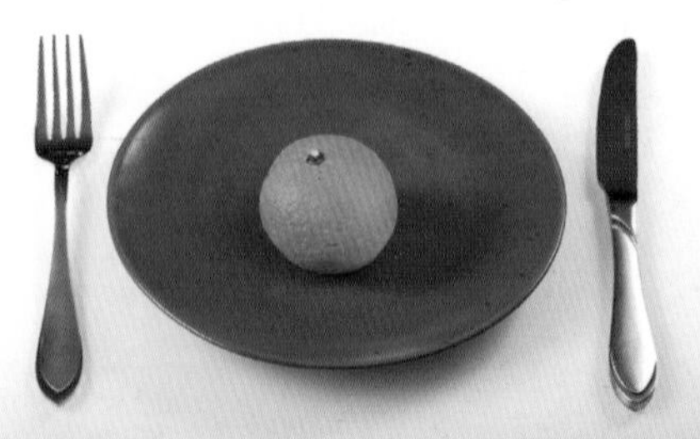

1g FIBRE	Weight: 80g	0g SAT FAT

10g CARBS	45 CALS	1g PROTEIN	0g FAT

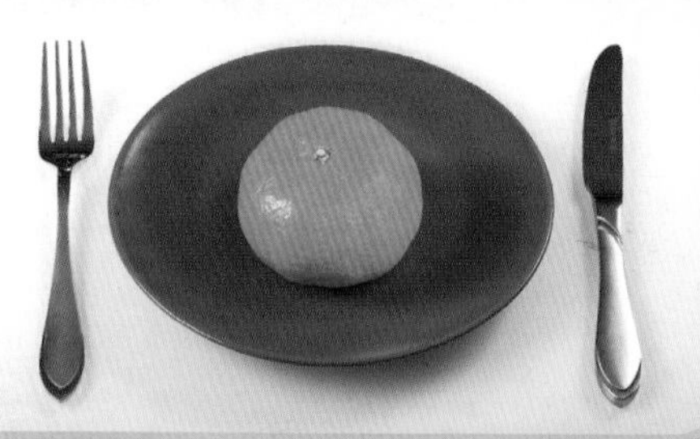

2g FIBRE	Weight: 160g	0g SAT FAT

Satsuma

5g CARBS	22 CALS	1g PROTEIN	0g FAT

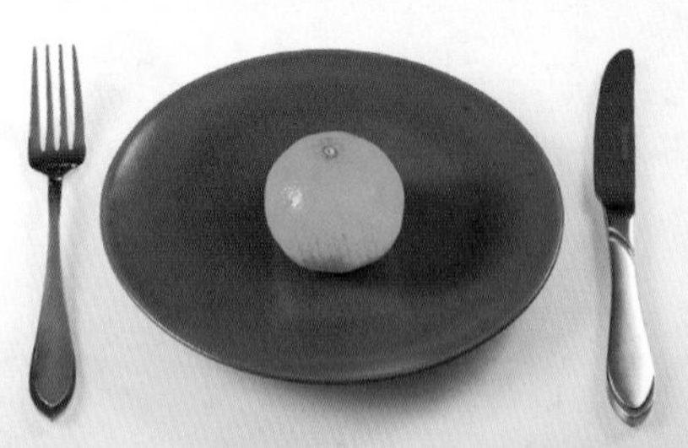

1g FIBRE	Weight: 85g	0g SAT FAT

Cranberries

1g CARBS	5 CALS	0g PROTEIN	0g FAT

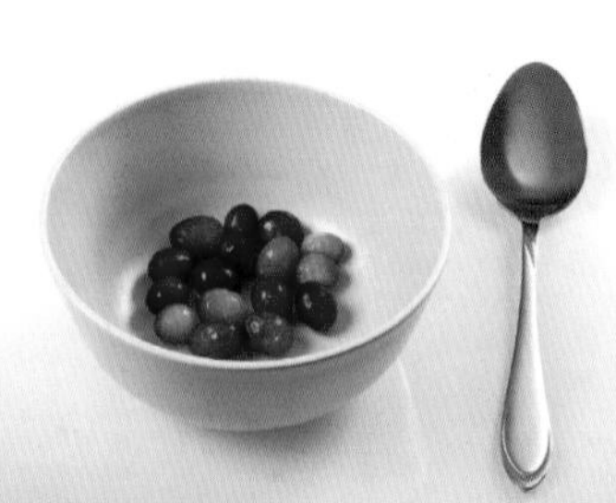

1g FIBRE	Weight: 30g	0g SAT FAT

3g CARBS	12 CALS	0g PROTEIN	0g FAT

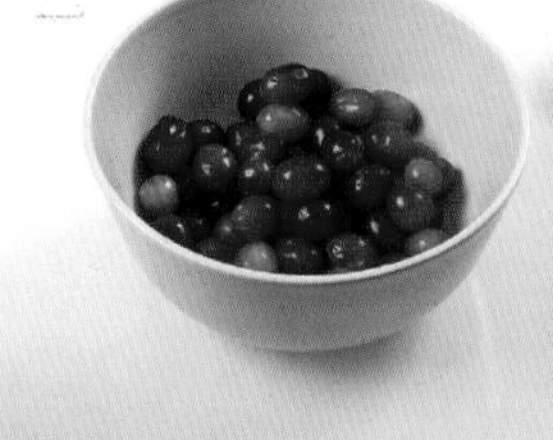

3g FIBRE	Weight: 80g	0g SAT FAT

5g CARBS	24 CALS	1g PROTEIN	0g FAT

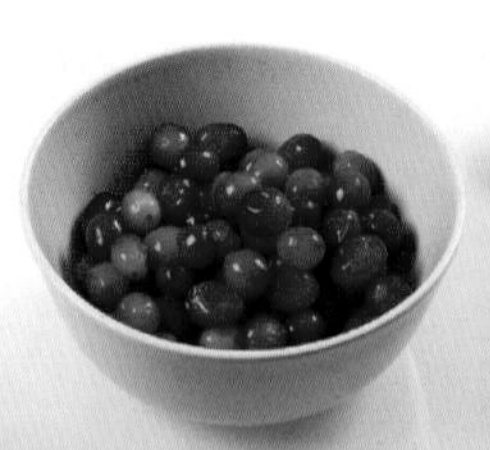

6g FIBRE	Weight: 160g	0g SAT FAT

Figs

3g CARBS	13 CALS	0g PROTEIN	0g FAT

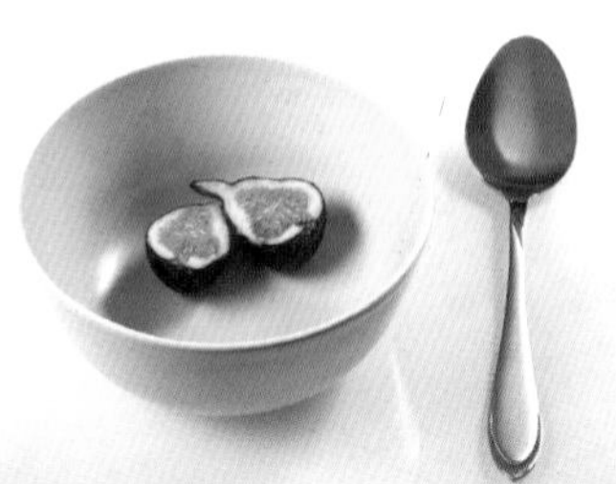

1g FIBRE	Weight: 30g	0g SAT FAT

5g CARBS	24 CALS	1g PROTEIN	0g FAT

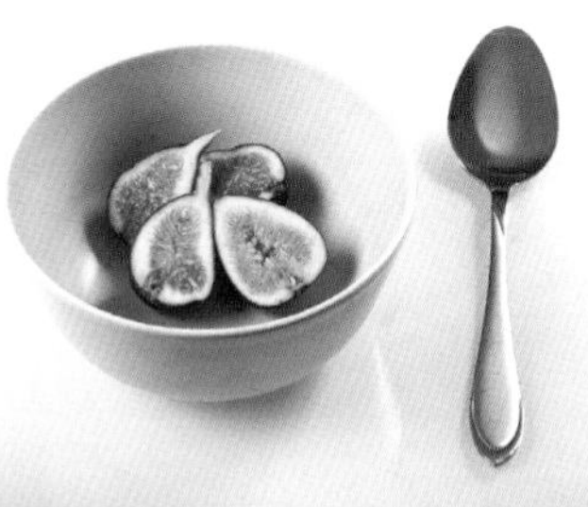

1g FIBRE	Weight: 55g	0g SAT FAT

8g CARBS	34 CALS	1g PROTEIN	0g FAT

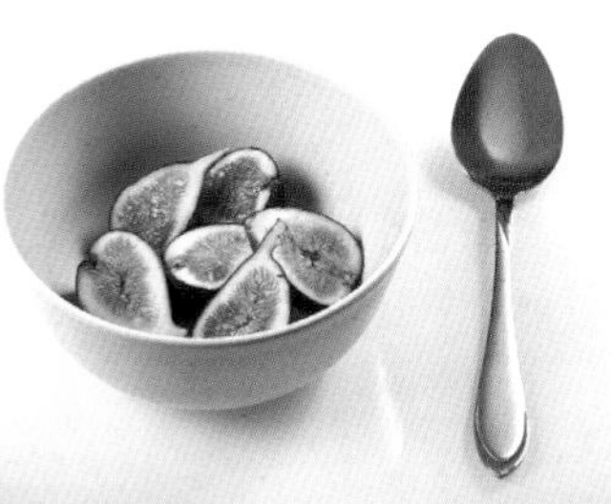

2g FIBRE	Weight: 80g	0g SAT FAT

Fruit Cocktail (tinned in juice)

6g CARBS	23 CALS	0g PROTEIN	0g FAT

1g FIBRE	Weight: 80g	0g SAT FAT

15g CARBS	61 CALS	1g PROTEIN	0g FAT

3g FIBRE	Weight: 210g	0g SAT FAT

30g CARBS	122 CALS	2g PROTEIN	0g FAT

6g FIBRE	Weight: 420g	0g SAT FAT

20cm Side Plate / 14cm Cereal Bowl

Grapefruit

CARBS	CALS	PROTEIN	FAT
6g	24	1g	0g

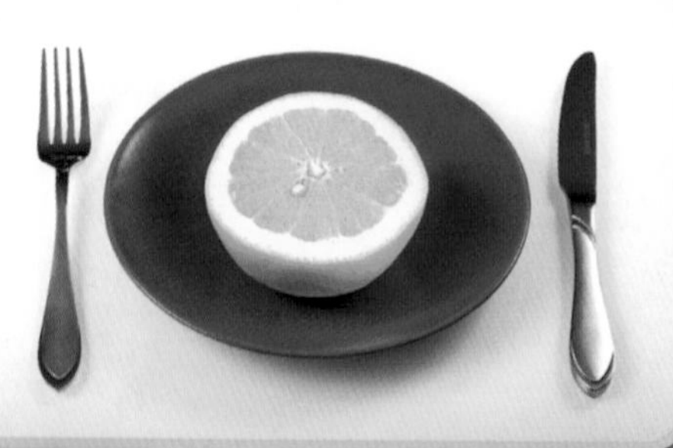

FIBRE		SAT FAT
1g	Weight: 119g	0g

CARBS	CALS	PROTEIN	FAT
11g	46	1g	0g

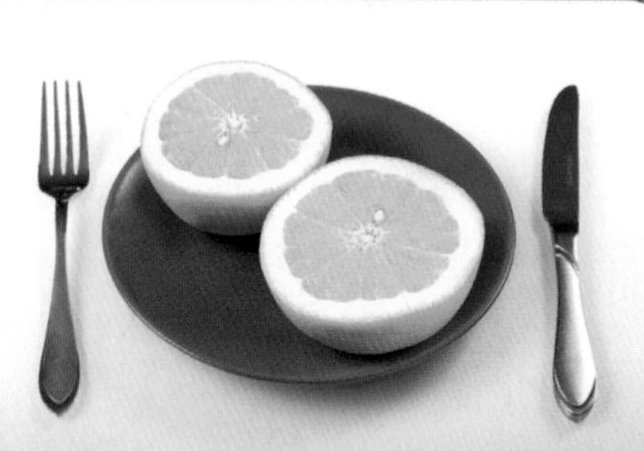

FIBRE		SAT FAT
3g	Weight: 228g	0g

CARBS	CALS	PROTEIN	FAT
11g	46	1g	0g

FIBRE		SAT FAT
3g	Weight: 140g (1 grapefruit)	0g

Grapes (seedless)

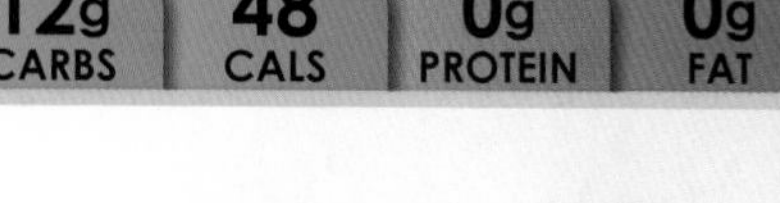

CARBS	CALS	PROTEIN	FAT
12g	48	0g	0g

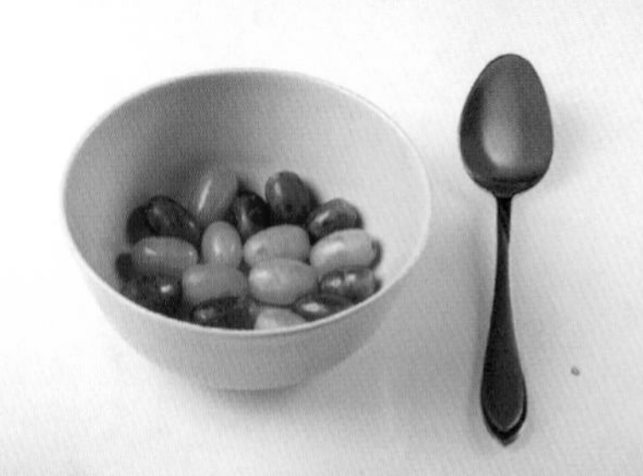

FIBRE		SAT FAT
1g	Weight: 80g	0g

CARBS	CALS	PROTEIN	FAT
25g	96	1g	0g

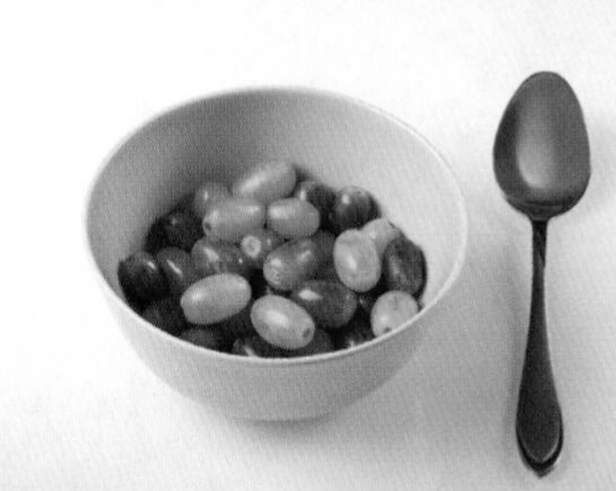

FIBRE		SAT FAT
1g	Weight: 160g	0g

CARBS	CALS	PROTEIN	FAT
37g	144	1g	0g

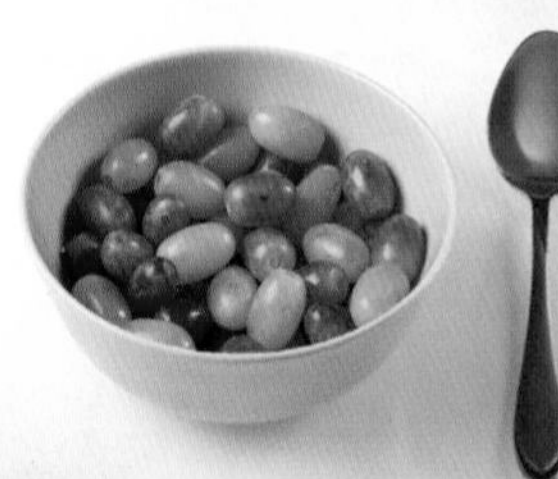

FIBRE		SAT FAT
2g	Weight: 240g	0g

Kiwi

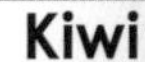

CARBS	CALS	PROTEIN	FAT	FIBRE	SAT FAT	Weight
5g	23	1g	0g	1g	0g	55g

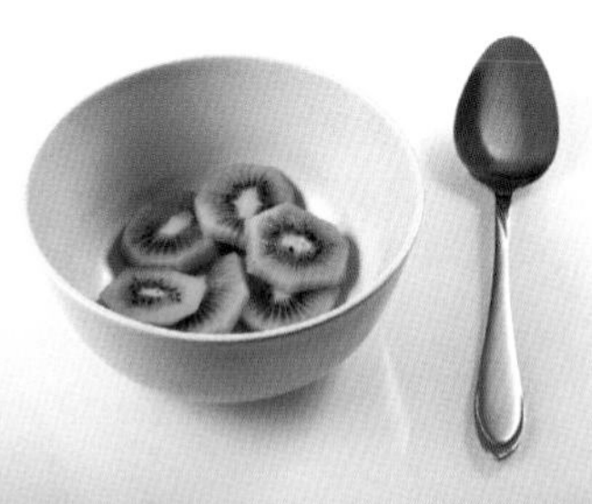

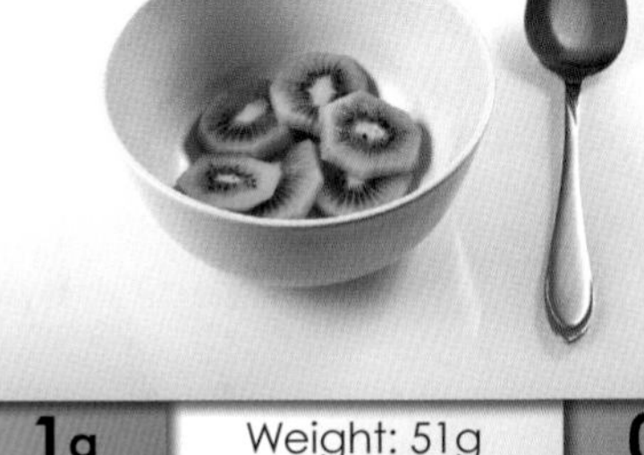

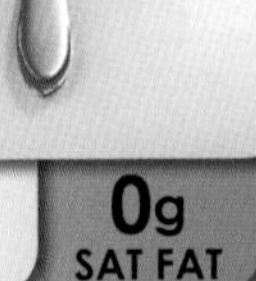

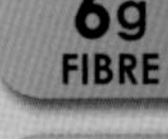

CARBS	CALS	PROTEIN	FAT	FIBRE	SAT FAT	Weight
5g	25	1g	0g	1g	0g	51g (1 kiwi)

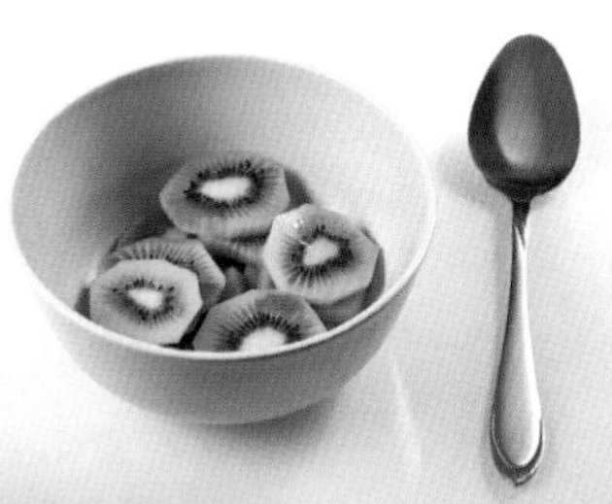

CARBS	CALS	PROTEIN	FAT	FIBRE	SAT FAT	Weight
10g	47	1g	1g	2g	0g	95g (2 kiwis)

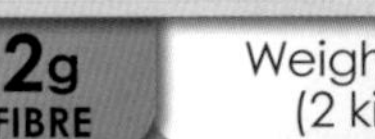

Mango

CARBS	CALS	PROTEIN	FAT	FIBRE	SAT FAT	Weight
11g	46	1g	0g	3g	0g	80g

CARBS	CALS	PROTEIN	FAT	FIBRE	SAT FAT	Weight
23g	91	1g	0g	6g	0g	160g

CARBS	CALS	PROTEIN	FAT	FIBRE	SAT FAT	Weight
34g	137	2g	1g	8g	0g	240g

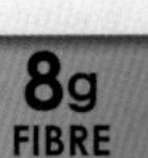

22cm Large Bowl / 20cm Side Plate

Melon (honeydew)

CARBS	CALS	PROTEIN	FAT
5g	22	1g	0g

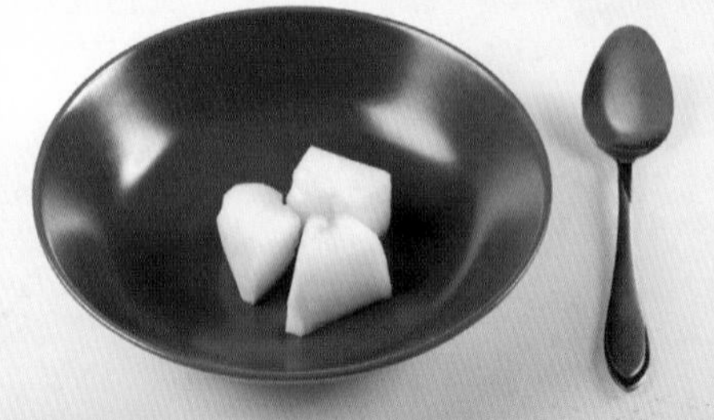

FIBRE	Weight	SAT FAT
1g	Weight: 80g	0g

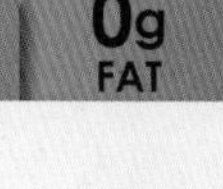

CARBS	CALS	PROTEIN	FAT
11g	45	1g	0g

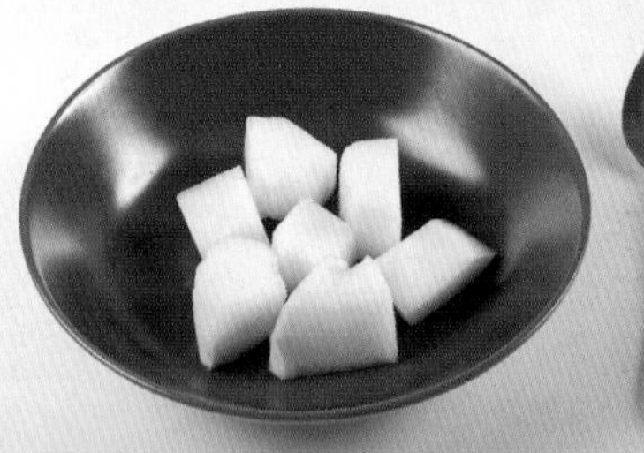

FIBRE	Weight	SAT FAT
1g	Weight: 160g	0g

CARBS	CALS	PROTEIN	FAT
16g	67	1g	0g

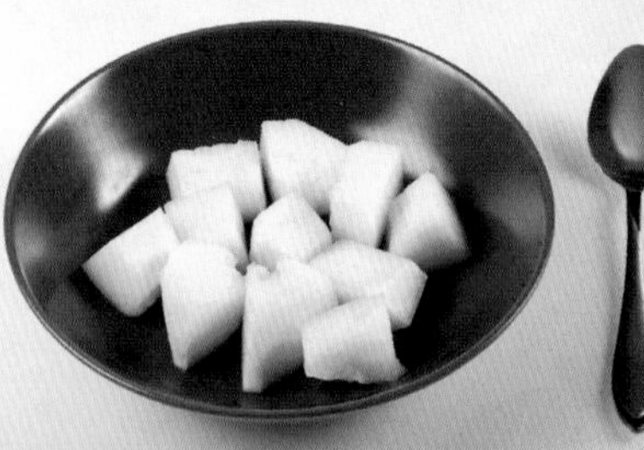

FIBRE	Weight	SAT FAT
2g	Weight: 240g	0g

Orange

CARBS	CALS	PROTEIN	FAT
4g	19	1g	0g

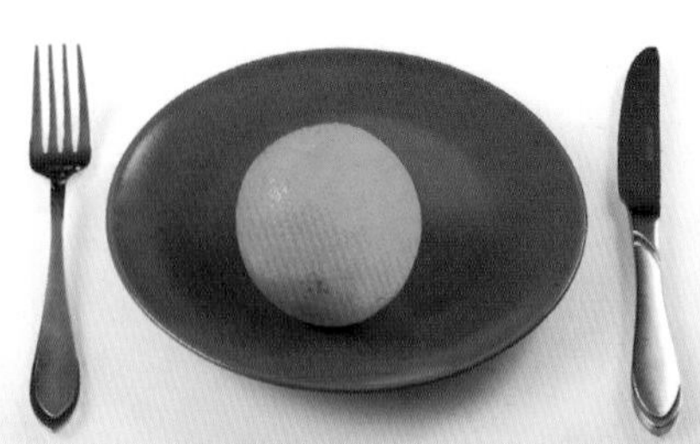

FIBRE	Weight	SAT FAT
1g	Weight: 71g	0g

CARBS	CALS	PROTEIN	FAT
7g	30	1g	0g

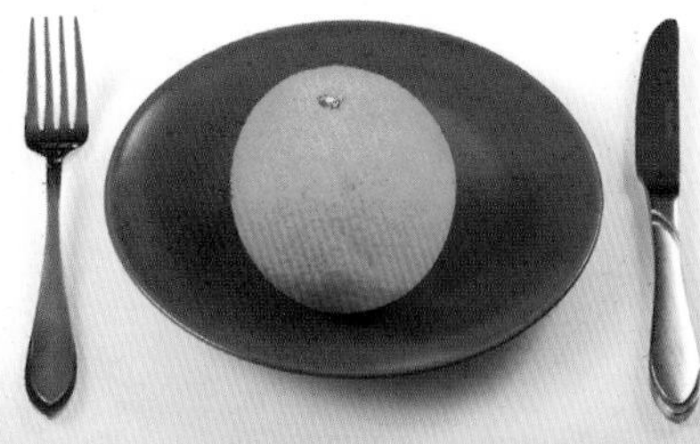

FIBRE	Weight	SAT FAT
2g	Weight: 115g	0g

CARBS	CALS	PROTEIN	FAT
10g	45	1g	0g

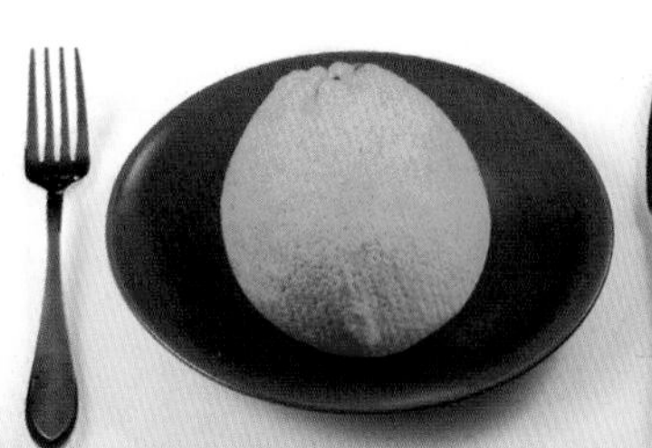

FIBRE	Weight	SAT FAT
3g	Weight: 172g	0g

Papaya

4g CARBS	22 CALS	1g PROTEIN	0g FAT

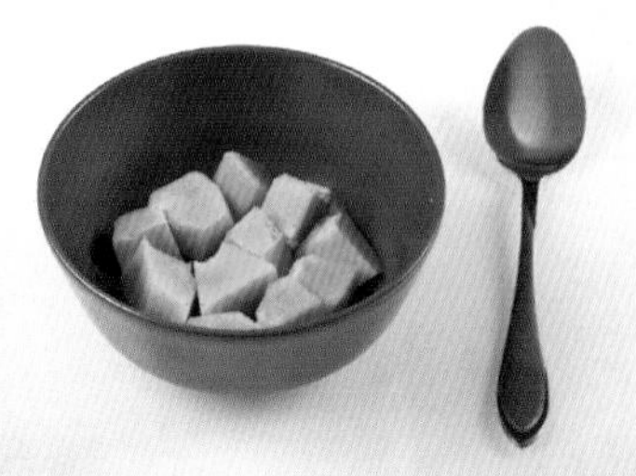

2g FIBRE	Weight: 80g	0g SAT FAT

9g CARBS	43 CALS	1g PROTEIN	0g FAT

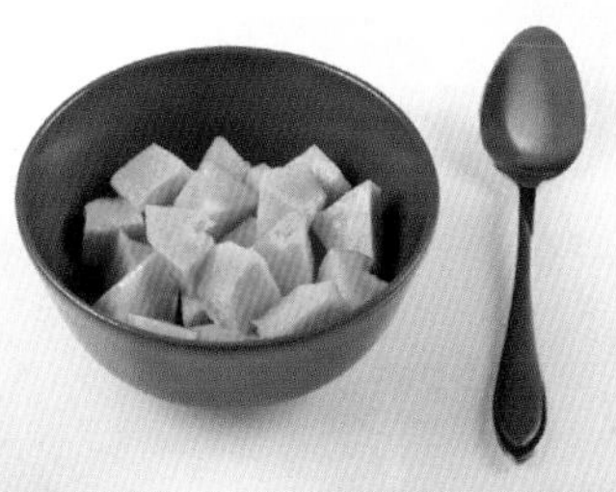

3g FIBRE	Weight: 160g	0g SAT FAT

13g CARBS	65 CALS	2g PROTEIN	0g FAT

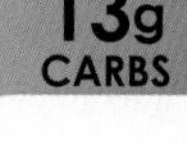

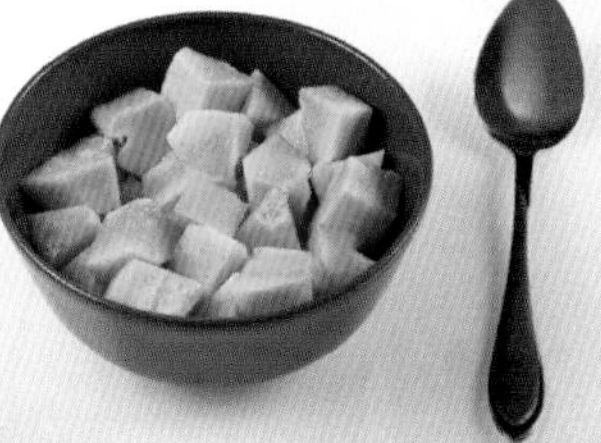

5g FIBRE	Weight: 240g	0g SAT FAT

Pomegranate

5g CARBS	20 CALS	1g PROTEIN	0g FAT

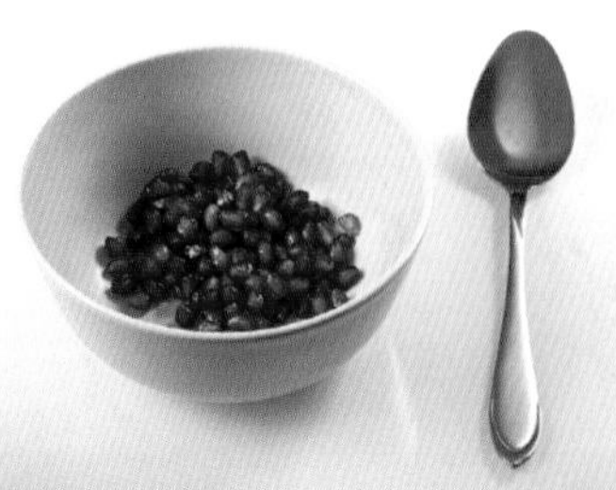

2g FIBRE	Weight: 40g	0g SAT FAT

9g CARBS	41 CALS	1g PROTEIN	0g FAT

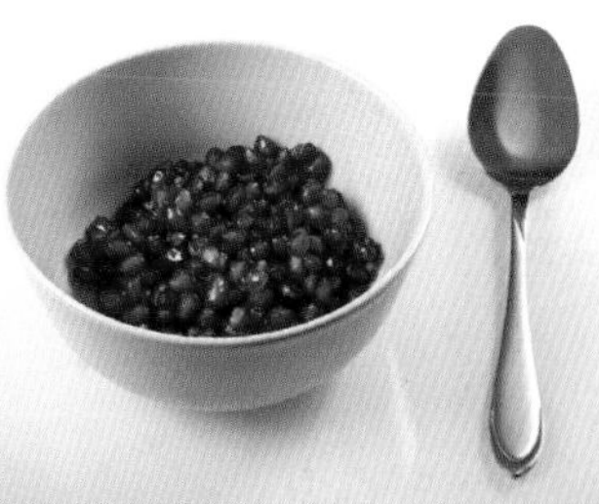

4g FIBRE	Weight: 80g	0g SAT FAT

15g CARBS	64 CALS	2g PROTEIN	0g FAT

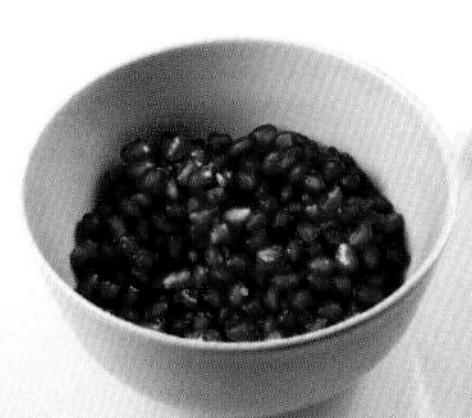

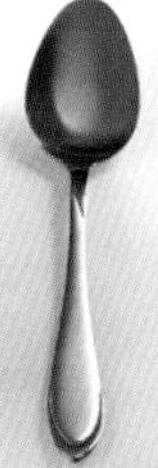

6g FIBRE	Weight: 125g	0g SAT FAT

Plum

CARBS	CALS	PROTEIN	FAT	FIBRE	Weight	SAT FAT
5g	20	0g	0g	1g	55g	0g
10g	40	1g	0g	2g	110g	0g

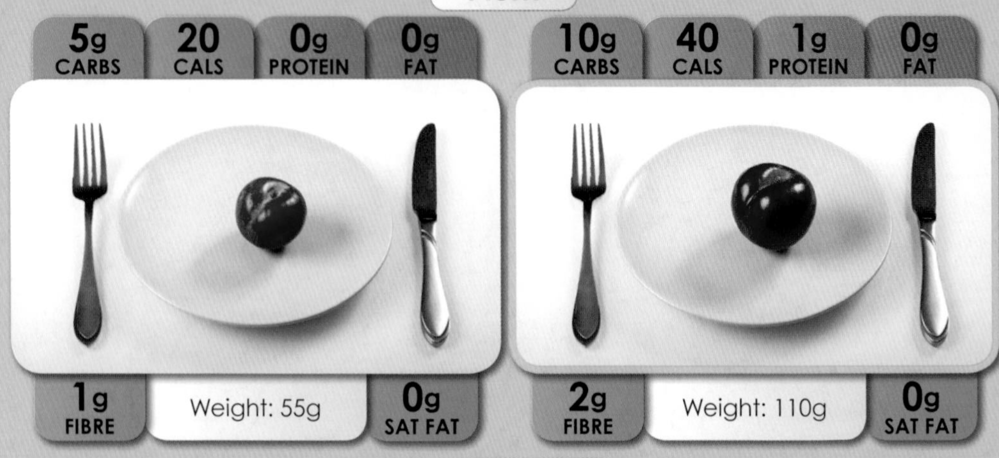

Persimmon

CARBS	CALS	PROTEIN	FAT	FIBRE	Weight	SAT FAT
14g	58	1g	0g	1g	70g	0g
27g	116	1g	0g	2g	140g	0g

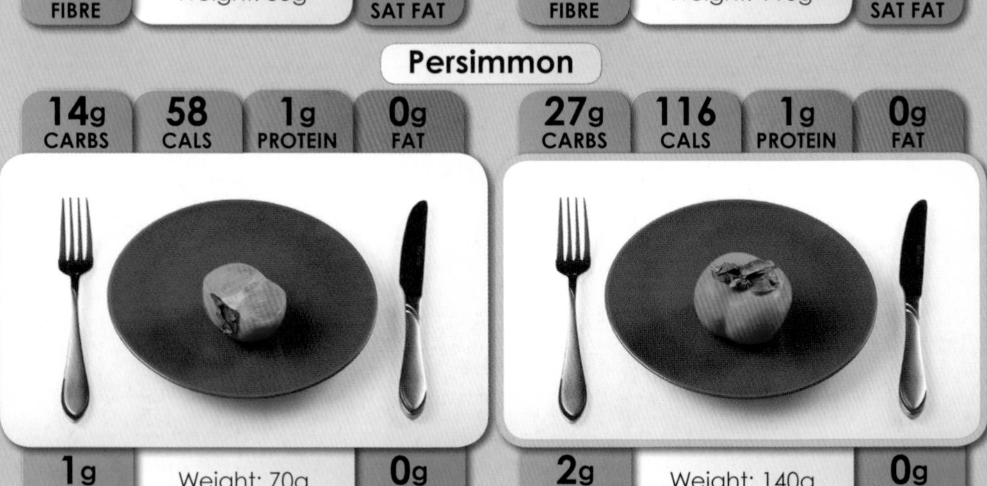

Nectarine

CARBS	CALS	PROTEIN	FAT	FIBRE	Weight	SAT FAT
7g	32	1g	0g	1g	80g	0g
15g	66	2g	0g	3g	165g	0g

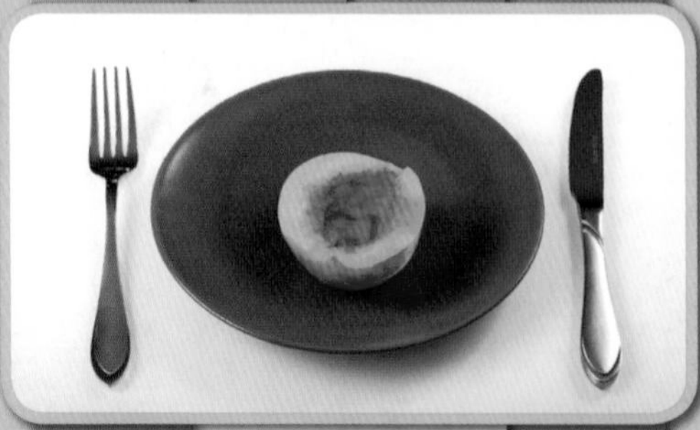

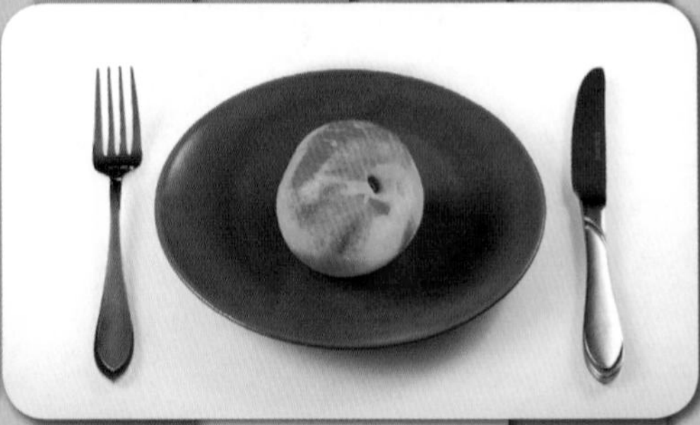

Peach

CARBS	CALS	PROTEIN	FAT
5g	23	1g	0g

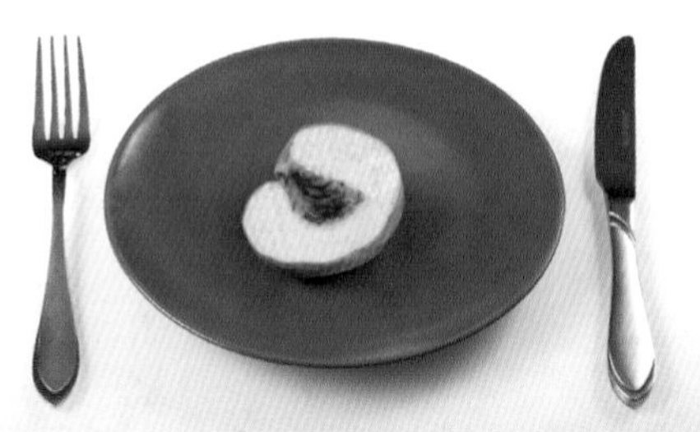

FIBRE	Weight	SAT FAT
1g	Weight: 70g	0g

CARBS	CALS	PROTEIN	FAT
11g	46	1g	0g

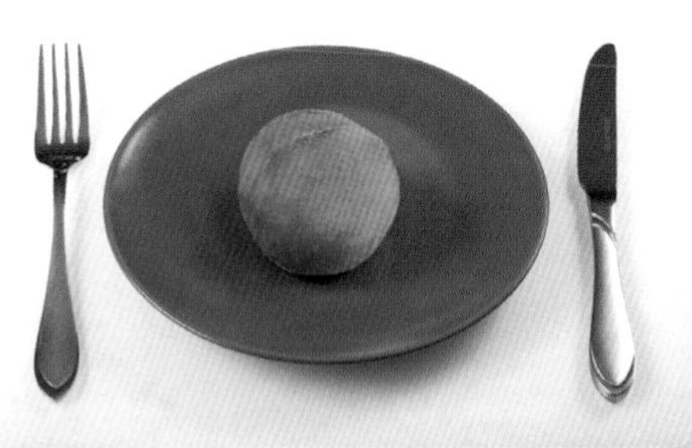

FIBRE	Weight	SAT FAT
3g	Weight: 138g	0g

CARBS	CALS	PROTEIN	FAT
15g	66	2g	0g

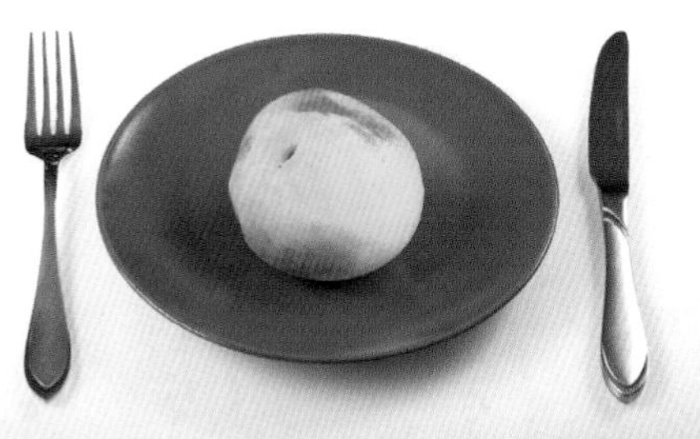

FIBRE	Weight	SAT FAT
4g	Weight: 200g	0g

Peaches (tinned in juice)

CARBS	CALS	PROTEIN	FAT
8g	31	1g	0g

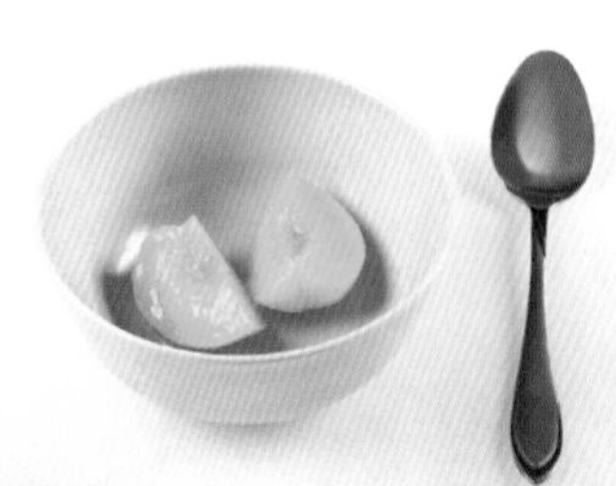

FIBRE	Weight	SAT FAT
1g	Weight: 80g	0g

CARBS	CALS	PROTEIN	FAT
16g	62	1g	0g

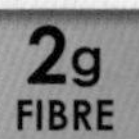

FIBRE	Weight	SAT FAT
2g	Weight: 160g	0g

CARBS	CALS	PROTEIN	FAT
39g	156	2g	0g

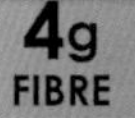

FIBRE	Weight	SAT FAT
4g	Weight: 400g	0g

Pear

CARBS	CALS	PROTEIN	FAT
10g	42	0g	0g

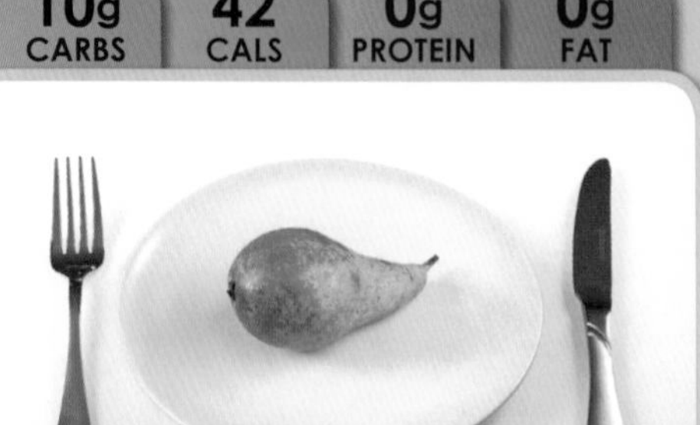

FIBRE	Weight	SAT FAT
3g	Weight: 104g	0g

CARBS	CALS	PROTEIN	FAT
20g	78	1g	0g

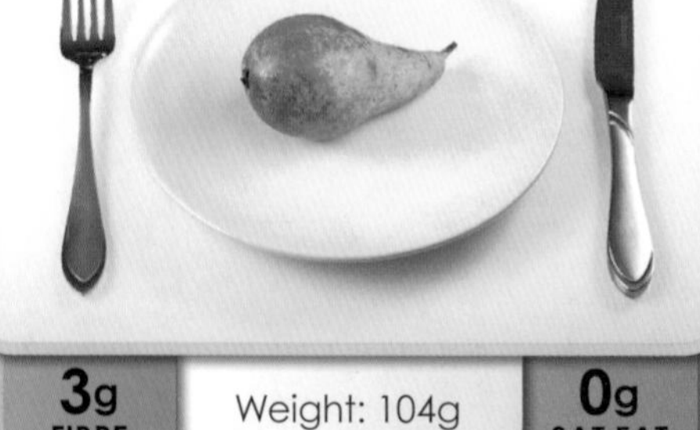

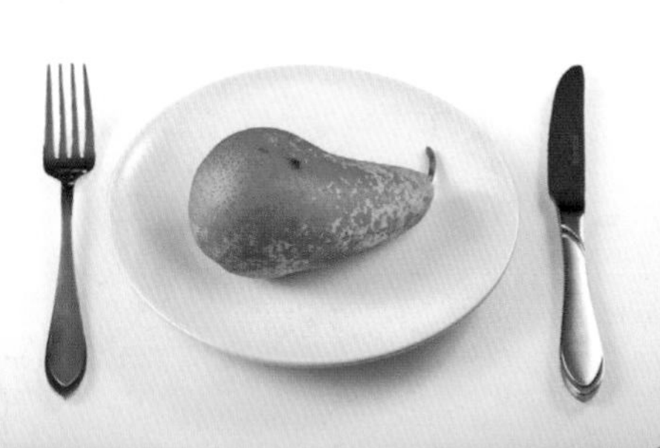

FIBRE	Weight	SAT FAT
6g	Weight: 195g	0g

CARBS	CALS	PROTEIN	FAT
30g	118	1g	0g

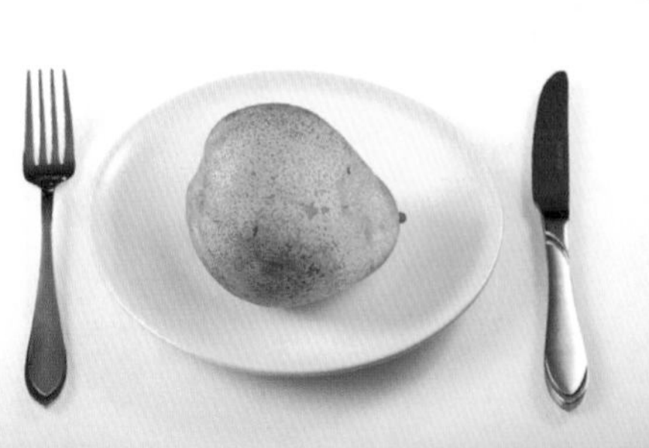

FIBRE	Weight	SAT FAT
9g	Weight: 295g	0g

Pears (tinned in juice)

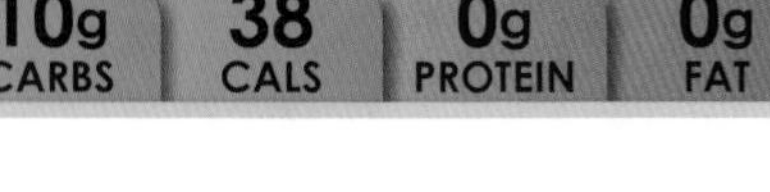

CARBS	CALS	PROTEIN	FAT
10g	38	0g	0g

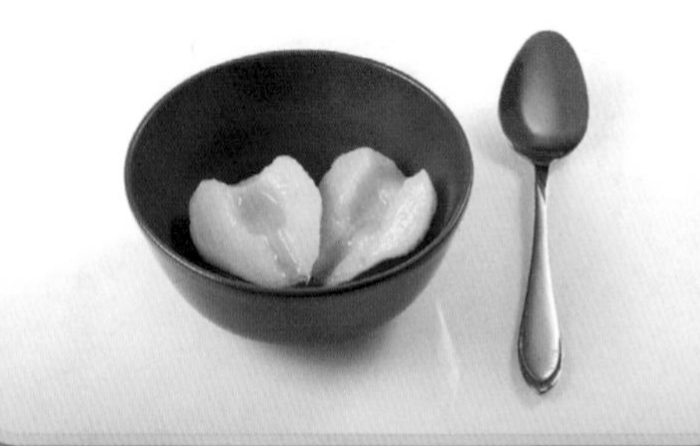

FIBRE	Weight	SAT FAT
2g	Weight: 115g	0g

CARBS	CALS	PROTEIN	FAT
20g	76	1g	0g

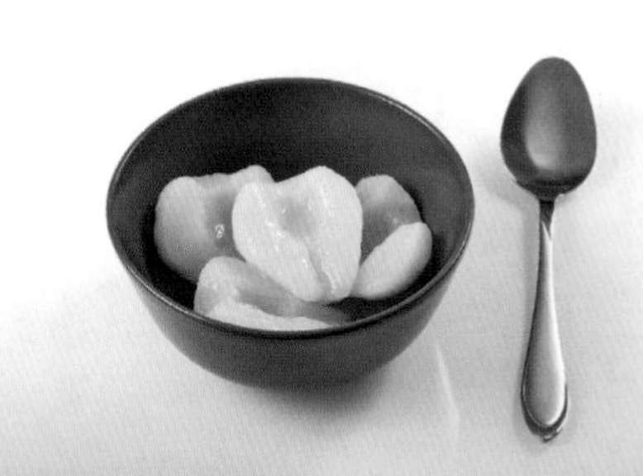

FIBRE	Weight	SAT FAT
4g	Weight: 230g	0g

CARBS	CALS	PROTEIN	FAT
30g	117	1g	0g

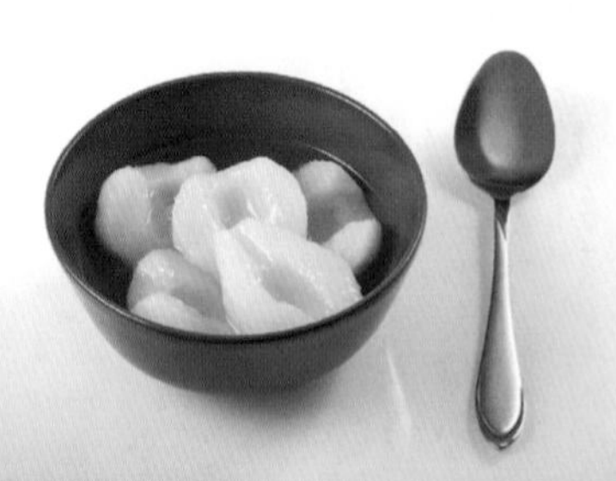

FIBRE	Weight	SAT FAT
7g	Weight: 355g	0g

Pineapple

CARBS	CALS	PROTEIN	FAT
4g	16	0g	0g

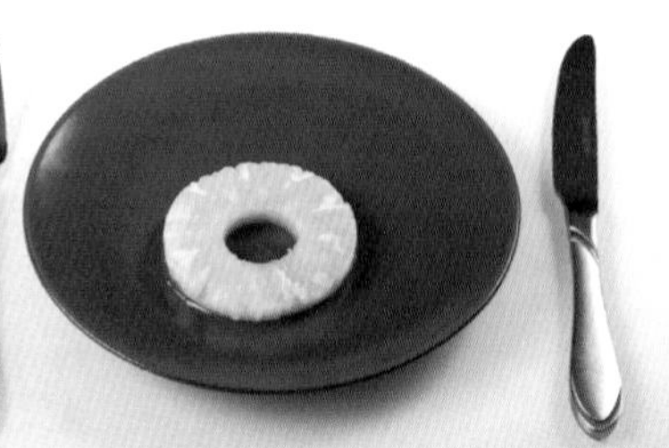

FIBRE	Weight	SAT FAT
1g	Weight: 40g	0g

CARBS	CALS	PROTEIN	FAT
8g	33	0g	0g

FIBRE	Weight	SAT FAT
1g	Weight: 80g	0g

CARBS	CALS	PROTEIN	FAT
12g	49	1g	0g

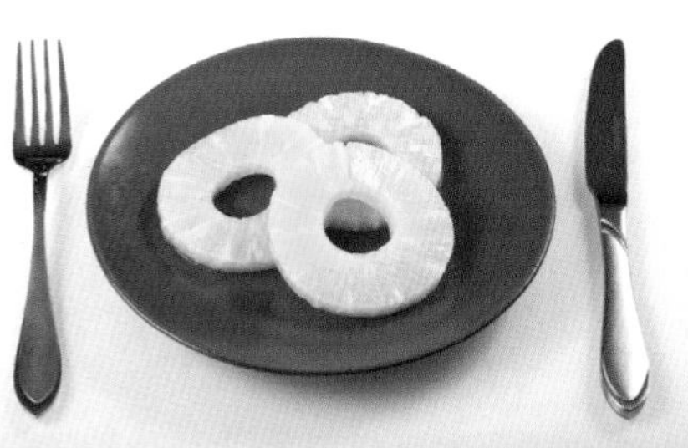

FIBRE	Weight	SAT FAT
2g	Weight: 120g	0g

Pineapple (tinned in juice)

CARBS	CALS	PROTEIN	FAT
10g	38	0g	0g

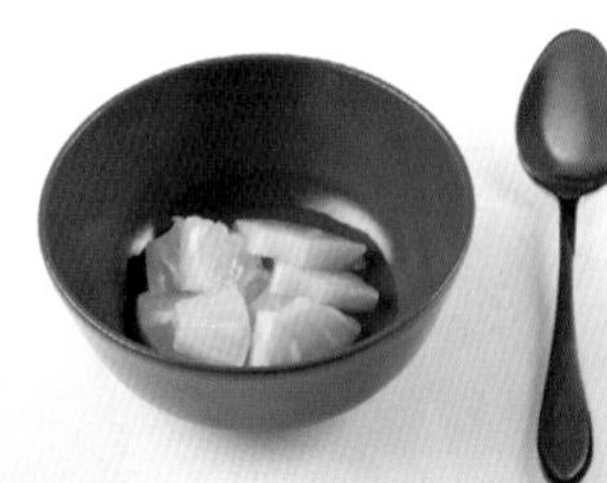

FIBRE	Weight	SAT FAT
1g	Weight: 80g	0g

CARBS	CALS	PROTEIN	FAT
24g	94	1g	0g

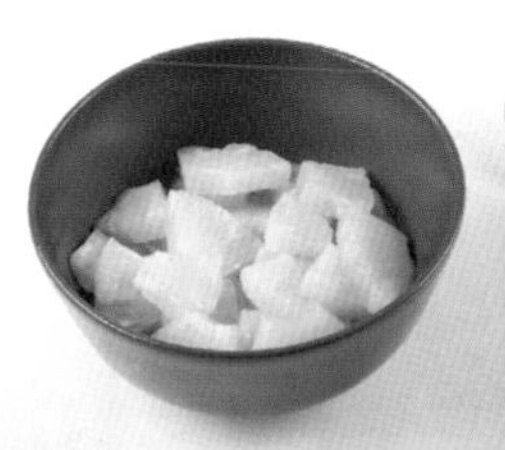

FIBRE	Weight	SAT FAT
1g	Weight: 200g	0g

CARBS	CALS	PROTEIN	FAT
49g	188	1g	0g

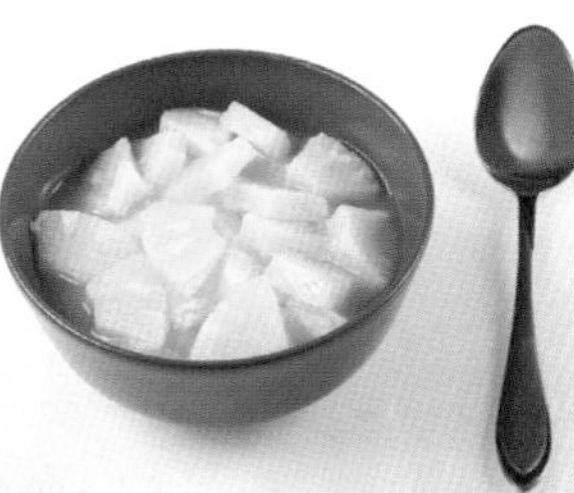

FIBRE	Weight	SAT FAT
3g	Weight: 400g	0g

Raspberries

2g CARBS	10 CALS	1g PROTEIN	0g FAT

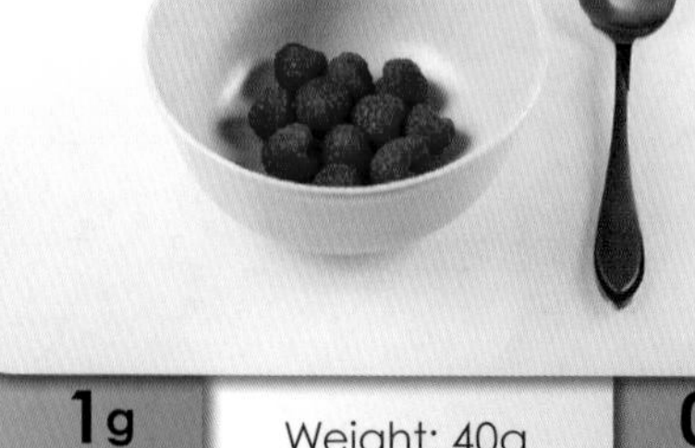

1g FIBRE	Weight: 40g	0g SAT FAT

4g CARBS	20 CALS	1g PROTEIN	0g FAT

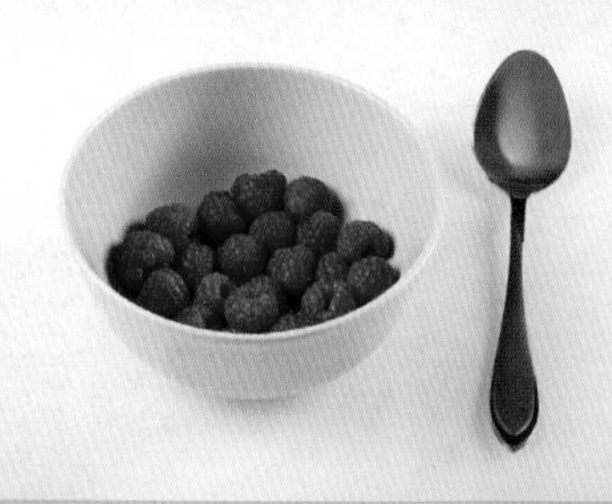

3g FIBRE	Weight: 80g	0g SAT FAT

7g CARBS	40 CALS	2g PROTEIN	1g FAT

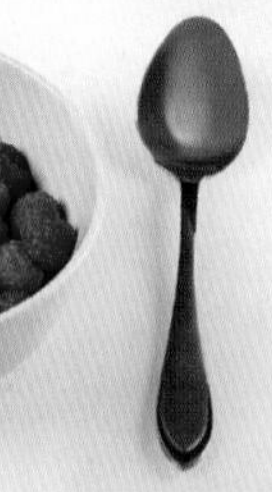

5g FIBRE	Weight: 160g	0g SAT FAT

Rhubarb (stewed)

9g CARBS	38 CALS	1g PROTEIN	0g FAT

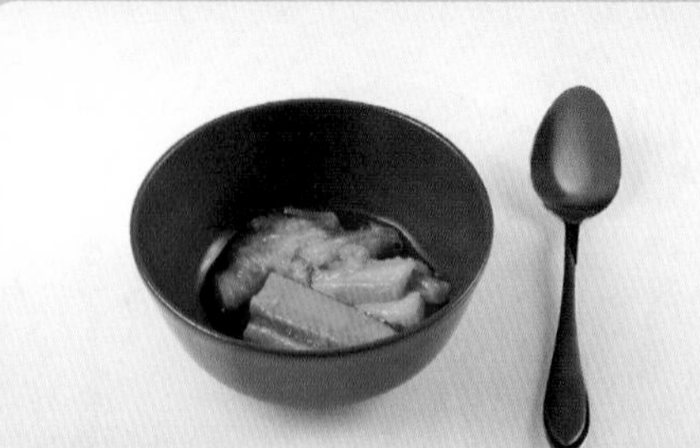

1g FIBRE	Weight: 80g	0g SAT FAT

18g CARBS	77 CALS	1g PROTEIN	0g FAT

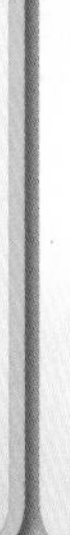

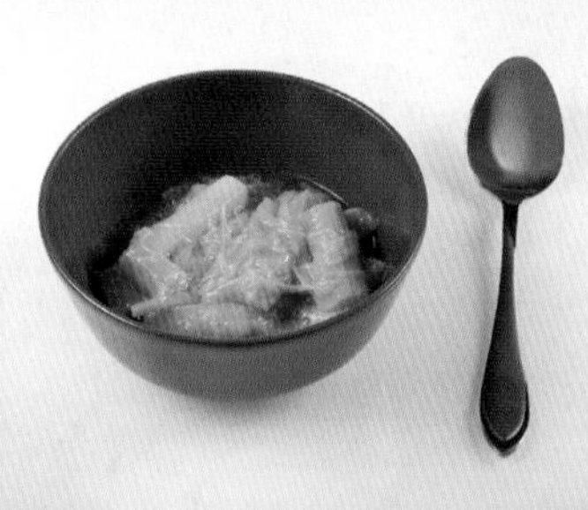

3g FIBRE	Weight: 160g	0g SAT FAT

37g CARBS	154 CALS	3g PROTEIN	0g FAT

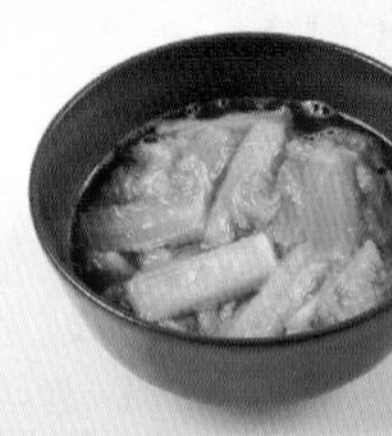

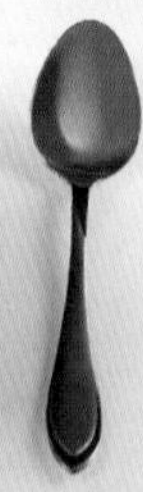

5g FIBRE	Weight: 320g	0g SAT FAT

Strawberries

5g CARBS	22 CALS	1g PROTEIN	0g FAT

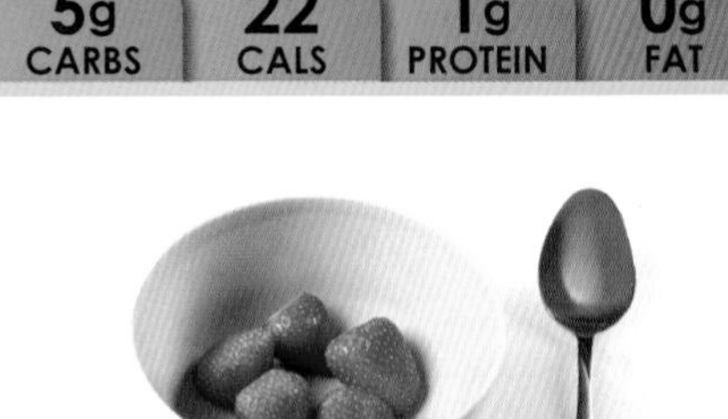

1g FIBRE	Weight: 80g	0g SAT FAT

8g CARBS	38 CALS	1g PROTEIN	0g FAT

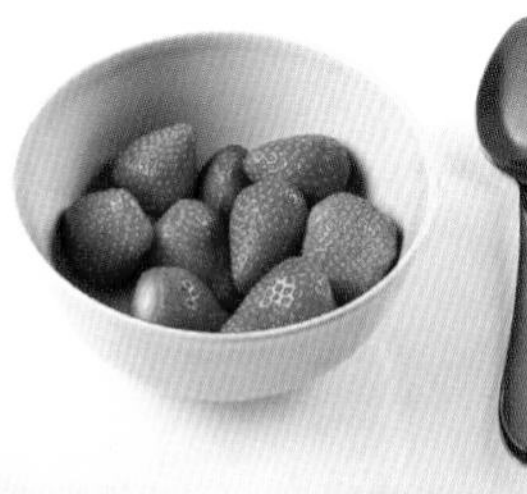

2g FIBRE	Weight: 140g	0g SAT FAT

17g CARBS	76 CALS	2g PROTEIN	0g FAT

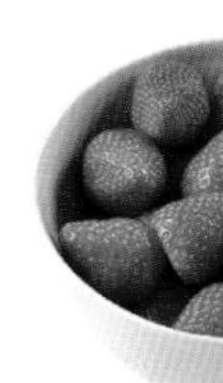

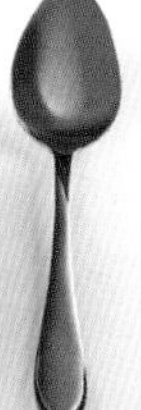

4g FIBRE	Weight: 280g	0g SAT FAT

Watermelon

6g CARBS	25 CALS	0g PROTEIN	0g FAT

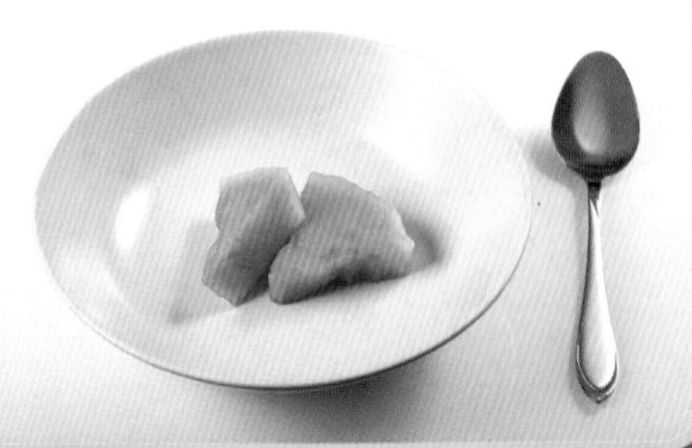

0g FIBRE	Weight: 80g	0g SAT FAT

10g CARBS	43 CALS	1g PROTEIN	0g FAT

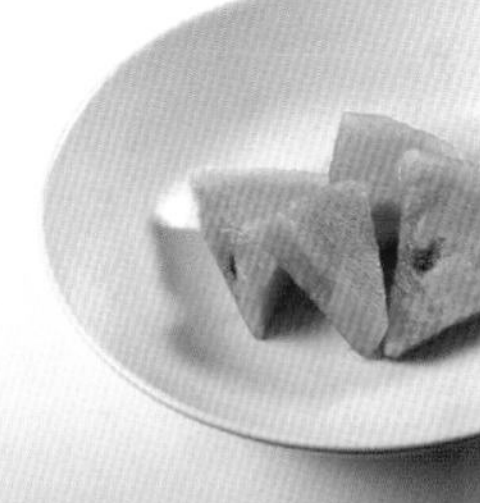

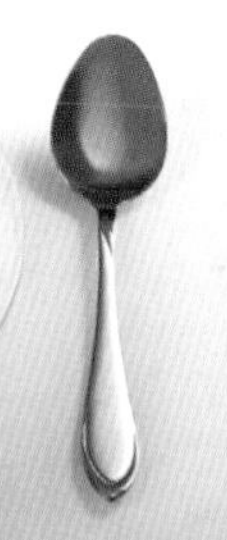

0g FIBRE	Weight: 140g	0g SAT FAT

20g CARBS	87 CALS	1g PROTEIN	1g FAT

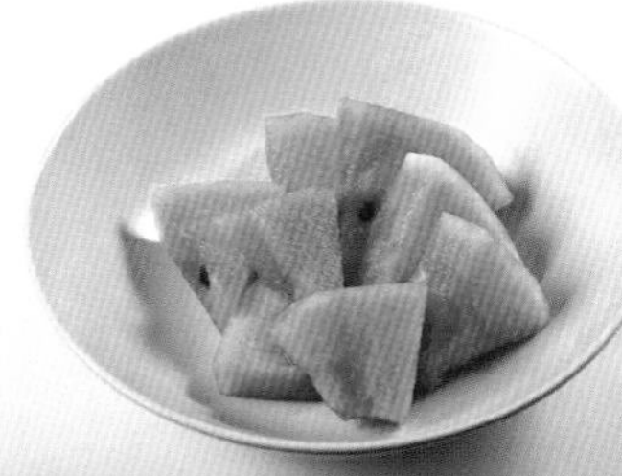

0g FIBRE	Weight: 280g	0g SAT FAT

Apple Rings

CARBS	CALS	PROTEIN	FAT	FIBRE	Weight	SAT FAT
9g	36	0g	0g	2g	Weight: 15g	0g
18g	71	1g	0g	4g	Weight: 30g	0g
36g	143	1g	0g	8g	Weight: 60g	0g

Apricots

13g CARBS | 56 CALS | 1g PROTEIN | 0g FAT

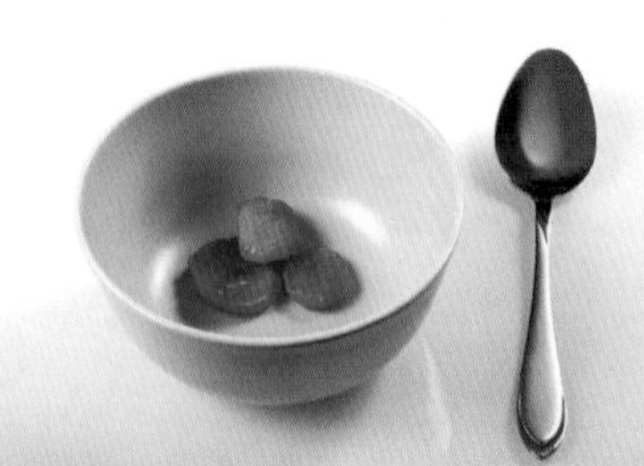

3g FIBRE | Weight: 30g | 0g SAT FAT

26g CARBS | 113 CALS | 3g PROTEIN | 0g FAT

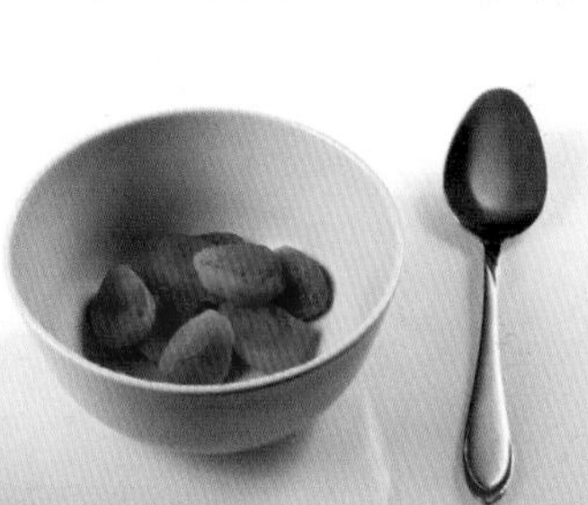

6g FIBRE | Weight: 60g | 0g SAT FAT

39g CARBS | 169 CALS | 4g PROTEIN | 1g FAT

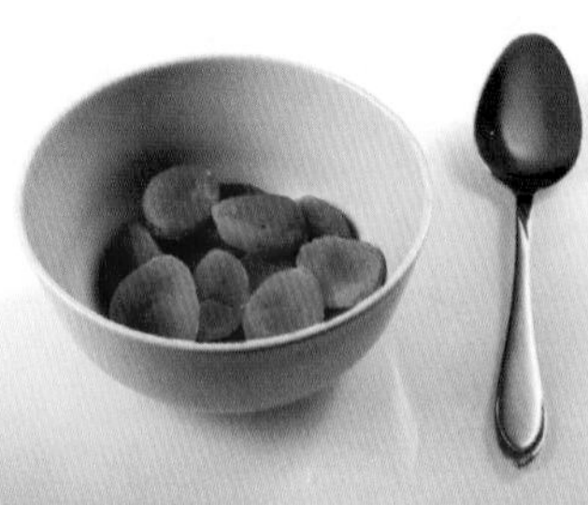

9g FIBRE | Weight: 90g | 0g SAT FAT

Banana Chips

CARBS	CALS	PROTEIN	FAT
17g	158	1g	9g

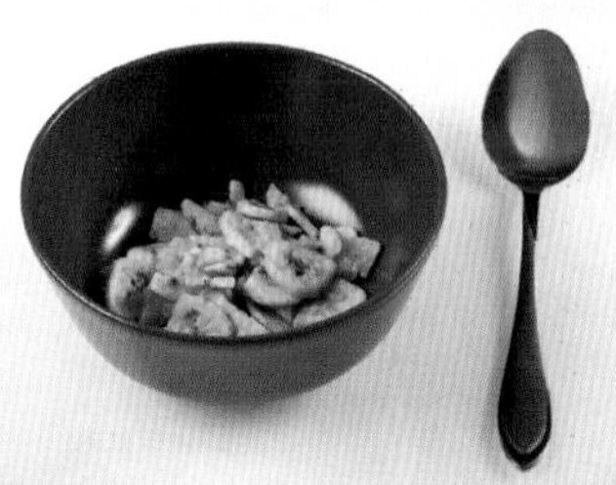

FIBRE	Weight	SAT FAT
1g	Weight: 30g	8g

CARBS	CALS	PROTEIN	FAT
35g	317	1g	19g

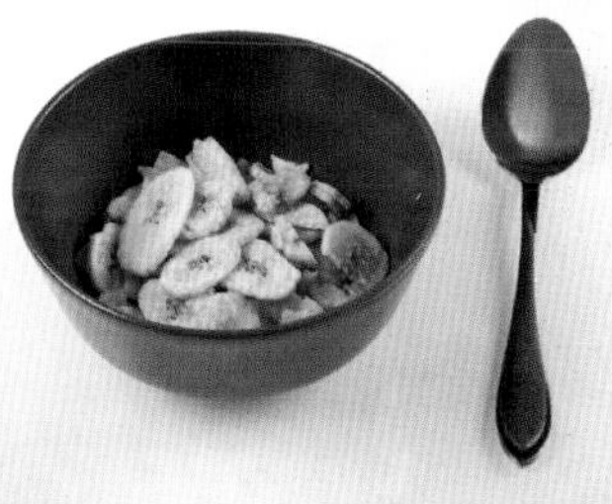

FIBRE	Weight	SAT FAT
2g	Weight: 60g	16g

CARBS	CALS	PROTEIN	FAT
52g	475	2g	28g

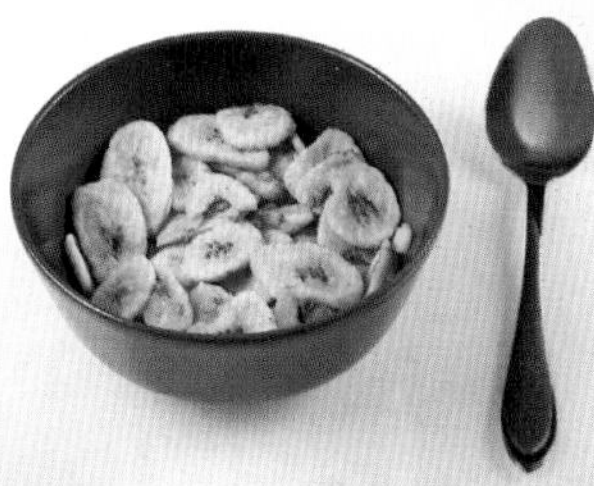

FIBRE	Weight	SAT FAT
3g	Weight: 90g	24g

Cranberries

CARBS	CALS	PROTEIN	FAT
25g	103	0g	0g

FIBRE	Weight	SAT FAT
2g	Weight: 30g	0g

CARBS	CALS	PROTEIN	FAT
49g	205	0g	1g

FIBRE	Weight	SAT FAT
3g	Weight: 60g	0g

CARBS	CALS	PROTEIN	FAT
74g	308	0g	1g

FIBRE	Weight	SAT FAT
5g	Weight: 90g	0g

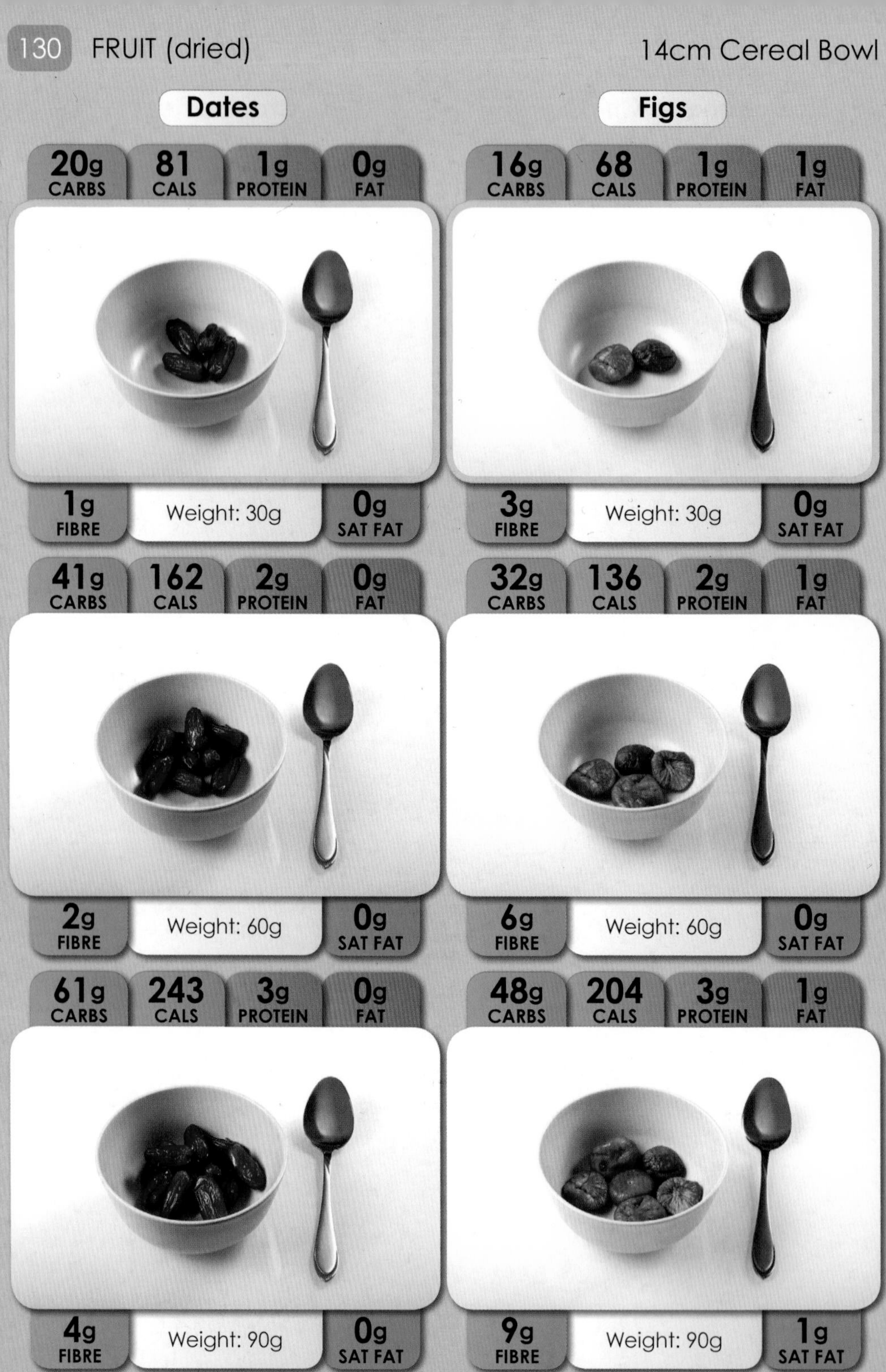
Dates
Figs
20g CARBS
81 CALS
1g PROTEIN
0g FAT
1g FIBRE
Weight: 30g
0g SAT FAT
16g CARBS
68 CALS
1g PROTEIN
1g FAT
3g FIBRE
Weight: 30g
0g SAT FAT
41g CARBS
162 CALS
2g PROTEIN
0g FAT
2g FIBRE
Weight: 60g
0g SAT FAT
32g CARBS
136 CALS
2g PROTEIN
1g FAT
6g FIBRE
Weight: 60g
0g SAT FAT
61g CARBS
243 CALS
3g PROTEIN
0g FAT
4g FIBRE
Weight: 90g
0g SAT FAT
48g CARBS
204 CALS
3g PROTEIN
1g FAT
9g FIBRE
Weight: 90g
1g SAT FAT

Pineapple

Weight	Carbs	Cals	Protein	Fat	Fibre	Sat Fat
30g	20g	83	1g	0g	3g	0g
60g	41g	166	2g	1g	7g	0g
90g	61g	248	2g	1g	10g	0g

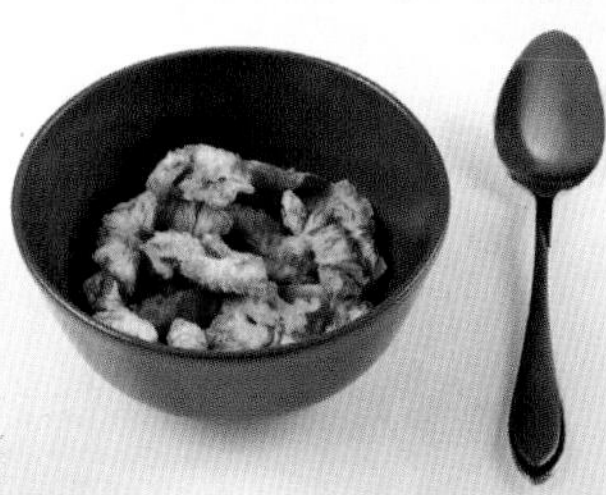

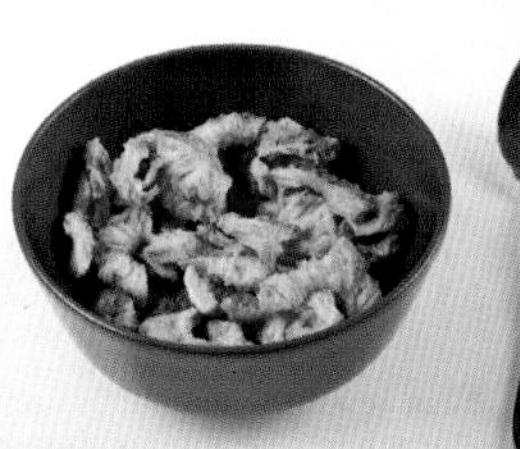

Prunes

Weight	Carbs	Cals	Protein	Fat	Fibre	Sat Fat
30g	10g	48	1g	0g	2g	0g
60g	21g	96	2g	0g	4g	0g
90g	31g	144	2g	0g	6g	0g

14cm Cereal Bowl

Raisins

8g CARBS	32 CALS	0g PROTEIN	0g FAT

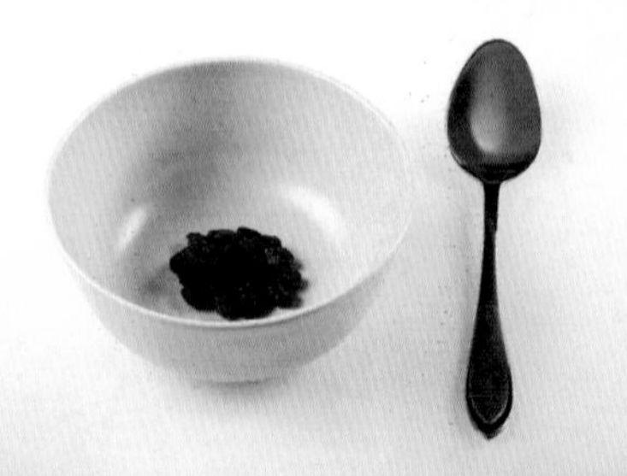

0g FIBRE	Weight: 11g (tablespoon)	0g SAT FAT

21g CARBS	87 CALS	1g PROTEIN	0g FAT

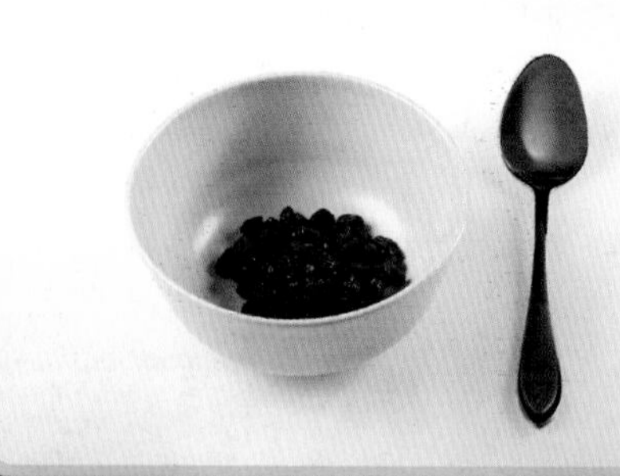

1g FIBRE	Weight: 30g	0g SAT FAT

41g CARBS	174 CALS	1g PROTEIN	0g FAT

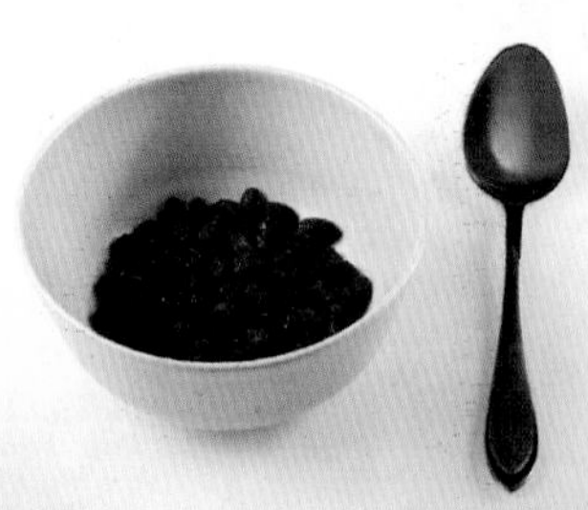

1g FIBRE	Weight: 60g	0g SAT FAT

Sultanas

9g CARBS	38 CALS	0g PROTEIN	0g FAT

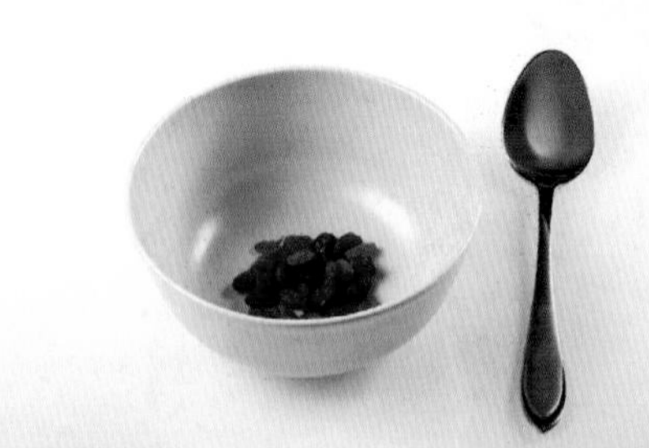

0g FIBRE	Weight: 13g (tablespoon)	0g SAT FAT

21g CARBS	88 CALS	1g PROTEIN	0g FAT

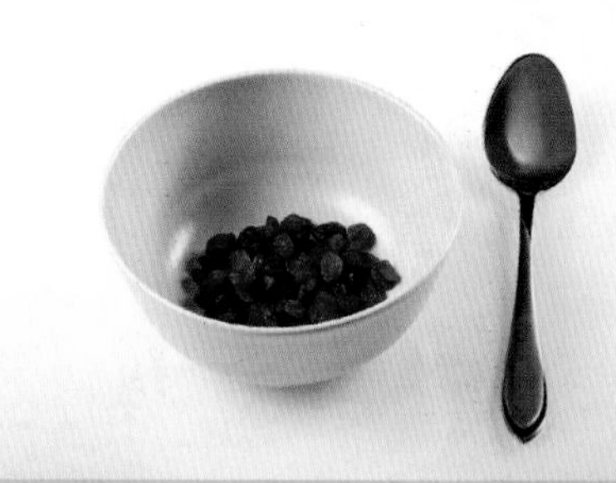

1g FIBRE	Weight: 30g	0g SAT FAT

41g CARBS	176 CALS	2g PROTEIN	0g FAT

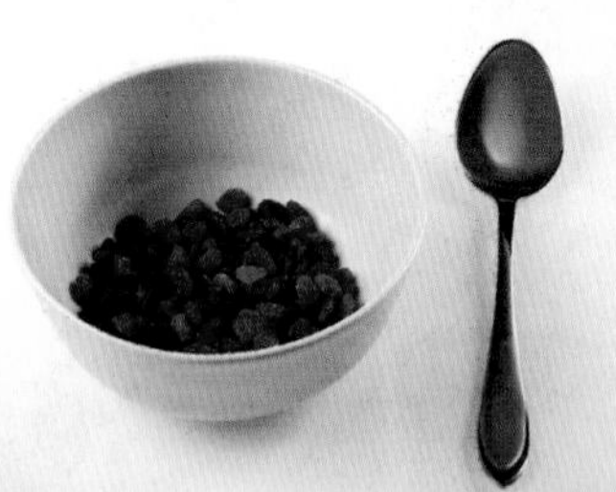

1g FIBRE	Weight: 60g	0g SAT FAT

Fibre Flakes GF

CARBS	CALS	PROTEIN	FAT
11g	53	1g	0g

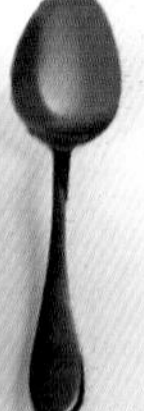

FIBRE	Weight	SAT FAT
2g	Weight: 15g	0g

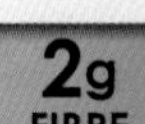

CARBS	CALS	PROTEIN	FAT
21g	106	2g	1g

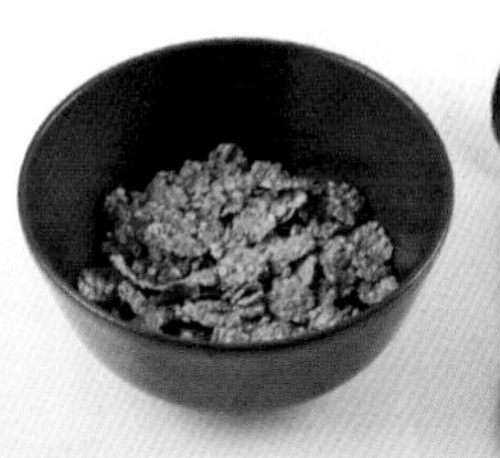
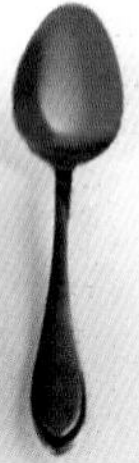

FIBRE	Weight	SAT FAT
5g	Weight: 30g	0g

CARBS	CALS	PROTEIN	FAT
42g	212	4g	1g

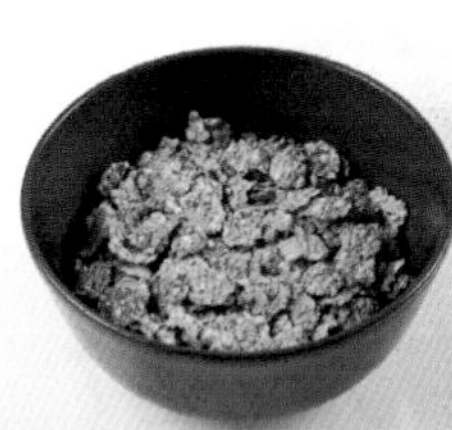
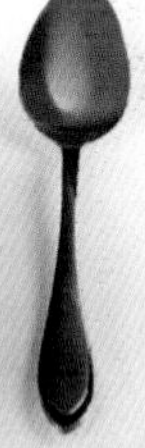

FIBRE	Weight	SAT FAT
9g	Weight: 60g	0g

Special Flakes GF

CARBS	CALS	PROTEIN	FAT
12g	56	1g	0g

FIBRE	Weight	SAT FAT
1g	Weight: 15g	0g

CARBS	CALS	PROTEIN	FAT
24g	111	2g	1g

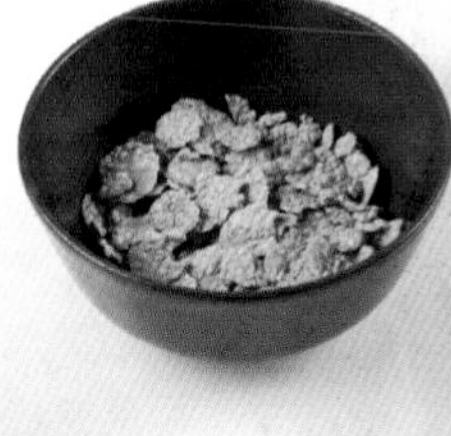
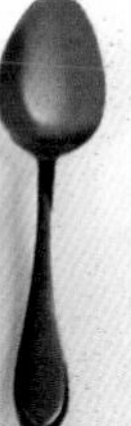

FIBRE	Weight	SAT FAT
1g	Weight: 30g	0g

CARBS	CALS	PROTEIN	FAT
48g	223	5g	1g

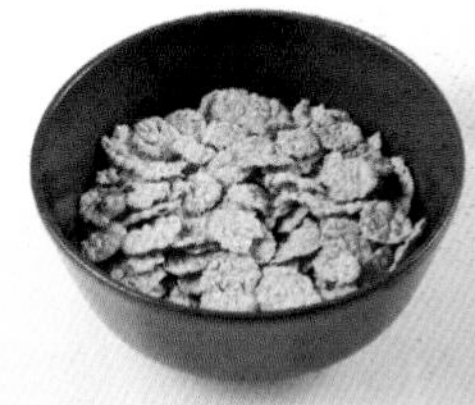
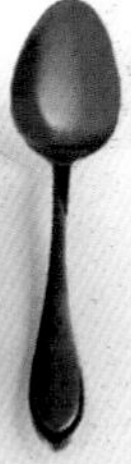

FIBRE	Weight	SAT FAT
3g	Weight: 60g	0g

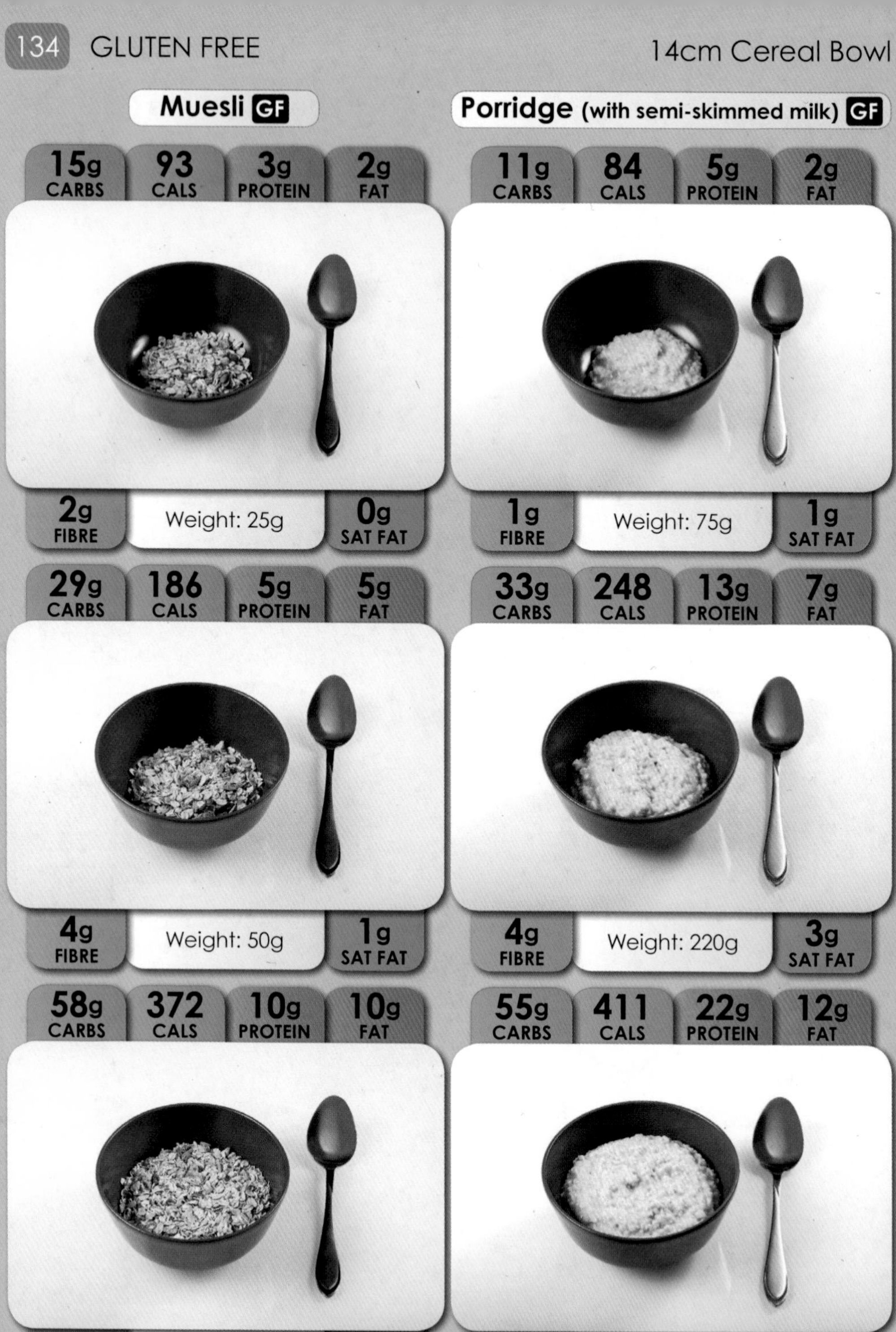
Muesli GF
15g CARBS
93 CALS
3g PROTEIN
2g FAT
2g FIBRE
Weight: 25g
0g SAT FAT
29g CARBS
186 CALS
5g PROTEIN
5g FAT
4g FIBRE
Weight: 50g
1g SAT FAT
58g CARBS
372 CALS
10g PROTEIN
10g FAT
8g FIBRE
Weight: 100g
1g SAT FAT
Porridge (with semi-skimmed milk) GF
11g CARBS
84 CALS
5g PROTEIN
2g FAT
1g FIBRE
Weight: 75g
1g SAT FAT
33g CARBS
248 CALS
13g PROTEIN
7g FAT
4g FIBRE
Weight: 220g
3g SAT FAT
55g CARBS
411 CALS
22g PROTEIN
12g FAT
6g FIBRE
Weight: 365g
6g SAT FAT

Brown Bread (home baked) GF

9g CARBS	60 CALS	1g PROTEIN	2g FAT

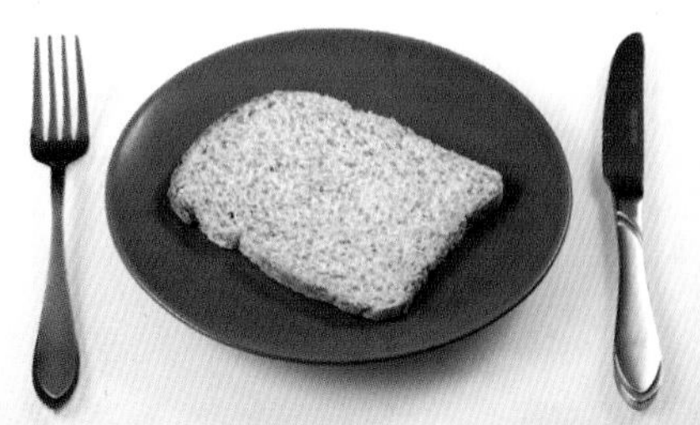

1g FIBRE	Weight: 22g (thin slice)	0g SAT FAT

14g CARBS	90 CALS	1g PROTEIN	3g FAT

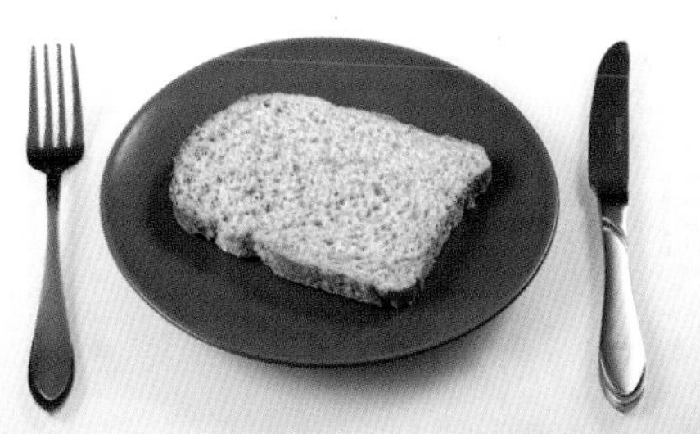

2g FIBRE	Weight: 33g (medium slice)	0g SAT FAT

19g CARBS	120 CALS	1g PROTEIN	4g FAT

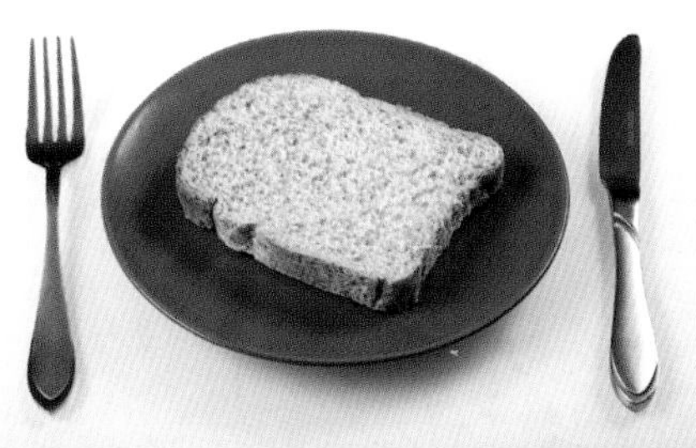

3g FIBRE	Weight: 44g (thick slice)	0g SAT FAT

White Bread (home baked) GF

10g CARBS	64 CALS	1g PROTEIN	2g FAT

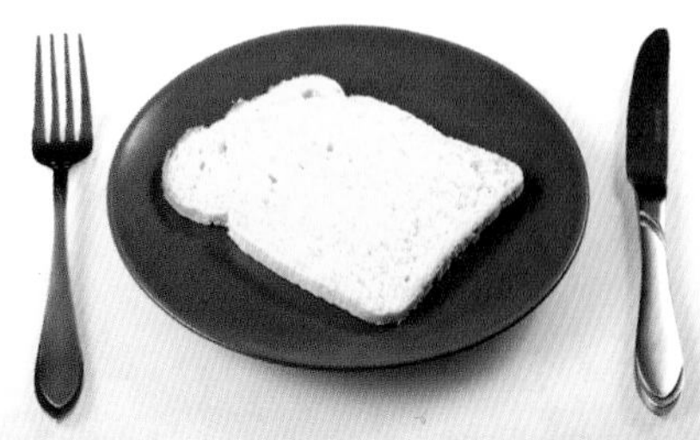

1g FIBRE	Weight: 22g (thin slice)	0g SAT FAT

15g CARBS	96 CALS	1g PROTEIN	3g FAT

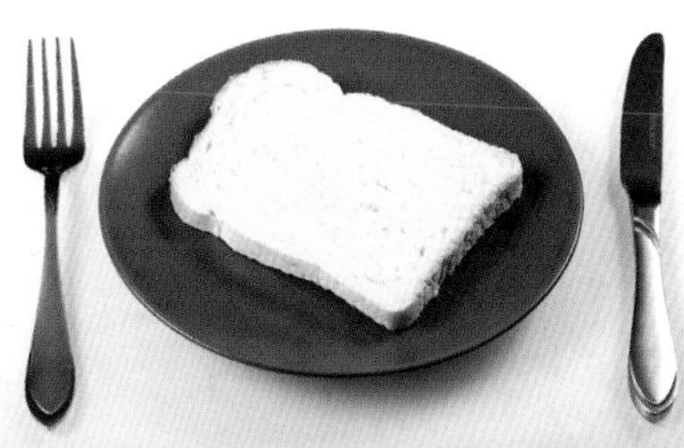

1g FIBRE	Weight: 33g (medium slice)	0g SAT FAT

20g CARBS	128 CALS	1g PROTEIN	4g FAT

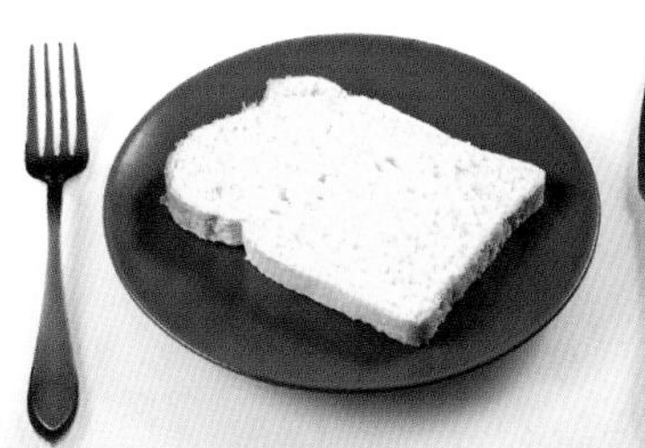

2g FIBRE	Weight: 44g (thick slice)	0g SAT FAT

Brown Bread (sliced) GF

12g CARBS	82 CALS	1g PROTEIN	3g FAT
2g FIBRE	Weight: 31g	0g SAT FAT	

White Bread (sliced) GF

13g CARBS	77 CALS	1g PROTEIN	2g FAT
2g FIBRE	Weight: 30g	0g SAT FAT	

Fibre Roll GF

32g CARBS	212 CALS	4g PROTEIN	7g FAT
8g FIBRE	Weight: 85g	2g SAT FAT	

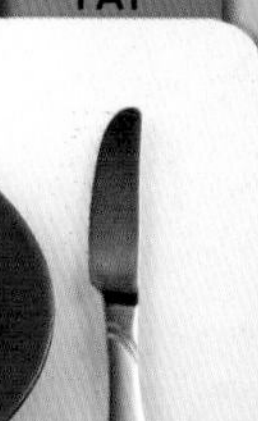

White Roll GF

38g CARBS	220 CALS	3g PROTEIN	6g FAT
4g FIBRE	Weight: 85g	1g SAT FAT	

Part Baked Roll (white) GF

38g CARBS	195 CALS	3g PROTEIN	3g FAT
5g FIBRE	Weight: 85g	1g SAT FAT	

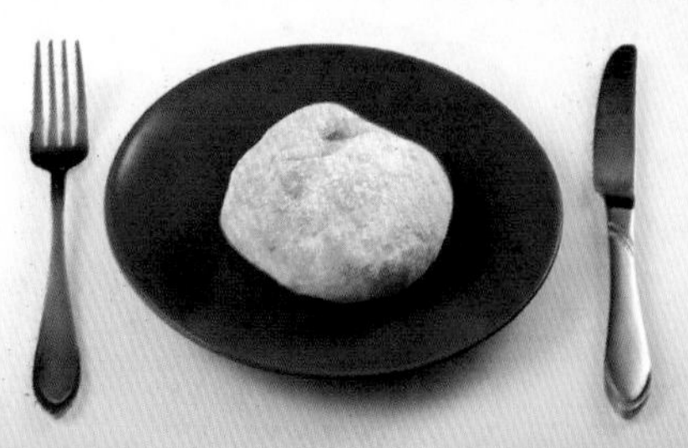

Part Baked Roll (brown) GF

36g CARBS	223 CALS	4g PROTEIN	6g FAT
6g FIBRE	Weight: 85g	1g SAT FAT	

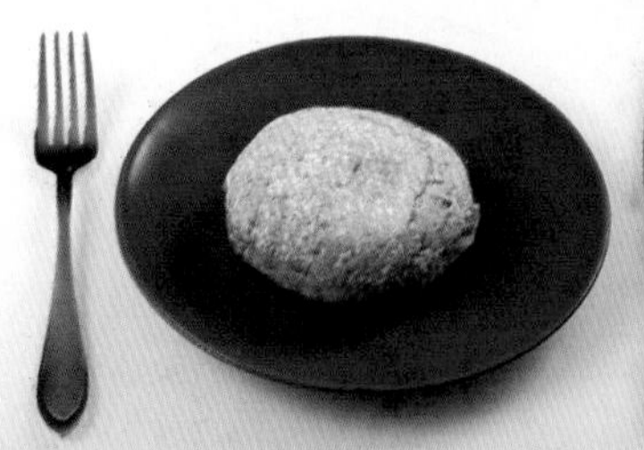

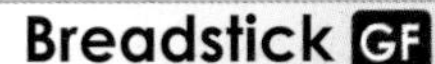

Breadstick GF

CARBS	CALS	PROTEIN	FAT
2g	10	0g	0g

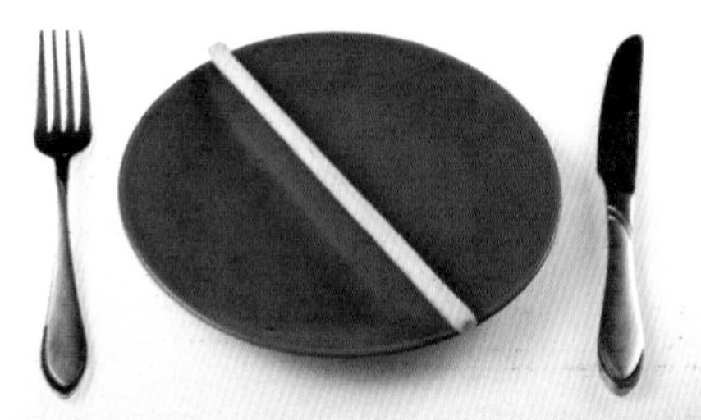

FIBRE	Weight	SAT FAT
0g	Weight: 5g	0g

Crispbread GF

CARBS	CALS	PROTEIN	FAT
10g	48	1g	0g

FIBRE	Weight	SAT FAT
1g	Weight: 14g	0g

Naan Bread GF

CARBS	CALS	PROTEIN	FAT
37g	220	4g	6g

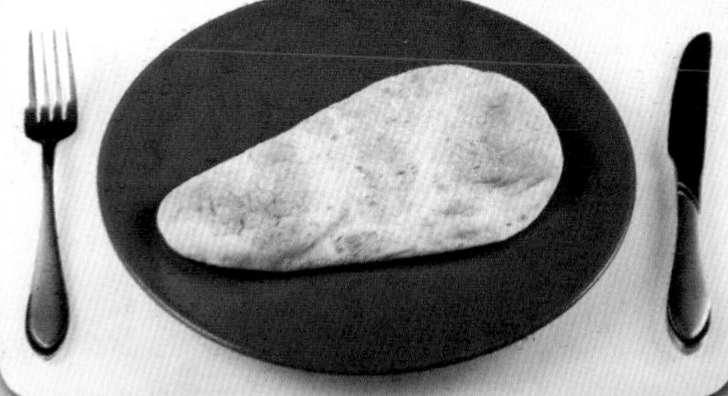

FIBRE	Weight	SAT FAT
3g	Weight: 84g	0g

Pitta Bread GF

CARBS	CALS	PROTEIN	FAT
33g	175	3g	3g

FIBRE	Weight	SAT FAT
3g	Weight: 66g	0g

Pizza Base GF

CARBS	CALS	PROTEIN	FAT
75g	367	5g	5g

FIBRE	Weight	SAT FAT
5g	Weight: 140g	1g

Rice Cake GF

CARBS	CALS	PROTEIN	FAT
6g	31	1g	0g

FIBRE	Weight	SAT FAT
0g	Weight: 8g	0g

Chocolate Chip Cookie GF

12g CARBS	95 CALS	1g PROTEIN	5g FAT

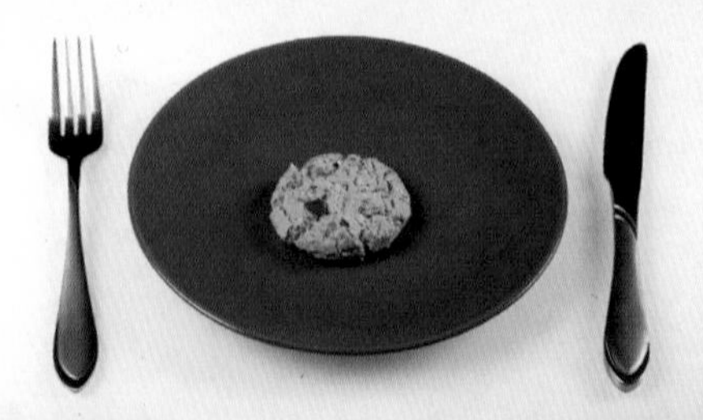

1g FIBRE	Weight: 19g	3g SAT FAT

Chocolate Digestive GF

8g CARBS	60 CALS	1g PROTEIN	3g FAT

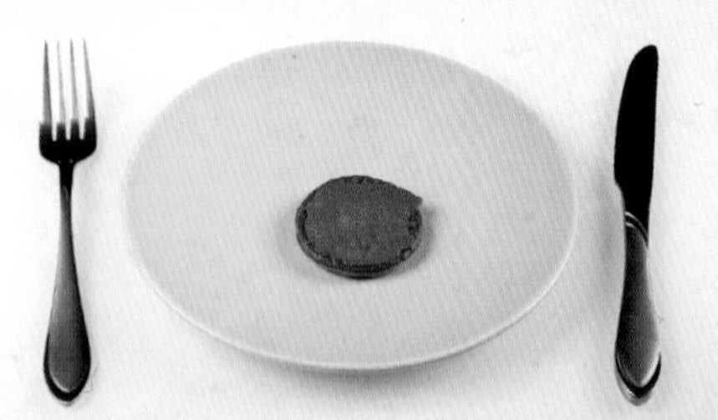

1g FIBRE	Weight: 12g	1g SAT FAT

Digestive GF

5g CARBS	38 CALS	0g PROTEIN	2g FAT

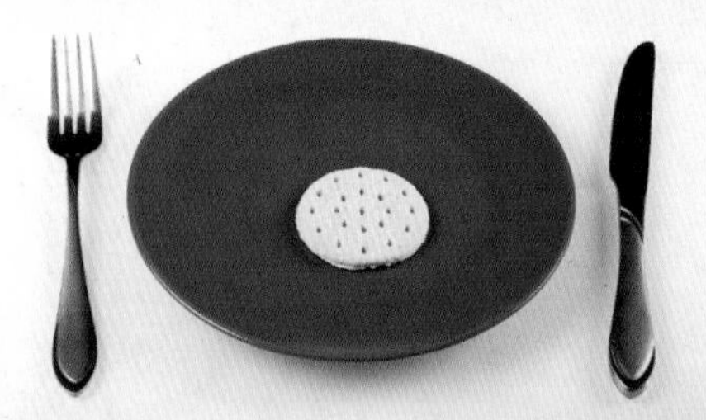

0g FIBRE	Weight: 8g	1g SAT FAT

Savoury Biscuit GF

5g CARBS	38 CALS	1g PROTEIN	2g FAT

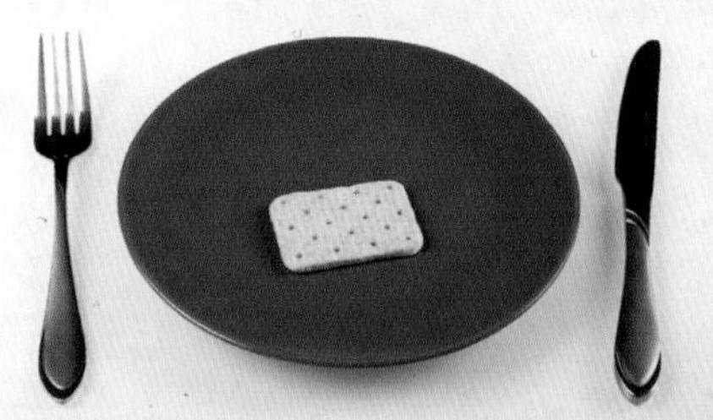

0g FIBRE	Weight: 8g	1g SAT FAT

Sweet Biscuit GF

8g CARBS	60 CALS	1g PROTEIN	3g FAT

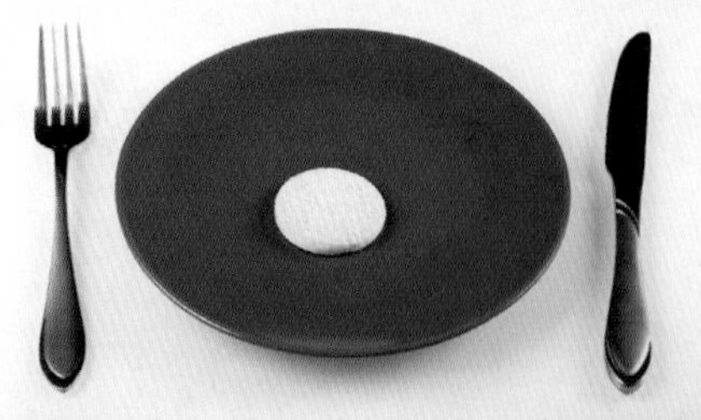

0g FIBRE	Weight: 12g	1g SAT FAT

Tea Biscuit GF

5g CARBS	38 CALS	0g PROTEIN	2g FAT

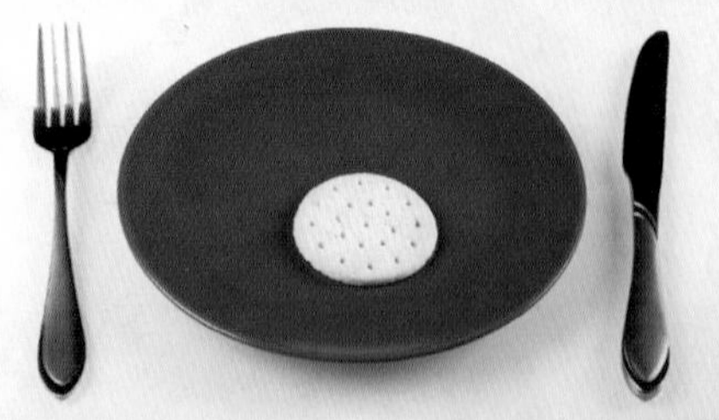

0g FIBRE	Weight: 8g	1g SAT FAT

Pasta Twists GF

10g CARBS | 47 CALS | 1g PROTEIN | 0g FAT

0g FIBRE | Weight: 30g | 0g SAT FAT

51g CARBS | 228 CALS | 4g PROTEIN | 1g FAT

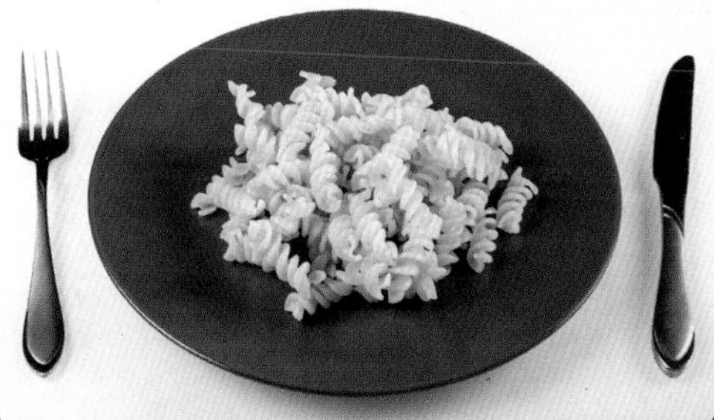

1g FIBRE | Weight: 145g | 0g SAT FAT

94g CARBS | 408 CALS | 8g PROTEIN | 2g FAT

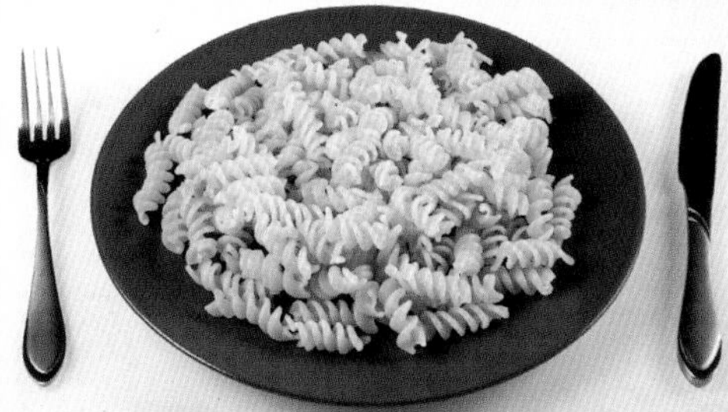

1g FIBRE | Weight: 260g | 0g SAT FAT

Penne (fibre) GF

10g CARBS | 47 CALS | 1g PROTEIN | 0g FAT

1g FIBRE | Weight: 30g | 0g SAT FAT

51g CARBS | 232 CALS | 4g PROTEIN | 1g FAT

5g FIBRE | Weight: 148g | 0g SAT FAT

91g CARBS | 416 CALS | 8g PROTEIN | 2g FAT

8g FIBRE | Weight: 265g | 0g SAT FAT

Spaghetti GF

11g	52	1g	0g
CARBS	CALS	PROTEIN	FAT

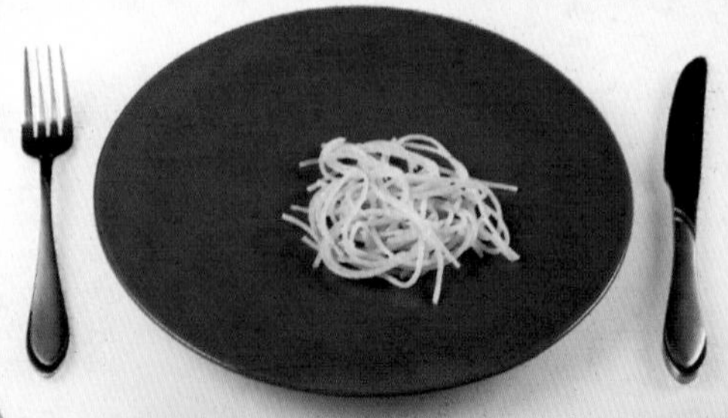

0g FIBRE	Weight: 33g	0g SAT FAT

54g	247	5g	1g
CARBS	CALS	PROTEIN	FAT

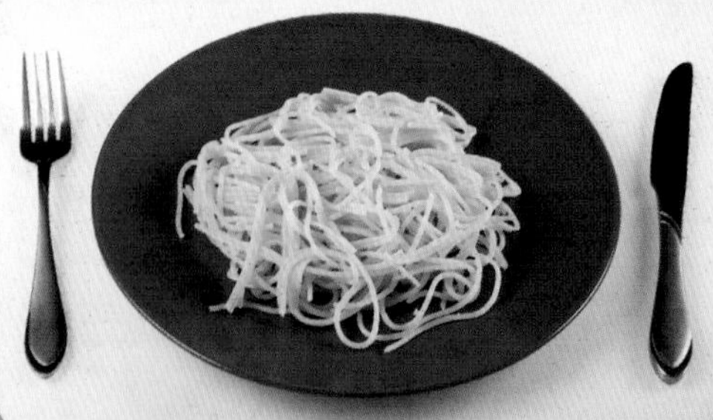

1g FIBRE	Weight: 158g	0g SAT FAT

98g	446	9g	2g
CARBS	CALS	PROTEIN	FAT

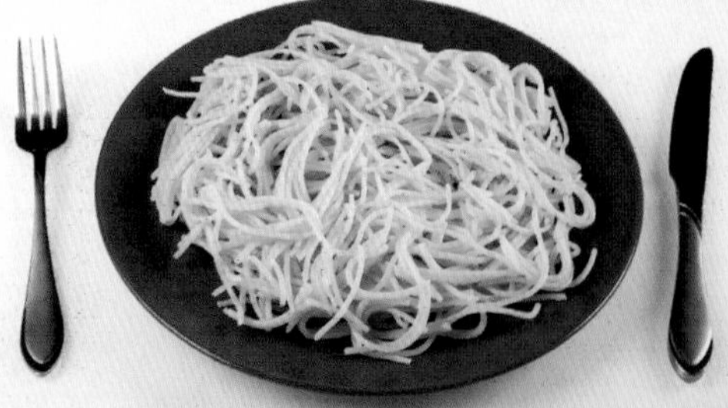

1g FIBRE	Weight: 285g	0g SAT FAT

Tagliatelle GF

11g	50	1g	1g
CARBS	CALS	PROTEIN	FAT

0g FIBRE	Weight: 30g	0g SAT FAT

53g	249	3g	3g
CARBS	CALS	PROTEIN	FAT

1g FIBRE	Weight: 150g	1g SAT FAT

96g	449	6g	5g
CARBS	CALS	PROTEIN	FAT

1g FIBRE	Weight: 270g	2g SAT FAT

Beans on Toast (with margarine)

Portion	Carbs	Cals	Protein	Fat	Fibre	Sat Fat
22g toast, 65g beans, 5g marg	22g	151	5g	4g	4g	1g
22g toast, 130g beans, 5g marg	32g	205	9g	5g	7g	1g
22g toast, 195g beans, 5g marg	42g	260	12g	5g	10g	1g
44g toast, 195g beans, 10g marg	55g	356	14g	10g	11g	2g
44g toast, 293g beans, 10g marg	70g	438	19g	11g	16g	2g
44g toast, 390g beans, 10g marg	85g	520	24g	11g	20g	2g

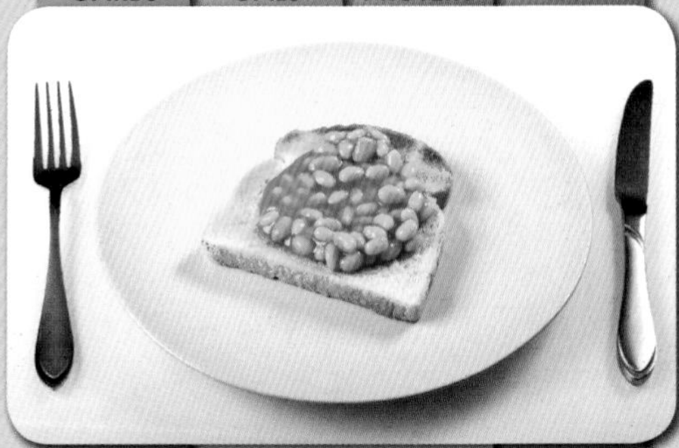

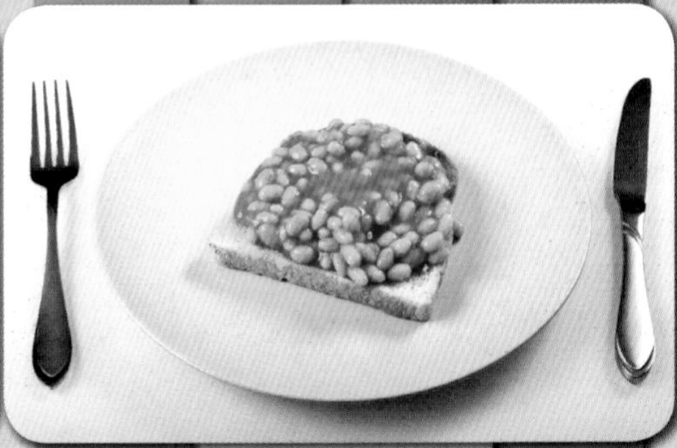

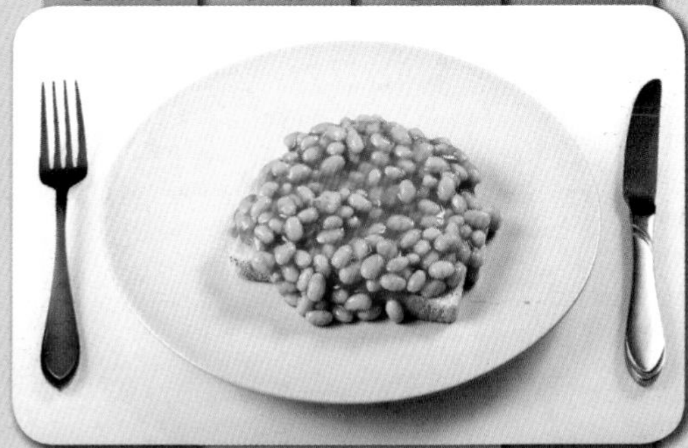

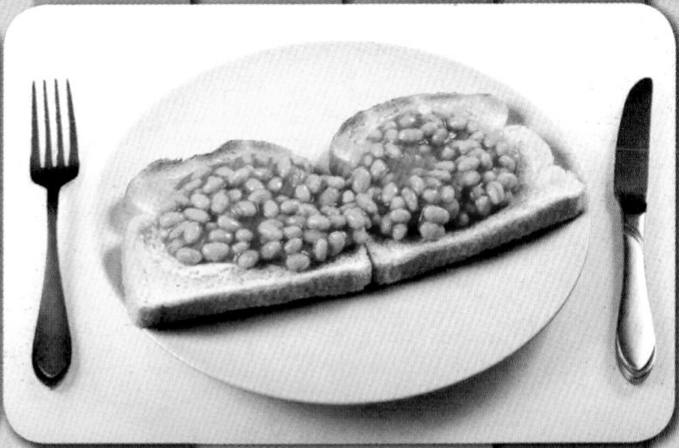

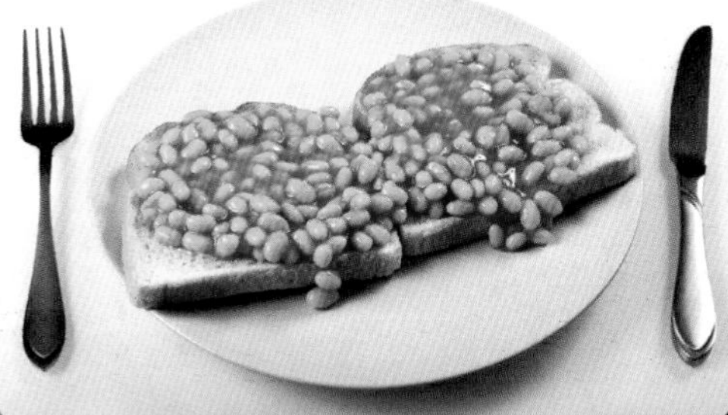

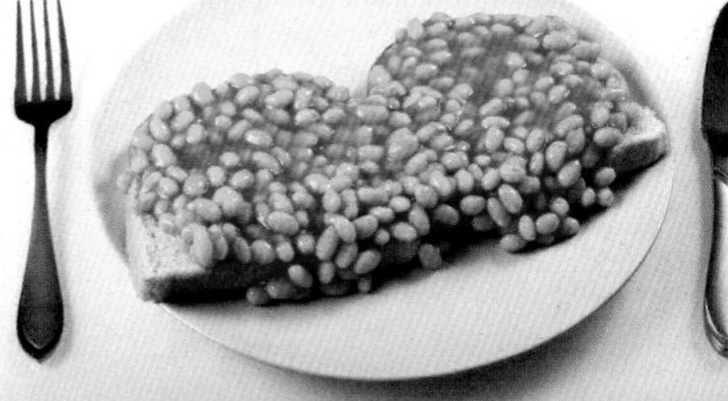

Chicken Goujons, Potato Smiles & Peas

CARBS	CALS	PROTEIN	FAT
18g	172	9g	7g

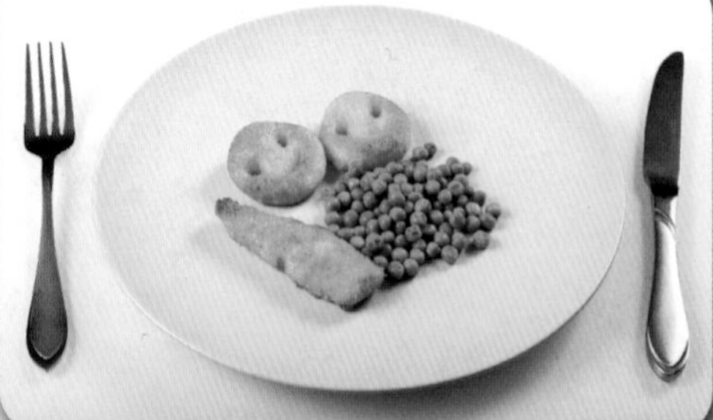

FIBRE		SAT FAT
3g	30g chicken, 34g smiles, 25g peas	1g

CARBS	CALS	PROTEIN	FAT
38g	346	17g	14g

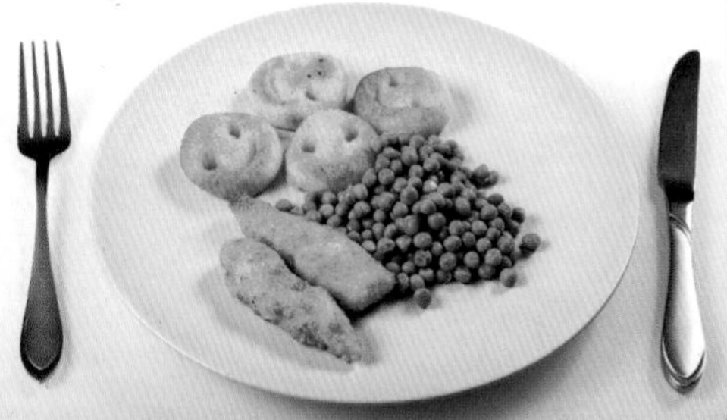

FIBRE		SAT FAT
6g	60g chicken, 68g smiles, 50g peas	3g

CARBS	CALS	PROTEIN	FAT
56g	518	25g	23g

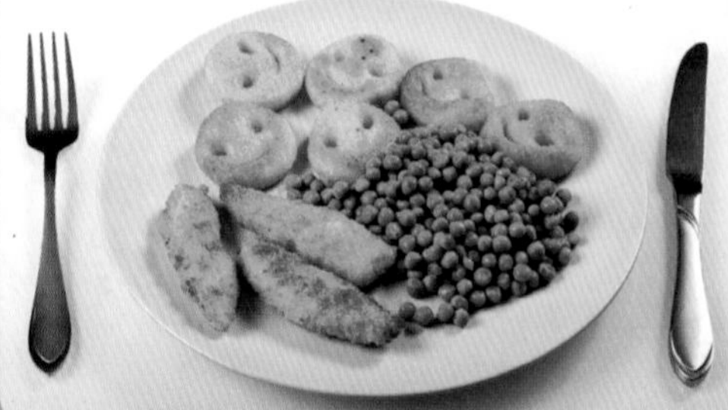

FIBRE		SAT FAT
8g	90g chicken, 102g smiles, 75g peas	5g

Fish Fingers, Chips & Beans

CARBS	CALS	PROTEIN	FAT
30g	185	7g	5g

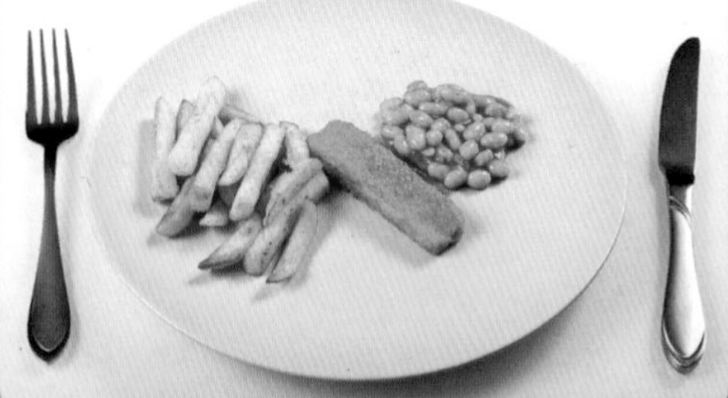

FIBRE		SAT FAT
4g	20g fish, 66g chips, 45g beans	2g

CARBS	CALS	PROTEIN	FAT
51g	316	14g	9g

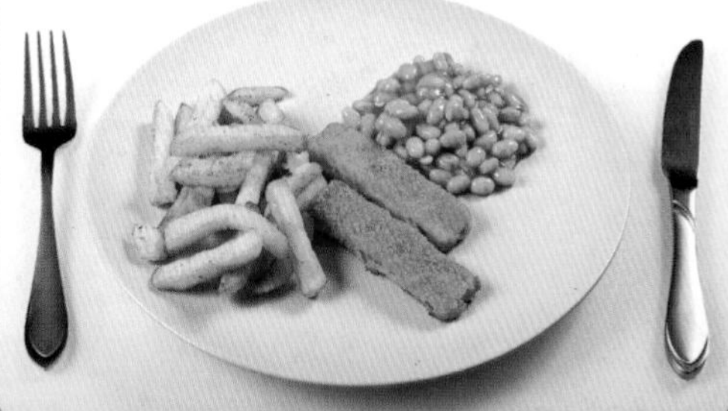

FIBRE		SAT FAT
7g	40g fish, 99g chips, 90g beans	3g

CARBS	CALS	PROTEIN	FAT
70g	444	20g	11g

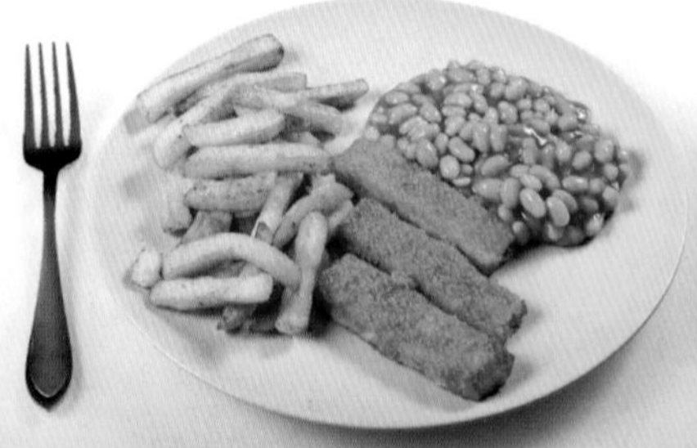

FIBRE		SAT FAT
12g	60g fish, 130g chips, 135g beans	4g

Chilli con Carne with White Rice

15g CARBS | **137** CALS | **8g** PROTEIN | **5g** FAT

2g FIBRE | 90g chilli, 32g rice | **2g** SAT FAT

40g CARBS | **307** CALS | **15g** PROTEIN | **10g** FAT

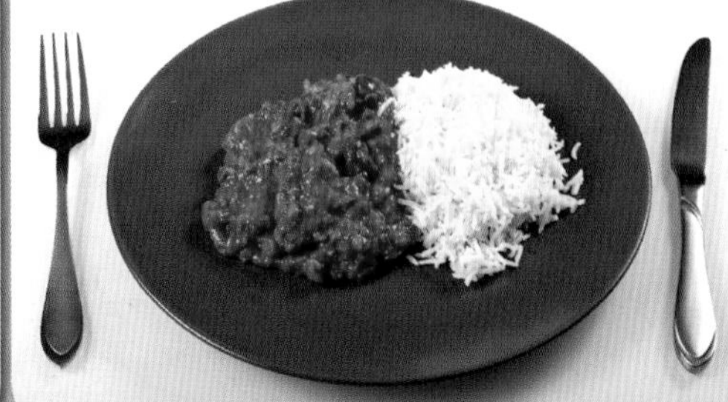

4g FIBRE | 170g chilli, 96g rice | **4g** SAT FAT

65g CARBS | **483** CALS | **23g** PROTEIN | **16g** FAT

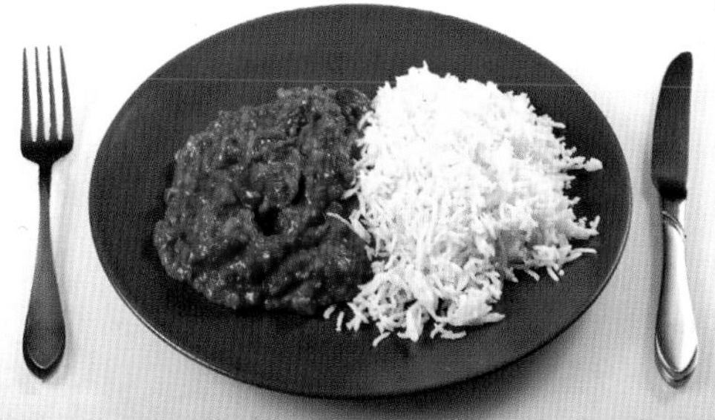

5g FIBRE | 250g chilli, 163g rice | **6g** SAT FAT

91g CARBS | **661** CALS | **32g** PROTEIN | **22g** FAT

7g FIBRE | 340g chilli, 225g rice | **8g** SAT FAT

116g CARBS | **843** CALS | **41g** PROTEIN | **28g** FAT

9g FIBRE | 430g chilli, 290g rice | **10g** SAT FAT

141g CARBS | **1015** CALS | **48g** PROTEIN | **33g** FAT

11g FIBRE | 510g chilli, 355g rice | **12g** SAT FAT

Corned Beef Hash

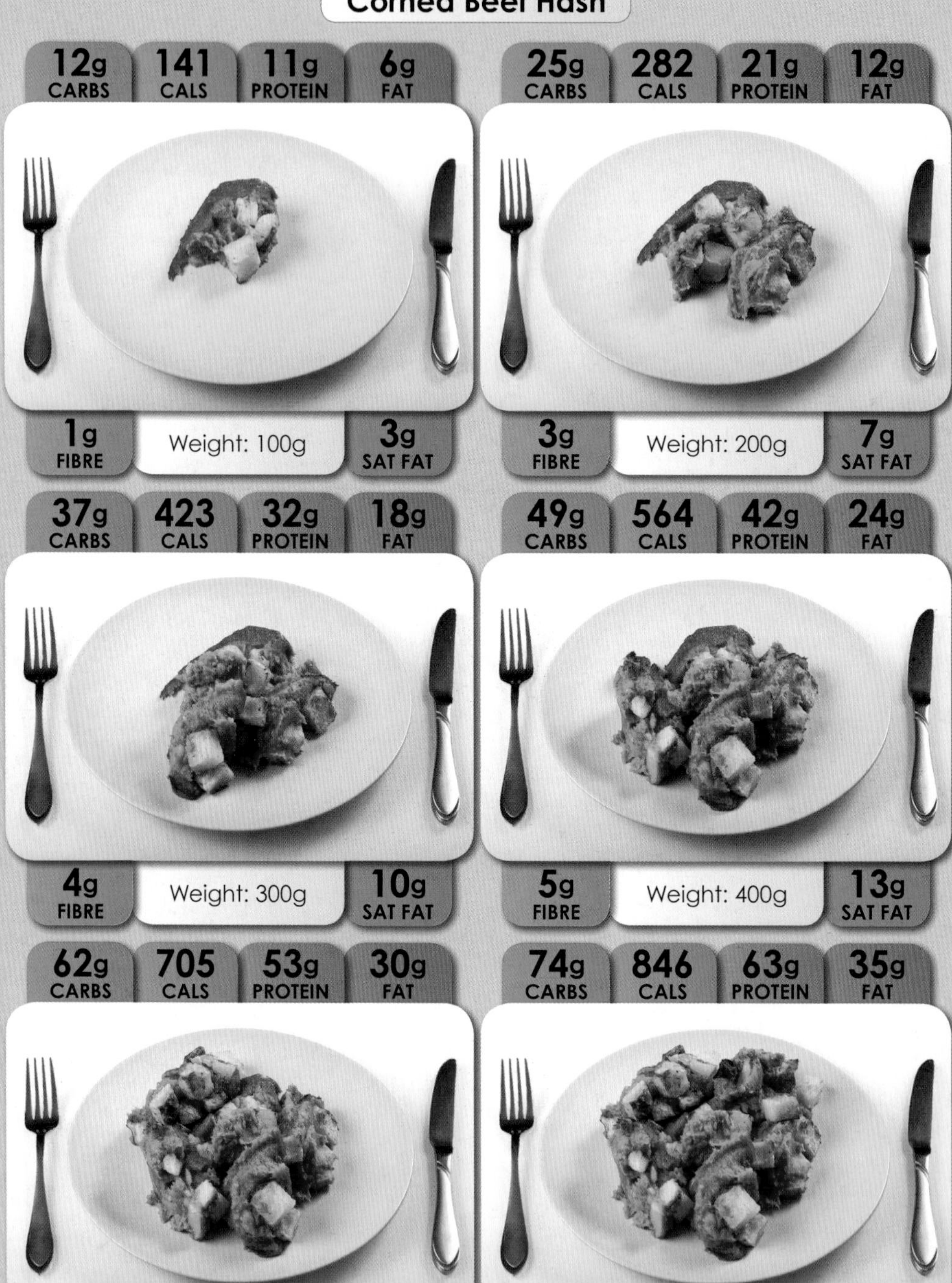

Weight	Carbs	Cals	Protein	Fat	Fibre	Sat Fat
Weight: 100g	12g	141	11g	6g	1g	3g
Weight: 200g	25g	282	21g	12g	3g	7g
Weight: 300g	37g	423	32g	18g	4g	10g
Weight: 400g	49g	564	42g	24g	5g	13g
Weight: 500g	62g	705	53g	30g	7g	17g
Weight: 600g	74g	846	63g	35g	8g	20g

Curry, Chicken (with White Rice)

Carbs	Cals	Protein	Fat	Fibre	Portion	Sat Fat
11g	146	11g	6g	0g	105g curry, 31g rice	2g
35g	390	29g	16g	1g	260g curry, 98g rice	4g
56g	579	41g	23g	2g	365g curry, 161g rice	5g
80g	809	57g	32g	2g	505g curry, 228g rice	7g
101g	1012	70g	39g	3g	625g curry, 290g rice	9g
125g	1266	88g	49g	3g	790g curry, 357g rice	12g

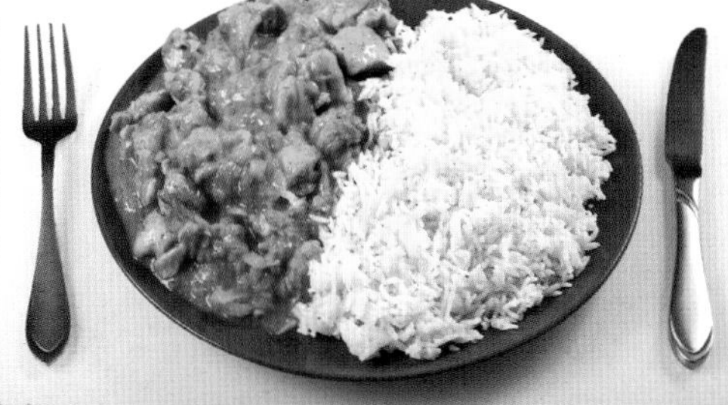

Curry, Lentil (with Brown Rice)

Portion	Carbs	Cals	Protein	Fat	Fibre	Sat Fat
95g curry, 30g rice	20g	179	5g	9g	3g	5g
185g curry, 95g rice	49g	400	11g	19g	6g	10g
280g curry, 157g rice	79g	624	17g	29g	10g	15g
380g curry, 219g rice	110g	856	23g	38g	13g	21g
475g curry, 281g rice	140g	1080	29g	49g	17g	26g
570g curry, 344g rice	170g	1306	35g	59g	20g	31g

Curry, Vegetable & Potato (with White Rice)

CARBS	CALS	PROTEIN	FAT
20g	122	3g	4g

FIBRE	Portion	SAT FAT
2g	90g curry, 32g rice	1g

CARBS	CALS	PROTEIN	FAT
49g	286	6g	8g

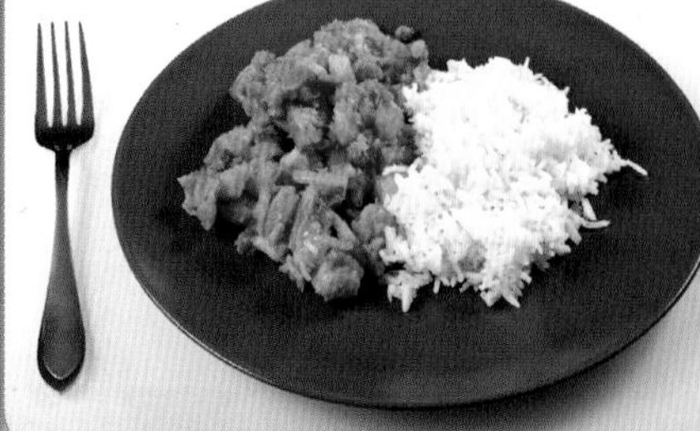

FIBRE	Portion	SAT FAT
4g	175g curry, 97g rice	1g

CARBS	CALS	PROTEIN	FAT
79g	451	9g	13g

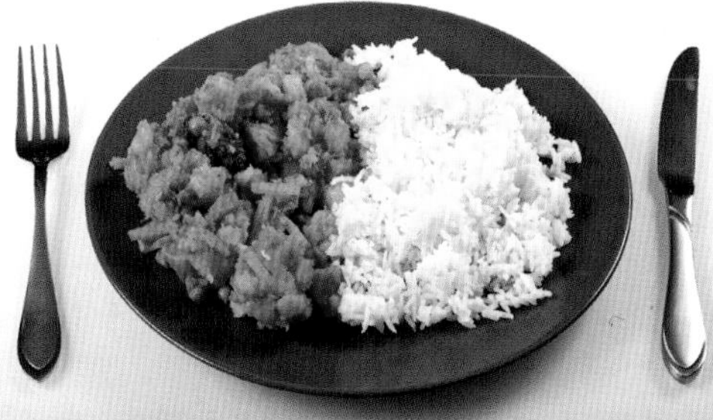

FIBRE	Portion	SAT FAT
5g	260g curry, 163g rice	2g

CARBS	CALS	PROTEIN	FAT
109g	608	13g	17g

FIBRE	Portion	SAT FAT
7g	350g curry, 227g rice	3g

CARBS	CALS	PROTEIN	FAT
138g	784	16g	22g

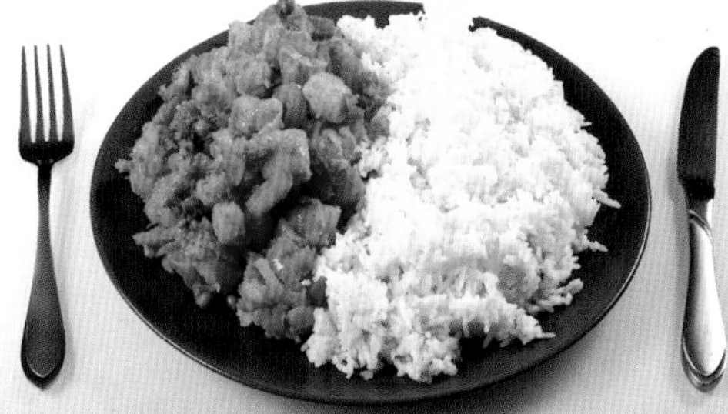

FIBRE	Portion	SAT FAT
9g	440g curry, 291g rice	3g

CARBS	CALS	PROTEIN	FAT
168g	951	20g	26g

FIBRE	Portion	SAT FAT
11g	530g curry, 355g rice	4g

Fish Stew with Jollof Rice

CARBS	CALS	PROTEIN	FAT	FIBRE	SAT FAT	Portion
46g	490	20g	26g	4g	9g	55g fish, 145g rice, 55g veg
96g	1024	42g	55g	9g	20g	115g fish, 303g rice, 115g veg

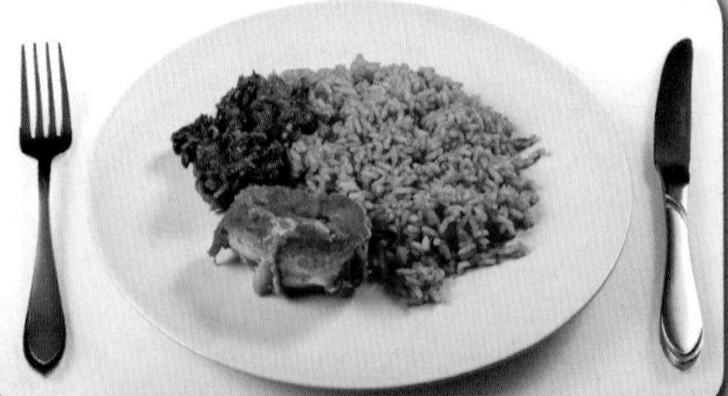

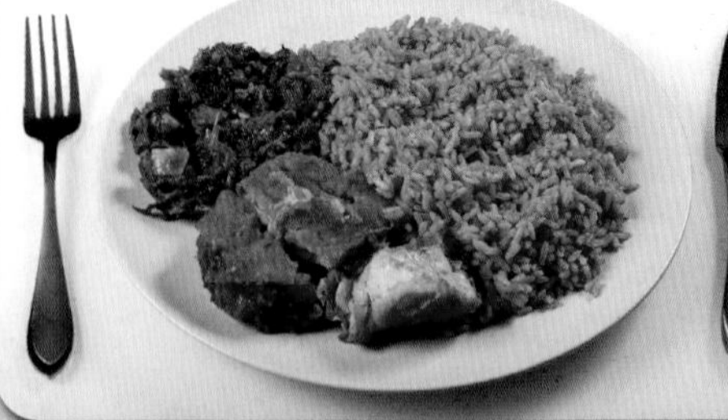

Caribbean Dumplings

CARBS	CALS	PROTEIN	FAT	FIBRE	SAT FAT	Portion
31g	210	4g	9g	1g	1g	Weight: 60g
63g	420	8g	17g	3g	2g	Weight: 120g

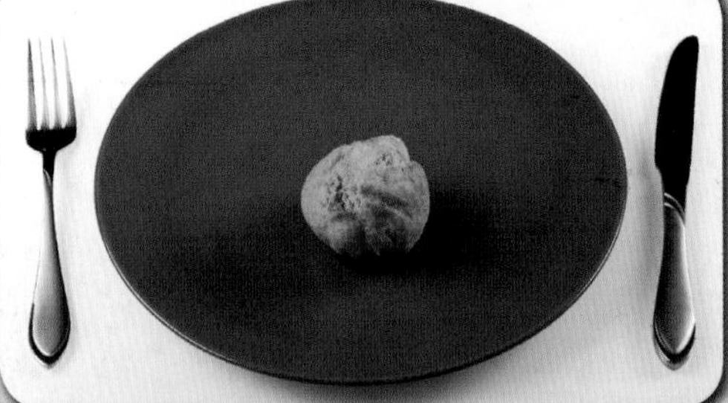

Jamaican Beef Patty

CARBS	CALS	PROTEIN	FAT	FIBRE	SAT FAT	Portion
26g	278	5g	16g	2g	7g	Weight: 85g
53g	556	11g	33g	4g	15g	Weight: 170g

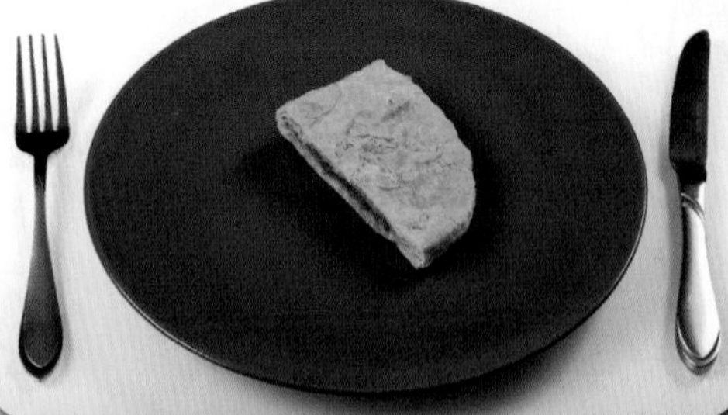

Goat & Potato Curry with Rice & Peas

CARBS	CALS	PROTEIN	FAT	FIBRE	SAT FAT	Portion
64g	445	19g	11g	9g	5g	225g curry, 150g rice & peas
127g	890	37g	22g	17g	9g	450g curry, 300g rice & peas

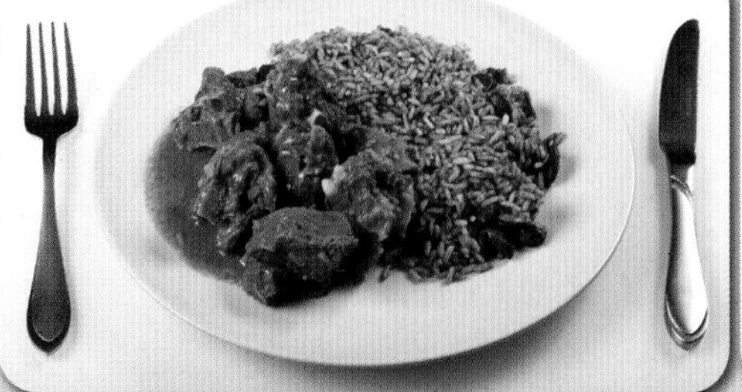

Jerk Chicken with Rice & Peas

CARBS	CALS	PROTEIN	FAT	FIBRE	SAT FAT	Portion
49g	511	30g	22g	5g	6g	210g chicken, 150g rice & peas
98g	1023	62g	45g	10g	13g	420g chicken, 300g rice & peas

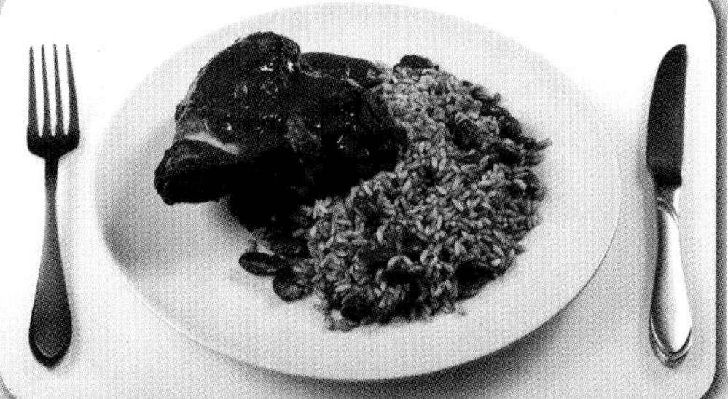

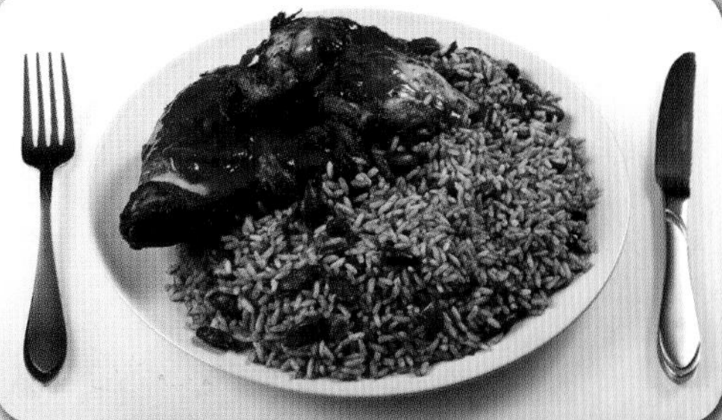

Fried Fish with Rice & Peas

CARBS	CALS	PROTEIN	FAT	FIBRE	SAT FAT	Portion
56g	555	24g	27g	6g	7g	115g fish, 150g rice & peas
113g	1110	48g	55g	11g	14g	230g fish, 300g rice & peas

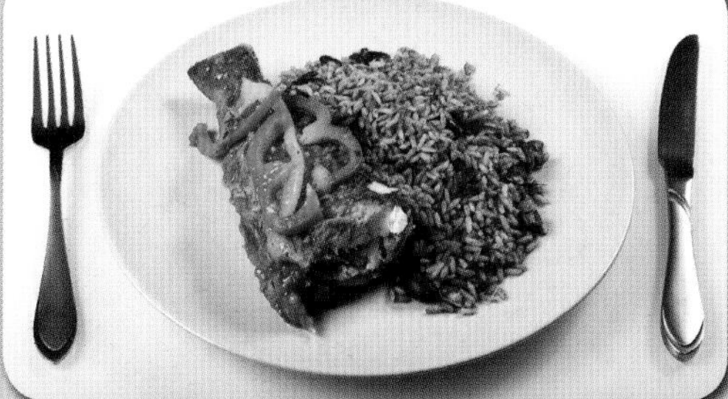

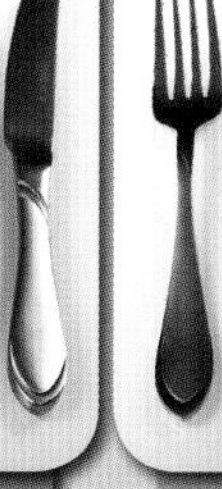

Fish Pie

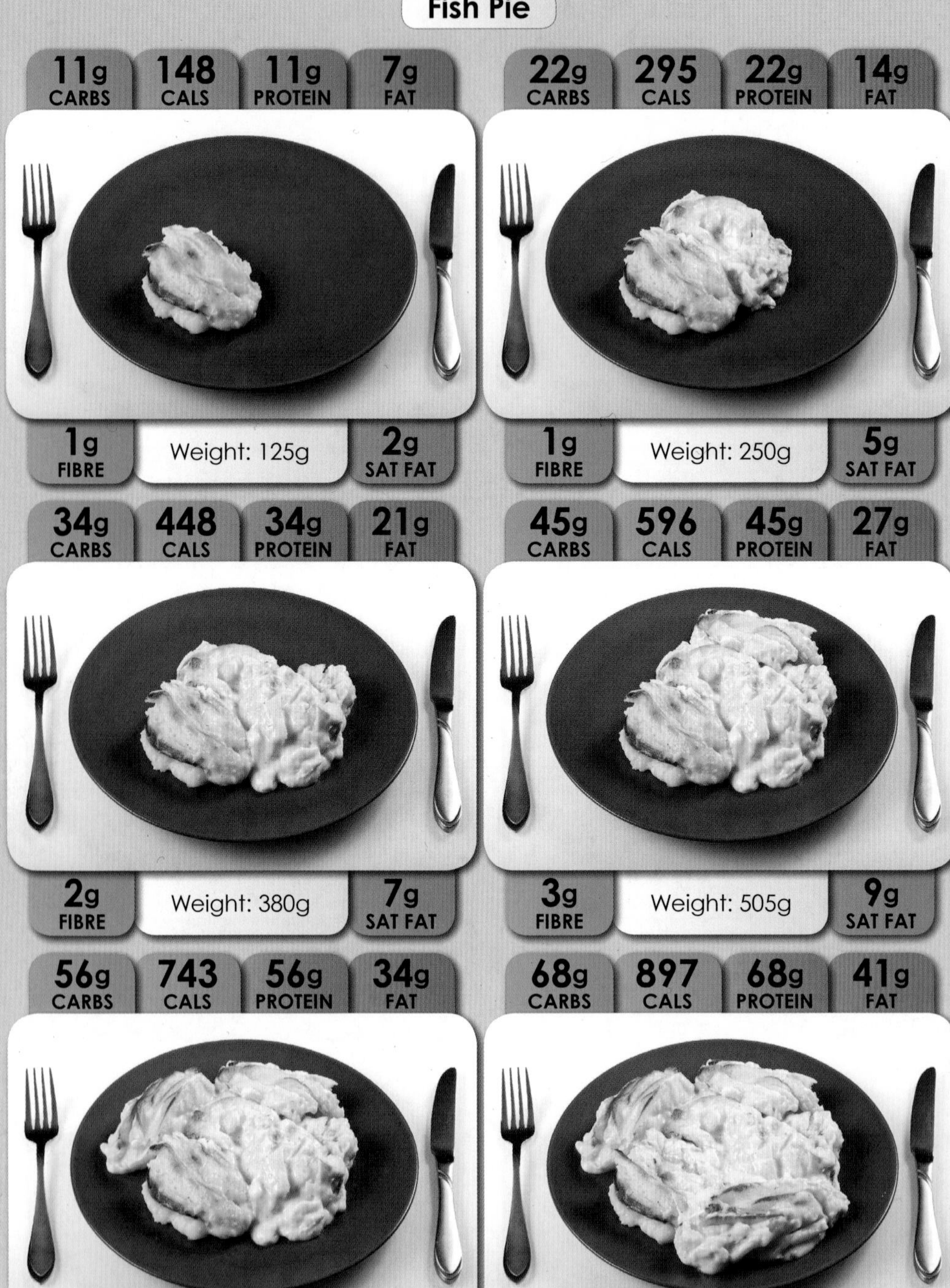

Weight	Carbs	Cals	Protein	Fat	Fibre	Sat Fat
125g	11g	148	11g	7g	1g	2g
250g	22g	295	22g	14g	1g	5g
380g	34g	448	34g	21g	2g	7g
505g	45g	596	45g	27g	3g	9g
630g	56g	743	56g	34g	3g	11g
760g	68g	897	68g	41g	4g	14g

Lasagne

15g CARBS | 211 CALS | 12g PROTEIN | 12g FAT

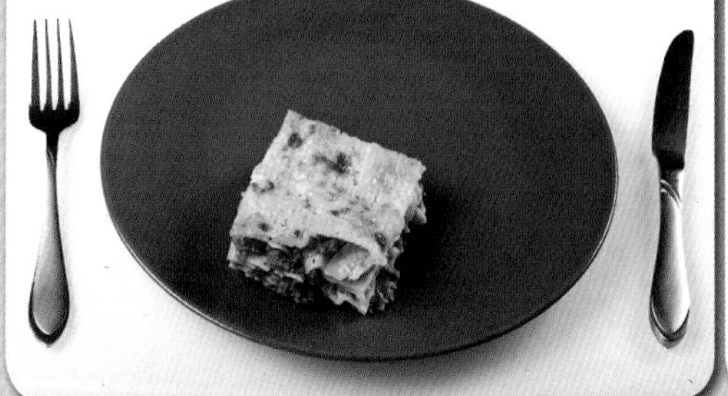

1g FIBRE | Weight: 115g | 6g SAT FAT

29g CARBS | 412 CALS | 24g PROTEIN | 23g FAT

2g FIBRE | Weight: 225g | 12g SAT FAT

44g CARBS | 622 CALS | 36g PROTEIN | 35g FAT

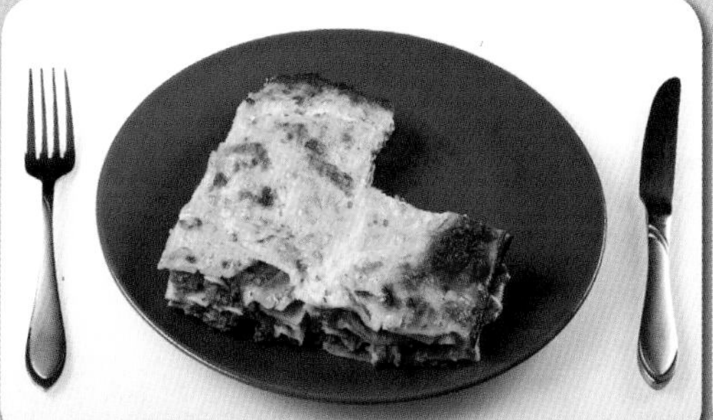

3g FIBRE | Weight: 340g | 19g SAT FAT

58g CARBS | 833 CALS | 48g PROTEIN | 47g FAT

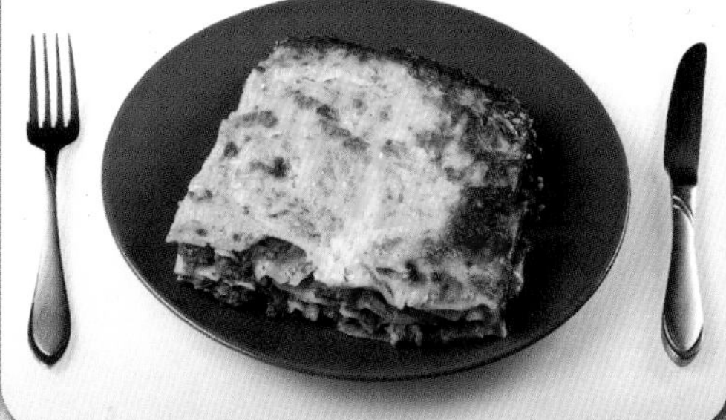

5g FIBRE | Weight: 455g | 25g SAT FAT

72g CARBS | 1034 CALS | 59g PROTEIN | 59g FAT

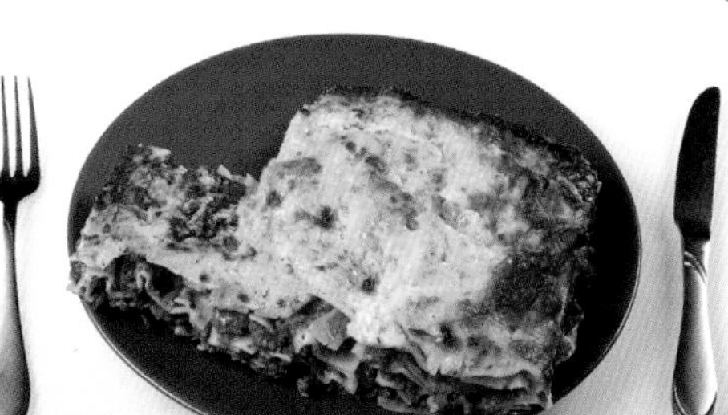

6g FIBRE | Weight: 565g | 31g SAT FAT

87g CARBS | 1244 CALS | 71g PROTEIN | 71g FAT

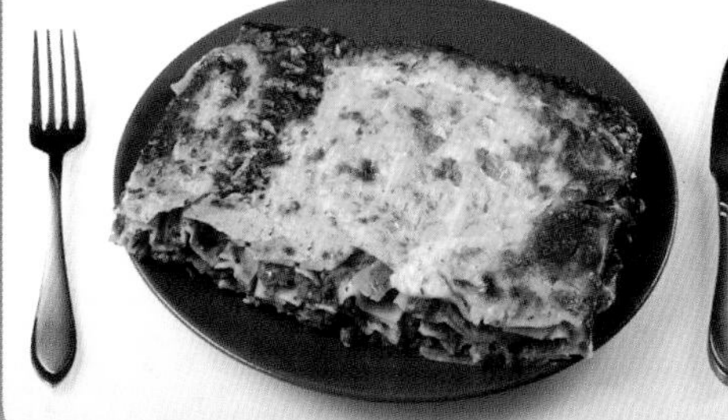

7g FIBRE | Weight: 680g | 37g SAT FAT

Macaroni Cheese

15g CARBS	166 CALS	7g PROTEIN	9g FAT

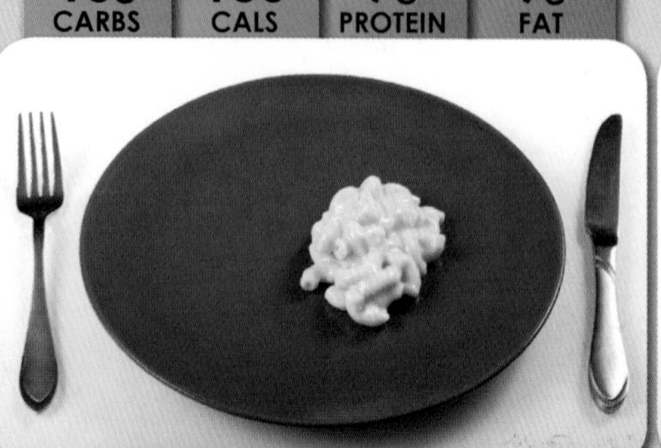

1g FIBRE	Weight: 80g	5g SAT FAT

30g CARBS	337 CALS	15g PROTEIN	18g FAT

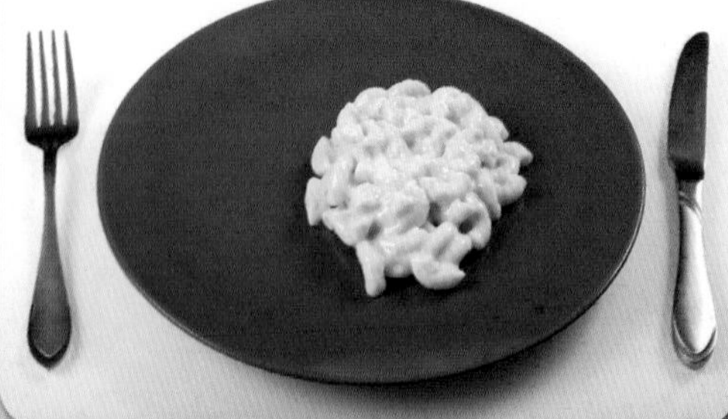

1g FIBRE	Weight: 163g	11g SAT FAT

40g CARBS	460 CALS	20g PROTEIN	24g FAT

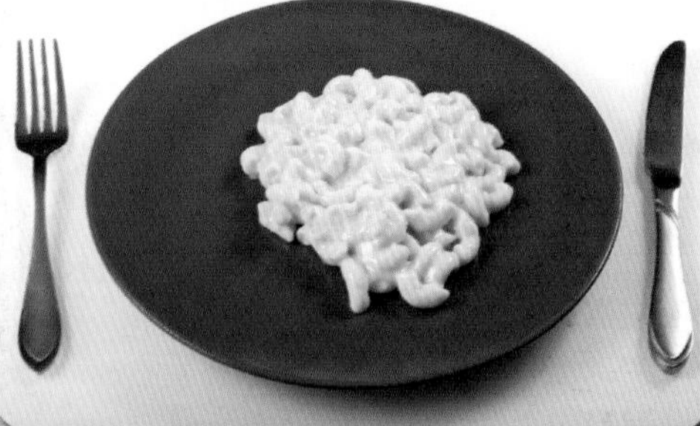

2g FIBRE	Weight: 222g	15g SAT FAT

55g CARBS	629 CALS	28g PROTEIN	33g FAT

2g FIBRE	Weight: 304g	20g SAT FAT

70g CARBS	797 CALS	35g PROTEIN	42g FAT

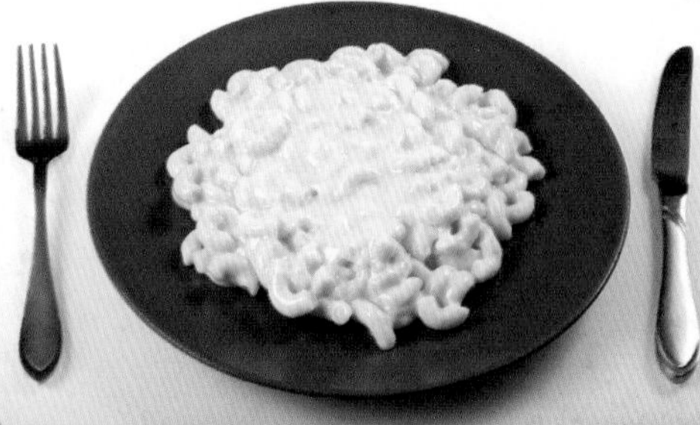

3g FIBRE	Weight: 385g	26g SAT FAT

84g CARBS	963 CALS	42g PROTEIN	51g FAT

3g FIBRE	Weight: 465g	31g SAT FAT

Mushroom Risotto

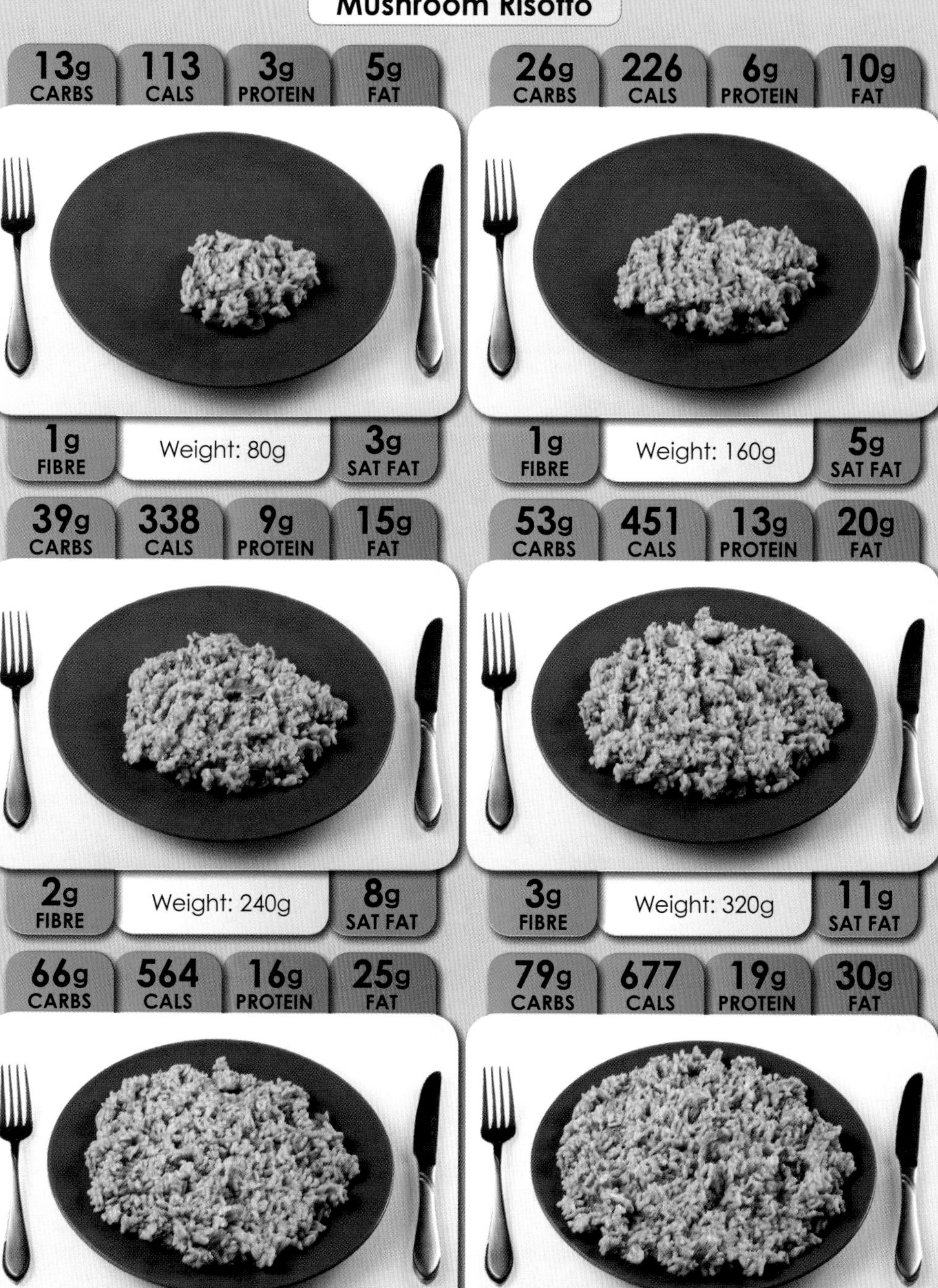

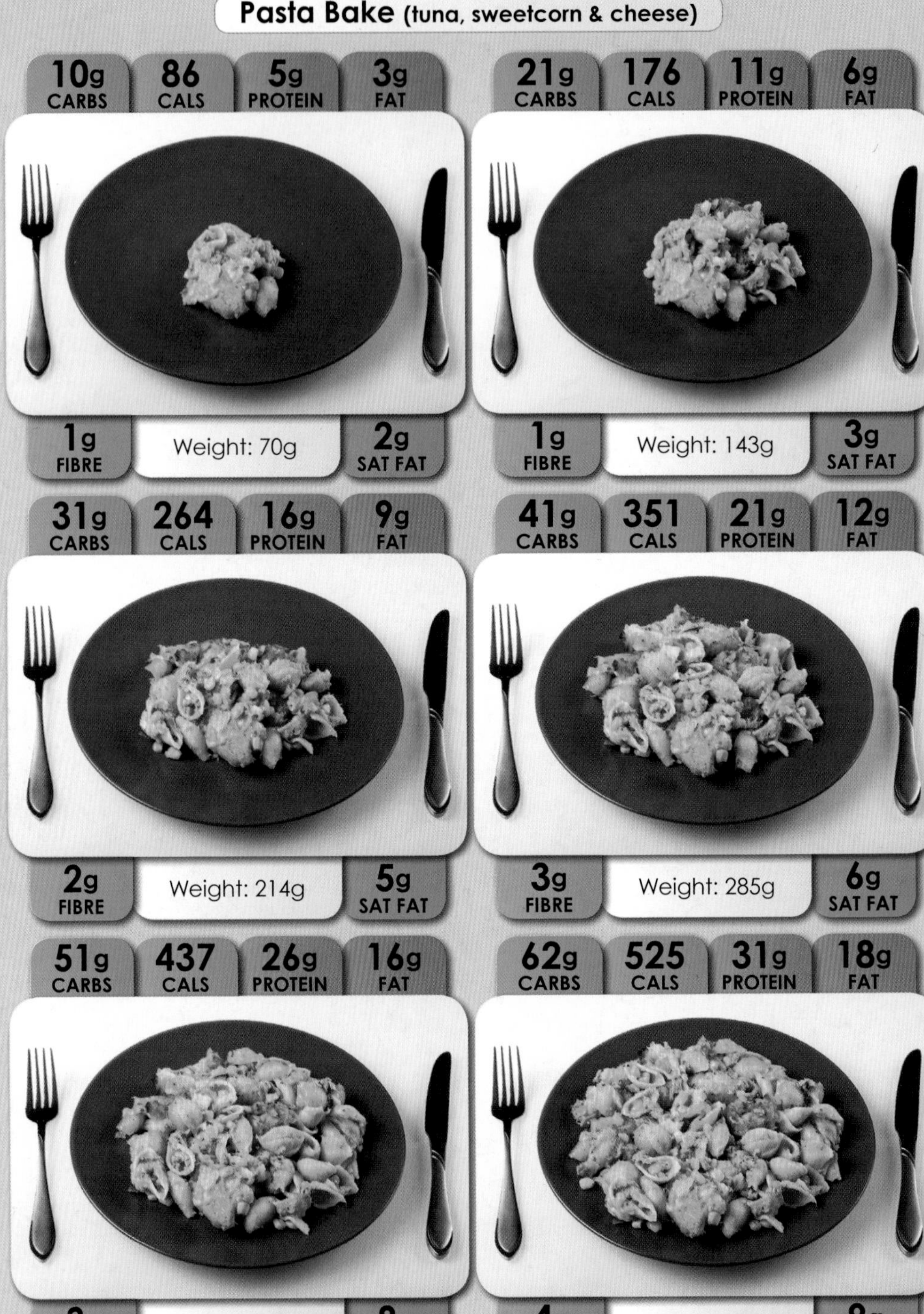
Pasta Bake (tuna, sweetcorn & cheese)
10g CARBS
86 CALS
5g PROTEIN
3g FAT
1g FIBRE
Weight: 70g
2g SAT FAT
21g CARBS
176 CALS
11g PROTEIN
6g FAT
1g FIBRE
Weight: 143g
3g SAT FAT
31g CARBS
264 CALS
16g PROTEIN
9g FAT
2g FIBRE
Weight: 214g
5g SAT FAT
41g CARBS
351 CALS
21g PROTEIN
12g FAT
3g FIBRE
Weight: 285g
6g SAT FAT
51g CARBS
437 CALS
26g PROTEIN
16g FAT
3g FIBRE
Weight: 355g
8g SAT FAT
62g CARBS
525 CALS
31g PROTEIN
18g FAT
4g FIBRE
Weight: 426g
9g SAT FAT

Pasta Meal (chicken, broccoli & mascarpone)

10g CARBS	117 CALS	5g PROTEIN	7g FAT
1g FIBRE	Weight: 65g		3g SAT FAT

24g CARBS	299 CALS	13g PROTEIN	17g FAT
3g FIBRE	Weight: 166g		7g SAT FAT

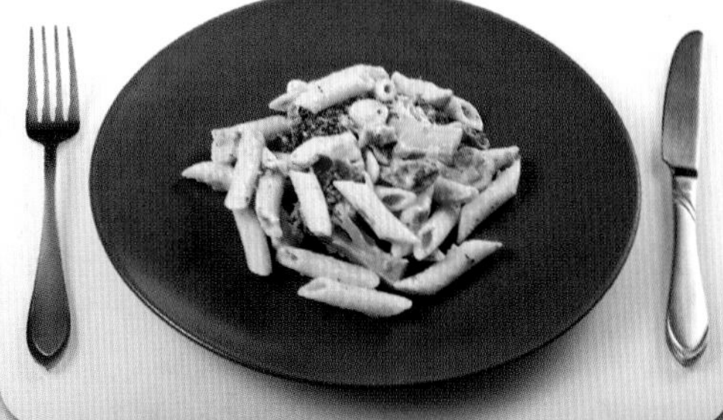

39g CARBS	481 CALS	20g PROTEIN	27g FAT
5g FIBRE	Weight: 267g		11g SAT FAT

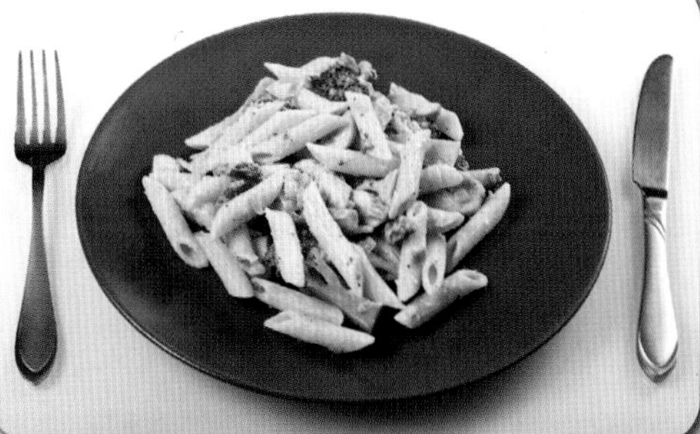

50g CARBS	615 CALS	26g PROTEIN	34g FAT
7g FIBRE	Weight: 341g		15g SAT FAT

65g CARBS	797 CALS	34g PROTEIN	45g FAT
9g FIBRE	Weight: 442g		19g SAT FAT

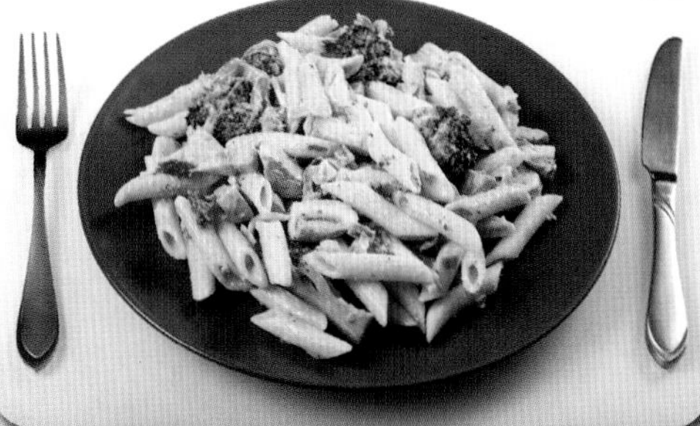

80g CARBS	979 CALS	41g PROTEIN	55g FAT
11g FIBRE	Weight: 543g		23g SAT FAT

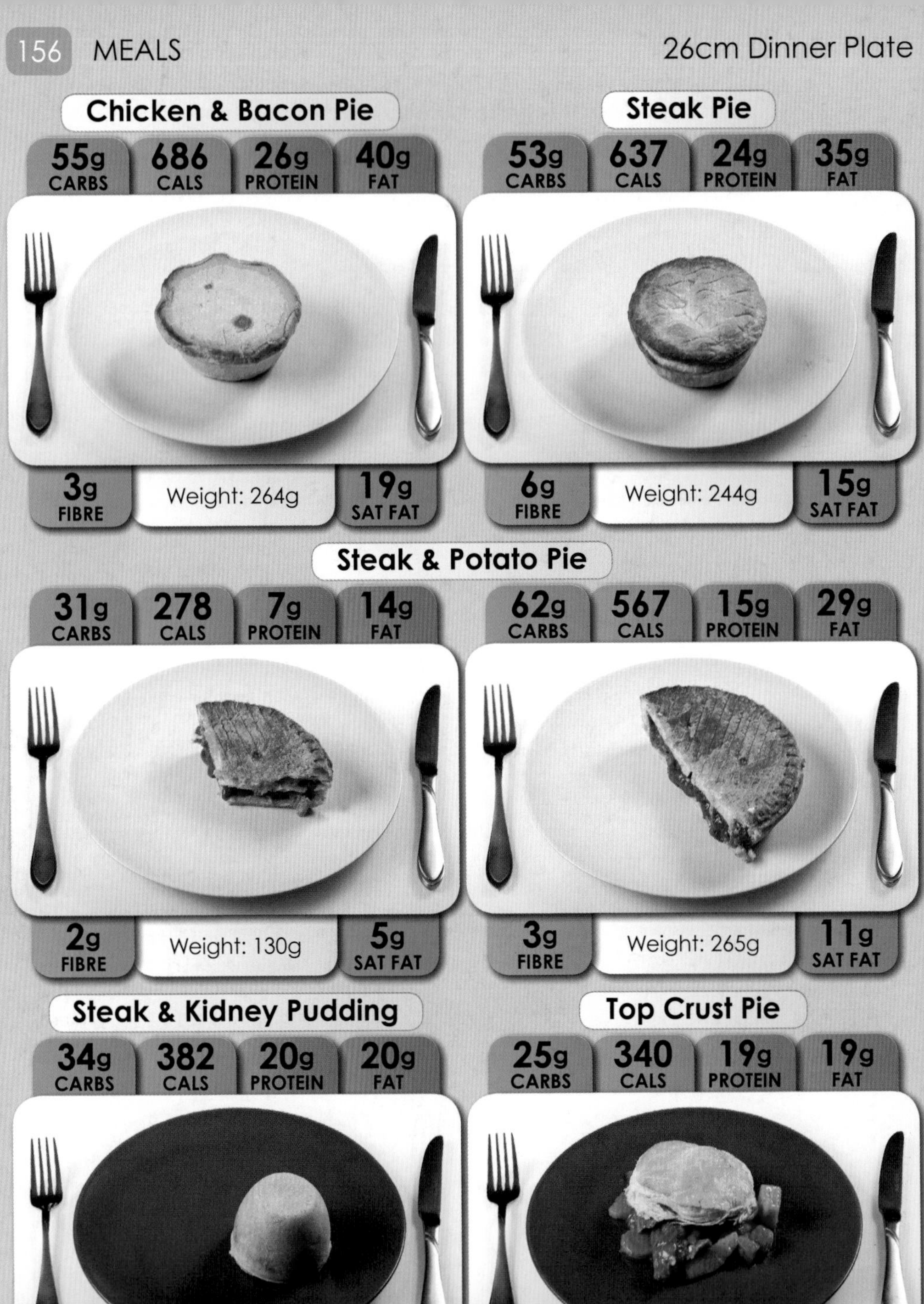
Chicken & Bacon Pie
55g CARBS
686 CALS
26g PROTEIN
40g FAT
3g FIBRE
Weight: 264g
19g SAT FAT
Steak Pie
53g CARBS
637 CALS
24g PROTEIN
35g FAT
6g FIBRE
Weight: 244g
15g SAT FAT
Steak & Potato Pie
31g CARBS
278 CALS
7g PROTEIN
14g FAT
2g FIBRE
Weight: 130g
5g SAT FAT
62g CARBS
567 CALS
15g PROTEIN
29g FAT
3g FIBRE
Weight: 265g
11g SAT FAT
Steak & Kidney Pudding
34g CARBS
382 CALS
20g PROTEIN
20g FAT
2g FIBRE
Weight: 182g
10g SAT FAT
Top Crust Pie
25g CARBS
340 CALS
19g PROTEIN
19g FAT
4g FIBRE
Weight: 264g
6g SAT FAT

Pizza (chicken, deep pan, oven baked)

20g CARBS	143 CALS	6g PROTEIN	4g FAT

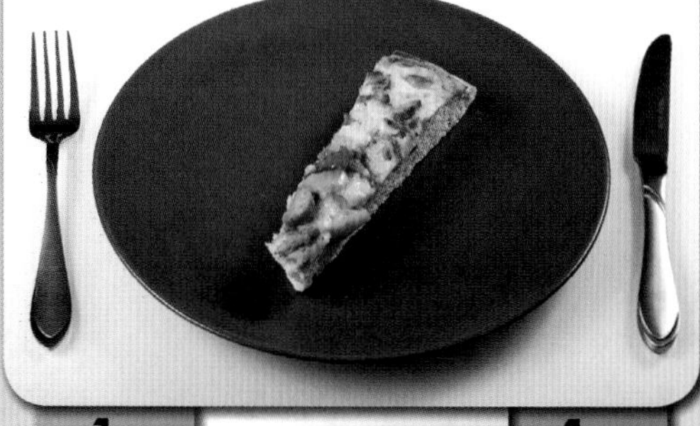

1g FIBRE	Weight: 65g	1g SAT FAT

40g CARBS	286 CALS	13g PROTEIN	8g FAT

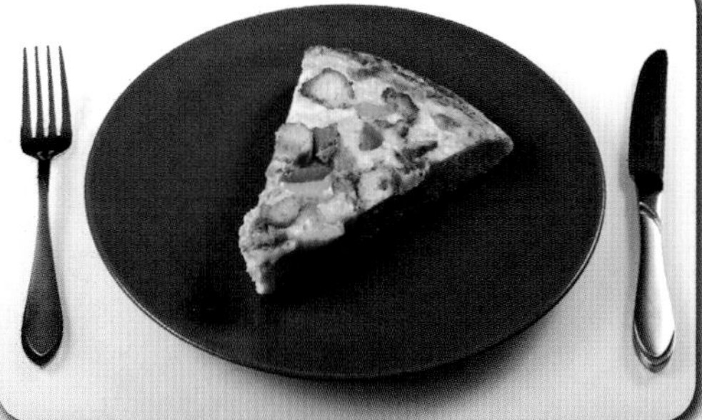

2g FIBRE	Weight: 130g	3g SAT FAT

61g CARBS	429 CALS	19g PROTEIN	12g FAT

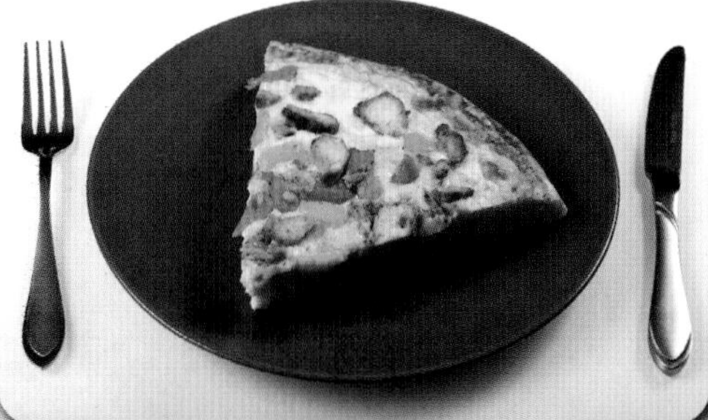

3g FIBRE	Weight: 195g	4g SAT FAT

Pizza (pepperoni, thin crust, oven baked)

12g CARBS	115 CALS	5g PROTEIN	5g FAT

1g FIBRE	Weight: 40g	2g SAT FAT

22g CARBS	215 CALS	9g PROTEIN	10g FAT

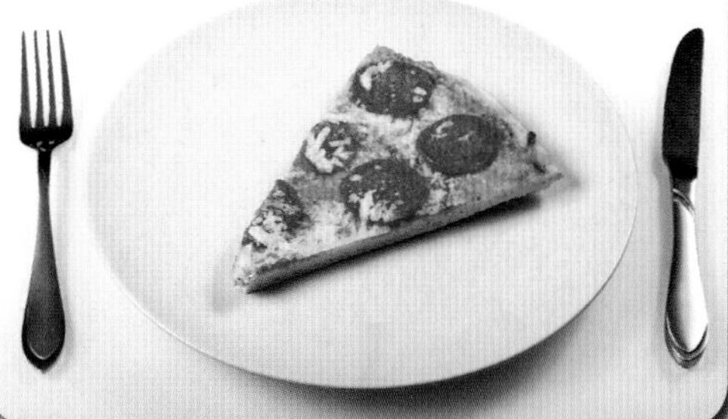

2g FIBRE	Weight: 75g	4g SAT FAT

34g CARBS	330 CALS	14g PROTEIN	15g FAT

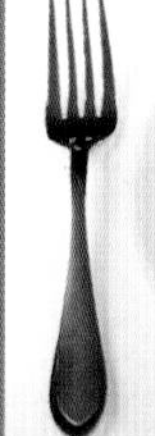

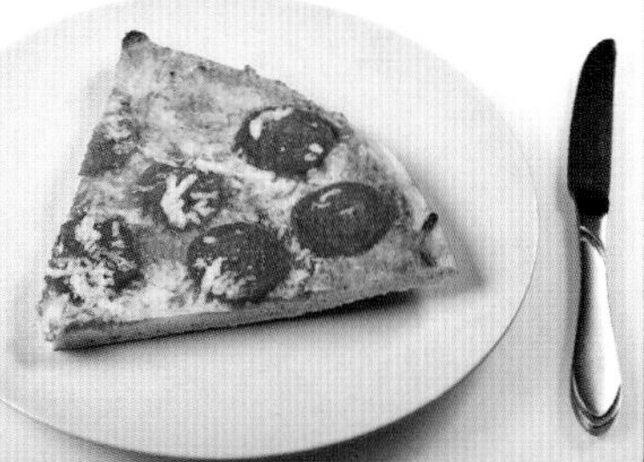

3g FIBRE	Weight: 115g	6g SAT FAT

Quiche Lorraine

CARBS	CALS	PROTEIN	FAT
20g	369	15g	26g

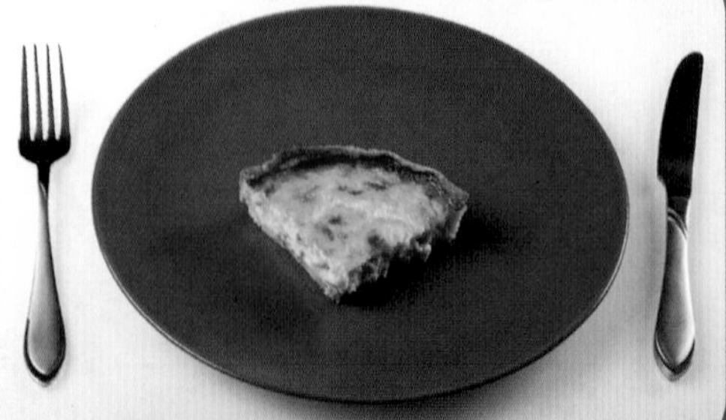

FIBRE		SAT FAT
1g	Weight: 100g	11g

CARBS	CALS	PROTEIN	FAT
39g	738	30g	52g

FIBRE		SAT FAT
1g	Weight: 200g	22g

CARBS	CALS	PROTEIN	FAT
78g	1476	61g	104g

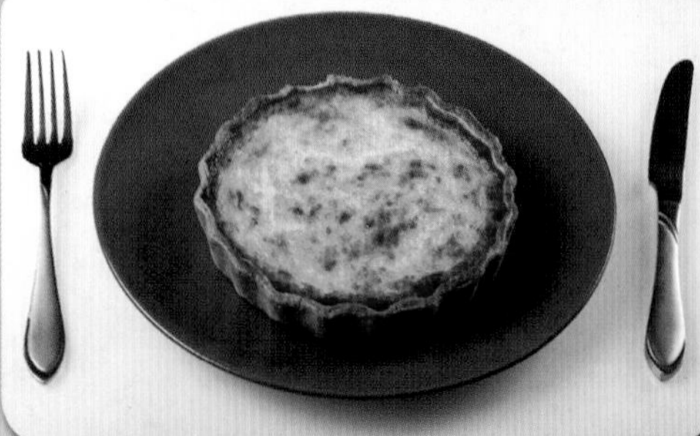

FIBRE		SAT FAT
3g	Weight: 400g	43g

Stew (beef) & Dumplings

CARBS	CALS	PROTEIN	FAT
20g	203	9g	10g

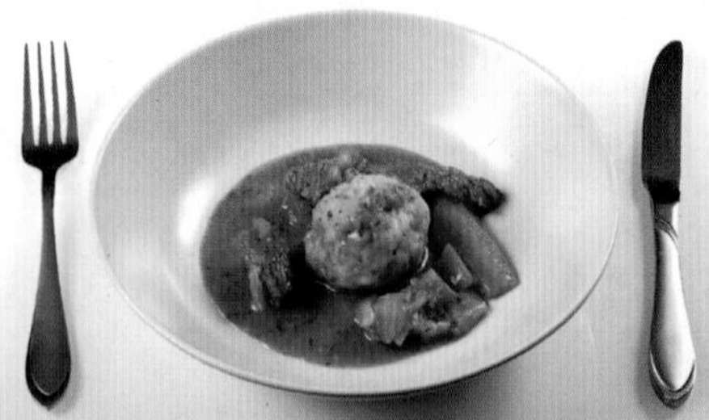

FIBRE		SAT FAT
2g	95g stew, 45g dumpling	6g

CARBS	CALS	PROTEIN	FAT
40g	396	17g	20g

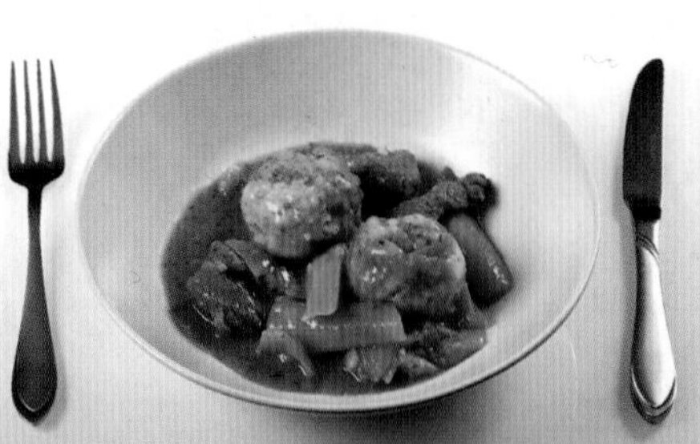

FIBRE		SAT FAT
4g	175g stew, 90g dumplings	11g

CARBS	CALS	PROTEIN	FAT
85g	852	41g	41g

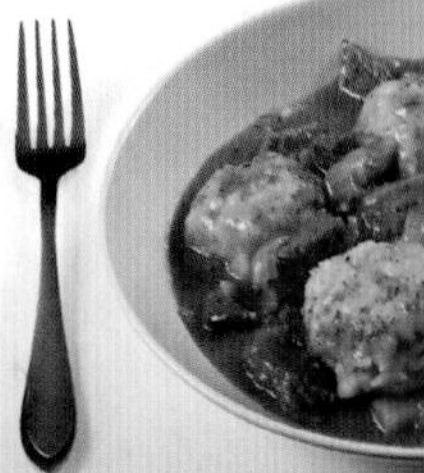

FIBRE		SAT FAT
10g	440g stew, 180g dumplings	22g

Sausage & Mash (with butter)

CARBS	CALS	PROTEIN	FAT
24g	287	10g	17g

FIBRE		SAT FAT
2g	55g sausage, 120g mash	7g

CARBS	CALS	PROTEIN	FAT
47g	568	20g	34g

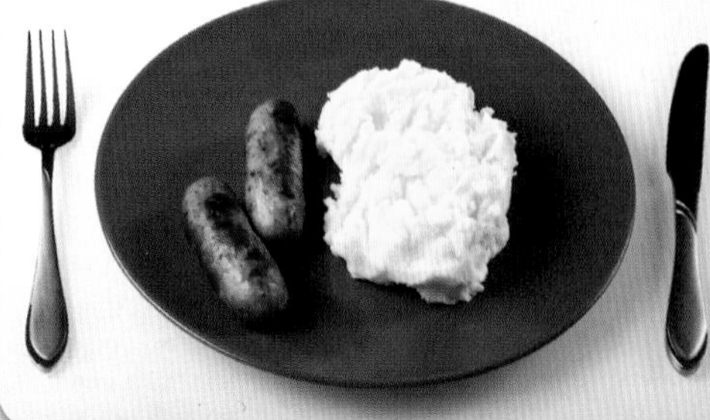

FIBRE		SAT FAT
5g	110g sausages, 235g mash	15g

CARBS	CALS	PROTEIN	FAT
71g	854	30g	51g

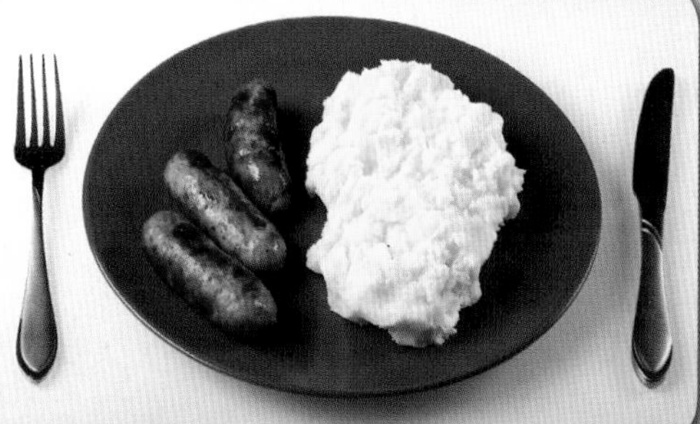

FIBRE		SAT FAT
7g	165g sausages, 355g mash	22g

CARBS	CALS	PROTEIN	FAT
94g	1136	40g	67g

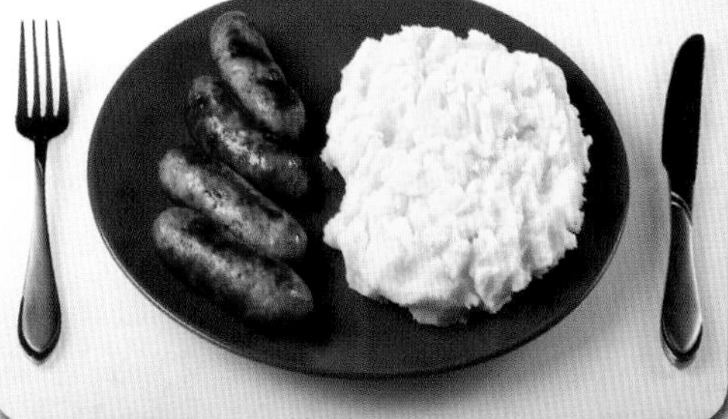

FIBRE		SAT FAT
9g	220g sausages, 470g mash	29g

CARBS	CALS	PROTEIN	FAT
118g	1422	51g	84g

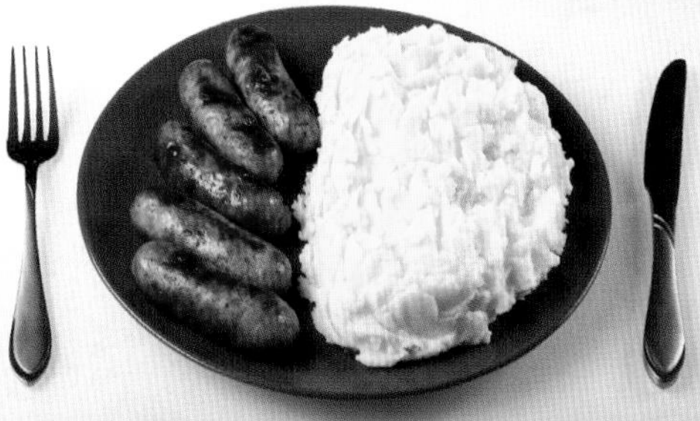

FIBRE		SAT FAT
11g	275g sausages, 590g mash	37g

CARBS	CALS	PROTEIN	FAT
142g	1703	61g	101g

FIBRE		SAT FAT
14g	330g sausages, 705g mash	44g

Shepherd's Pie

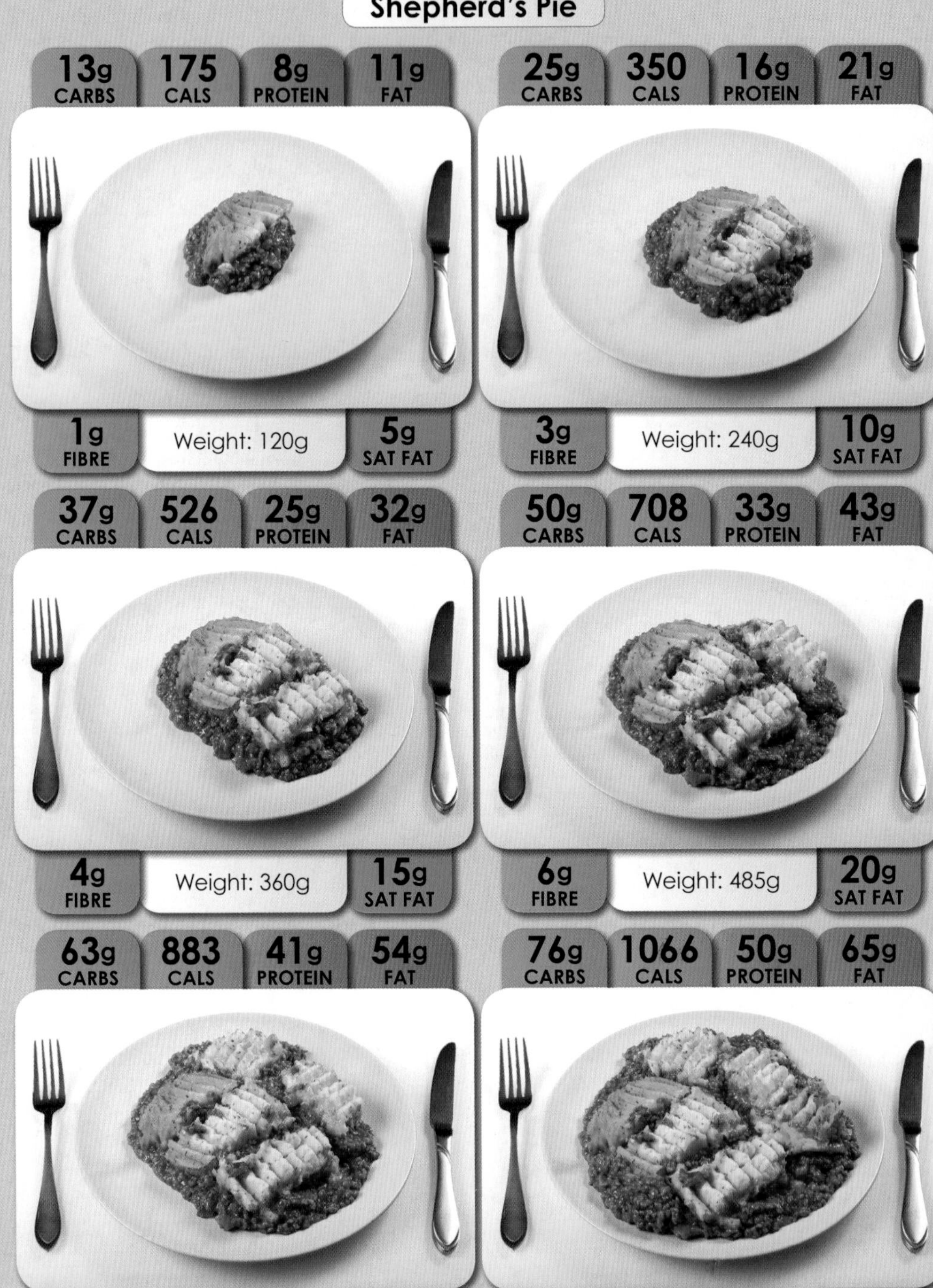

Weight	Carbs	Cals	Protein	Fat	Fibre	Sat Fat
120g	13g	175	8g	11g	1g	5g
240g	25g	350	16g	21g	3g	10g
360g	37g	526	25g	32g	4g	15g
485g	50g	708	33g	43g	6g	20g
605g	63g	883	41g	54g	7g	25g
730g	76g	1066	50g	65g	9g	30g

Spaghetti Bolognese

CARBS	CALS	PROTEIN	FAT
23g	164	8g	5g

FIBRE	Portion	SAT FAT
2g	60g spaghetti, 90g bolognese	2g

CARBS	CALS	PROTEIN	FAT
45g	327	16g	9g

FIBRE	Portion	SAT FAT
4g	120g spaghetti, 180g bolognese	3g

CARBS	CALS	PROTEIN	FAT
68g	491	24g	14g

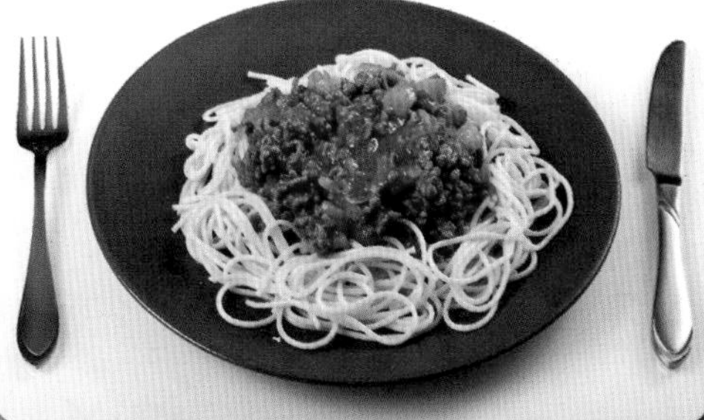

FIBRE	Portion	SAT FAT
7g	180g spaghetti, 270g bolognese	5g

CARBS	CALS	PROTEIN	FAT
91g	654	32g	18g

FIBRE	Portion	SAT FAT
9g	240g spaghetti, 360g bolognese	6g

CARBS	CALS	PROTEIN	FAT
113g	818	40g	23g

FIBRE	Portion	SAT FAT
11g	300g spaghetti, 450g bolognese	8g

CARBS	CALS	PROTEIN	FAT
136g	981	48g	28g

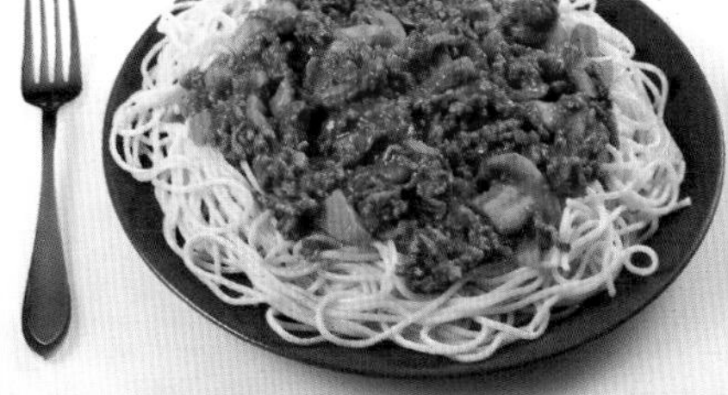

FIBRE	Portion	SAT FAT
13g	360g spaghetti, 540g bolognese	10g

Stir-fry (chicken & noodles)

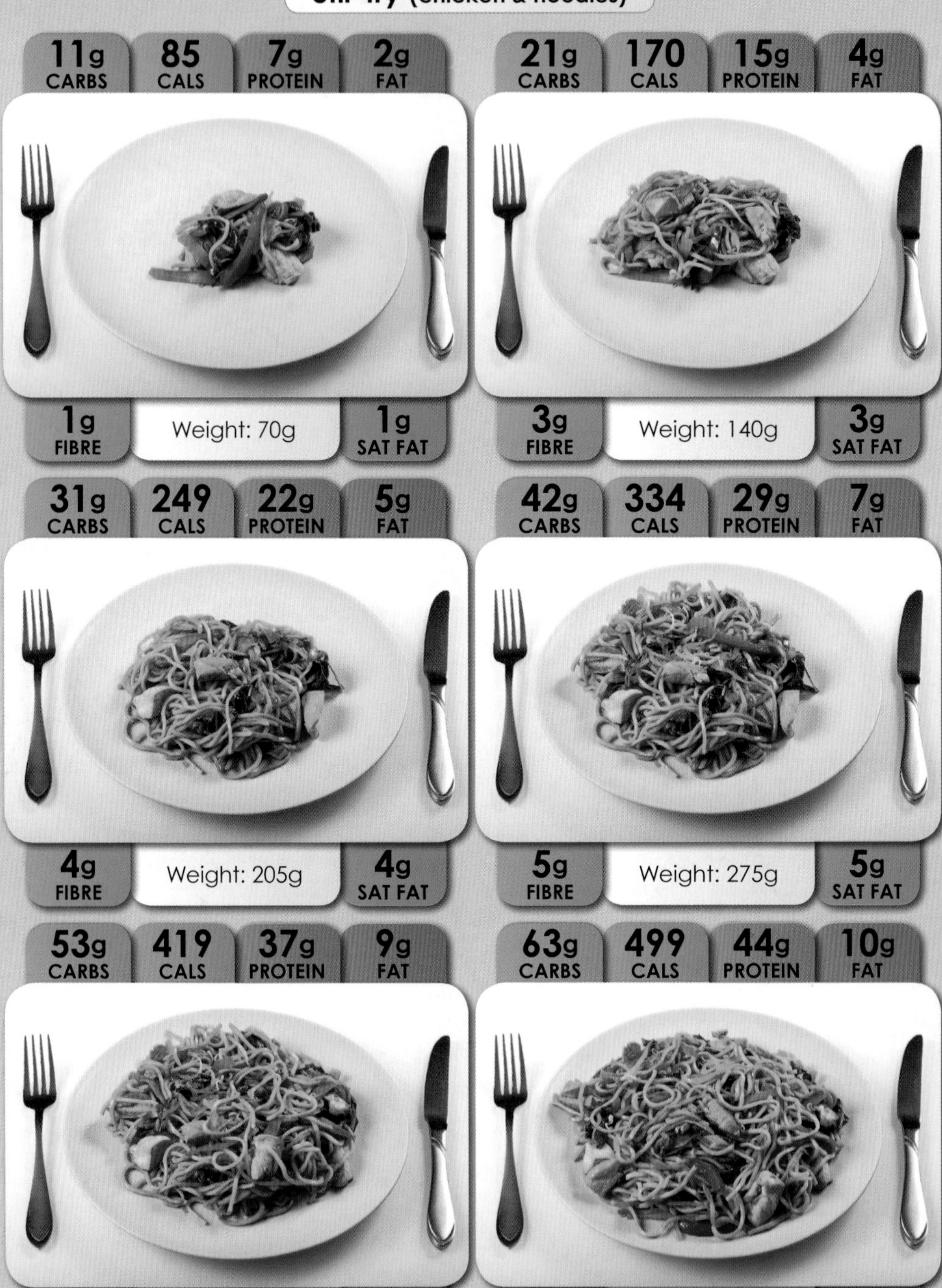

Toad in the Hole

CARBS	CALS	PROTEIN	FAT	FIBRE	Portion	SAT FAT
20g	269	12g	16g	1g	55g sausage, 37g yorkshire	5g
40g	534	24g	32g	2g	110g sausages, 73g yorkshire	11g
60g	803	37g	48g	4g	165g sausages, 110g yorkshire	16g
80g	1069	49g	65g	5g	220g sausages, 146g yorkshire	22g
100g	1335	61g	81g	6g	275g sausages, 182g yorkshire	27g
119g	1603	73g	97g	7g	330g sausages, 219g yorkshire	32g

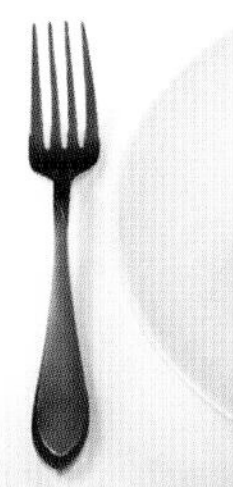

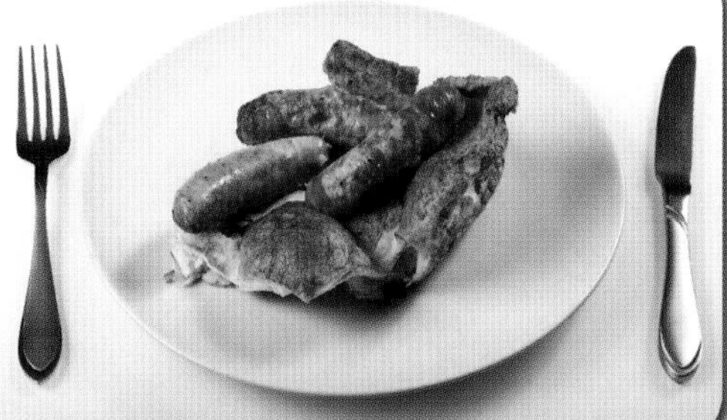

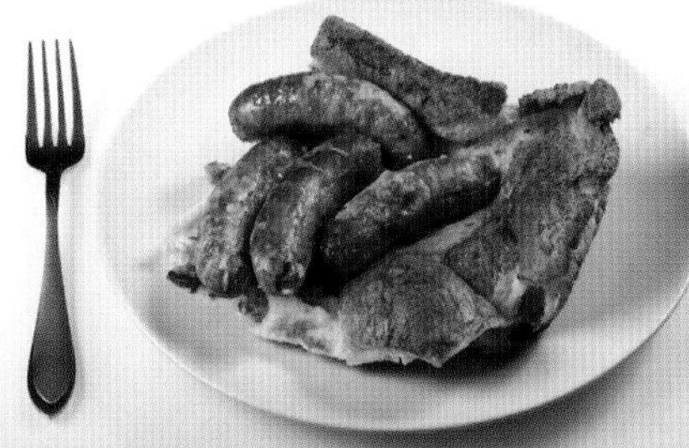

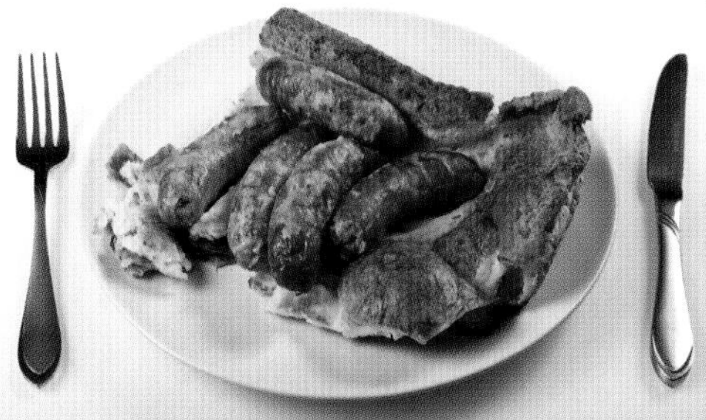

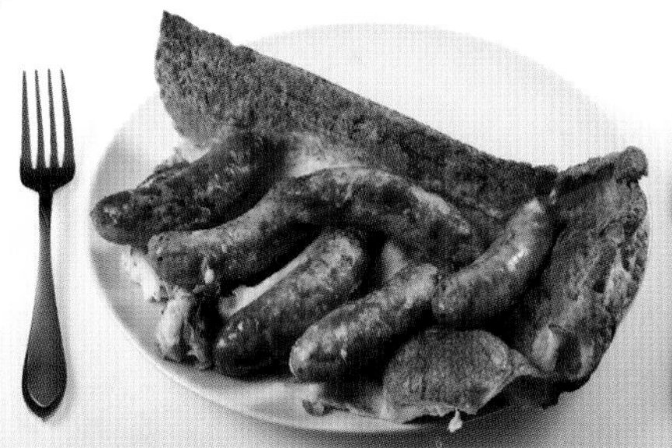

Coleslaw

	Carbs	Cals	Protein	Fat	Fibre	Weight	Sat Fat
Small	3g	168	1g	17g	1g	65g	3g
Large	6g	335	2g	34g	3g	130g	5g

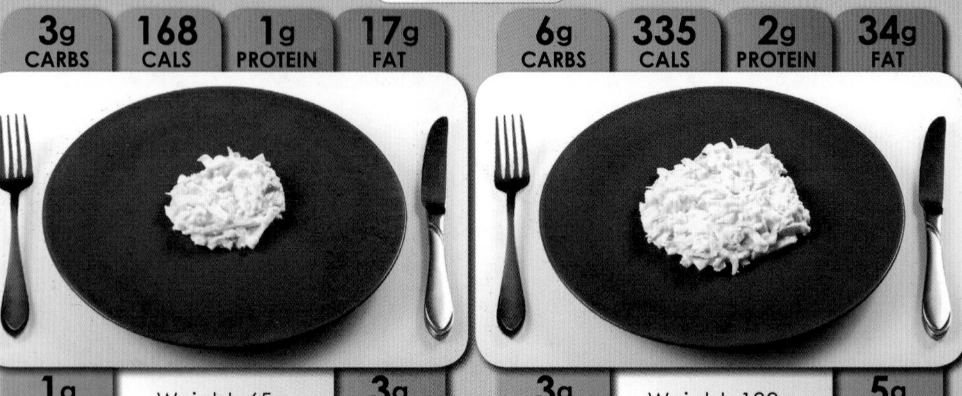

Gherkins

	Carbs	Cals	Protein	Fat	Fibre	Weight	Sat Fat
Small	1g	8	1g	0g	1g	55g	0g
Large	3g	16	1g	0g	2g	115g	0g

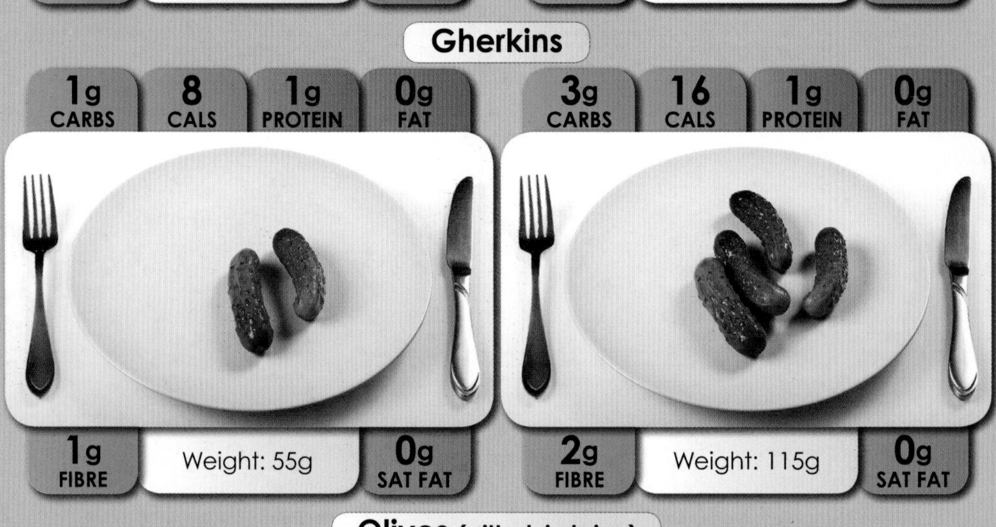

Olives (pitted, in brine)

	Carbs	Cals	Protein	Fat	Fibre	Weight	Sat Fat
Small	0g	26	0g	3g	1g	25g	0g
Large	0g	52	1g	6g	2g	50g	1g

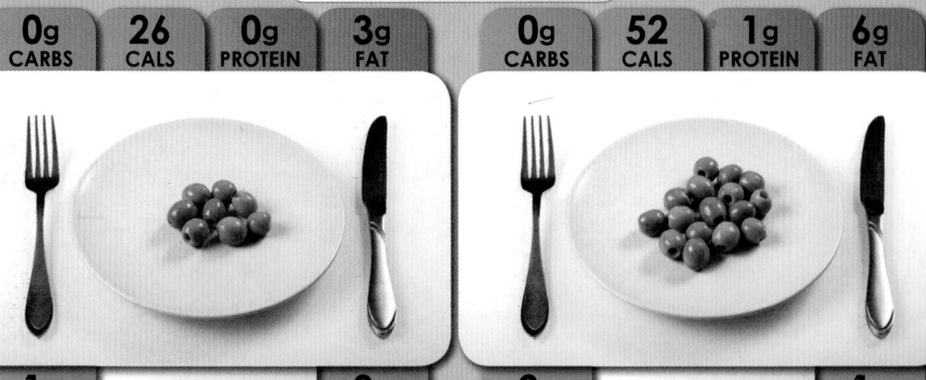

Onion Rings (battered)

	Carbs	Cals	Protein	Fat	Fibre	Weight	Sat Fat
Left	7g	65	1g	4g	1g	26g	0g
Right	13g	130	2g	7g	1g	52g	1g

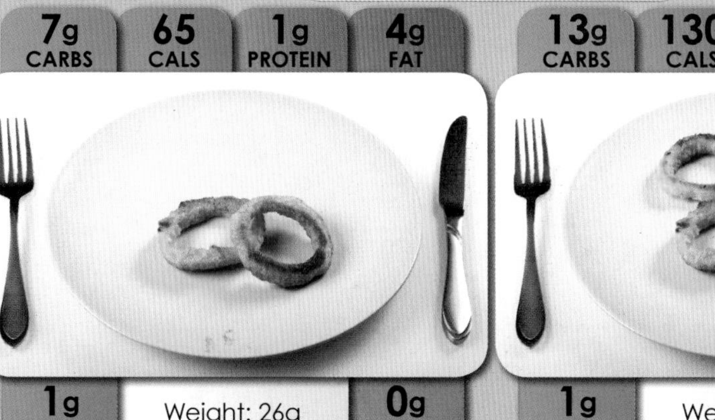
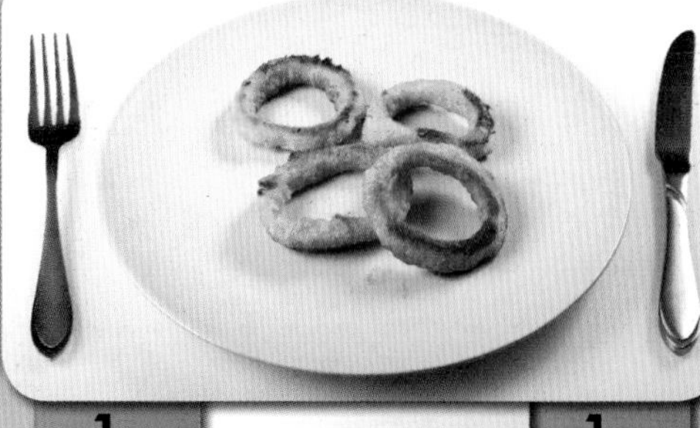

Pickled Onions

	Carbs	Cals	Protein	Fat	Fibre	Weight	Sat Fat
Left	2g	8	0g	0g	1g	35g	0g
Right	3g	17	1g	0g	1g	70g	0g

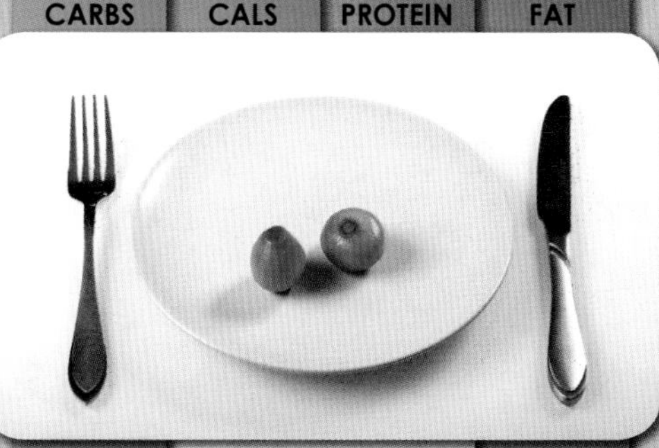
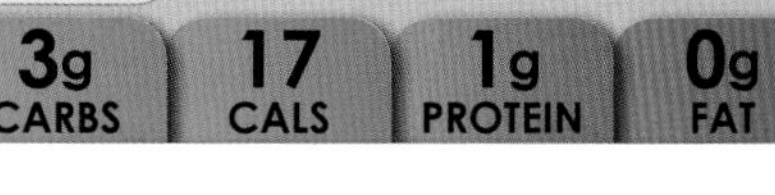
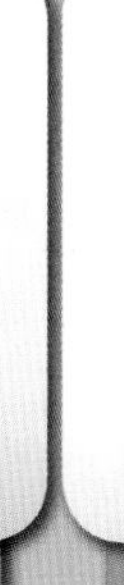
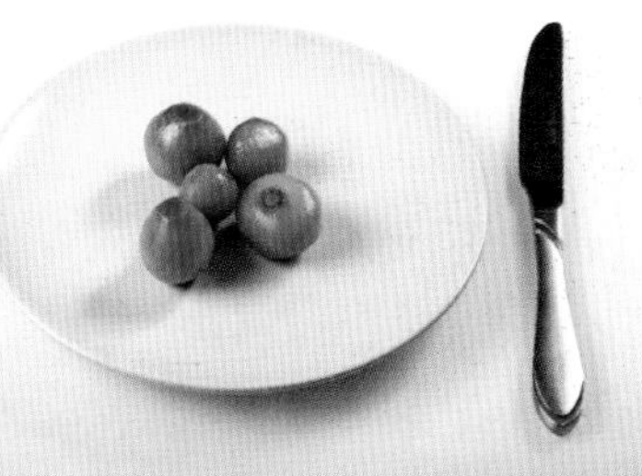

Sun-dried Tomatoes (in oil)

	Carbs	Cals	Protein	Fat	Fibre	Weight	Sat Fat
Left	1g	124	1g	13g	2g	25g	2g
Right	3g	248	2g	26g	4g	50g	3g

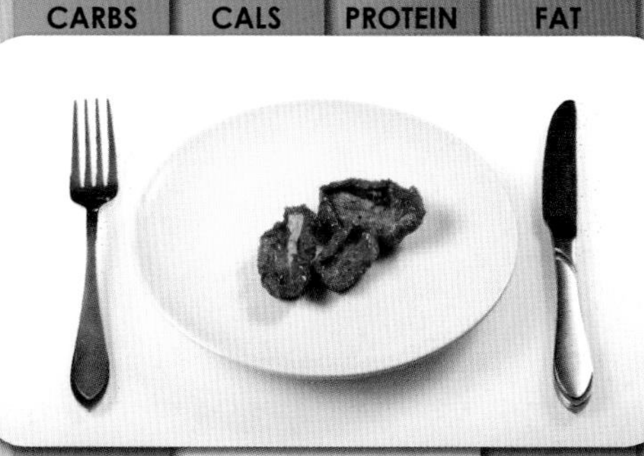
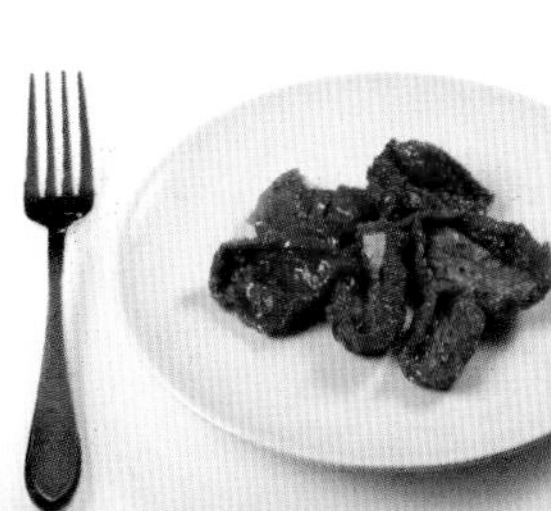
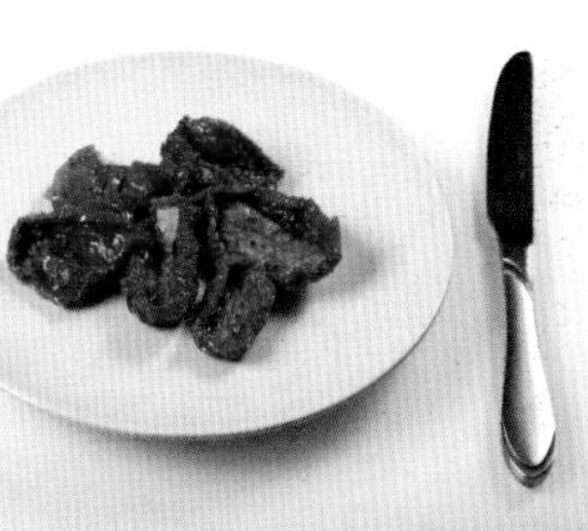

Stuffing (packet mix)

CARBS	CALS	PROTEIN	FAT
13g	63	2g	1g

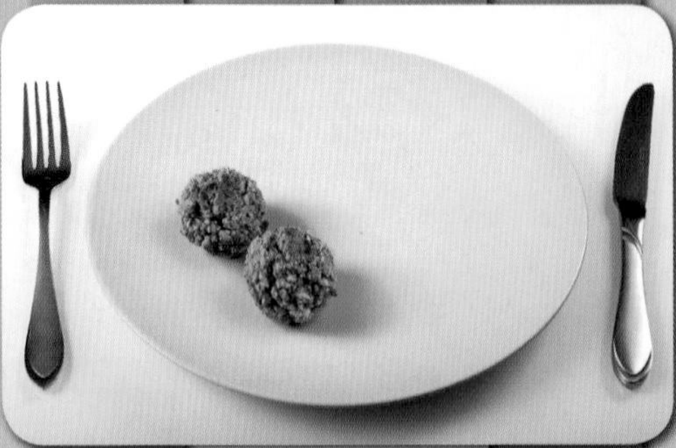

FIBRE		SAT FAT
1g	Weight: 65g	1g

CARBS	CALS	PROTEIN	FAT
25g	126	4g	2g

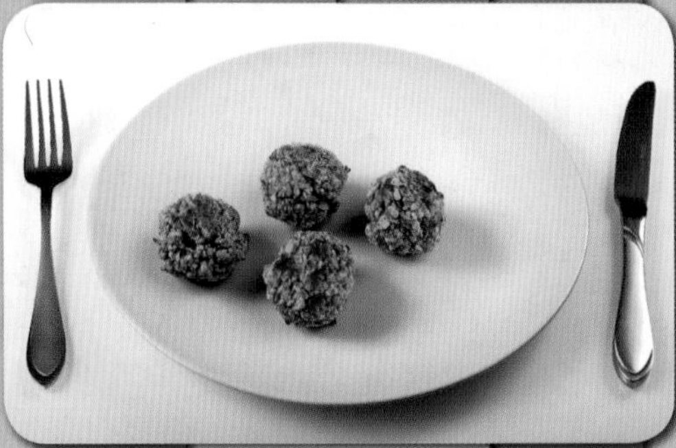

FIBRE		SAT FAT
2g	Weight: 130g	1g

CARBS	CALS	PROTEIN	FAT
38g	189	6g	3g

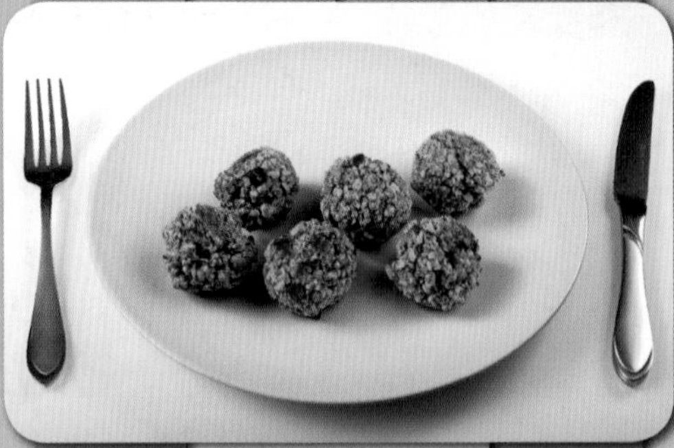

FIBRE		SAT FAT
3g	Weight: 195g	2g

Yorkshire Pudding

CARBS	CALS	PROTEIN	FAT
10g	84	3g	4g

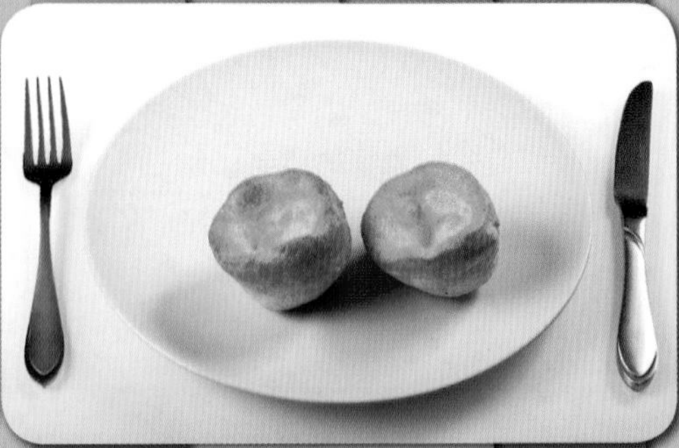

FIBRE		SAT FAT
1g	Weight: 40g	2g

CARBS	CALS	PROTEIN	FAT
20g	168	5g	8g

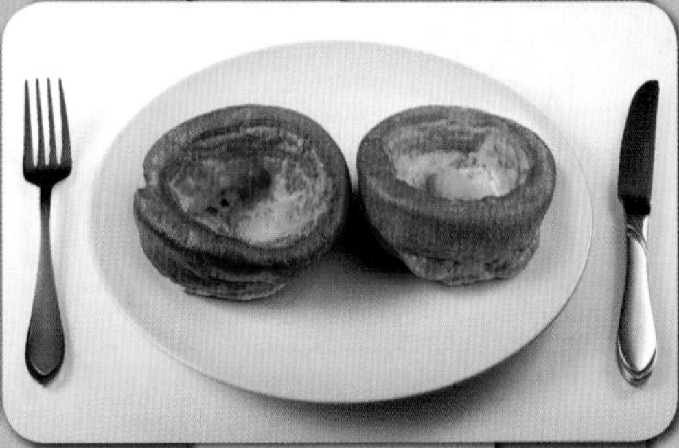

FIBRE		SAT FAT
1g	Weight: 80g	4g

CARBS	CALS	PROTEIN	FAT
30g	252	8g	12g

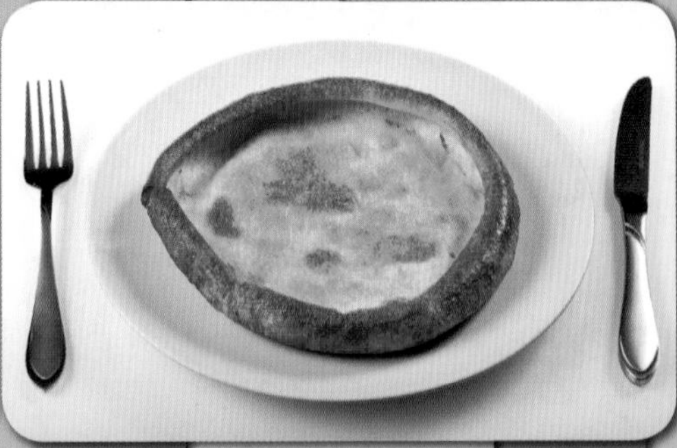

FIBRE		SAT FAT
1g	Weight: 120g	6g

Cornish Pasty

CARBS	CALS	PROTEIN	FAT	FIBRE	Weight	SAT FAT
8g	83	2g	5g	0g	31g (mini)	2g
41g	433	11g	26g	2g	162g	10g

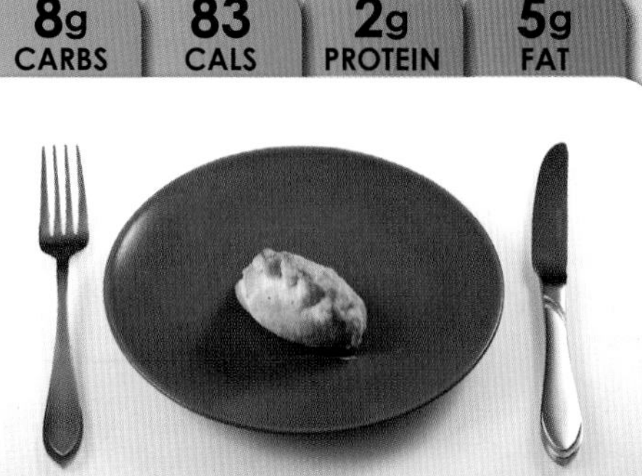

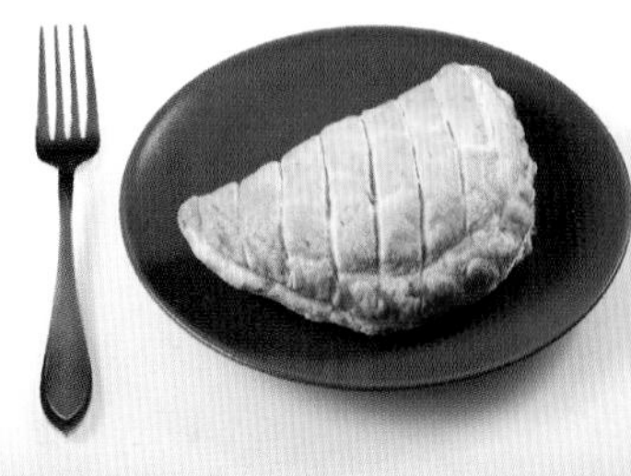

Pork Pie

CARBS	CALS	PROTEIN	FAT	FIBRE	Weight	SAT FAT
28g	432	13g	31g	1g	119g	12g
76g	1162	35g	82g	4g	320g	31g

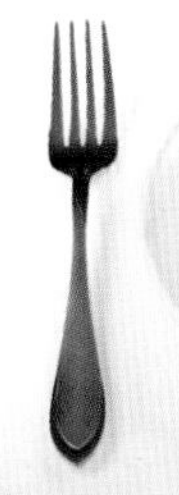

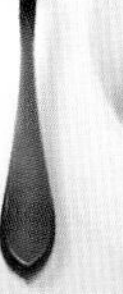

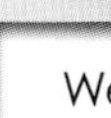

Sausage Roll

CARBS	CALS	PROTEIN	FAT	FIBRE	Weight	SAT FAT
16g	241	6g	17g	1g	63g	7g
32g	475	12g	34g	2g	124g	14g

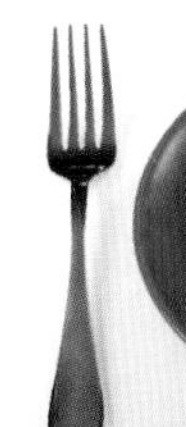

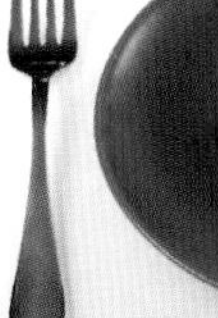

Sausages & Beans (tinned)

Weight	Carbs	Cals	Protein	Fat	Fibre	Sat Fat
Weight: 70g	9g	76	5g	2g	3g	1g
Weight: 210g (half tin)	27g	229	13g	7g	8g	2g
Weight: 425g (full tin)	54g	463	27g	14g	16g	5g

Haggis

Weight	Carbs	Cals	Protein	Fat	Fibre	Sat Fat
Weight: 105g	20g	326	11g	23g	0g	8g
Weight: 210g	40g	651	23g	46g	1g	16g
Weight: 315g	61g	977	34g	68g	1g	24g

Black Pudding (fried without oil)

10g CARBS	172 CALS	6g PROTEIN	12g FAT

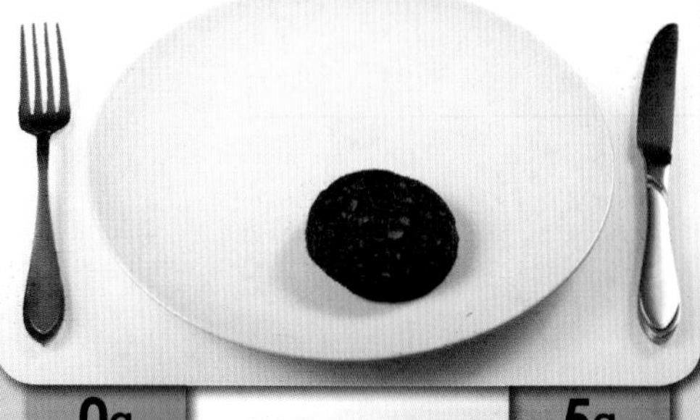

0g FIBRE	Weight: 58g	5g SAT FAT

Chicken Goujon (baked)

6g CARBS	83 CALS	6g PROTEIN	4g FAT

0g FIBRE	Weight: 30g	1g SAT FAT

Brussels Pâté

1g CARBS	99 CALS	3g PROTEIN	9g FAT

0g FIBRE	Weight: 30g	3g SAT FAT

2g CARBS	197 CALS	6g PROTEIN	18g FAT

1g FIBRE	Weight: 60g	7g SAT FAT

BBQ Ribs

5g CARBS	302 CALS	21g PROTEIN	22g FAT

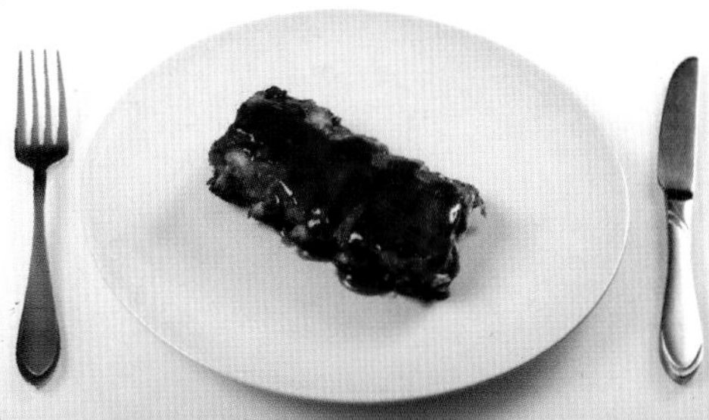

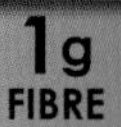

1g FIBRE	Weight: 200g (100g edible)	6g SAT FAT

10g CARBS	604 CALS	42g PROTEIN	44g FAT

2g FIBRE	Weight: 400g (200g edible)	13g SAT FAT

Gammon (grilled)

CARBS	CALS	PROTEIN	FAT	FIBRE	Weight	SAT FAT
0g	169	23g	8g	0g	85g	3g
0g	338	47g	17g	0g	170g	6g

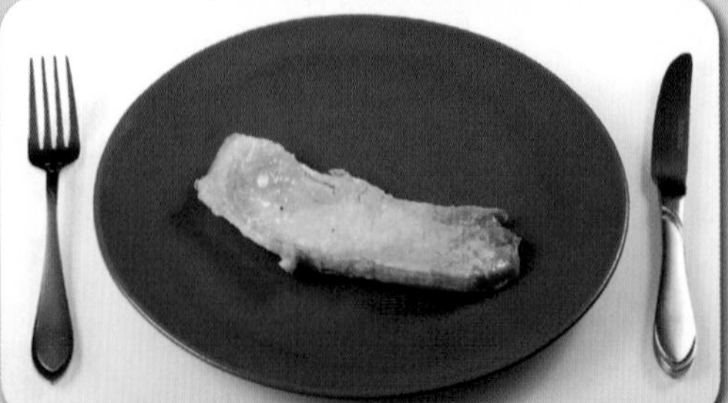

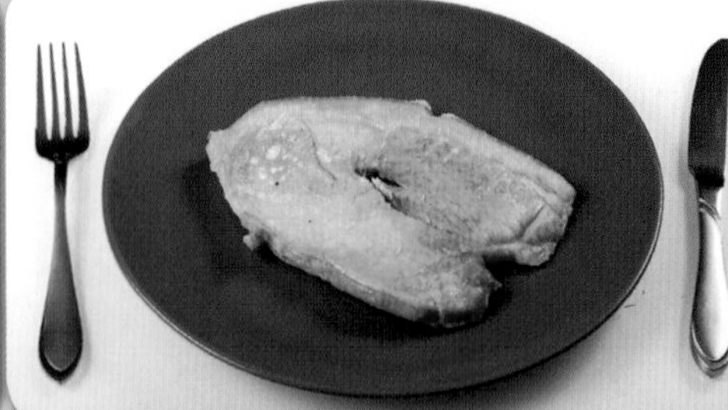

Pork Chop (grilled)

CARBS	CALS	PROTEIN	FAT	FIBRE	Weight	SAT FAT
0g	175	20g	11g	0g	68g	4g
0g	514	58g	31g	0g	200g	11g

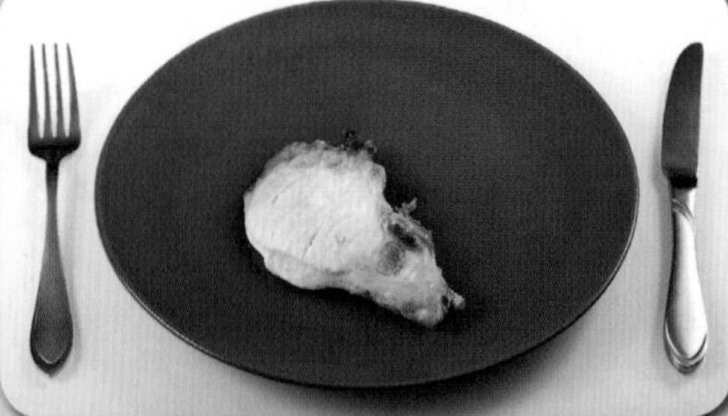

Roast Pork

CARBS	CALS	PROTEIN	FAT	FIBRE	Weight	SAT FAT
0g	161	23g	8g	0g	75g	3g
0g	269	39g	13g	0g	125g	5g

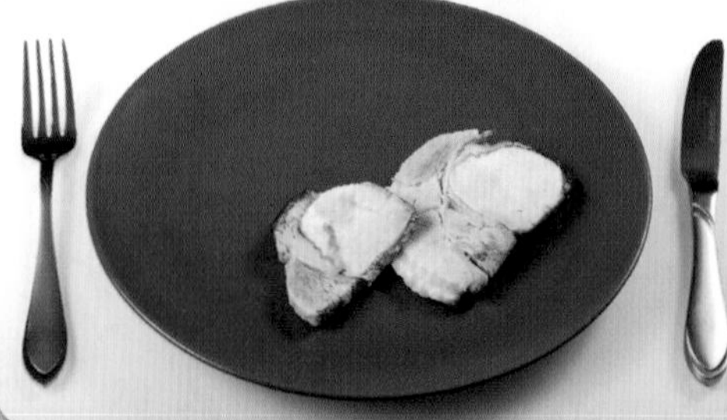

Back Bacon (fried)

0g CARBS	84 CALS	5g PROTEIN	7g FAT

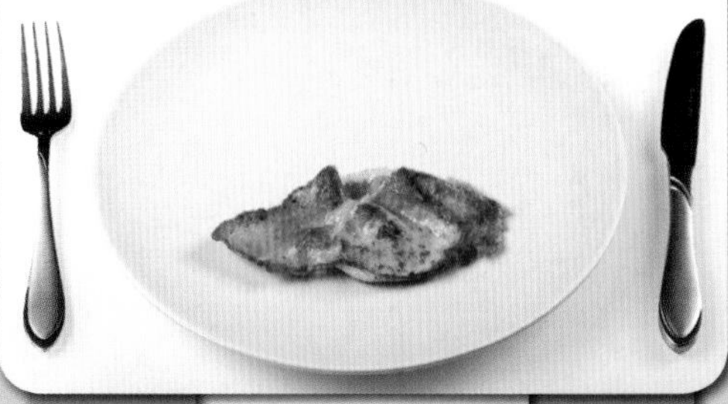

0g FIBRE	Weight: 18g	3g SAT FAT

Back Bacon (grilled)

0g CARBS	52 CALS	4g PROTEIN	4g FAT

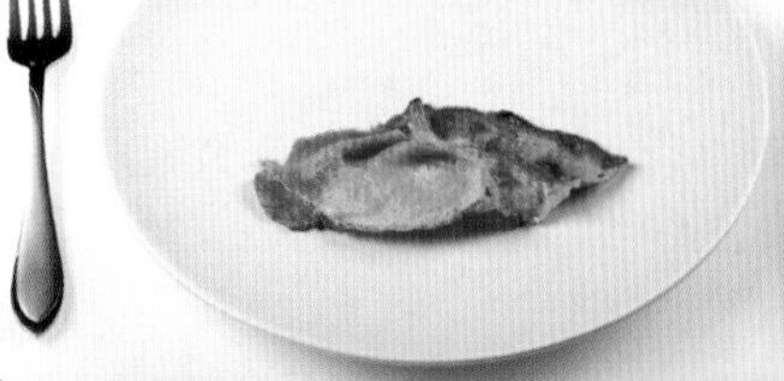

0g FIBRE	Weight: 18g	2g SAT FAT

Streaky Bacon (fried)

0g CARBS	30 CALS	2g PROTEIN	2g FAT

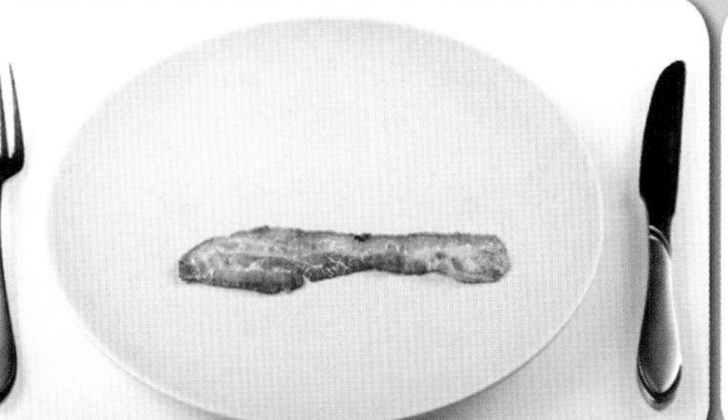

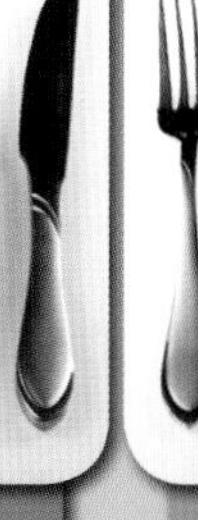

0g FIBRE	Weight: 9g	1g SAT FAT

Streaky Bacon (grilled)

0g CARBS	30 CALS	2g PROTEIN	2g FAT

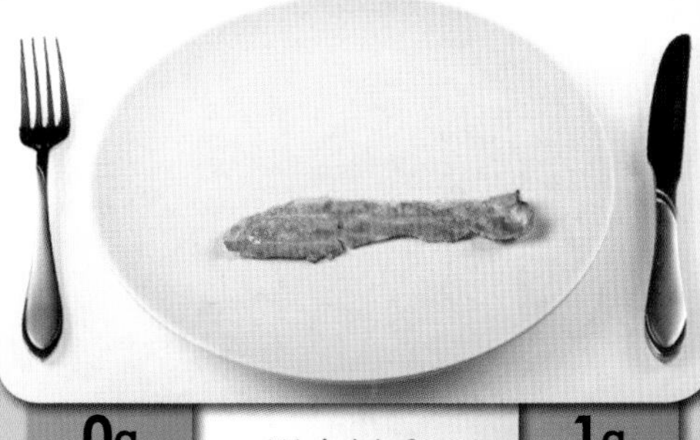

0g FIBRE	Weight: 9g	1g SAT FAT

Sausage (grilled)

2g CARBS	59 CALS	3g PROTEIN	4g FAT

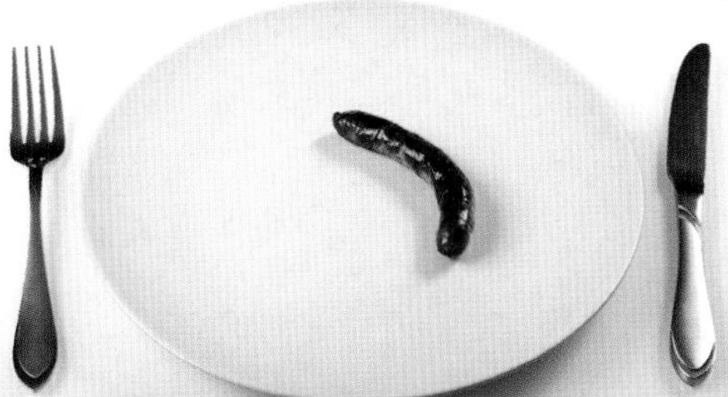

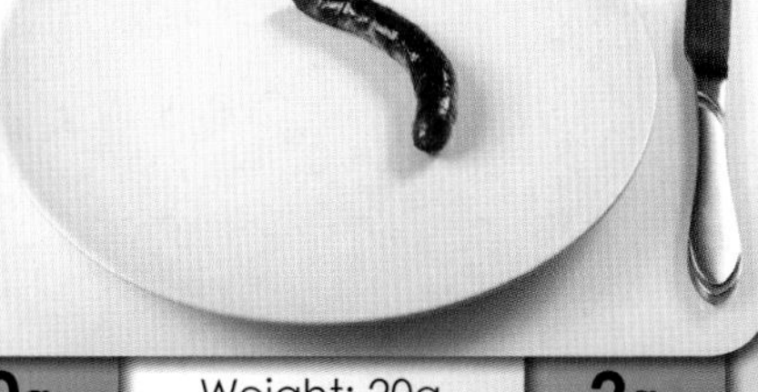

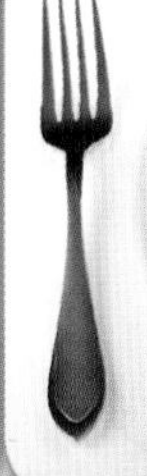

0g FIBRE	Weight: 20g (thin)	2g SAT FAT

5g CARBS	162 CALS	8g PROTEIN	12g FAT

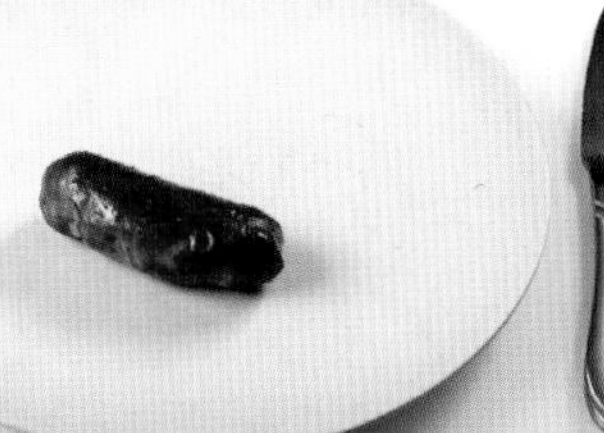

1g FIBRE	Weight: 55g (thick)	4g SAT FAT

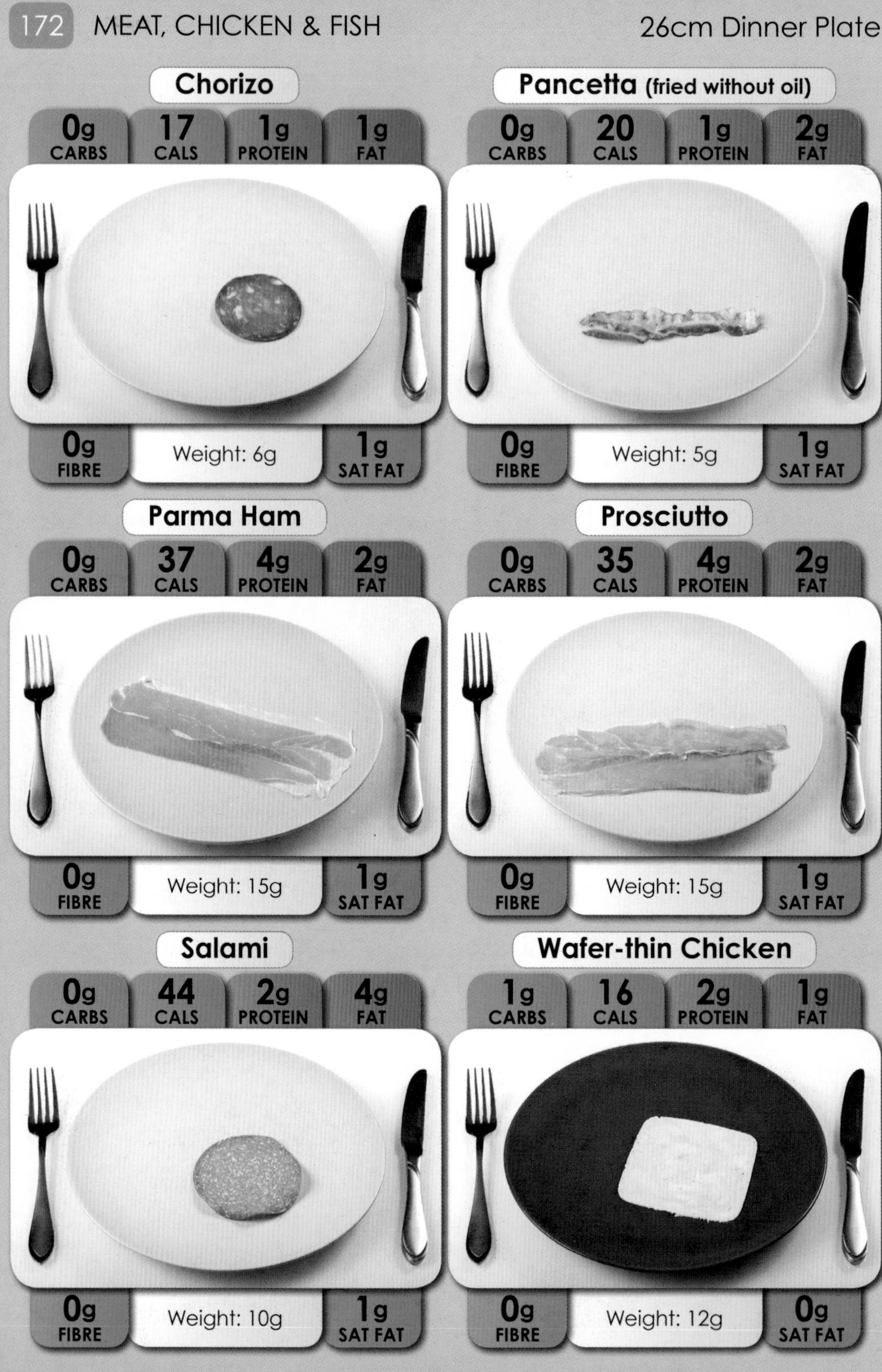

Chorizo

CARBS	CALS	PROTEIN	FAT	FIBRE	SAT FAT
0g	17	1g	1g	0g	1g

Weight: 6g

Pancetta (fried without oil)

CARBS	CALS	PROTEIN	FAT	FIBRE	SAT FAT
0g	20	1g	2g	0g	1g

Weight: 5g

Parma Ham

CARBS	CALS	PROTEIN	FAT	FIBRE	SAT FAT
0g	37	4g	2g	0g	1g

Weight: 15g

Prosciutto

CARBS	CALS	PROTEIN	FAT	FIBRE	SAT FAT
0g	35	4g	2g	0g	1g

Weight: 15g

Salami

CARBS	CALS	PROTEIN	FAT	FIBRE	SAT FAT
0g	44	2g	4g	0g	1g

Weight: 10g

Wafer-thin Chicken

CARBS	CALS	PROTEIN	FAT	FIBRE	SAT FAT
1g	16	2g	1g	0g	0g

Weight: 12g

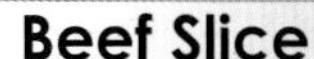

Beef Slice

CARBS	CALS	PROTEIN	FAT
0g	69	13g	2g

FIBRE	Weight	SAT FAT
0g	Weight: 50g	1g

Wafer-thin Beef

CARBS	CALS	PROTEIN	FAT
0g	16	3g	0g

FIBRE	Weight	SAT FAT
0g	Weight: 12g	0g

Ham Slice

CARBS	CALS	PROTEIN	FAT
0g	32	6g	1g

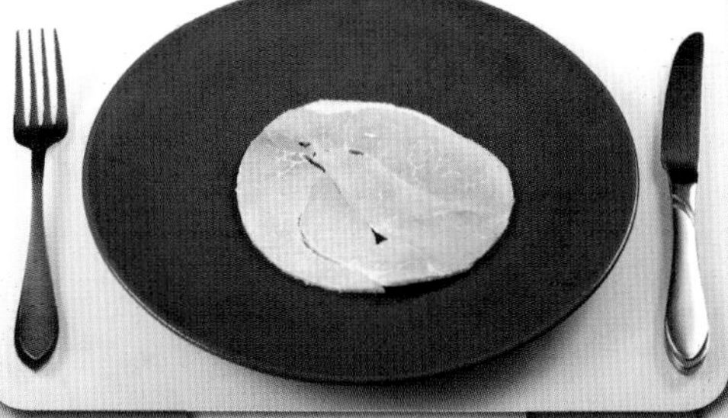

FIBRE	Weight	SAT FAT
0g	Weight: 30g	0g

Wafer-thin Ham

CARBS	CALS	PROTEIN	FAT
0g	13	2g	0g

FIBRE	Weight	SAT FAT
0g	Weight: 12g	0g

Turkey Slice

CARBS	CALS	PROTEIN	FAT
0g	49	9g	1g

FIBRE	Weight	SAT FAT
0g	Weight: 40g	1g

Wafer-thin Turkey

CARBS	CALS	PROTEIN	FAT
0g	8	1g	0g

FIBRE	Weight	SAT FAT
0g	Weight: 8g	0g

Beef Burger (fried)

Carbs	Cals	Protein	Fat	Fibre	Weight	Sat Fat
0g	329	29g	24g	0g	100g	11g

Beef Burger (grilled)

Carbs	Cals	Protein	Fat	Fibre	Weight	Sat Fat
0g	326	27g	24g	0g	100g	11g

Corned Beef

Carbs	Cals	Protein	Fat	Fibre	Weight	Sat Fat
0g	62	8g	3g	0g	30g	2g

Roast Beef

Carbs	Cals	Protein	Fat	Fibre	Weight	Sat Fat
0g	89	12g	5g	0g	40g	2g
0g	167	22g	9g	0g	75g	4g
0g	278	37g	14g	0g	125g	6g

Rump Steak (fried)

Carbs	Cals	Protein	Fat	Fibre	Sat Fat	Weight
0g	155	19g	9g	0g	3g	68g

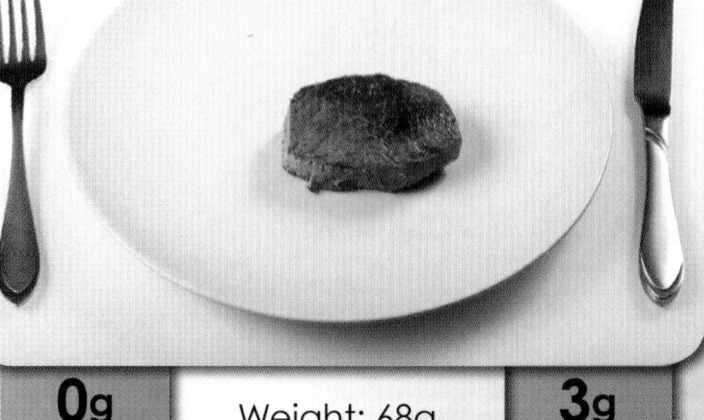

Carbs	Cals	Protein	Fat	Fibre	Sat Fat	Weight
0g	442	55g	25g	0g	10g	194g

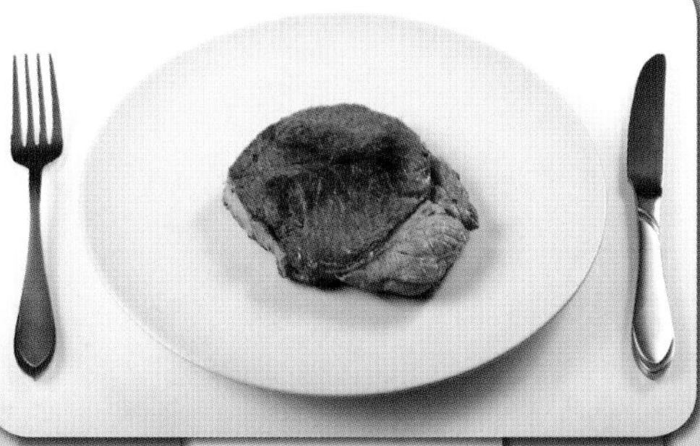

Carbs	Cals	Protein	Fat	Fibre	Sat Fat	Weight
0g	951	118g	53g	0g	20g	417g

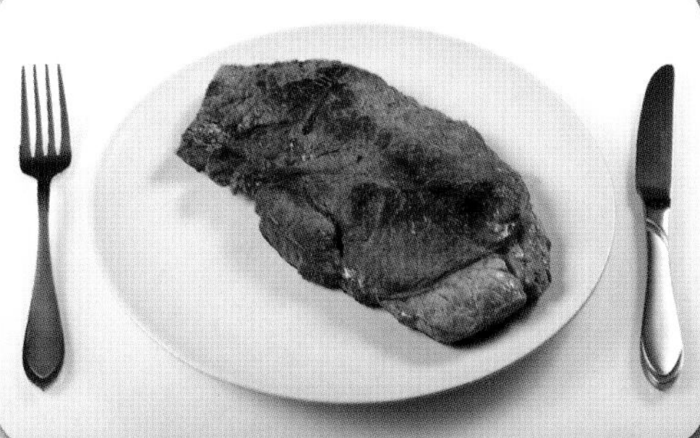

Sirloin Steak (fried)

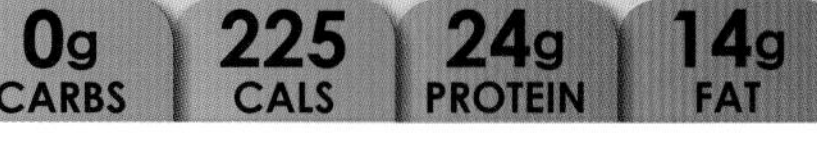

Carbs	Cals	Protein	Fat	Fibre	Sat Fat	Weight
0g	225	24g	14g	0g	6g	112g

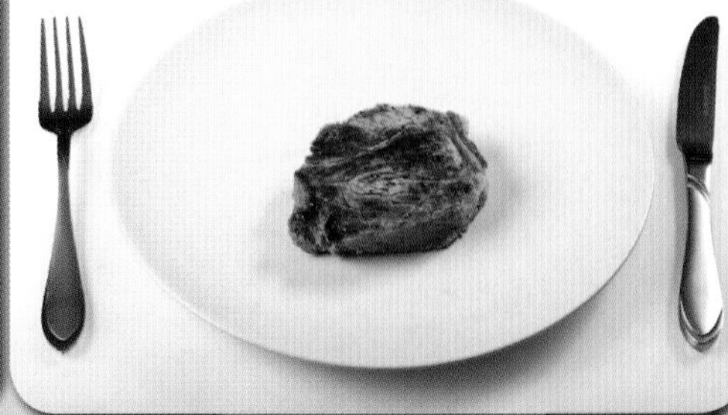

Carbs	Cals	Protein	Fat	Fibre	Sat Fat	Weight
0g	394	42g	25g	0g	11g	196g

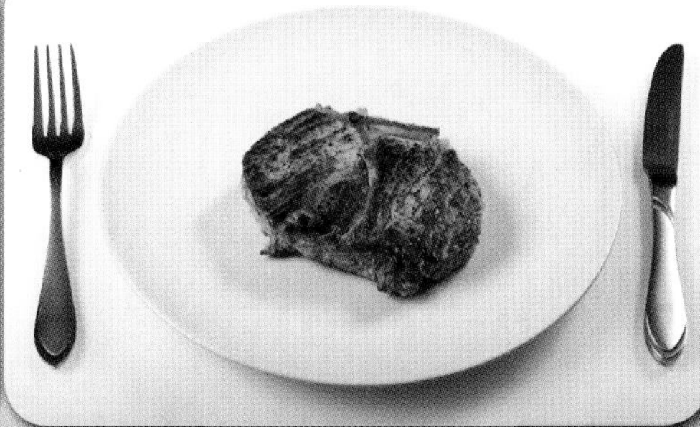

Carbs	Cals	Protein	Fat	Fibre	Sat Fat	Weight
0g	527	57g	33g	0g	15g	262g

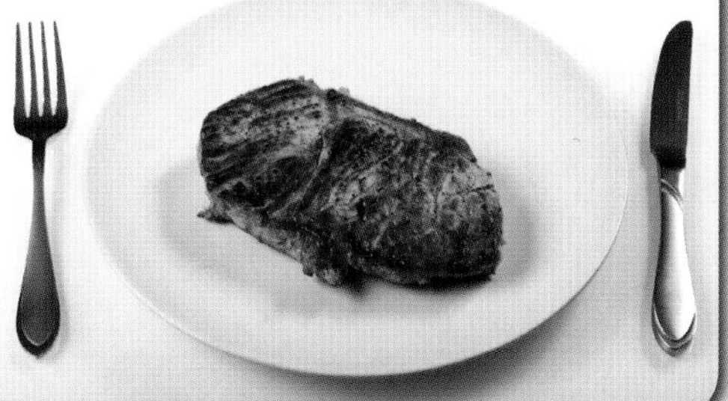

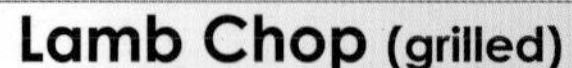

Lamb Chop (grilled)

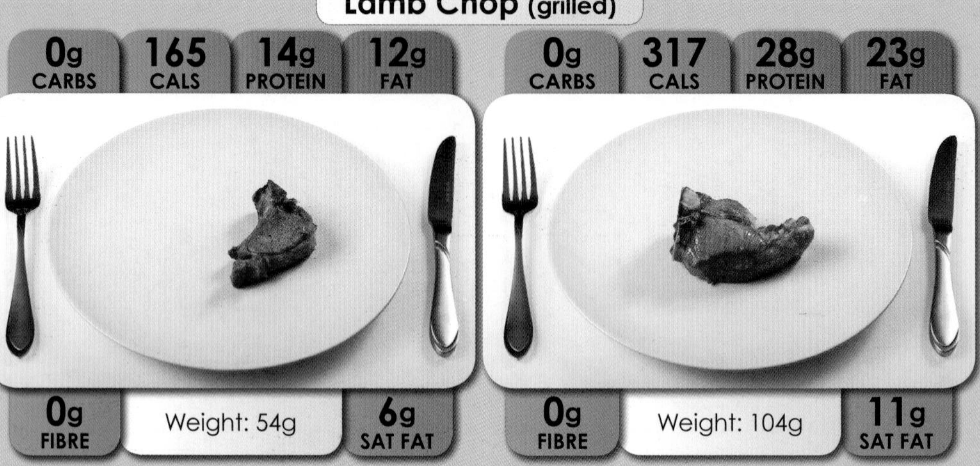

	CARBS	CALS	PROTEIN	FAT	FIBRE	Weight	SAT FAT
Left	0g	165	14g	12g	0g	Weight: 54g	6g
Right	0g	317	28g	23g	0g	Weight: 104g	11g

Lamb Steak (grilled)

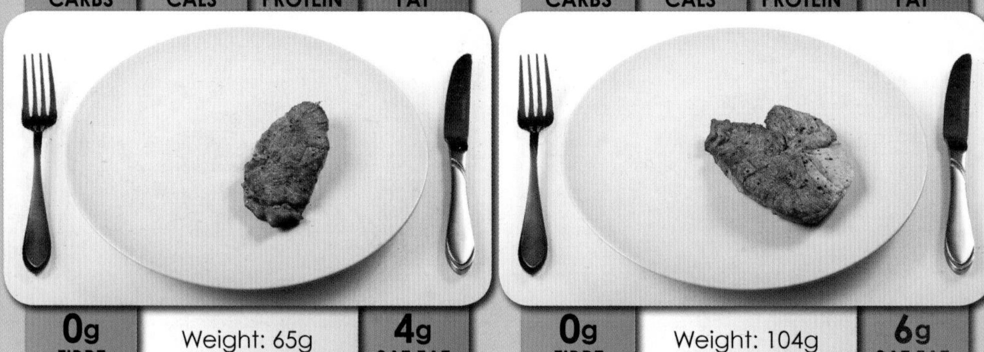

	CARBS	CALS	PROTEIN	FAT	FIBRE	Weight	SAT FAT
Left	0g	150	18g	9g	0g	Weight: 65g	4g
Right	0g	240	29g	14g	0g	Weight: 104g	6g

Roast Lamb

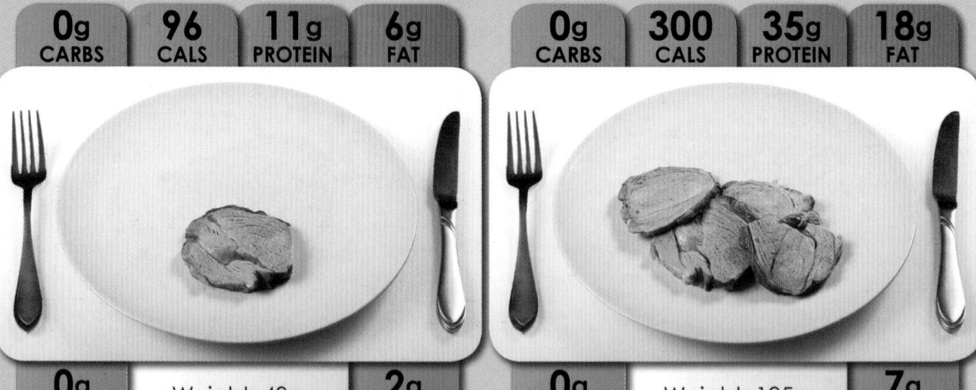

	CARBS	CALS	PROTEIN	FAT	FIBRE	Weight	SAT FAT
Left	0g	96	11g	6g	0g	Weight: 40g	2g
Right	0g	300	35g	18g	0g	Weight: 125g	7g

BBQ Chicken Wings

CARBS	CALS	PROTEIN	FAT
3g	192	19g	12g

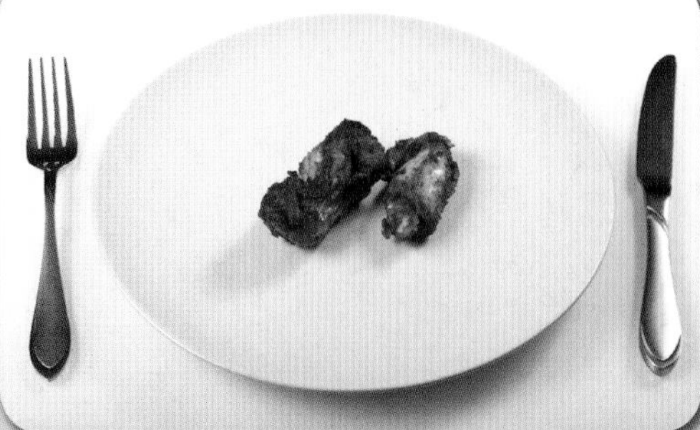

FIBRE	Weight	SAT FAT
0g	Weight: 70g	3g

CARBS	CALS	PROTEIN	FAT
6g	370	37g	22g

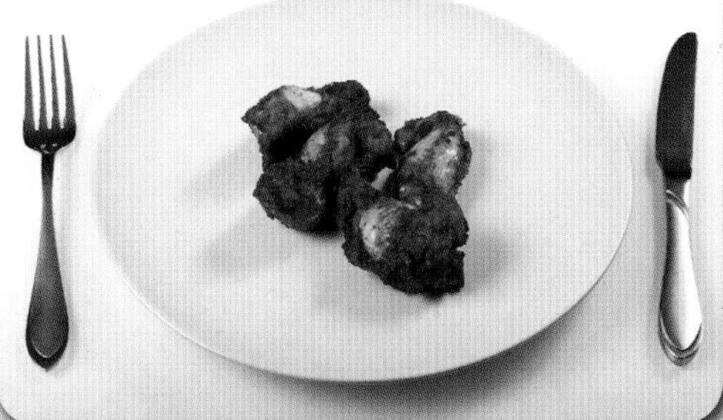

FIBRE	Weight	SAT FAT
0g	Weight: 135g	6g

CARBS	CALS	PROTEIN	FAT
8g	548	55g	33g

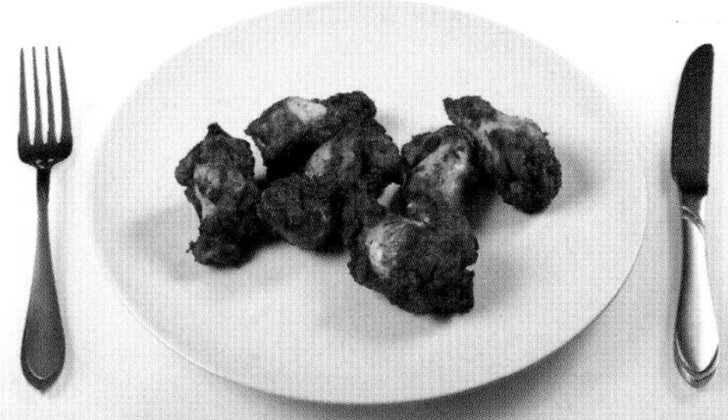

FIBRE	Weight	SAT FAT
0g	Weight: 200g	9g

Chicken Drumsticks (roasted)

CARBS	CALS	PROTEIN	FAT
0g	139	19g	7g

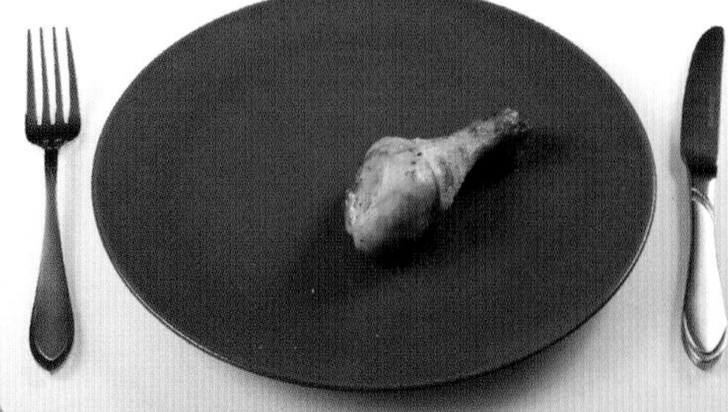

FIBRE	Weight	SAT FAT
0g	Weight: 75g	2g

CARBS	CALS	PROTEIN	FAT
0g	259	36g	13g

FIBRE	Weight	SAT FAT
0g	Weight: 140g	4g

CARBS	CALS	PROTEIN	FAT
0g	389	54g	19g

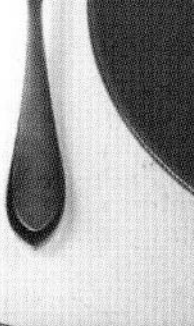

FIBRE	Weight	SAT FAT
0g	Weight: 210g	5g

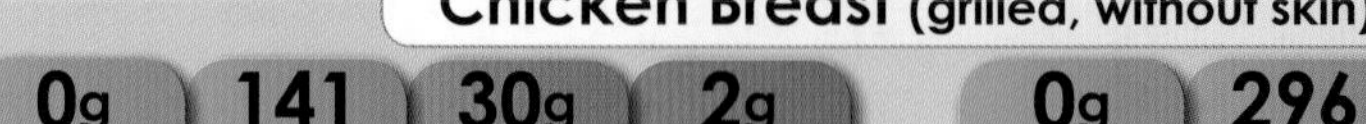

Chicken Breast (grilled, without skin)

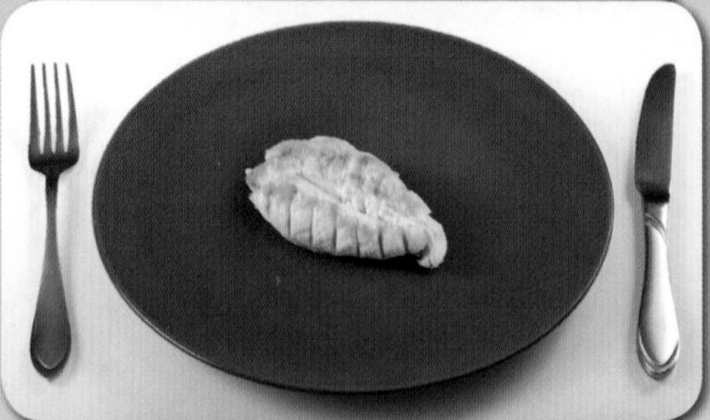

	Portion 1	Portion 2
CARBS	0g	0g
CALS	141	296
PROTEIN	30g	64g
FAT	2g	4g
FIBRE	0g	0g
Weight	95g	200g
SAT FAT	1g	1g

Chicken Breast (grilled, with skin)

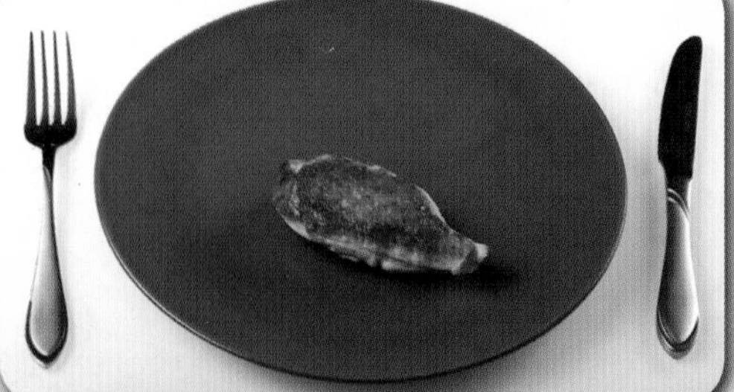

	Portion 1	Portion 2
CARBS	0g	0g
CALS	118	199
PROTEIN	24g	40g
FAT	3g	4g
FIBRE	0g	0g
Weight	80g	135g
SAT FAT	1g	1g

Roast Chicken (with skin)

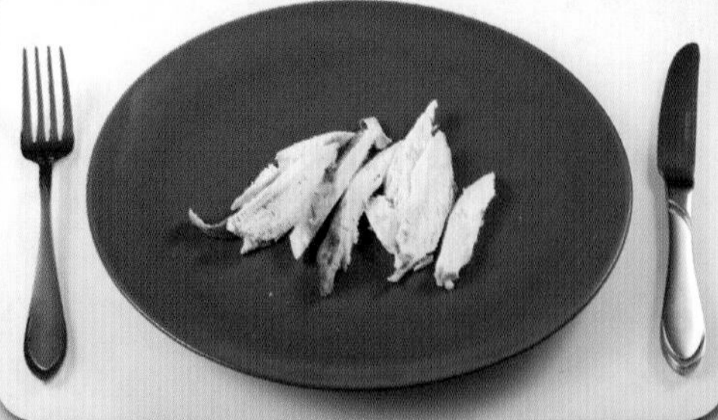

	Portion 1	Portion 2
CARBS	0g	0g
CALS	106	221
PROTEIN	16g	34g
FAT	5g	9g
FIBRE	0g	0g
Weight	60g	125g
SAT FAT	1g	3g

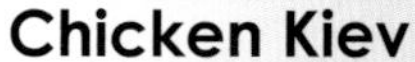

Chicken Kiev

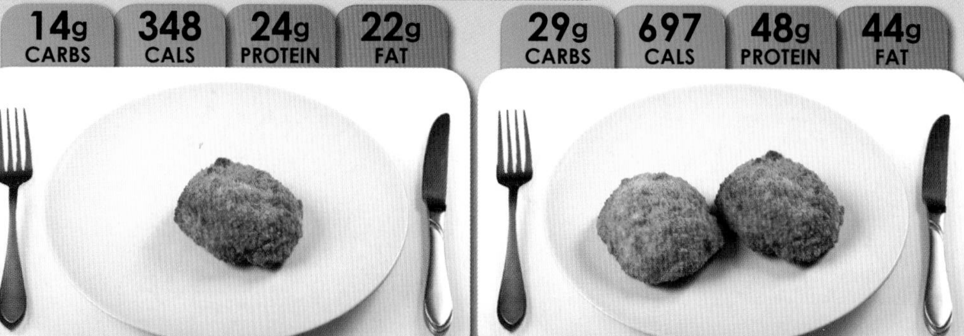

	Weight	Carbs	Cals	Protein	Fat	Fibre	Sat Fat
Left	130g	14g	348	24g	22g	1g	9g
Right	260g	29g	697	48g	44g	2g	19g

Roast Turkey (with skin)

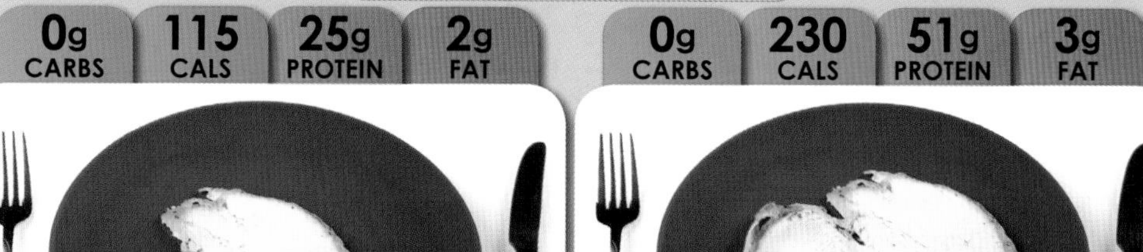

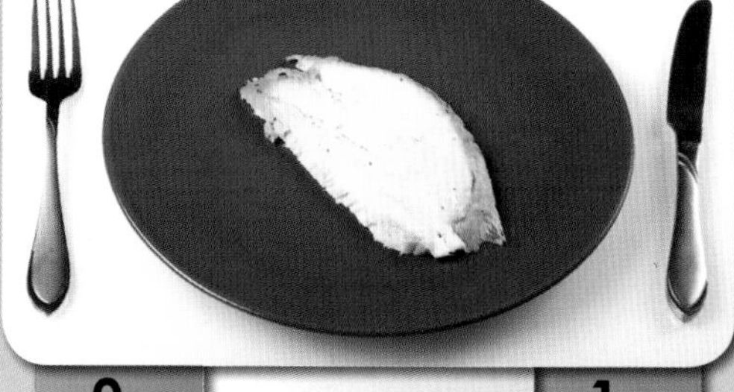

	Weight	Carbs	Cals	Protein	Fat	Fibre	Sat Fat
Left	75g	0g	115	25g	2g	0g	1g
Right	150g	0g	230	51g	3g	0g	1g

Turkey Breast (grilled)

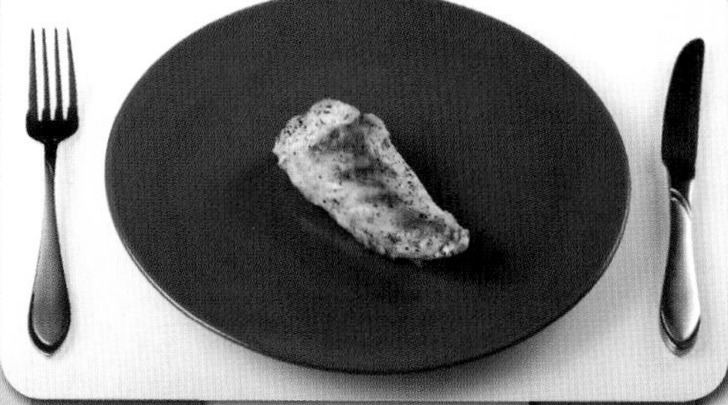

	Weight	Carbs	Cals	Protein	Fat	Fibre	Sat Fat
Left	85g	0g	132	30g	1g	0g	1g
Right	200g	0g	310	70g	3g	0g	1g

Fish (battered, baked)

CARBS	CALS	PROTEIN	FAT	FIBRE	Weight	SAT FAT
9g	137	8g	8g	1g	65g	2g

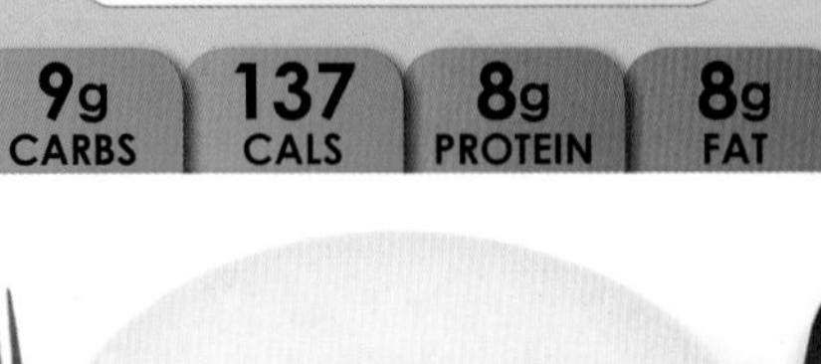
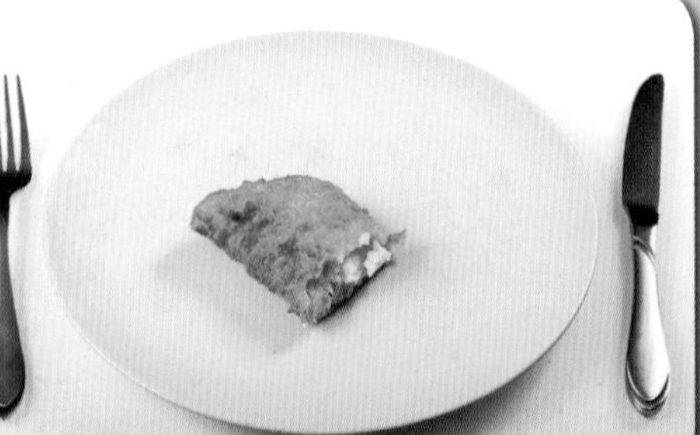
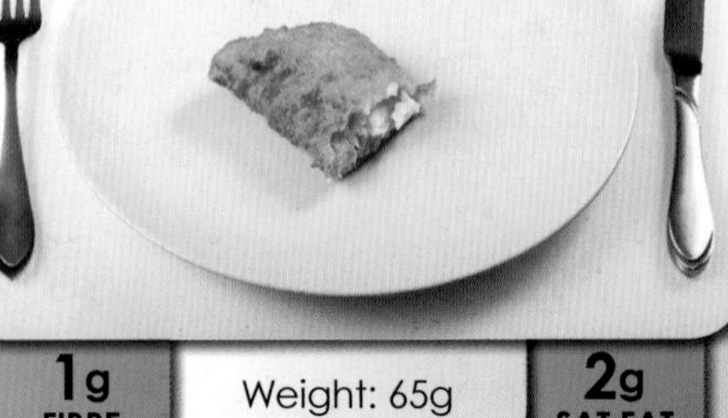

CARBS	CALS	PROTEIN	FAT	FIBRE	Weight	SAT FAT
19g	274	17g	15g	1g	130g	5g

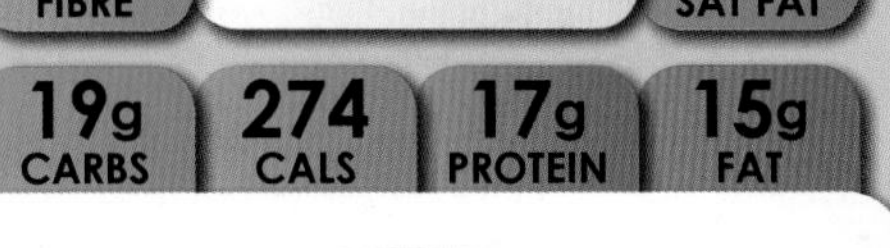
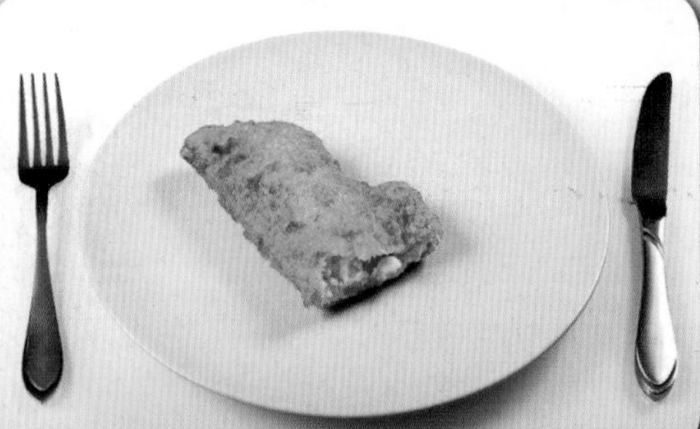

CARBS	CALS	PROTEIN	FAT	FIBRE	Weight	SAT FAT
38g	559	34g	31g	2g	265g	10g

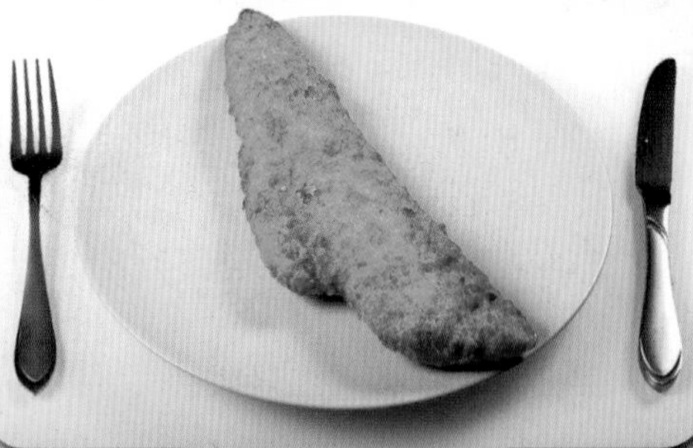
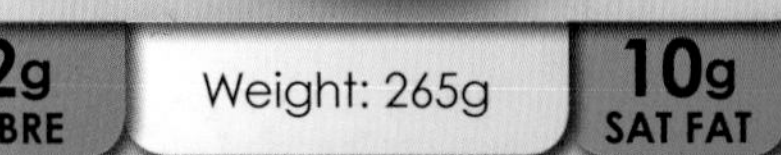

Fish (breaded, baked)

CARBS	CALS	PROTEIN	FAT	FIBRE	Weight	SAT FAT
10g	108	7g	4g	1g	53g	1g

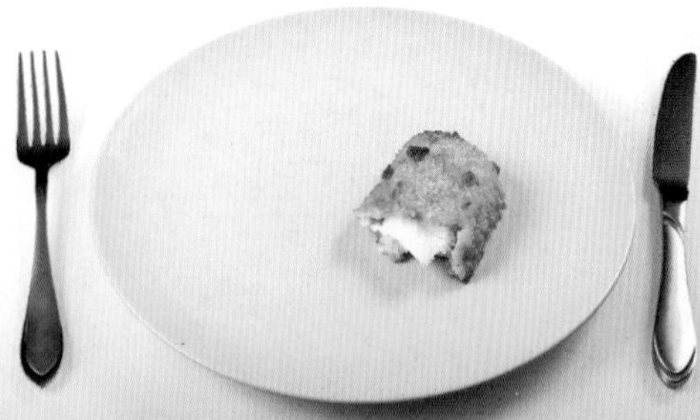

CARBS	CALS	PROTEIN	FAT	FIBRE	Weight	SAT FAT
20g	215	14g	9g	1g	106g	1g

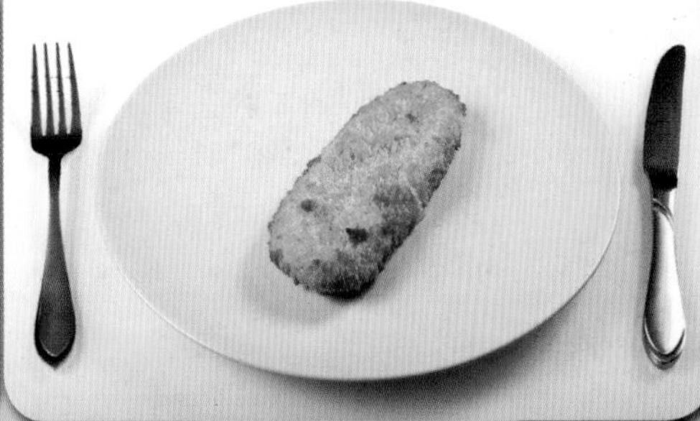

CARBS	CALS	PROTEIN	FAT	FIBRE	Weight	SAT FAT
30g	317	20g	13g	1g	156g	1g

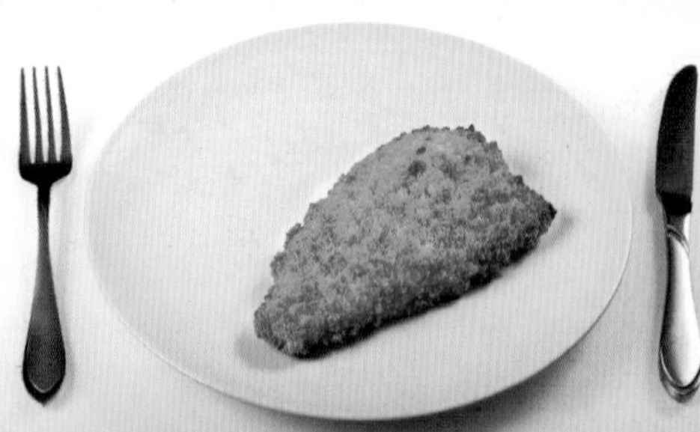

Fish Cake (baked)

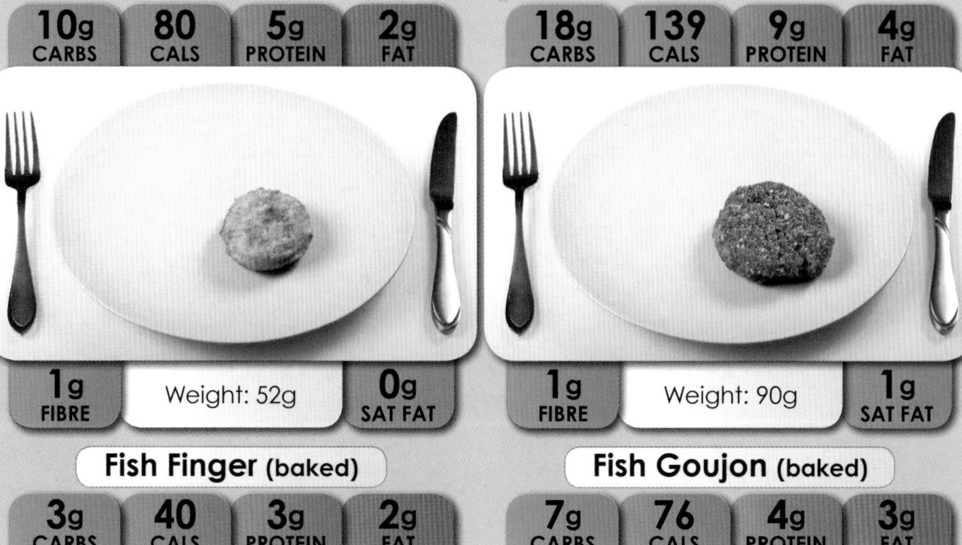

	Portion 1	Portion 2
Carbs	10g	18g
Cals	80	139
Protein	5g	9g
Fat	2g	4g
Fibre	1g	1g
Weight	52g	90g
Sat Fat	0g	1g

Fish Finger (baked)

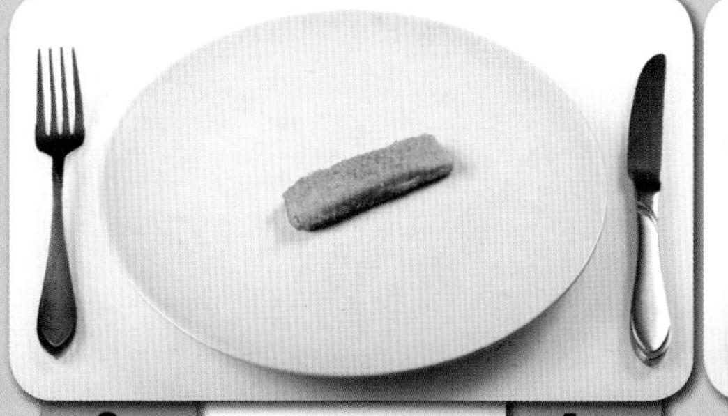

Carbs	Cals	Protein	Fat	Fibre	Weight	Sat Fat
3g	40	3g	2g	0g	20g	1g

Fish Goujon (baked)

Carbs	Cals	Protein	Fat	Fibre	Weight	Sat Fat
7g	76	4g	3g	1g	30g	0g

Scampi (fried)

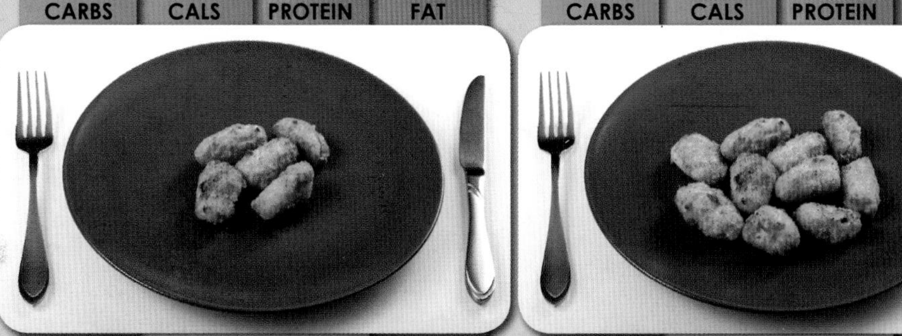

	Portion 1	Portion 2
Carbs	14g	29g
Cals	166	332
Protein	7g	13g
Fat	10g	19g
Fibre	1g	2g
Weight	70g	140g
Sat Fat	1g	2g

Prawns (boiled)

CARBS	CALS	PROTEIN	FAT
0g	50	11g	1g

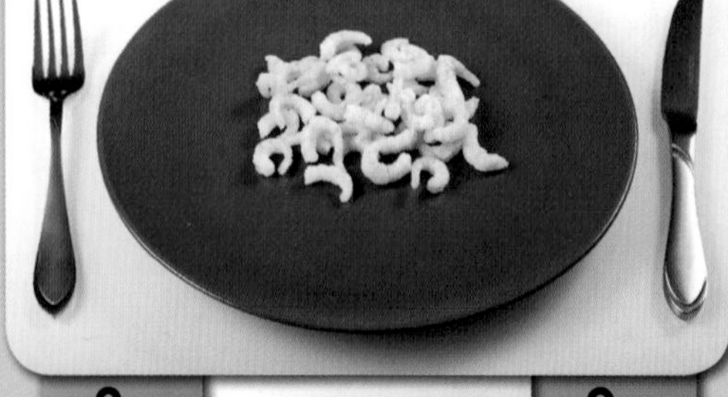

FIBRE	Weight	SAT FAT
0g	Weight: 50g	0g

CARBS	CALS	PROTEIN	FAT
0g	99	23g	1g

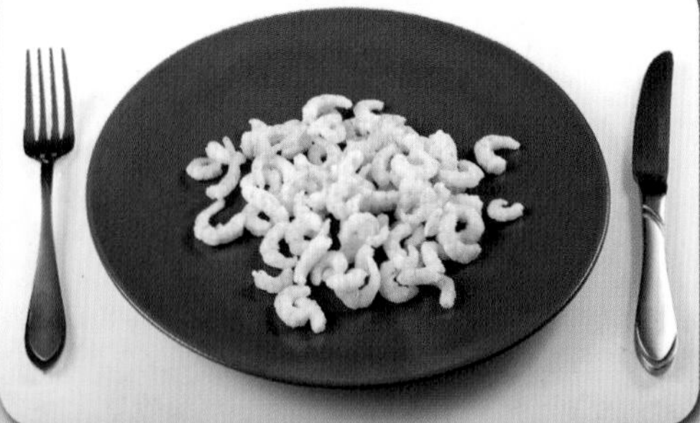

FIBRE	Weight	SAT FAT
0g	Weight: 100g	0g

CARBS	CALS	PROTEIN	FAT
0g	149	34g	1g

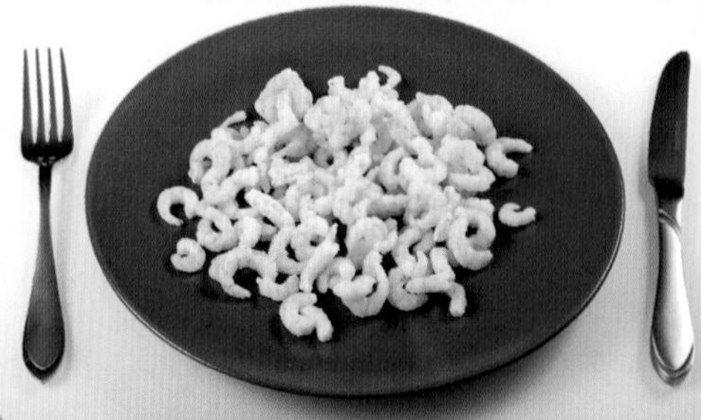

FIBRE	Weight	SAT FAT
0g	Weight: 150g	0g

King Prawns (boiled)

CARBS	CALS	PROTEIN	FAT
0g	50	11g	1g

FIBRE	Weight	SAT FAT
0g	Weight: 50g	0g

CARBS	CALS	PROTEIN	FAT
0g	99	23g	1g

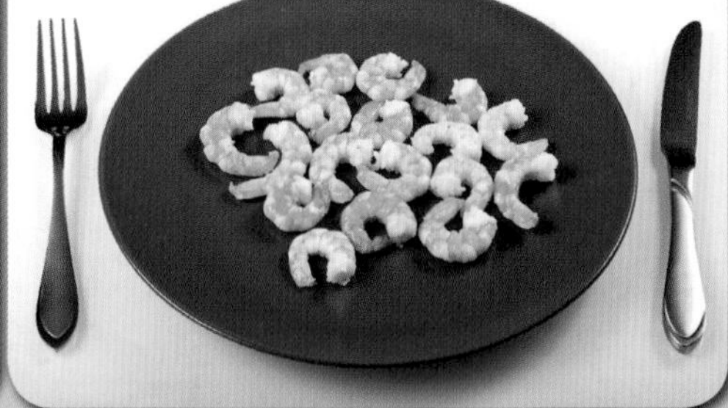

FIBRE	Weight	SAT FAT
0g	Weight: 100g	0g

CARBS	CALS	PROTEIN	FAT
0g	149	34g	1g

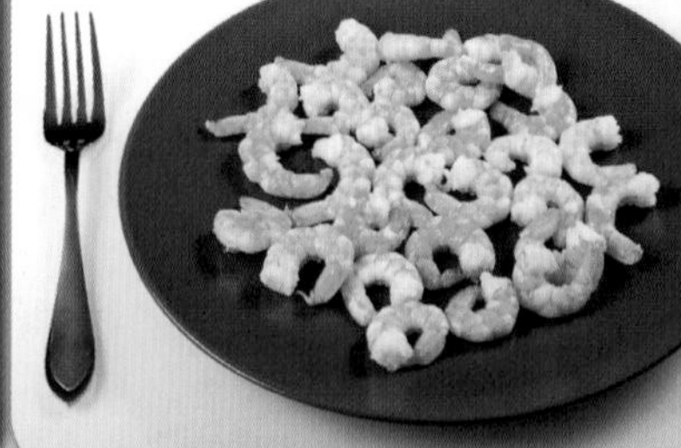

FIBRE	Weight	SAT FAT
0g	Weight: 150g	0g

Salmon (tinned in brine)

CARBS	CALS	PROTEIN	FAT
0g	142	18g	8g

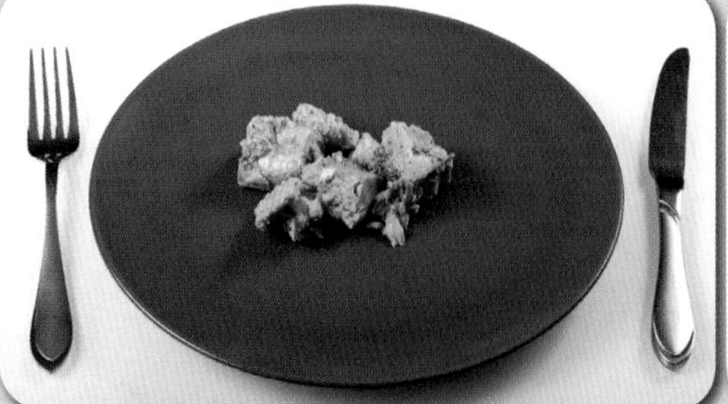

FIBRE		SAT FAT
0g	Weight: 85g (half tin)	1g

CARBS	CALS	PROTEIN	FAT
0g	284	37g	15g

FIBRE		SAT FAT
0g	Weight: 170g (full tin)	3g

Tuna (tinned in brine)

CARBS	CALS	PROTEIN	FAT
0g	69	17g	0g

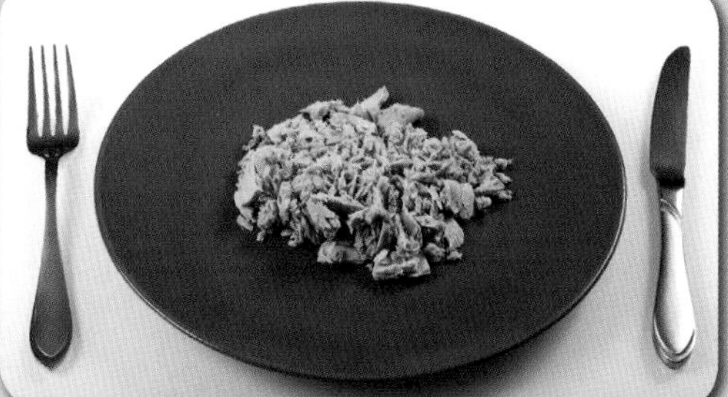

FIBRE		SAT FAT
0g	Weight: 70g (half tin)	0g

CARBS	CALS	PROTEIN	FAT
0g	139	33g	1g

FIBRE		SAT FAT
0g	Weight: 140g (full tin)	0g

Tuna (tinned in oil)

CARBS	CALS	PROTEIN	FAT
0g	132	19g	6g

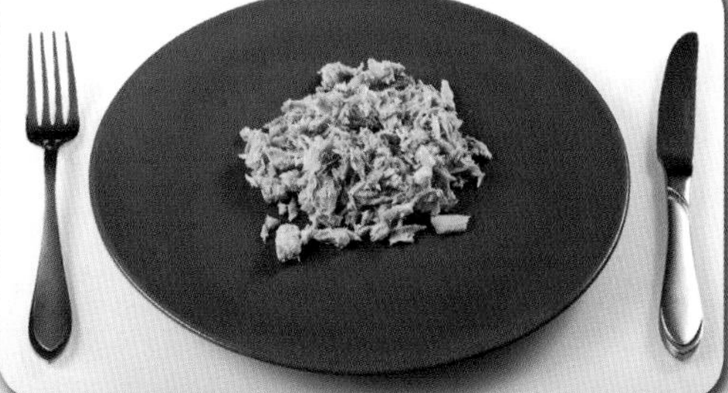

FIBRE		SAT FAT
0g	Weight: 70g (half tin)	1g

CARBS	CALS	PROTEIN	FAT
0g	265	38g	13g

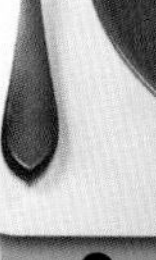

FIBRE		SAT FAT
0g	Weight: 140g (full tin)	2g

Sardines (tinned in brine)

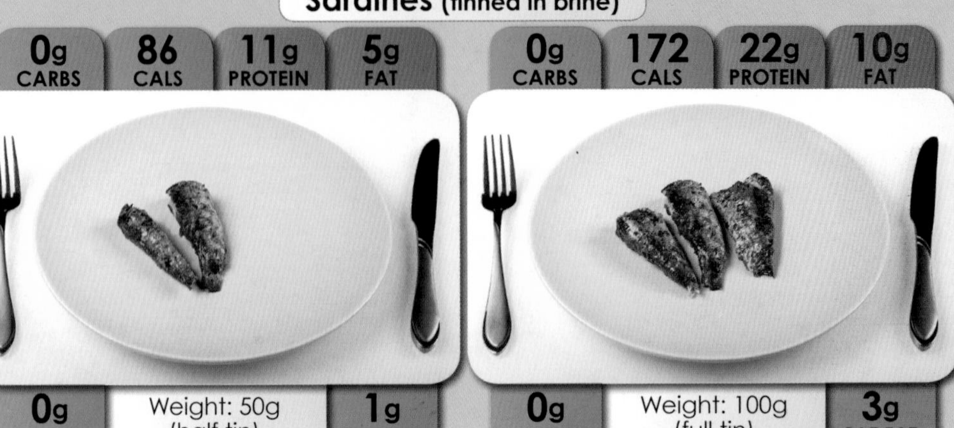

Weight	Carbs	Cals	Protein	Fat	Fibre	Sat Fat
Weight: 50g (half tin)	0g	86	11g	5g	0g	1g
Weight: 100g (full tin)	0g	172	22g	10g	0g	3g

Sardines (tinned in oil)

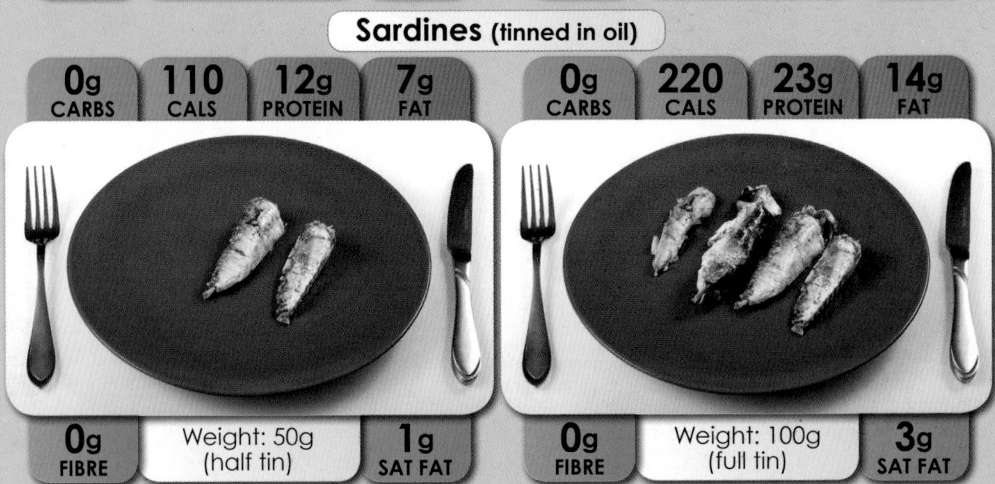

Weight	Carbs	Cals	Protein	Fat	Fibre	Sat Fat
Weight: 50g (half tin)	0g	110	12g	7g	0g	1g
Weight: 100g (full tin)	0g	220	23g	14g	0g	3g

Sardines (tinned in tomato sauce)

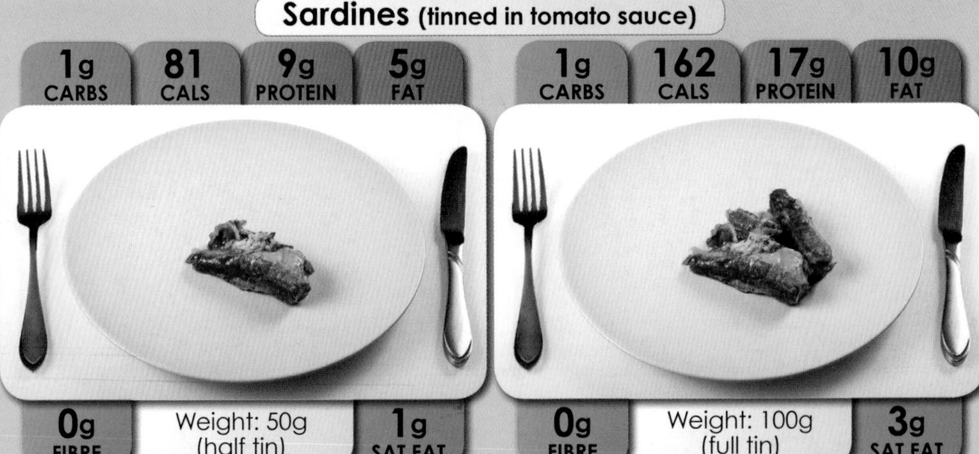

Weight	Carbs	Cals	Protein	Fat	Fibre	Sat Fat
Weight: 50g (half tin)	1g	81	9g	5g	0g	1g
Weight: 100g (full tin)	1g	162	17g	10g	0g	3g

Smoked Mackerel

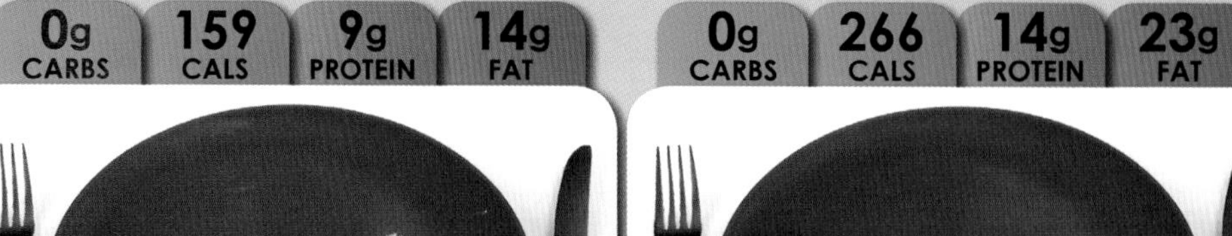

	CARBS	CALS	PROTEIN	FAT	FIBRE	Weight	SAT FAT
Left	0g	159	9g	14g	0g	45g	3g
Right	0g	266	14g	23g	0g	75g	5g

Smoked Salmon

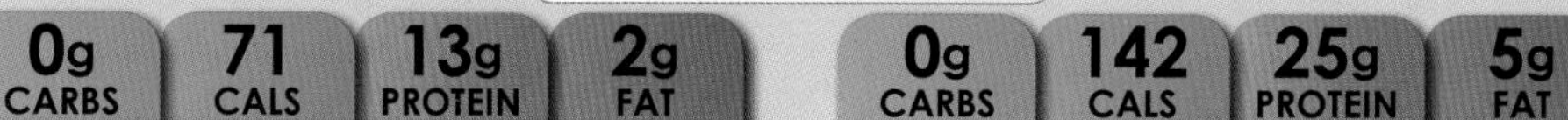

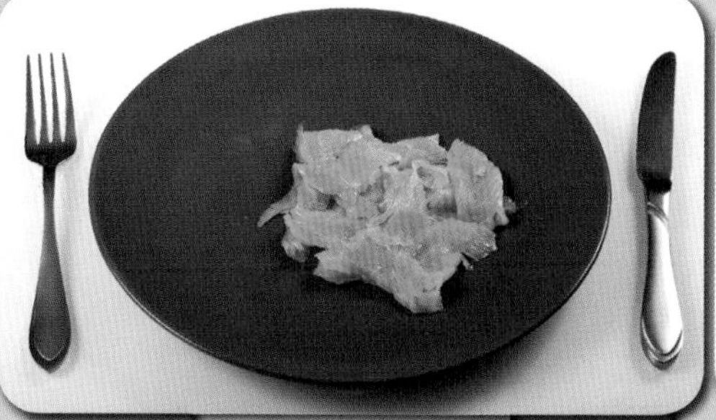

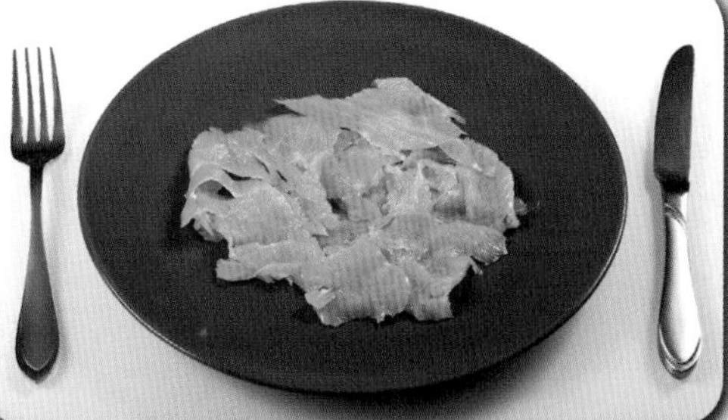

	CARBS	CALS	PROTEIN	FAT	FIBRE	Weight	SAT FAT
Left	0g	71	13g	2g	0g	50g	0g
Right	0g	142	25g	5g	0g	100g	1g

Saltfish (boiled)

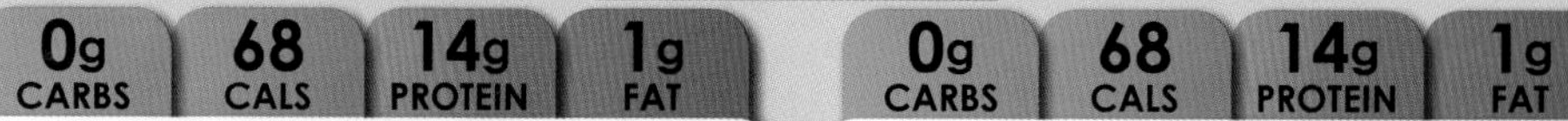

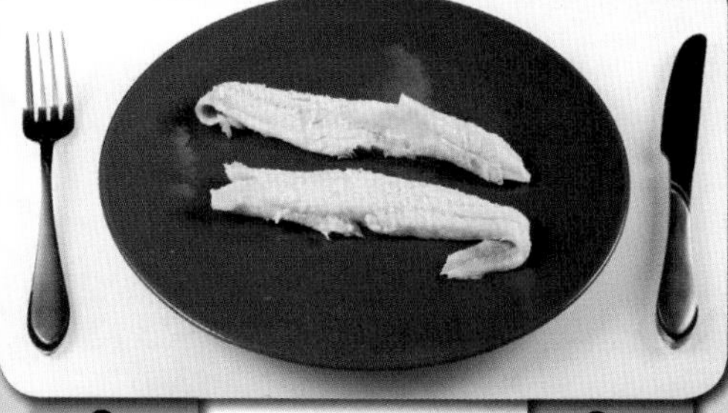

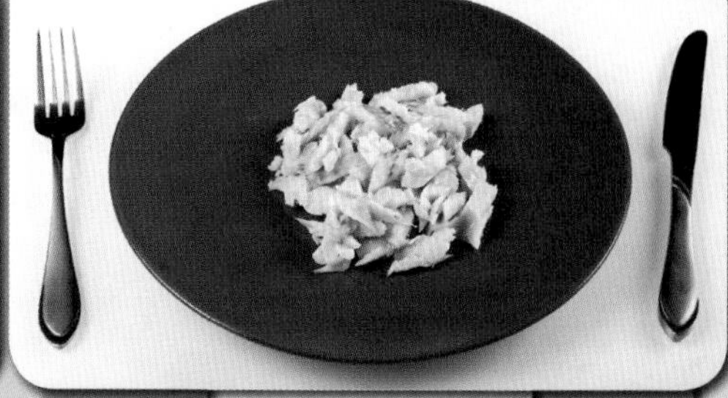

	CARBS	CALS	PROTEIN	FAT	FIBRE	Weight	SAT FAT
Left	0g	68	14g	1g	0g	80g	0g
Right	0g	68	14g	1g	0g	80g	0g

Cod / Haddock (baked)

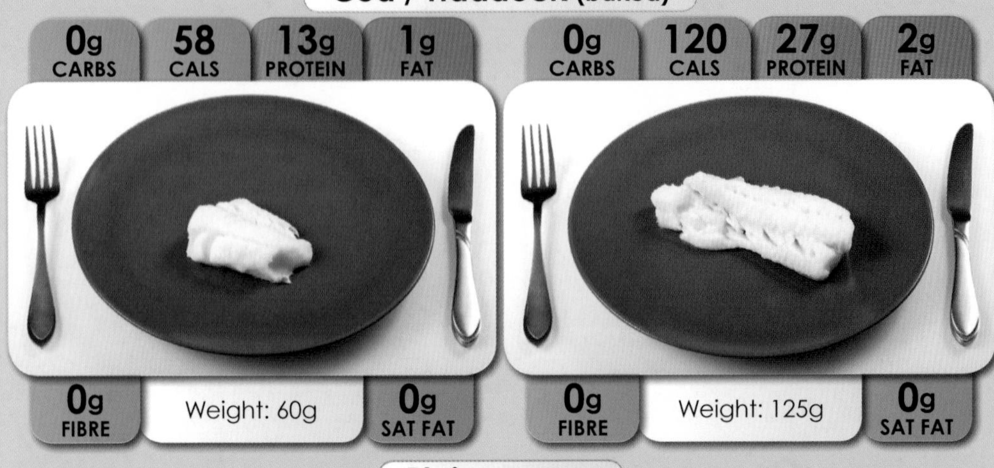

Weight	Carbs	Cals	Protein	Fat	Fibre	Sat Fat
60g	0g	58	13g	1g	0g	0g
125g	0g	120	27g	2g	0g	0g

Plaice (grilled)

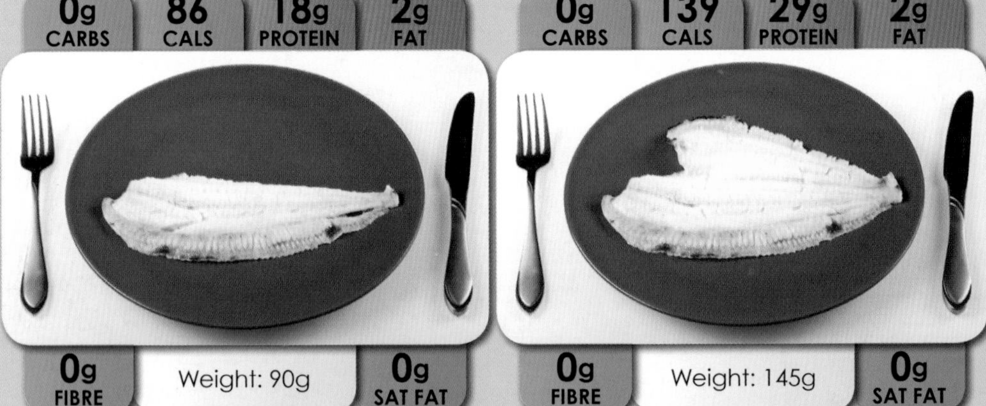

Weight	Carbs	Cals	Protein	Fat	Fibre	Sat Fat
90g	0g	86	18g	2g	0g	0g
145g	0g	139	29g	2g	0g	0g

Scallops (fried)

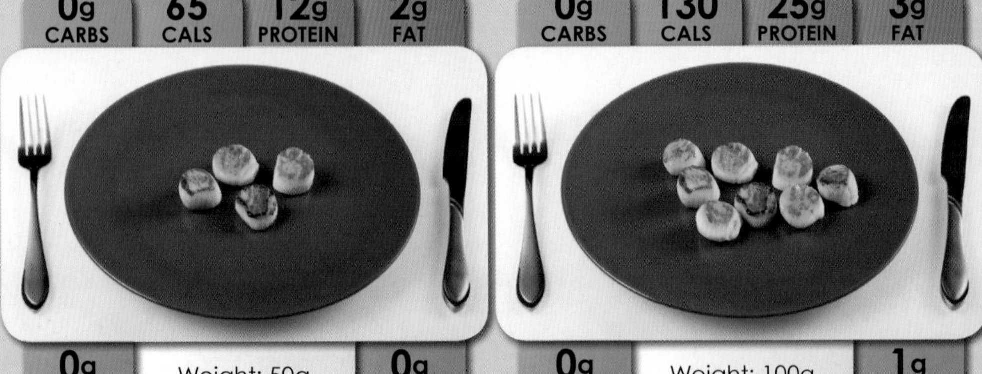

Weight	Carbs	Cals	Protein	Fat	Fibre	Sat Fat
50g	0g	65	12g	2g	0g	0g
100g	0g	130	25g	3g	0g	1g

Salmon Steak (grilled)

CARBS	CALS	PROTEIN	FAT	FIBRE	Weight	SAT FAT
0g	129	15g	8g	0g	60g	2g
0g	280	32g	17g	0g	130g	3g

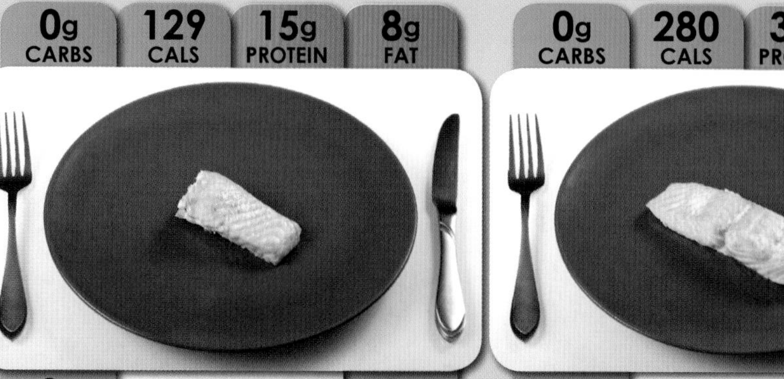

Trout Fillet (grilled)

CARBS	CALS	PROTEIN	FAT	FIBRE	Weight	SAT FAT
0g	81	13g	3g	0g	60g	1g
0g	142	23g	6g	0g	105g	1g

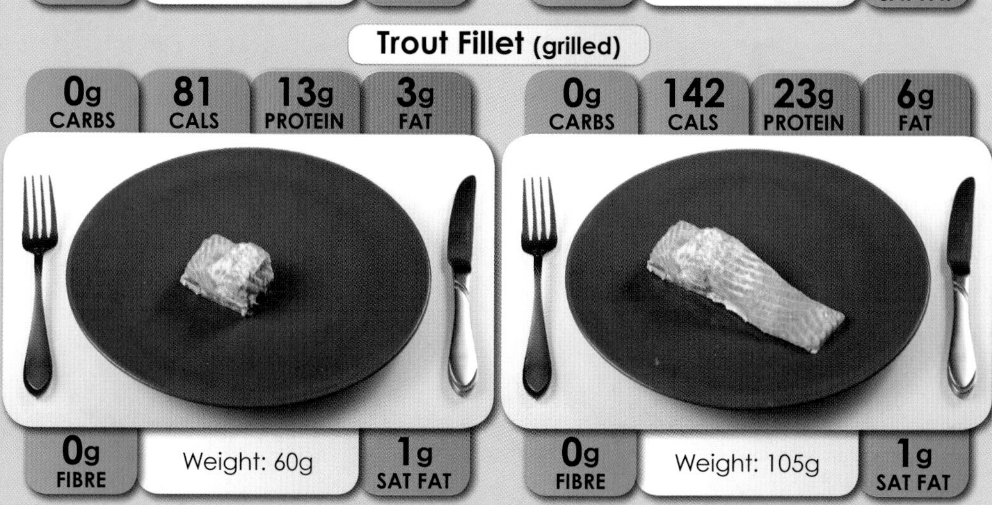

Tuna Steak (grilled)

CARBS	CALS	PROTEIN	FAT	FIBRE	Weight	SAT FAT
0g	102	18g	4g	0g	75g	1g
0g	177	31g	6g	0g	130g	2g

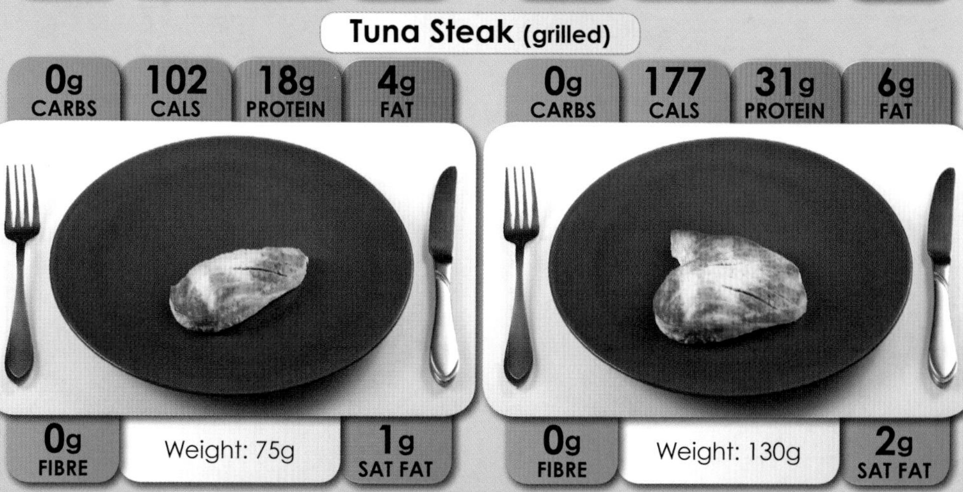

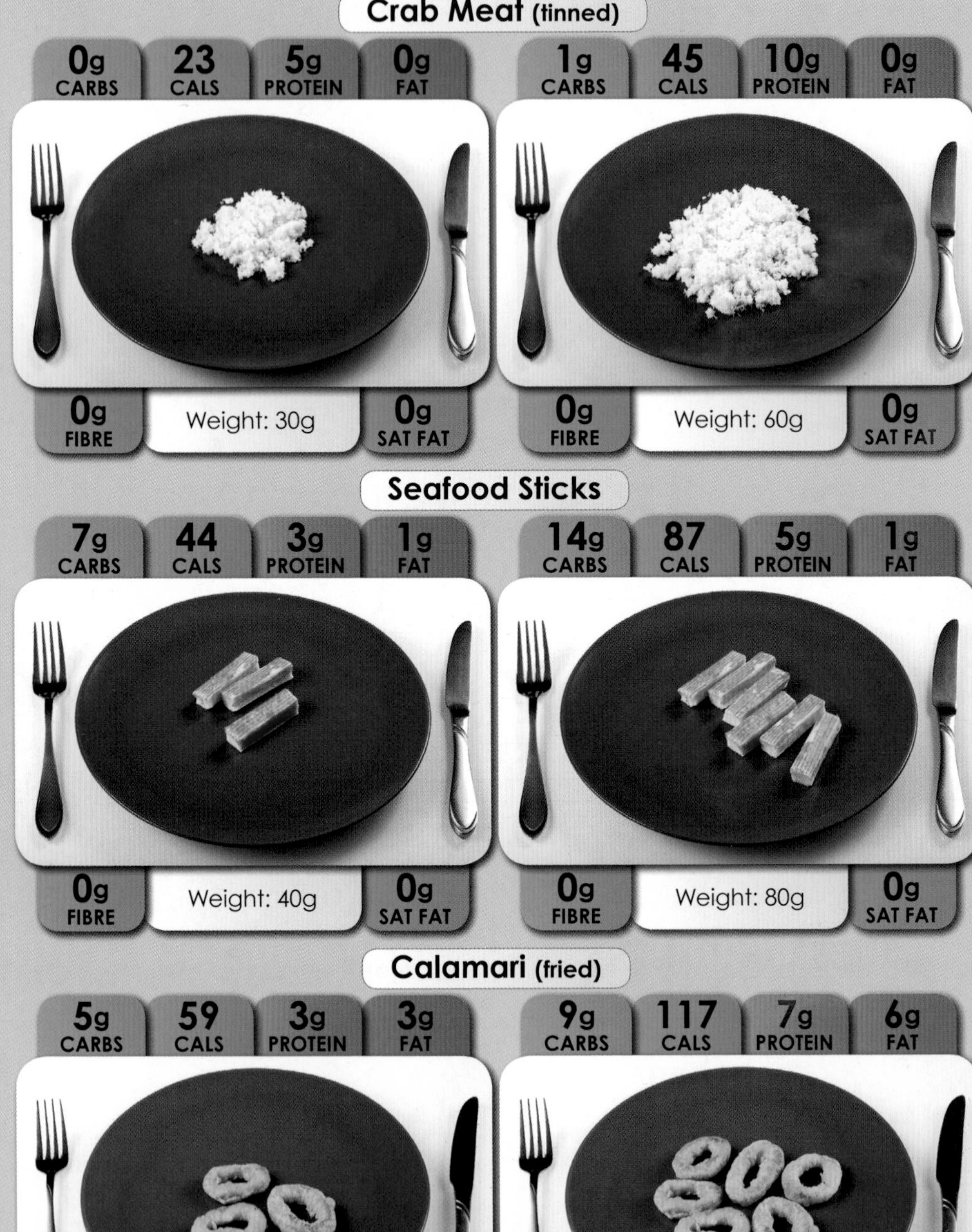

Crab Meat (tinned)

Weight	Carbs	Cals	Protein	Fat	Fibre	Sat Fat
30g	0g	23	5g	0g	0g	0g
60g	1g	45	10g	0g	0g	0g

Seafood Sticks

Weight	Carbs	Cals	Protein	Fat	Fibre	Sat Fat
40g	7g	44	3g	1g	0g	0g
80g	14g	87	5g	1g	0g	0g

Calamari (fried)

Weight	Carbs	Cals	Protein	Fat	Fibre	Sat Fat
30g	5g	59	3g	3g	0g	1g
60g	9g	117	7g	6g	0g	1g

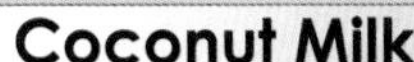

Coconut Milk

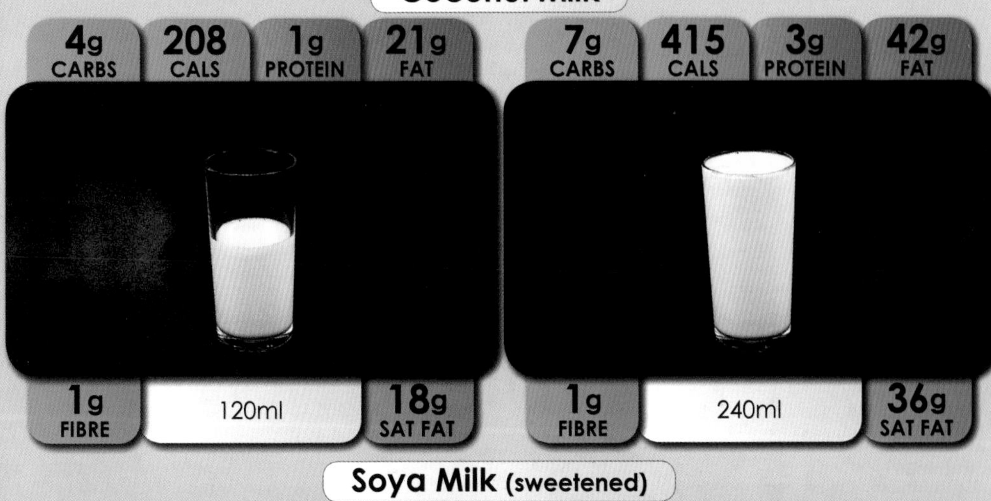

Serving	Carbs	Cals	Protein	Fat	Fibre	Sat Fat
120ml	4g	208	1g	21g	1g	18g
240ml	7g	415	3g	42g	1g	36g

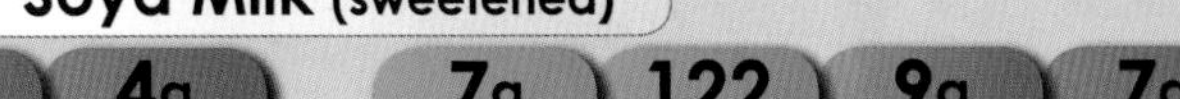

Soya Milk (sweetened)

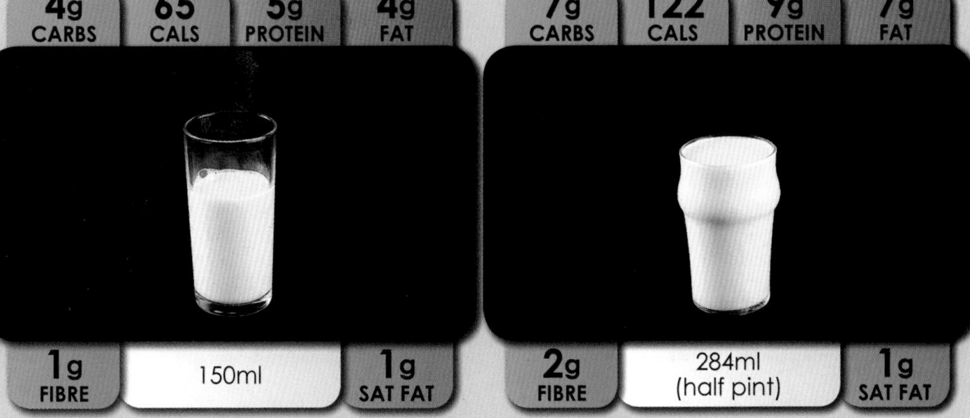

Serving	Carbs	Cals	Protein	Fat	Fibre	Sat Fat
150ml	4g	65	5g	4g	1g	1g
284ml (half pint)	7g	122	9g	7g	2g	1g

Soya Milk (unsweetened)

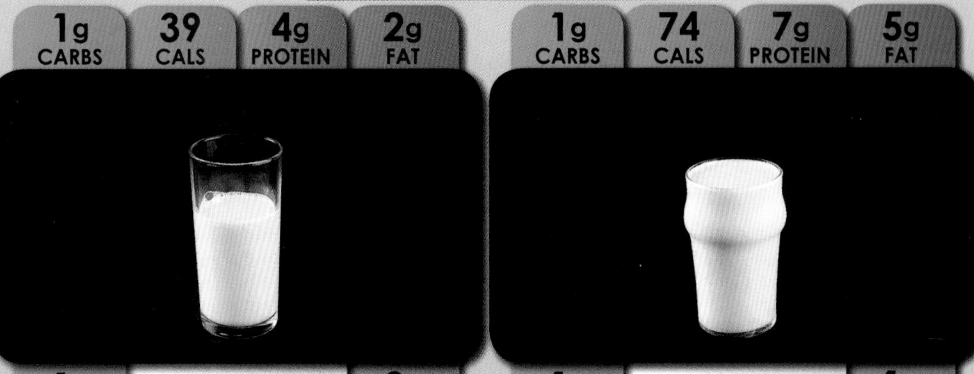

Serving	Carbs	Cals	Protein	Fat	Fibre	Sat Fat
150ml	1g	39	4g	2g	1g	0g
284ml (half pint)	1g	74	7g	5g	1g	1g

Milk (whole)

Portion	Carbs	Cals	Protein	Fat	Fibre	Sat Fat
150ml	7g	99	5g	6g	0g	4g
284ml (half pint)	13g	187	9g	11g	0g	7g
568ml (pint)	26g	375	19g	22g	0g	14g

Milk (semi-skimmed)

Portion	Carbs	Cals	Protein	Fat	Fibre	Sat Fat
150ml	7g	69	5g	3g	0g	2g
284ml (half pint)	13g	131	10g	5g	0g	3g
568ml (pint)	27g	261	19g	10g	0g	6g

Milk (1%)

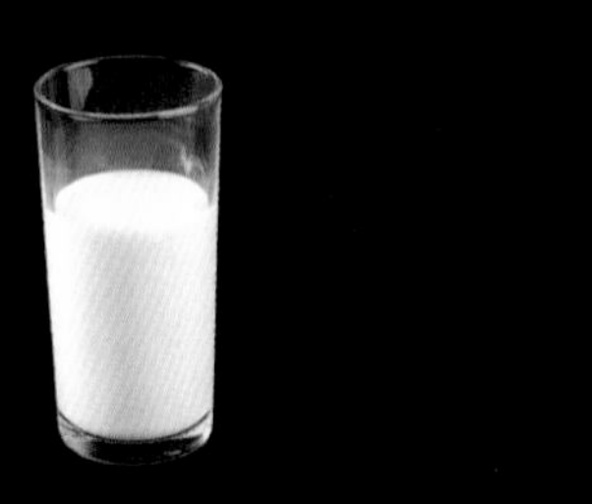

Serving	Carbs	Cals	Protein	Fat	Fibre	Sat Fat
150ml	7g	61	5g	2g	0g	1g
284ml (half pint)	13g	116	9g	3g	0g	2g
568ml (pint)	27g	232	18g	6g	0g	4g

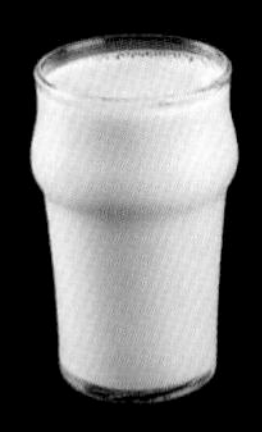

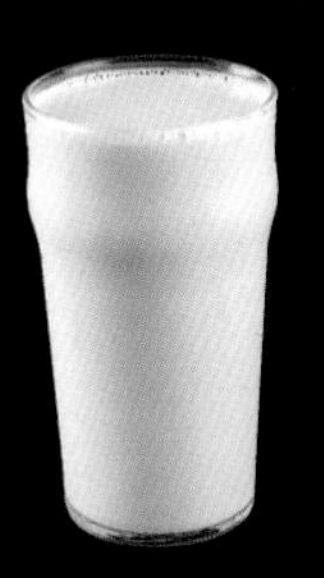

Milk (skimmed)

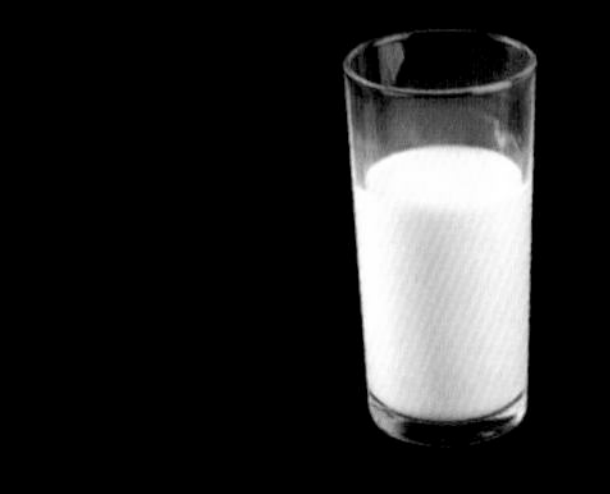

Serving	Carbs	Cals	Protein	Fat	Fibre	Sat Fat
150ml	7g	48	5g	0g	0g	0g
284ml (half pint)	13g	91	10g	1g	0g	0g
568ml (pint)	25g	182	19g	1g	0g	1g

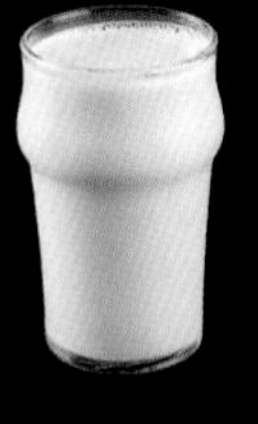

Milkshake (powder & semi-skimmed milk)

Serving	Carbs	Cals	Protein	Fat	Fibre	Sat fat
150ml	18g	107	5g	2g	0g	1g
150ml	15g	104	5g	3g	0g	2g
284ml (half pint)	33g	203	9g	4g	0g	3g
284ml (half pint)	29g	196	9g	5g	0g	3g
568ml (pint)	66g	407	18g	9g	0g	6g
568ml (pint)	57g	392	18g	10g	0g	7g

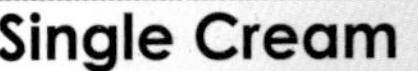

Single Cream

Weight	Carbs	Cals	Protein	Fat	Fibre	Sat Fat
5g (teaspoon)	0g	10	0g	1g	0g	1g
15g (tablespoon)	0g	29	1g	3g	0g	2g

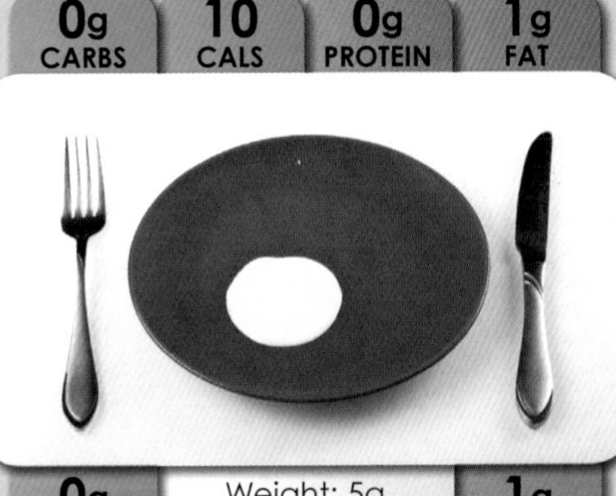

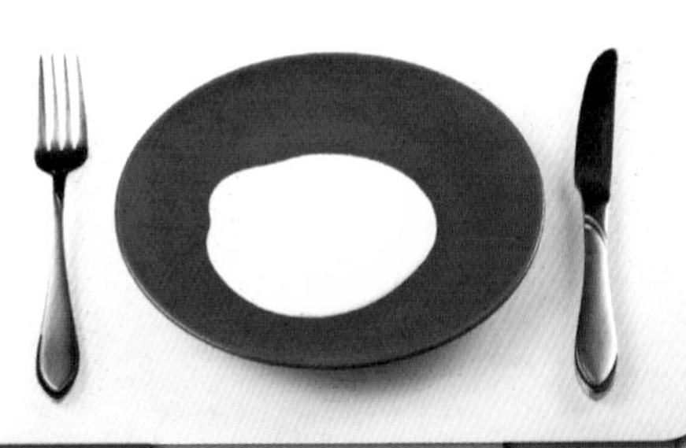

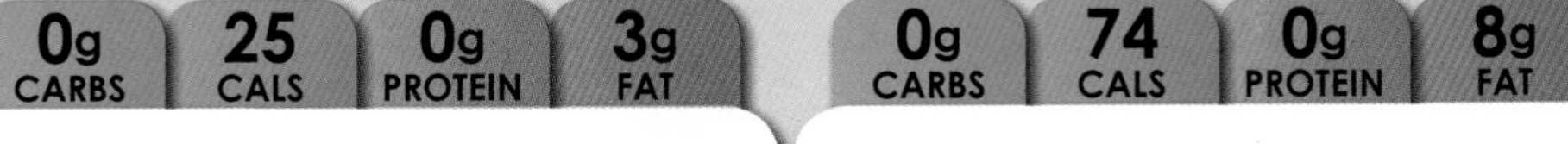

Double Cream

Weight	Carbs	Cals	Protein	Fat	Fibre	Sat Fat
5g (teaspoon)	0g	25	0g	3g	0g	2g
15g (tablespoon)	0g	74	0g	8g	0g	5g

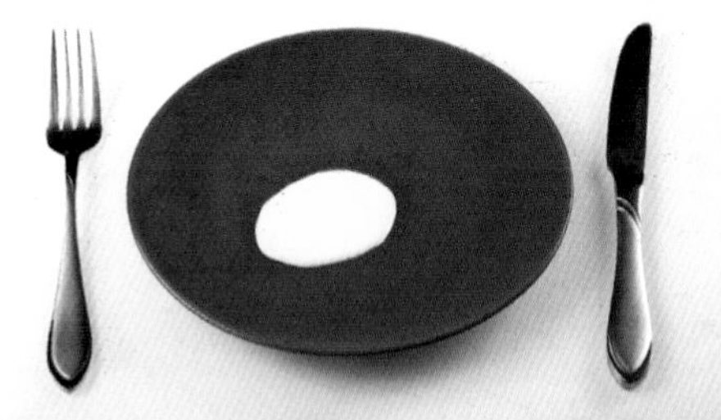

Clotted Cream

Weight	Carbs	Cals	Protein	Fat	Fibre	Sat Fat
15g (tablespoon)	0g	88	0g	10g	0g	6g
30g (2 tablespoons)	1g	176	1g	19g	0g	12g

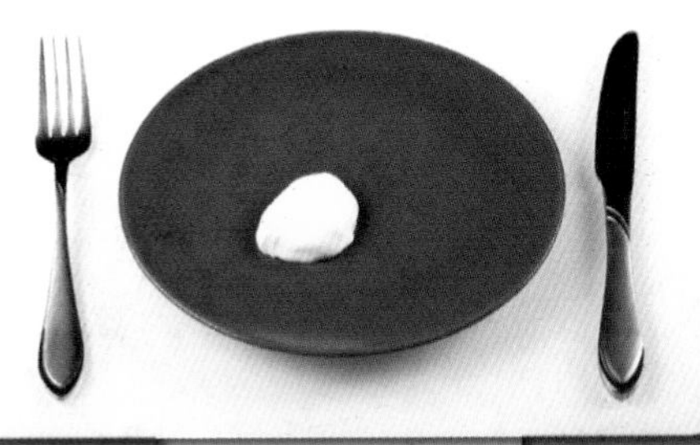

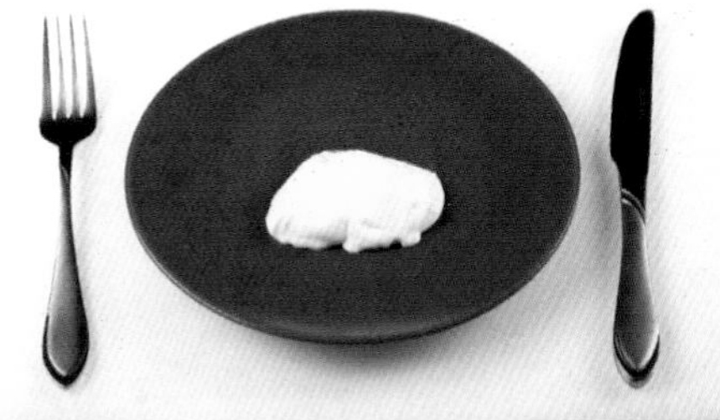

20cm Side Plate

Crème Fraîche

Weight	Carbs	Cals	Protein	Fat	Fibre	Sat Fat
Weight: 30g (2 tablespoons)	1g	113	1g	12g	0g	8g
Weight: 60g (4 tablespoons)	1g	227	1g	24g	0g	16g

Soured Cream

Weight	Carbs	Cals	Protein	Fat	Fibre	Sat Fat
Weight: 30g (2 tablespoons)	1g	62	1g	6g	0g	4g
Weight: 60g (4 tablespoons)	2g	123	2g	12g	0g	8g

Whipped Cream

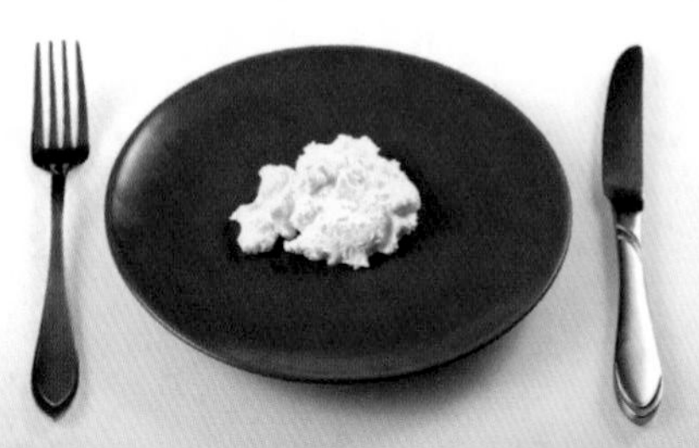

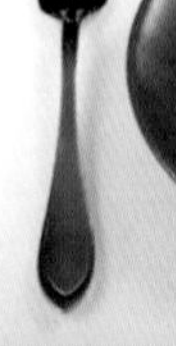

Weight	Carbs	Cals	Protein	Fat	Fibre	Sat Fat
Weight: 30g	1g	112	1g	12g	0g	7g
Weight: 60g	2g	224	1g	24g	0g	15g

Almonds

Carbs	Cals	Protein	Fat	Fibre	Weight	Sat Fat
1g	62	2g	5g	1g	Weight: 10g (tablespoon)	0g
2g	185	7g	16g	3g	Weight: 30g	1g

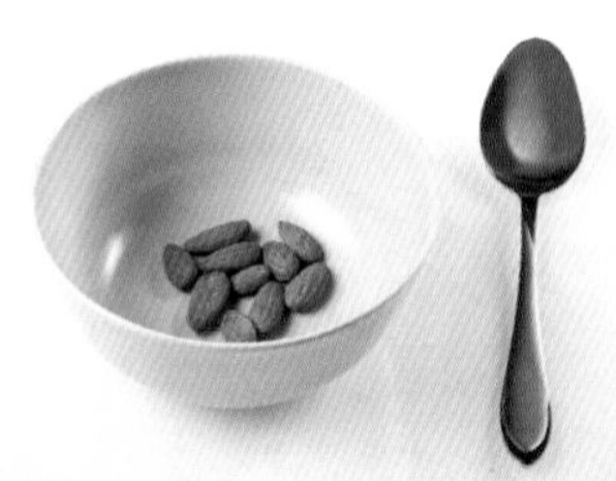

Brazil Nuts

Carbs	Cals	Protein	Fat	Fibre	Weight	Sat Fat
0g	68	1g	7g	1g	Weight: 10g (tablespoon)	2g
1g	205	4g	20g	2g	Weight: 30g	5g

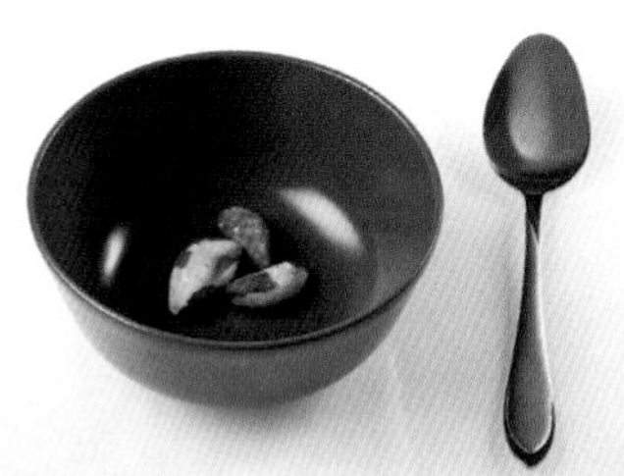

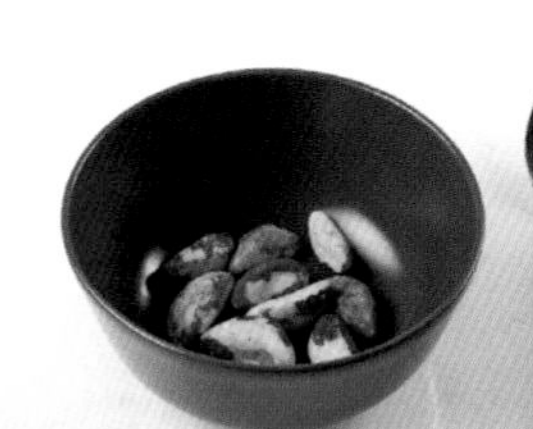

Cashew Nuts

Carbs	Cals	Protein	Fat	Fibre	Weight	Sat Fat
2g	61	2g	5g	0g	Weight: 10g (tablespoon)	1g
6g	183	6g	15g	1g	Weight: 30g	3g

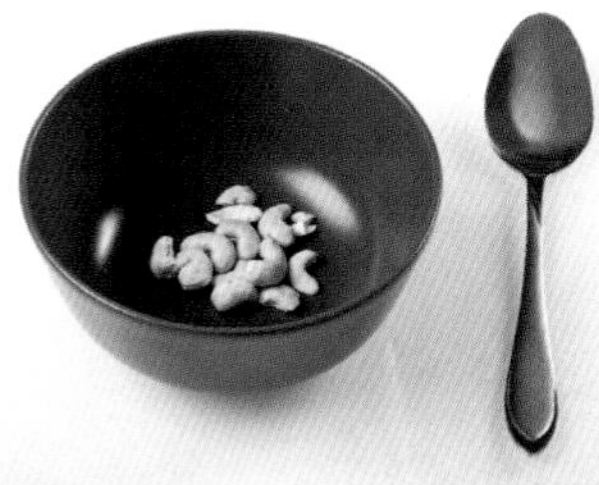

Dried Fruit & Nuts

CARBS	CALS	PROTEIN	FAT	FIBRE	Weight	SAT FAT
5g	44	1g	2g	1g	10g	0g
14g	133	3g	7g	1g	30g	1g

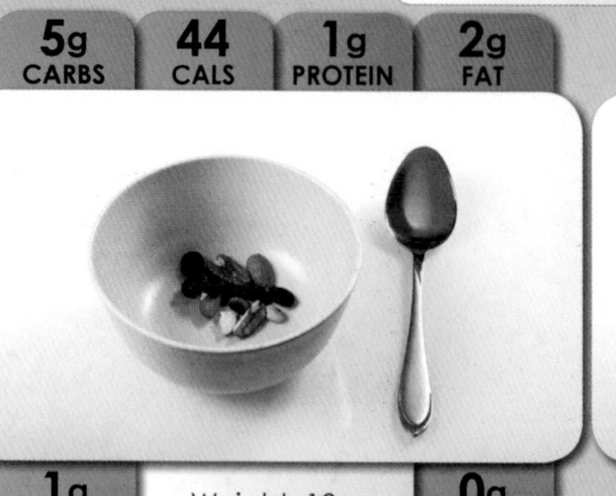

Hazelnuts

CARBS	CALS	PROTEIN	FAT	FIBRE	Weight	SAT FAT
1g	65	1g	6g	1g	10g (tablespoon)	0g
2g	195	4g	19g	3g	30g	1g

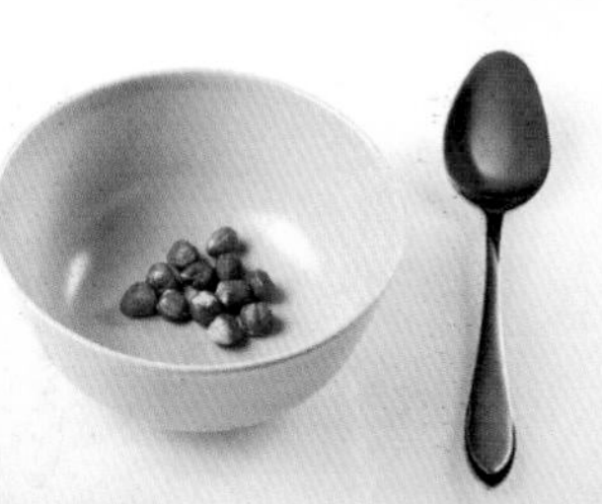

Macadamia Nuts

CARBS	CALS	PROTEIN	FAT	FIBRE	Weight	SAT FAT
0g	75	1g	8g	1g	10g	1g
1g	224	2g	23g	2g	30g	3g

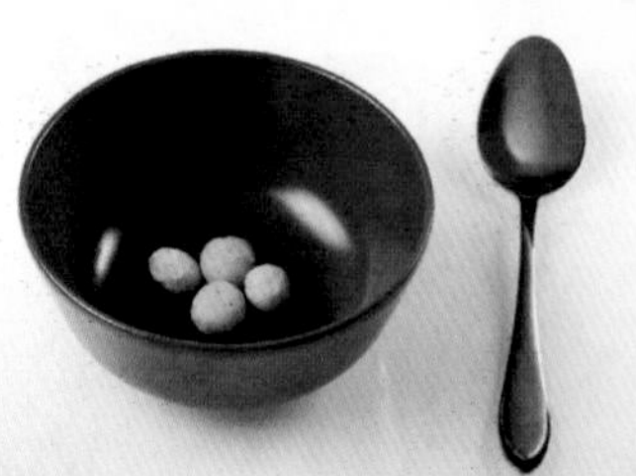

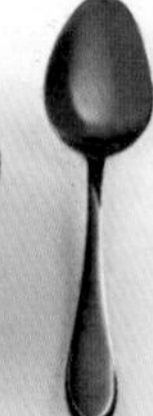

Peanuts (roasted)

Weight	Carbs	Cals	Protein	Fat	Fibre	Sat Fat
10g (tablespoon)	1g	60	3g	5g	1g	1g
30g	2g	181	7g	16g	2g	3g

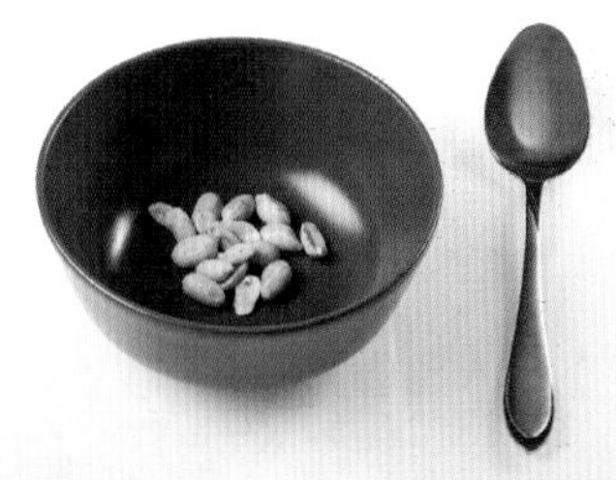

Pecan Nuts

Weight	Carbs	Cals	Protein	Fat	Fibre	Sat Fat
10g (tablespoon)	1g	69	1g	7g	1g	1g
30g	2g	207	3g	21g	2g	2g

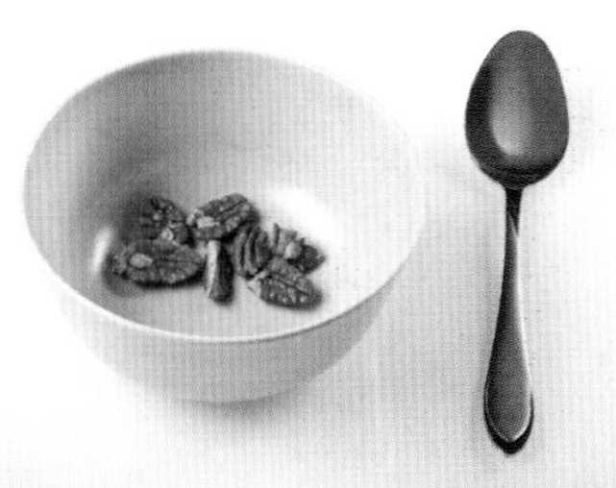

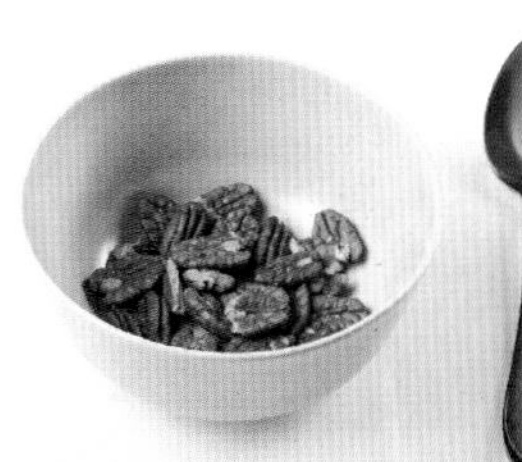

Pine Nuts

Weight	Carbs	Cals	Protein	Fat	Fibre	Sat Fat
10g (tablespoon)	0g	69	1g	7g	0g	1g
30g	1g	206	4g	21g	1g	1g

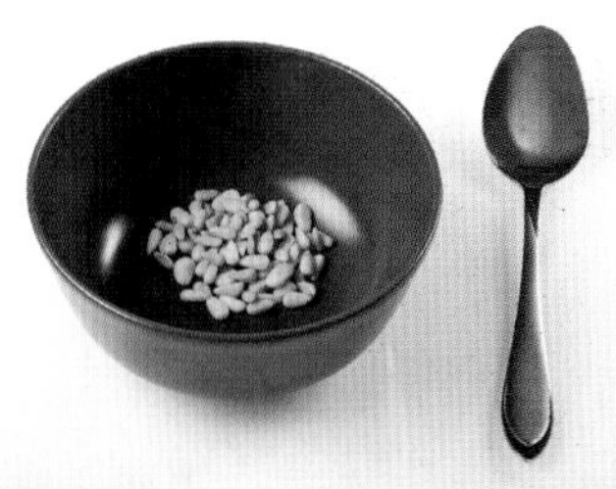

Pistachio Nuts

CARBS	CALS	PROTEIN	FAT	FIBRE	SAT FAT	Weight
2g	180	5g	17g	2g	2g	Weight: 60g (with shells)
2g	180	5g	17g	2g	2g	Weight: 30g (without shells)

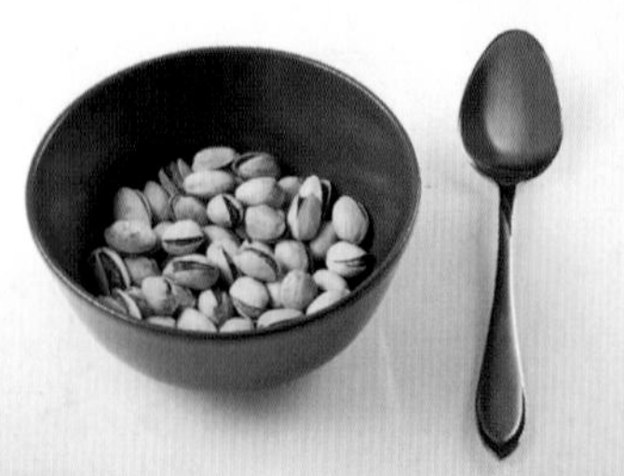

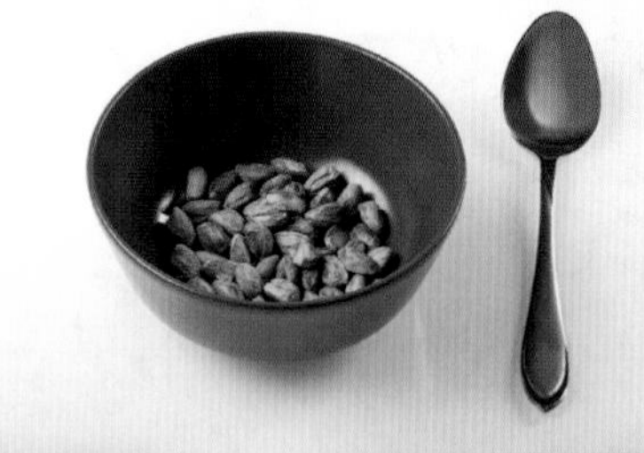

Soya Nuts

CARBS	CALS	PROTEIN	FAT	FIBRE	SAT FAT	Weight
1g	22	2g	1g	1g	0g	Weight: 6g (tablespoon)
5g	111	11g	6g	6g	1g	Weight: 30g

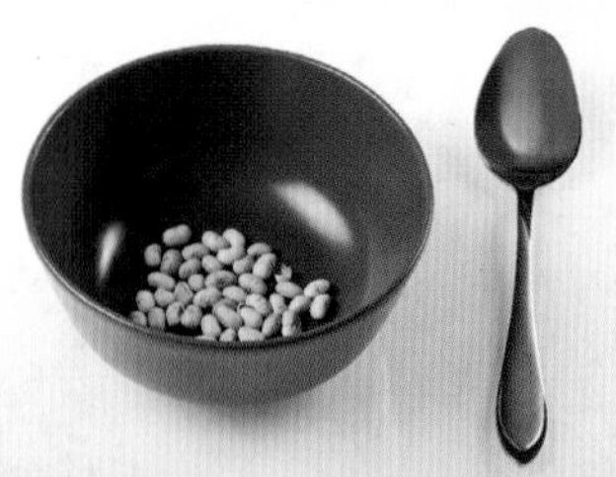

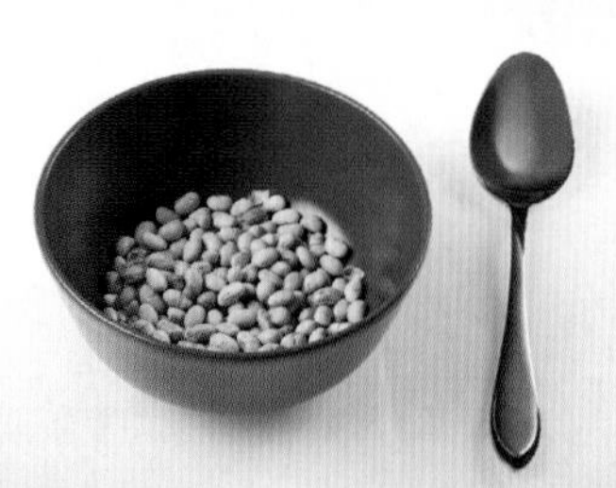

Walnuts

CARBS	CALS	PROTEIN	FAT	FIBRE	SAT FAT	Weight
0g	69	1g	7g	0g	1g	Weight: 10g (tablespoon)
1g	206	4g	21g	1g	2g	Weight: 30g

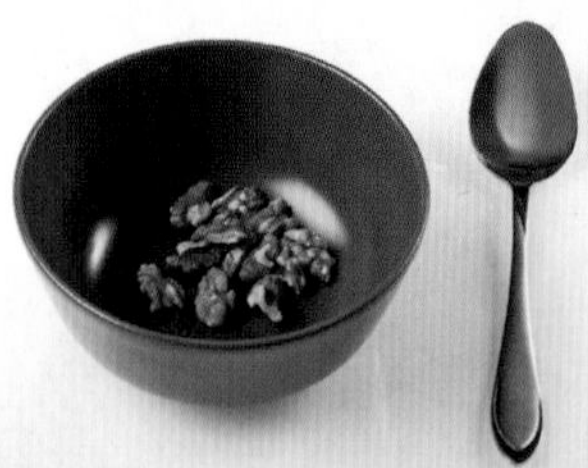

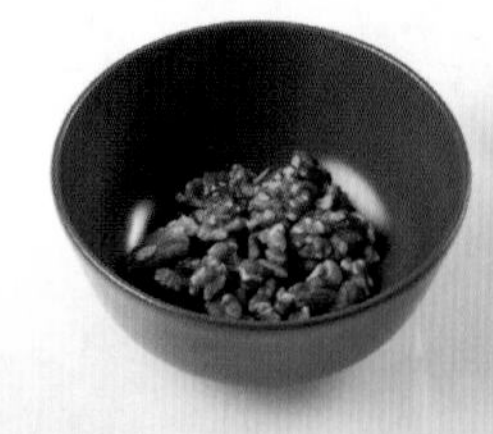

Linseeds

	Weight: 11g (tablespoon)	Weight: 30g
CARBS	2g	5g
CALS	55	151
PROTEIN	2g	6g
FAT	4g	11g
FIBRE	3g	8g
SAT FAT	0g	1g

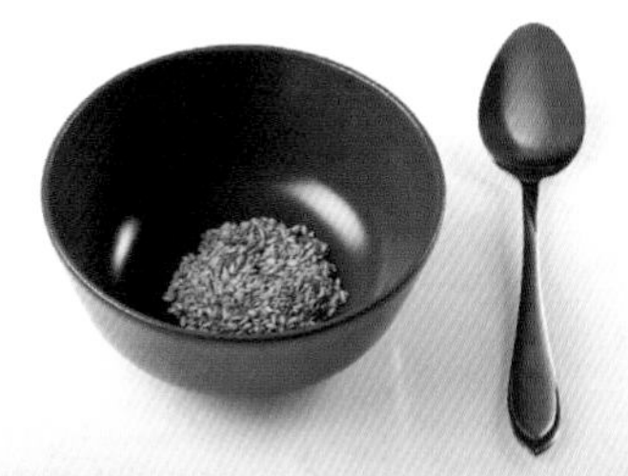

Pumpkin Seeds

	Weight: 10g (tablespoon)	Weight: 30g
CARBS	2g	5g
CALS	57	171
PROTEIN	2g	7g
FAT	5g	14g
FIBRE	1g	2g
SAT FAT	1g	2g

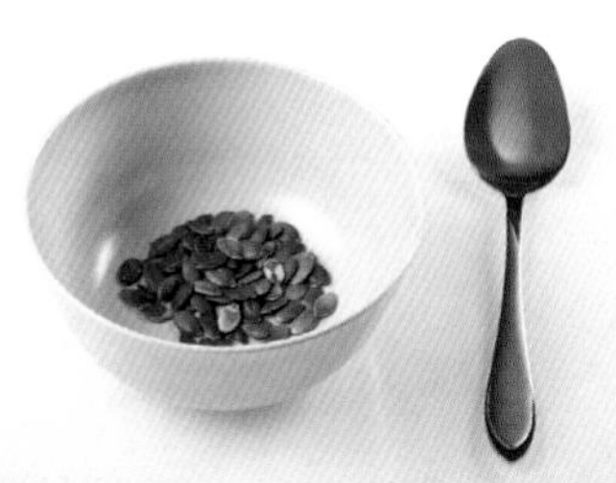

Sunflower Seeds

	Weight: 10g (tablespoon)	Weight: 30g
CARBS	2g	6g
CALS	58	174
PROTEIN	2g	6g
FAT	5g	14g
FIBRE	1g	2g
SAT FAT	1g	2g

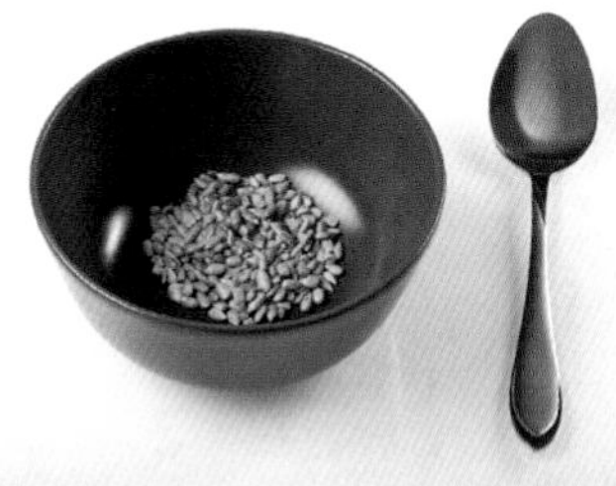

26cm Dinner Plate

Macaroni

10g CARBS	49 CALS	2g PROTEIN	0g FAT

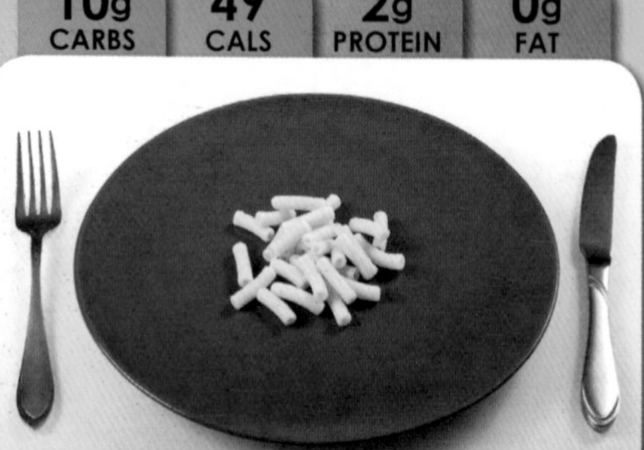
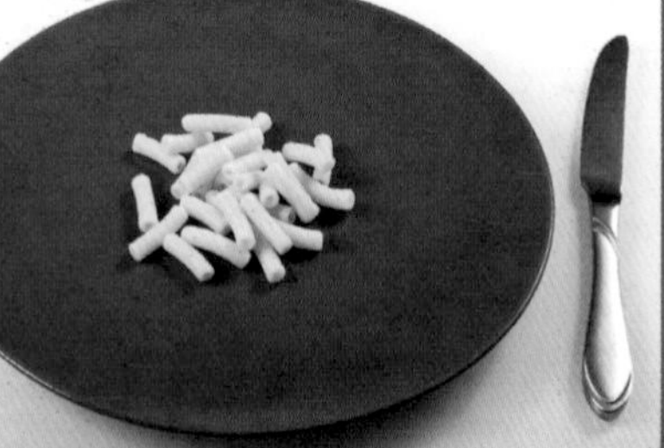

0g FIBRE	Weight: 32g	0g SAT FAT

30g CARBS	152 CALS	5g PROTEIN	1g FAT

1g FIBRE	Weight: 100g	0g SAT FAT

50g CARBS	252 CALS	9g PROTEIN	2g FAT

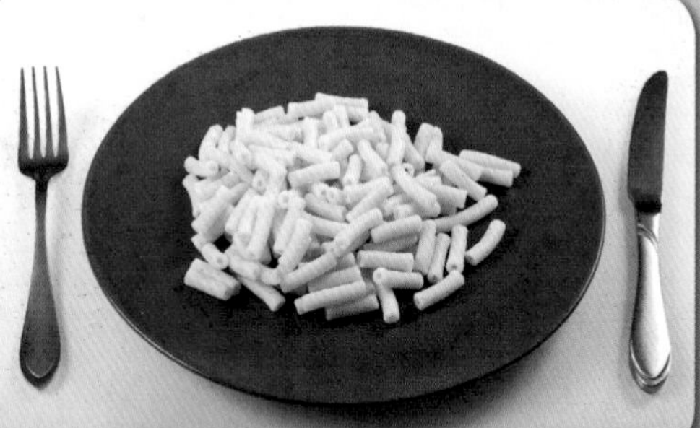

2g FIBRE	Weight: 166g	0g SAT FAT

70g CARBS	354 CALS	12g PROTEIN	2g FAT

3g FIBRE	Weight: 233g	0g SAT FAT

90g CARBS	456 CALS	16g PROTEIN	3g FAT

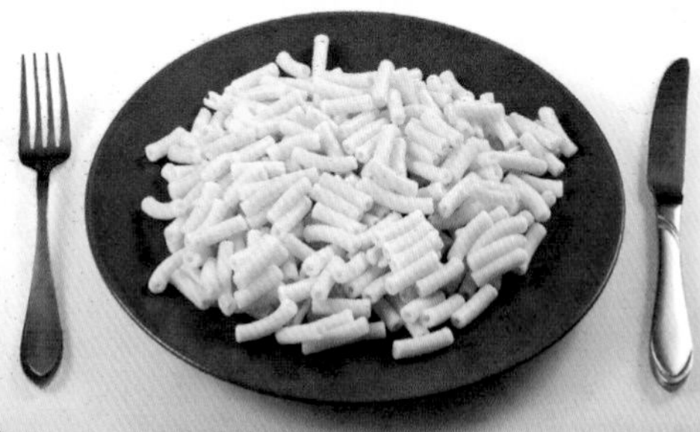

4g FIBRE	Weight: 300g	0g SAT FAT

110g CARBS	556 CALS	19g PROTEIN	4g FAT

4g FIBRE	Weight: 366g	0g SAT FAT

Pasta Bows

10g CARBS	50 CALS	2g PROTEIN	0g FAT
1g FIBRE	Weight: 30g		0g SAT FAT

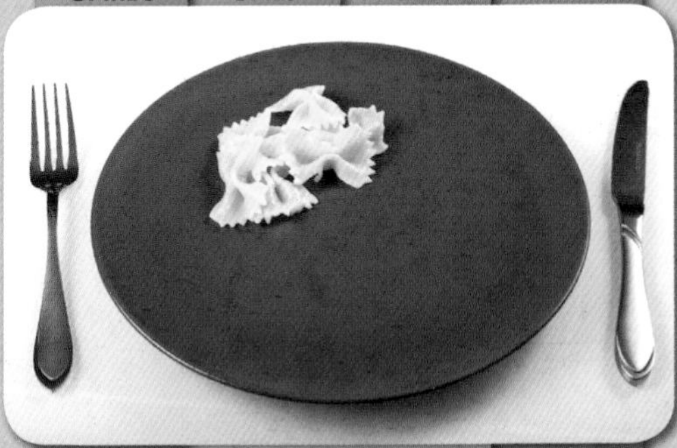

30g CARBS	148 CALS	5g PROTEIN	1g FAT
2g FIBRE	Weight: 88g		0g SAT FAT

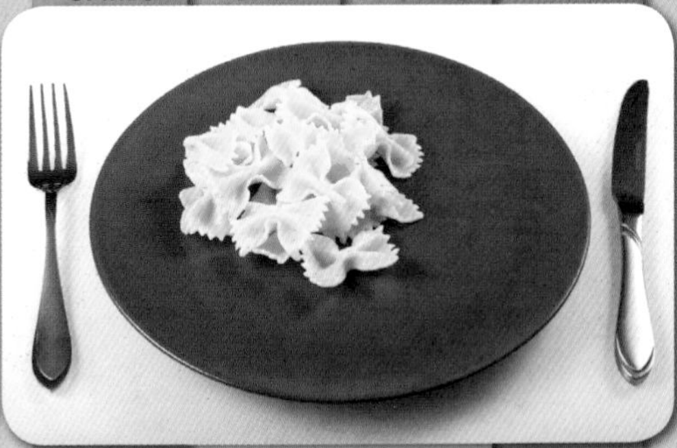

51g CARBS	249 CALS	8g PROTEIN	2g FAT
3g FIBRE	Weight: 148g		0g SAT FAT

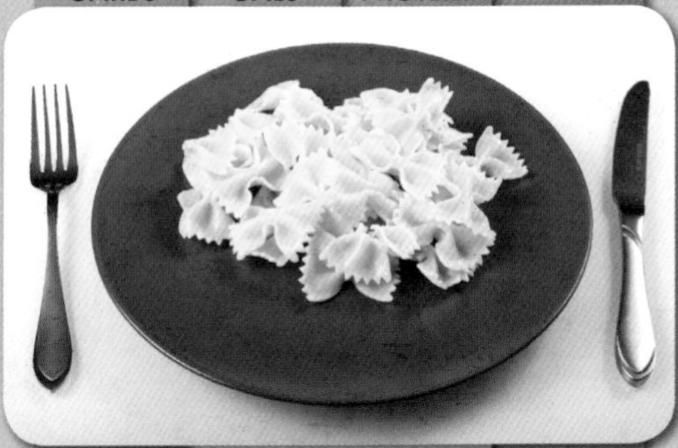

70g CARBS	344 CALS	11g PROTEIN	2g FAT
4g FIBRE	Weight: 205g		0g SAT FAT

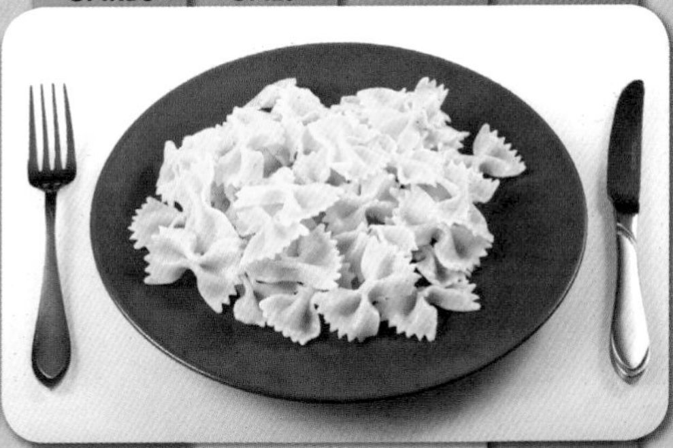

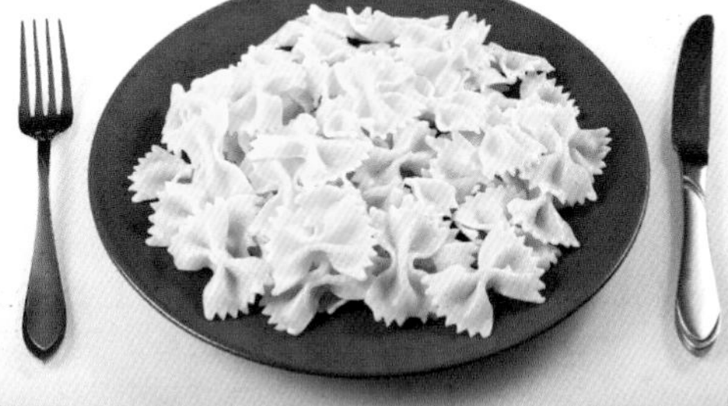

90g CARBS	445 CALS	14g PROTEIN	3g FAT
5g FIBRE	Weight: 265g		0g SAT FAT

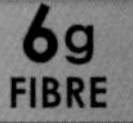

110g CARBS	543 CALS	17g PROTEIN	3g FAT
6g FIBRE	Weight: 323g		0g SAT FAT

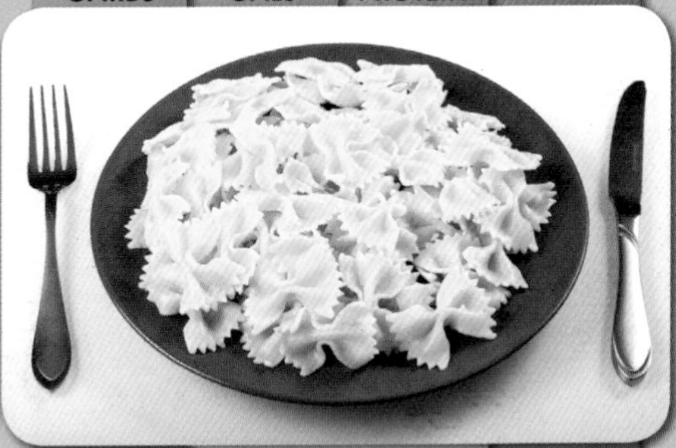

Pasta Shells

10g CARBS	50 CALS	2g PROTEIN	0g FAT

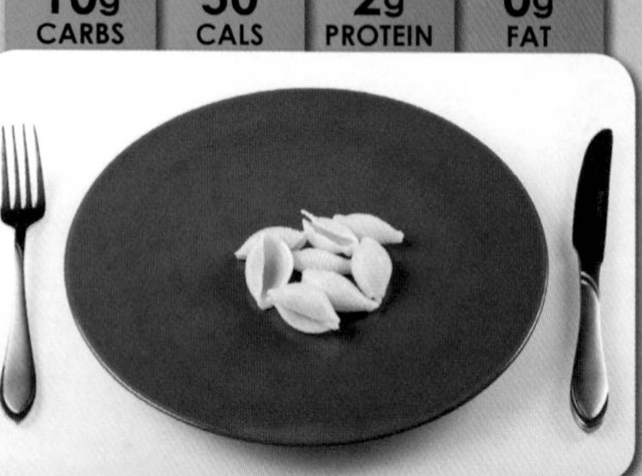

1g FIBRE	Weight: 30g	0g SAT FAT

30g CARBS	147 CALS	5g PROTEIN	1g FAT

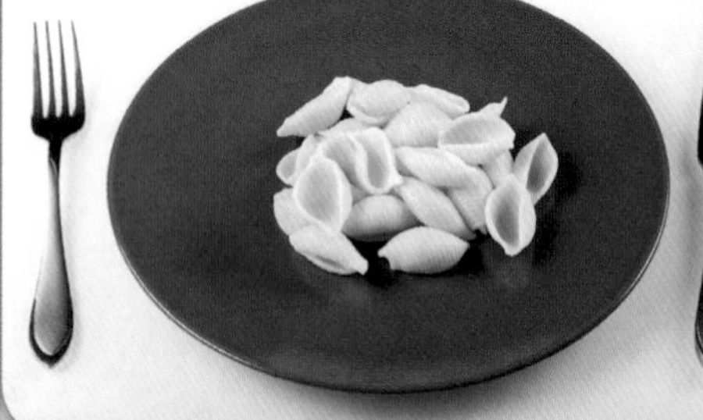

2g FIBRE	Weight: 88g	0g SAT FAT

50g CARBS	247 CALS	8g PROTEIN	2g FAT

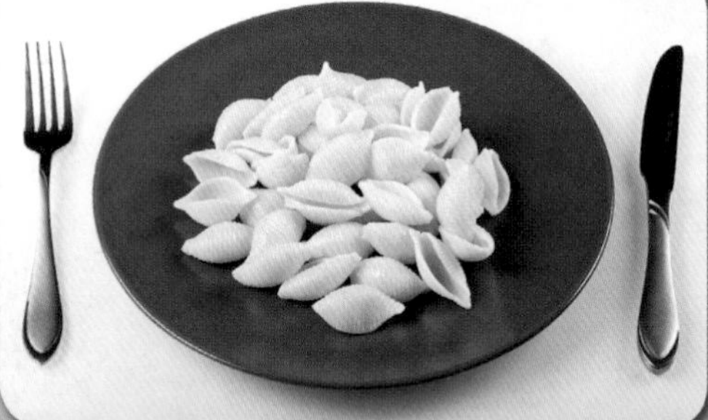

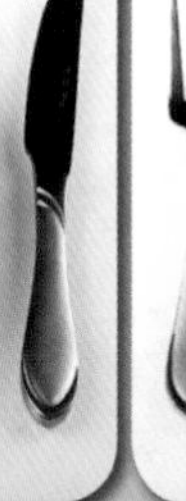

3g FIBRE	Weight: 148g	0g SAT FAT

70g CARBS	342 CALS	11g PROTEIN	2g FAT

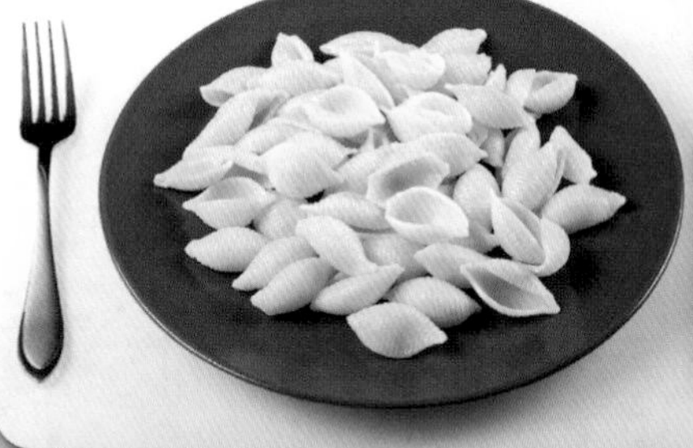

4g FIBRE	Weight: 205g	0g SAT FAT

90g CARBS	443 CALS	14g PROTEIN	3g FAT

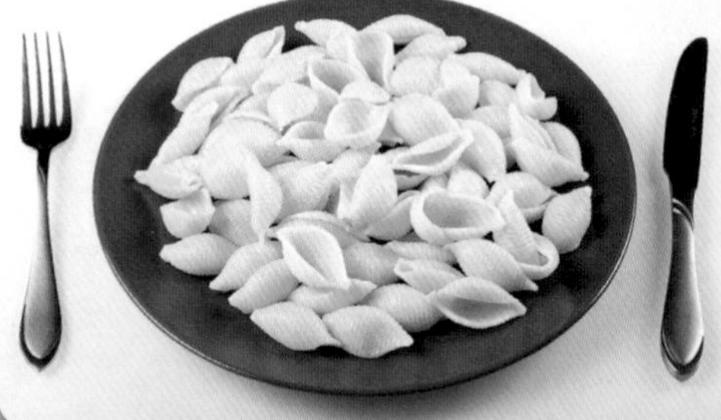

5g FIBRE	Weight: 265g	0g SAT FAT

110g CARBS	539 CALS	17g PROTEIN	3g FAT

6g FIBRE	Weight: 323g	0g SAT FAT

Pasta Twists

CARBS	CALS	PROTEIN	FAT
10g	51	2g	0g

FIBRE	Weight	SAT FAT
1g	Weight: 30g	0g

CARBS	CALS	PROTEIN	FAT
30g	149	5g	1g

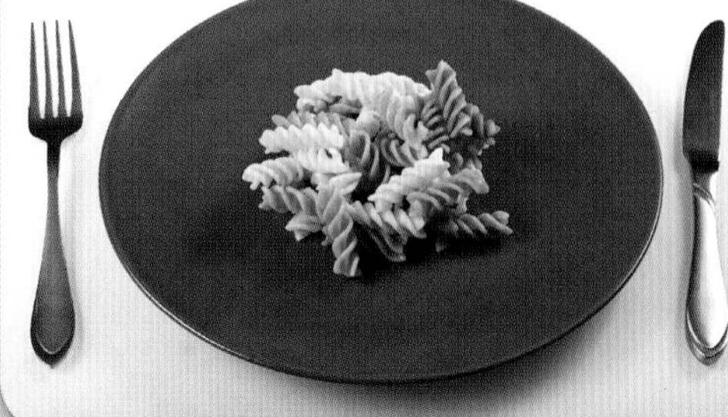

FIBRE	Weight	SAT FAT
2g	Weight: 88g	0g

CARBS	CALS	PROTEIN	FAT
50g	245	8g	2g

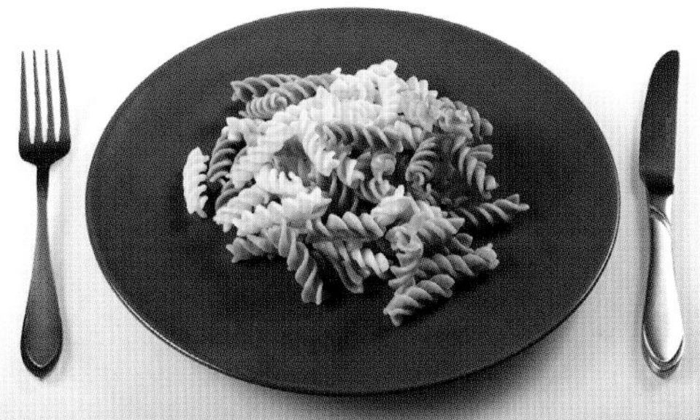

FIBRE	Weight	SAT FAT
3g	Weight: 145g	0g

CARBS	CALS	PROTEIN	FAT
70g	343	11g	2g

FIBRE	Weight	SAT FAT
4g	Weight: 203g	1g

CARBS	CALS	PROTEIN	FAT
90g	439	14g	3g

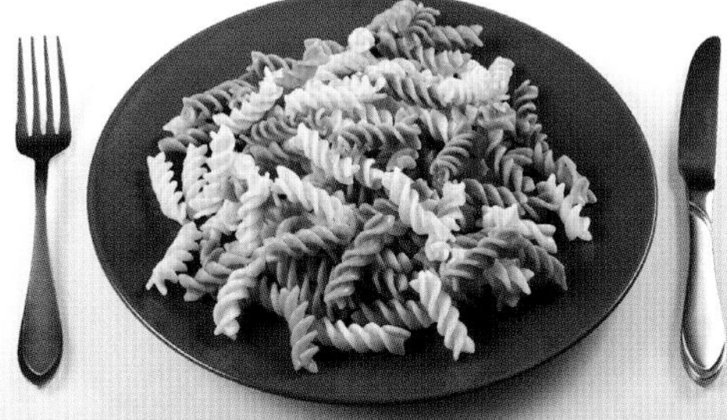

FIBRE	Weight	SAT FAT
4g	Weight: 260g	1g

CARBS	CALS	PROTEIN	FAT
110g	537	17g	3g

FIBRE	Weight	SAT FAT
5g	Weight: 318g	1g

Penne

CARBS	CALS	PROTEIN	FAT
10g	50	2g	0g

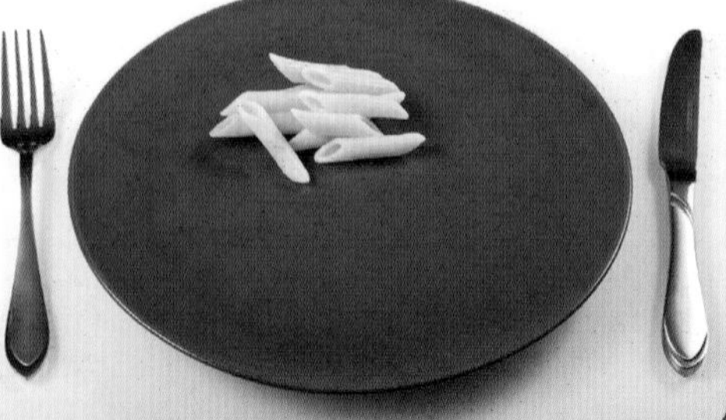

FIBRE	Weight	SAT FAT
1g	Weight: 30g	0g

CARBS	CALS	PROTEIN	FAT
30g	150	5g	1g

FIBRE	Weight	SAT FAT
2g	Weight: 90g	0g

CARBS	CALS	PROTEIN	FAT
50g	247	8g	2g

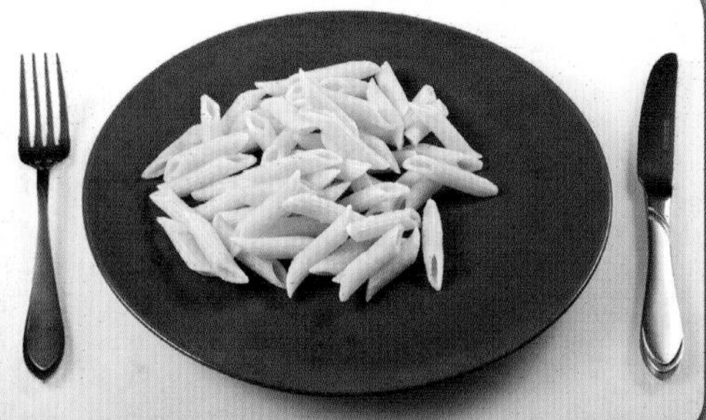

FIBRE	Weight	SAT FAT
3g	Weight: 148g	0g

CARBS	CALS	PROTEIN	FAT
70g	347	11g	2g

FIBRE	Weight	SAT FAT
4g	Weight: 208g	0g

CARBS	CALS	PROTEIN	FAT
90g	443	14g	3g

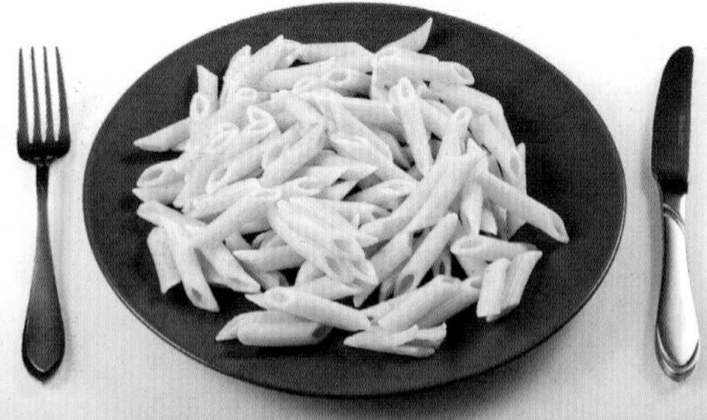

FIBRE	Weight	SAT FAT
5g	Weight: 265g	0g

CARBS	CALS	PROTEIN	FAT
110g	543	17g	3g

FIBRE	Weight	SAT FAT
6g	Weight: 325g	0g

Ravioli (fresh, meat-filled)

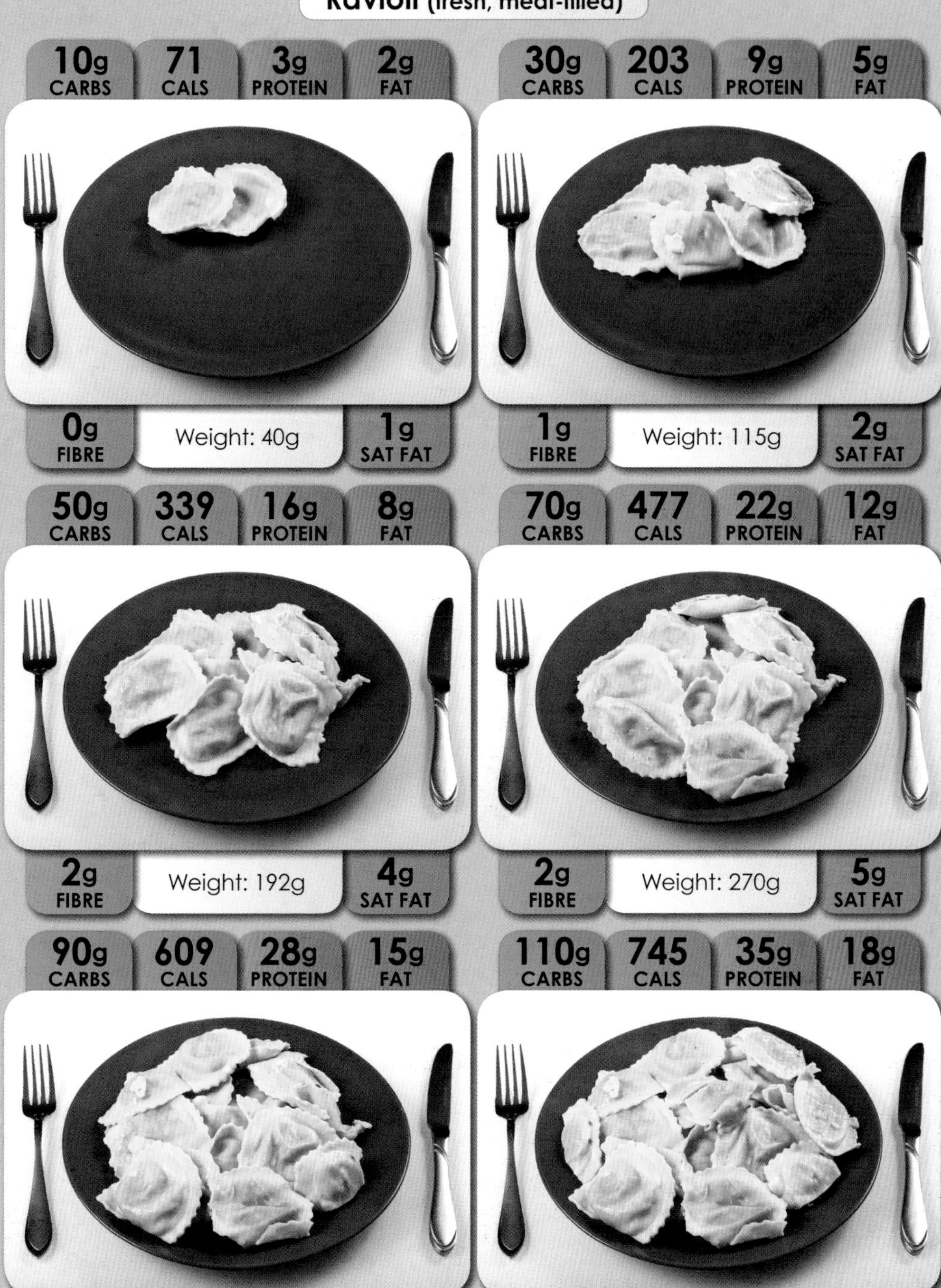

Weight	Carbs	Cals	Protein	Fat	Fibre	Sat Fat
40g	10g	71	3g	2g	0g	1g
115g	30g	203	9g	5g	1g	2g
192g	50g	339	16g	8g	2g	4g
270g	70g	477	22g	12g	2g	5g
345g	90g	609	28g	15g	3g	7g
422g	110g	745	35g	18g	4g	8g

Spaghetti (white)

10g CARBS	52 CALS	2g PROTEIN	0g FAT

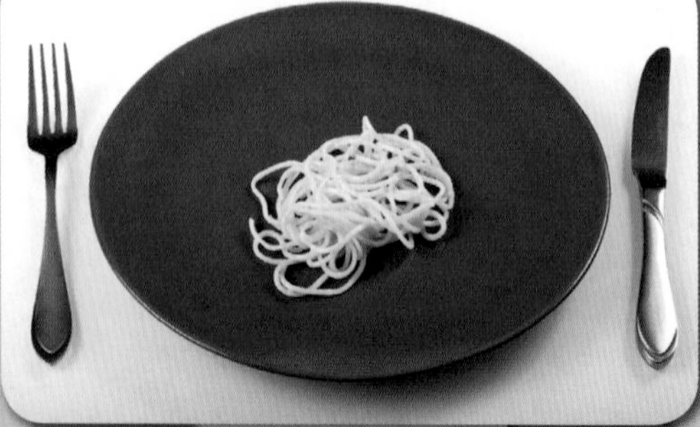

1g FIBRE	Weight: 33g	0g SAT FAT

30g CARBS	149 CALS	5g PROTEIN	1g FAT

2g FIBRE	Weight: 95g	0g SAT FAT

50g CARBS	248 CALS	8g PROTEIN	2g FAT

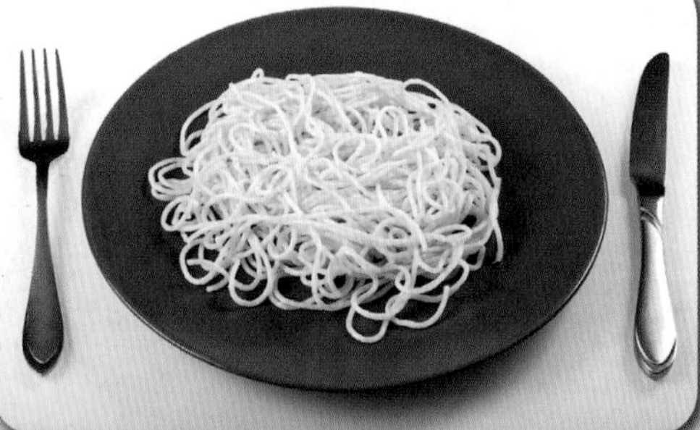

3g FIBRE	Weight: 158g	0g SAT FAT

70g CARBS	345 CALS	12g PROTEIN	2g FAT

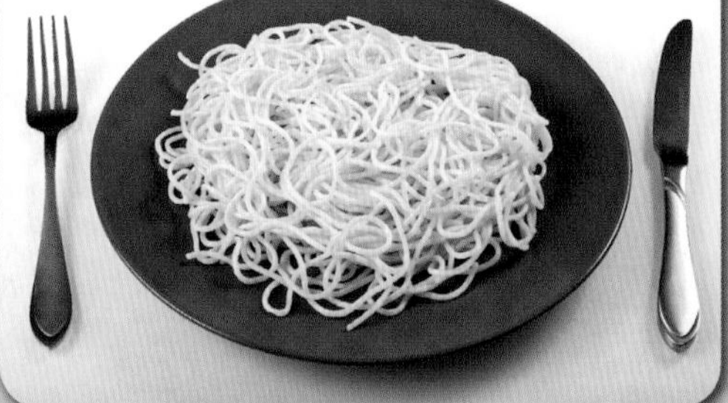

4g FIBRE	Weight: 220g	0g SAT FAT

90g CARBS	448 CALS	15g PROTEIN	3g FAT

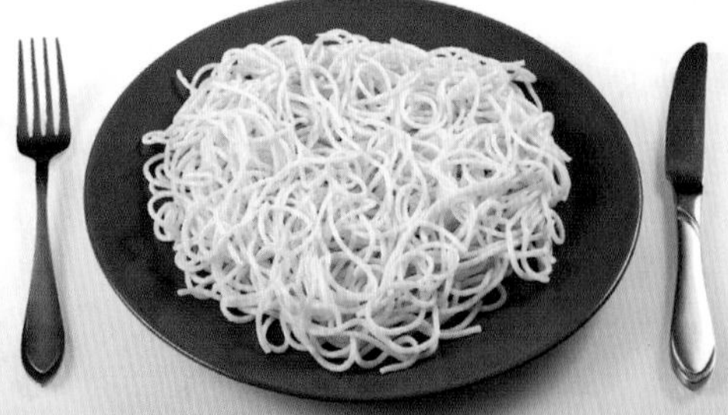

5g FIBRE	Weight: 285g	0g SAT FAT

110g CARBS	546 CALS	18g PROTEIN	4g FAT

6g FIBRE	Weight: 348g	0g SAT FAT

Spaghetti (wholemeal)

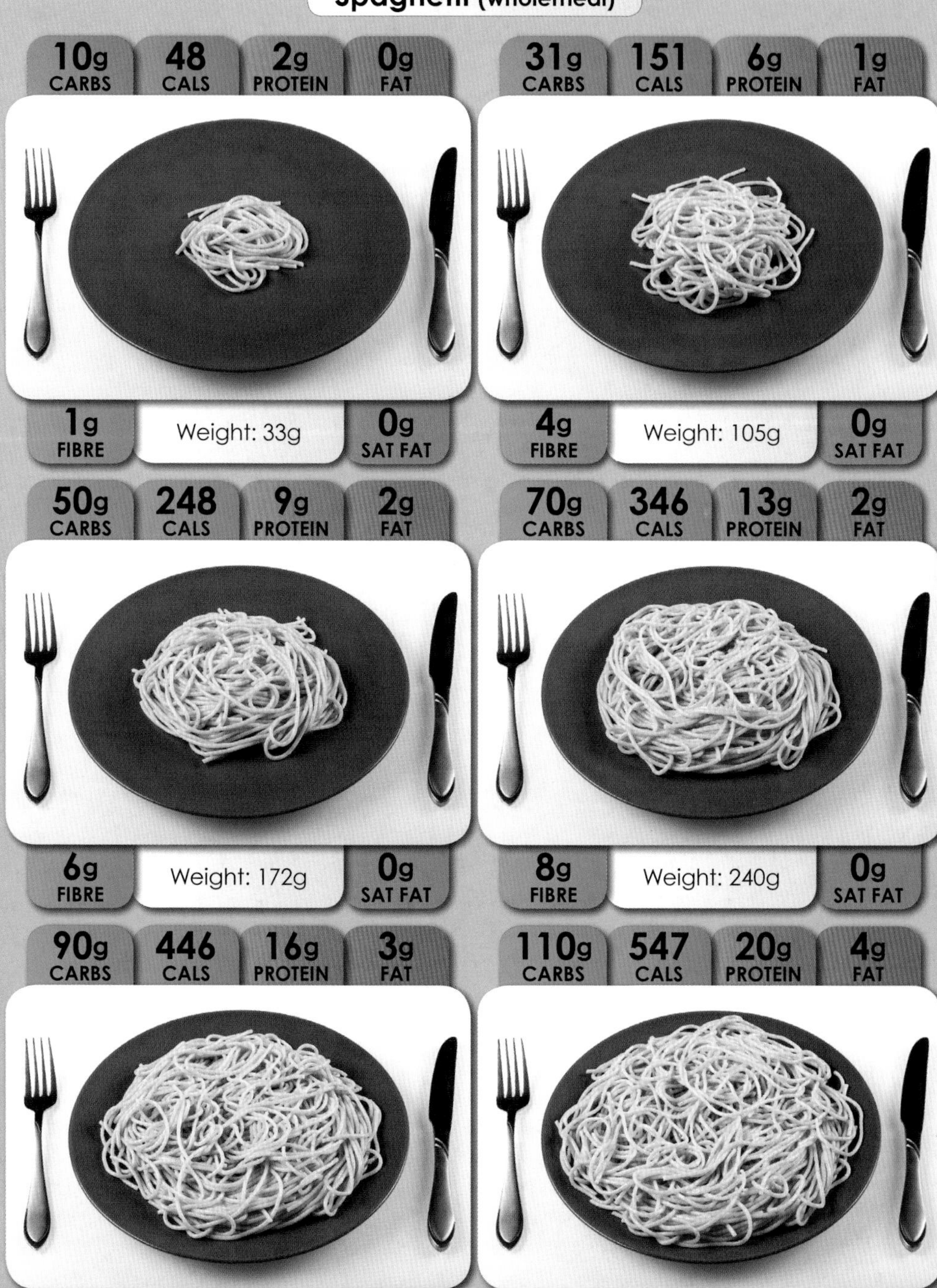

Tagliatelle

Carbs	Cals	Protein	Fat
10g	53	2g	0g

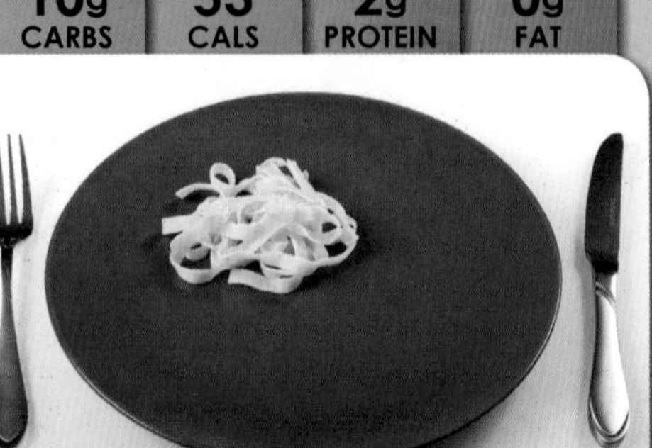
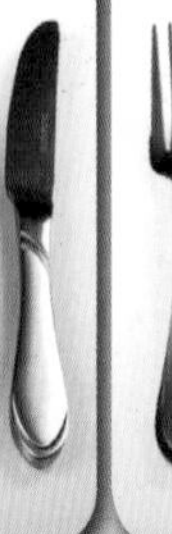

Fibre	Weight	Sat Fat
1g	Weight: 30g	0g

Carbs	Cals	Protein	Fat
30g	158	5g	1g

Fibre	Weight	Sat Fat
2g	Weight: 90g	0g

Carbs	Cals	Protein	Fat
50g	263	8g	2g

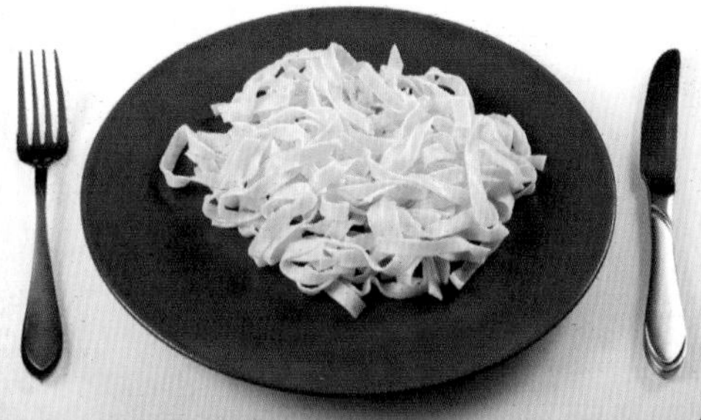

Fibre	Weight	Sat Fat
3g	Weight: 150g	0g

Carbs	Cals	Protein	Fat
70g	368	11g	2g

Fibre	Weight	Sat Fat
4g	Weight: 210g	0g

Carbs	Cals	Protein	Fat
90g	473	14g	3g

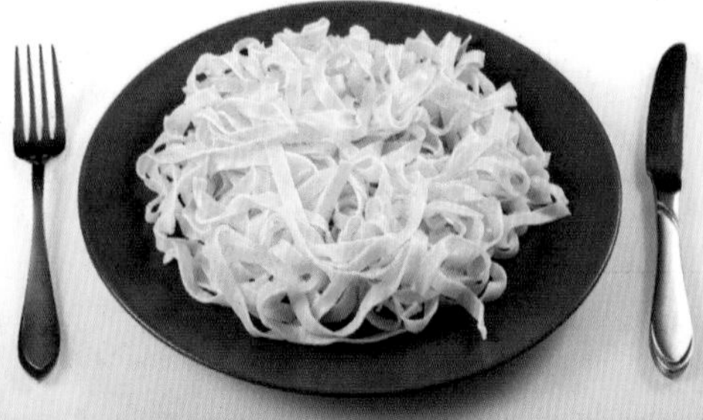

Fibre	Weight	Sat Fat
5g	Weight: 270g	0g

Carbs	Cals	Protein	Fat
110g	578	18g	3g

Fibre	Weight	Sat Fat
6g	Weight: 330g	0g

Tortellini (fresh, cheese-filled)

CARBS	CALS	PROTEIN	FAT
16g	108	5g	3g

FIBRE	Weight	SAT FAT
1g	Weight: 50g	2g

CARBS	CALS	PROTEIN	FAT
39g	271	12g	8g

FIBRE	Weight	SAT FAT
4g	Weight: 125g	5g

CARBS	CALS	PROTEIN	FAT
63g	433	19g	12g

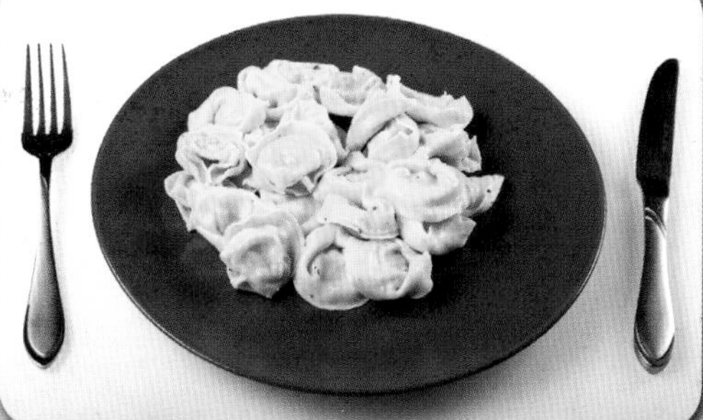

FIBRE	Weight	SAT FAT
6g	Weight: 200g	8g

CARBS	CALS	PROTEIN	FAT
86g	596	26g	16g

FIBRE	Weight	SAT FAT
8g	Weight: 275g	11g

CARBS	CALS	PROTEIN	FAT
110g	758	33g	21g

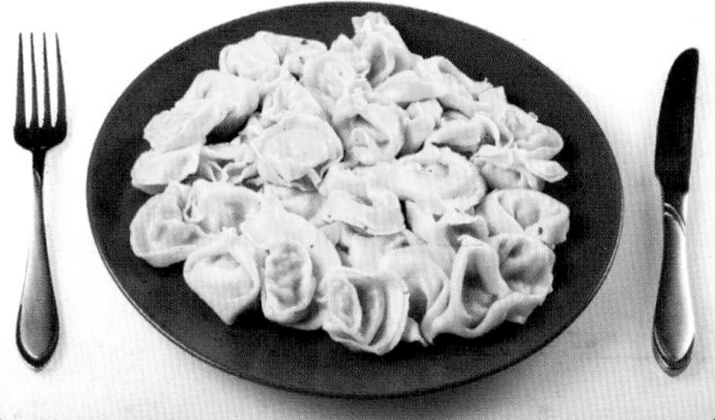

FIBRE	Weight	SAT FAT
10g	Weight: 350g	15g

CARBS	CALS	PROTEIN	FAT
133g	921	40g	25g

FIBRE	Weight	SAT FAT
12g	Weight: 425g	18g

Vermicelli

Carbs	Cals	Protein	Fat
10g	52	2g	1g

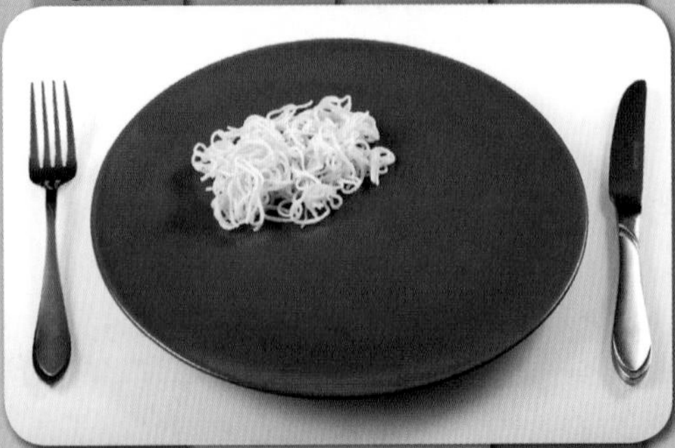

Fibre	Weight	Sat Fat
0g	Weight: 40g	0g

Carbs	Cals	Protein	Fat
30g	161	6g	2g

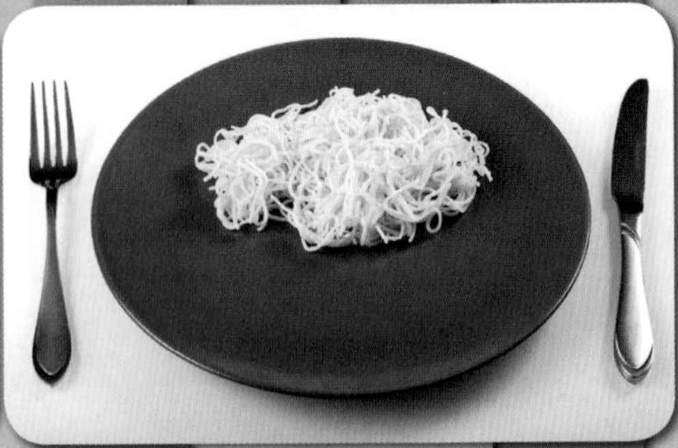

Fibre	Weight	Sat Fat
1g	Weight: 125g	0g

Carbs	Cals	Protein	Fat
50g	271	11g	3g

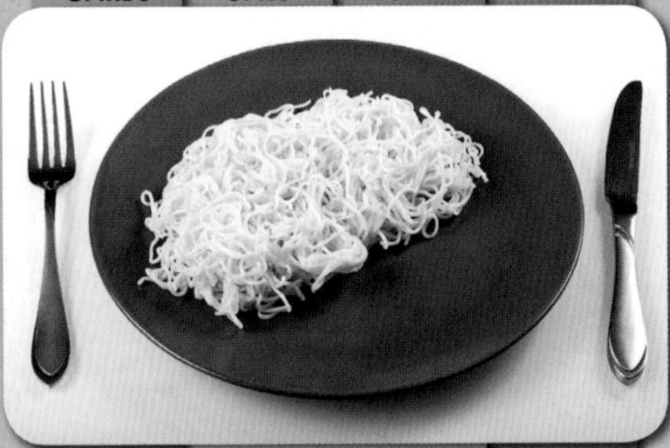

Fibre	Weight	Sat Fat
2g	Weight: 210g	0g

Carbs	Cals	Protein	Fat
70g	374	15g	4g

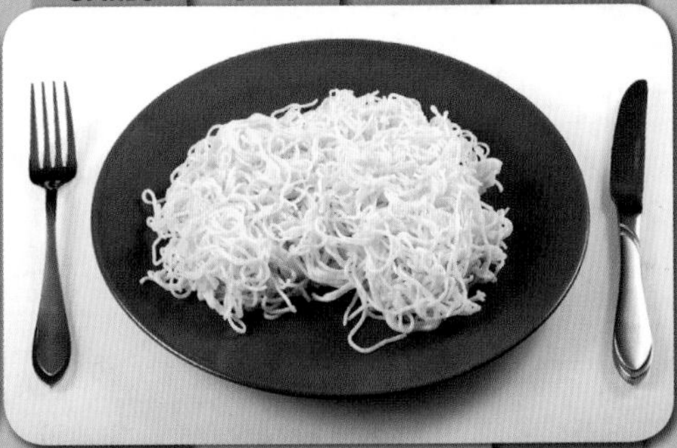

Fibre	Weight	Sat Fat
3g	Weight: 290g	1g

Carbs	Cals	Protein	Fat
90g	484	19g	5g

Fibre	Weight	Sat Fat
4g	Weight: 375g	1g

Carbs	Cals	Protein	Fat
110g	593	23g	6g

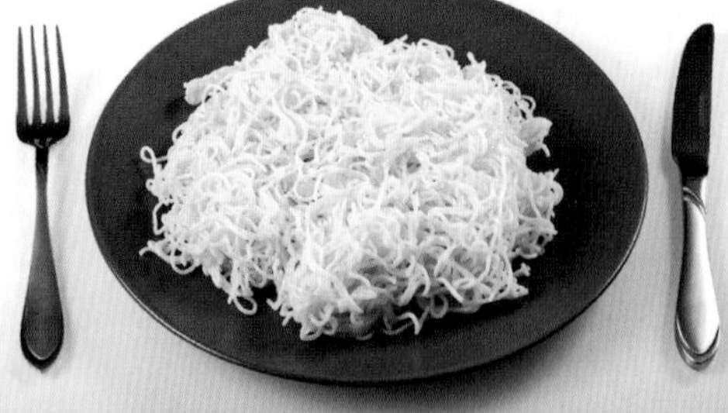

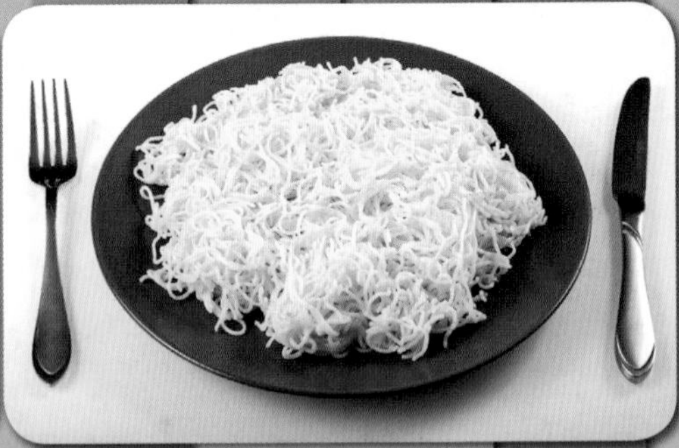

Fibre	Weight	Sat Fat
5g	Weight: 460g	1g

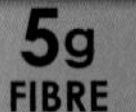

Pasta Shapes (tinned)

Carbs	Cals	Protein	Fat
9g	42	1g	0g

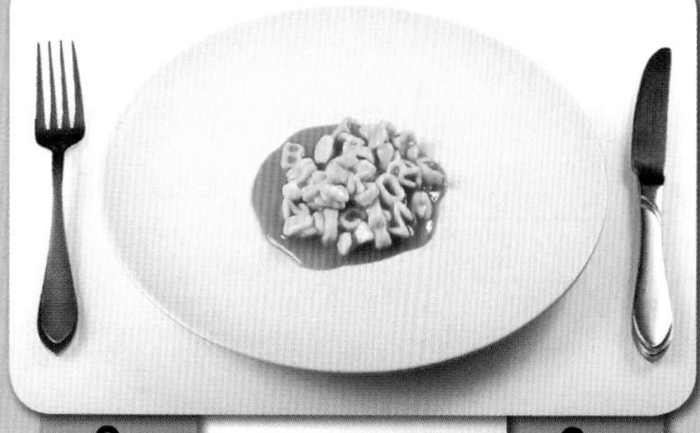

Fibre	Weight	Sat Fat
0g	Weight: 70g	0g

Carbs	Cals	Protein	Fat
27g	126	4g	1g

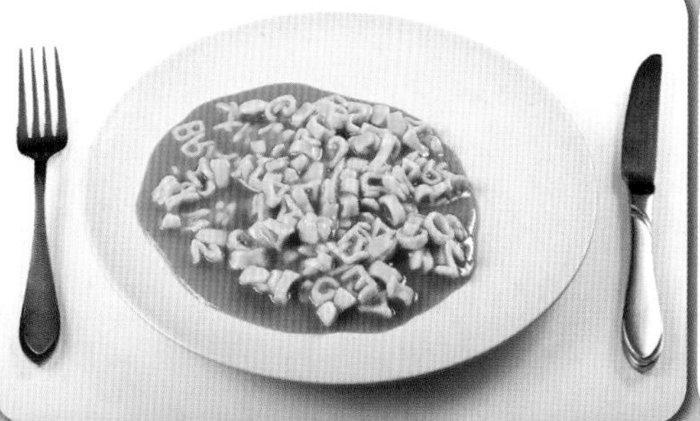

Fibre	Weight	Sat Fat
1g	Weight: 210g (half tin)	0g

Carbs	Cals	Protein	Fat
54g	255	8g	1g

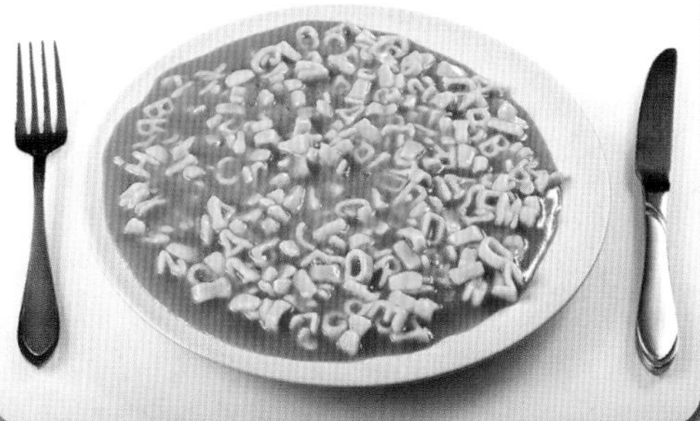

Fibre	Weight	Sat Fat
3g	Weight: 425g (full tin)	0g

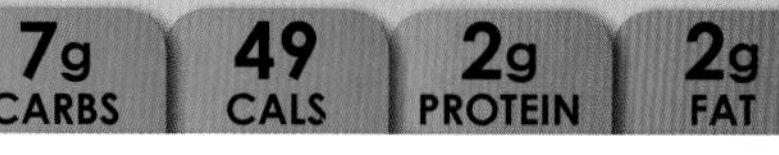

Ravioli (tinned)

Carbs	Cals	Protein	Fat
7g	49	2g	2g

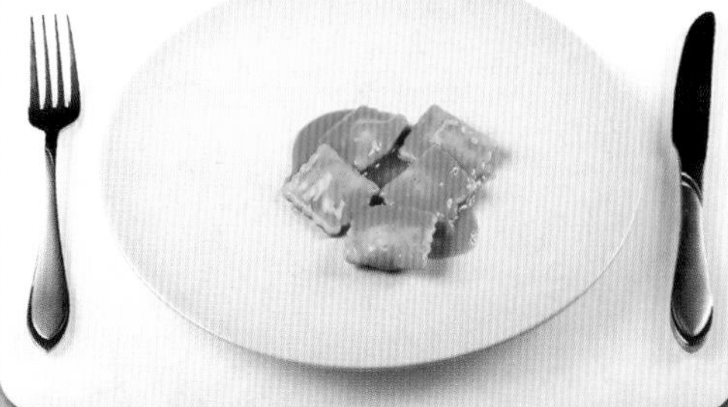

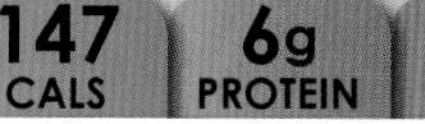

Fibre	Weight	Sat Fat
1g	Weight: 70g	1g

Carbs	Cals	Protein	Fat
22g	147	6g	5g

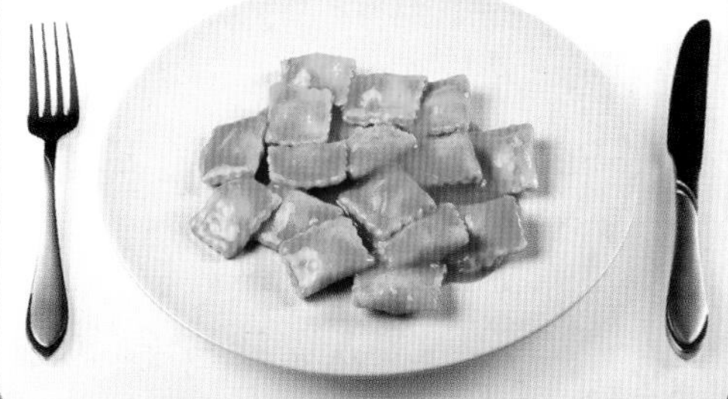

Fibre	Weight	Sat Fat
3g	Weight: 210g (half tin)	2g

Carbs	Cals	Protein	Fat
44g	298	13g	9g

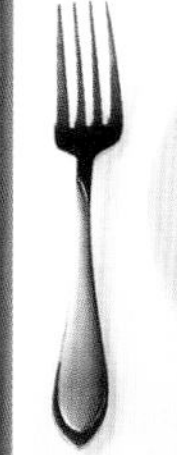

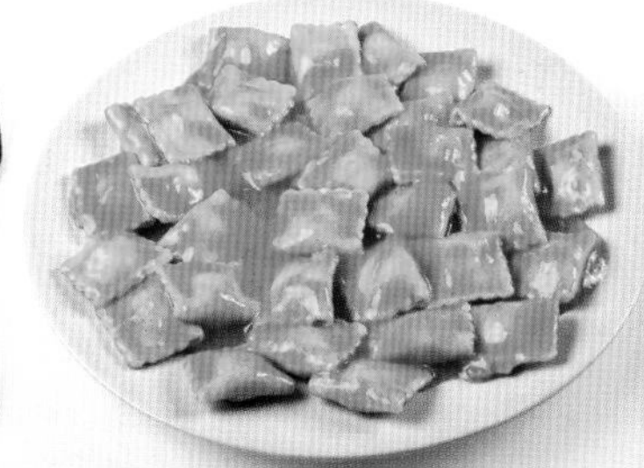

Fibre	Weight	Sat Fat
5g	Weight: 425g (full tin)	3g

Spaghetti (tinned)

CARBS	CALS	PROTEIN	FAT
10g	45	1g	0g

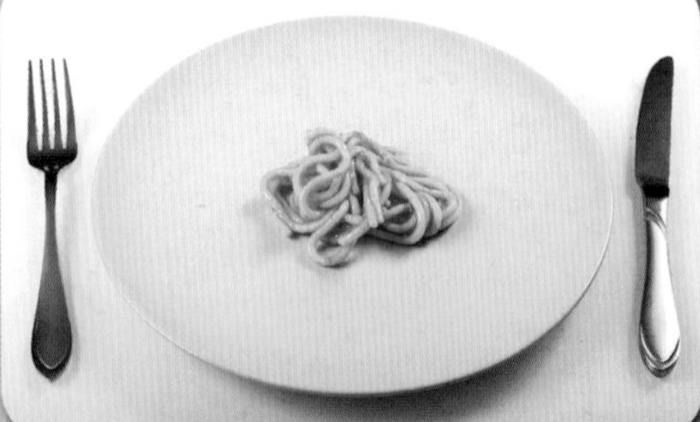

FIBRE		SAT FAT
1g	Weight: 70g	0g

CARBS	CALS	PROTEIN	FAT
30g	134	4g	1g

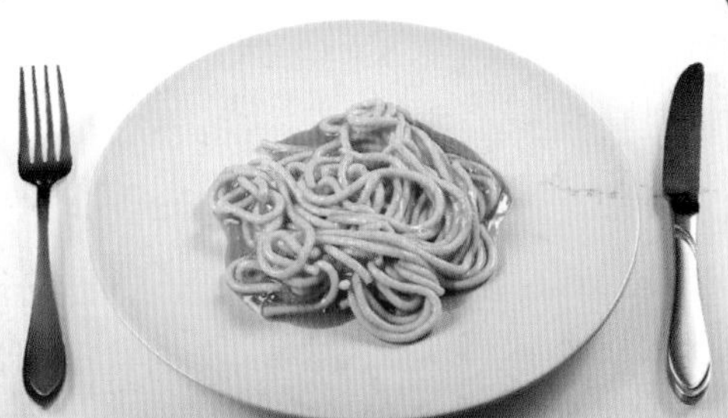

FIBRE		SAT FAT
2g	Weight: 210g (half tin)	0g

CARBS	CALS	PROTEIN	FAT
60g	272	8g	2g

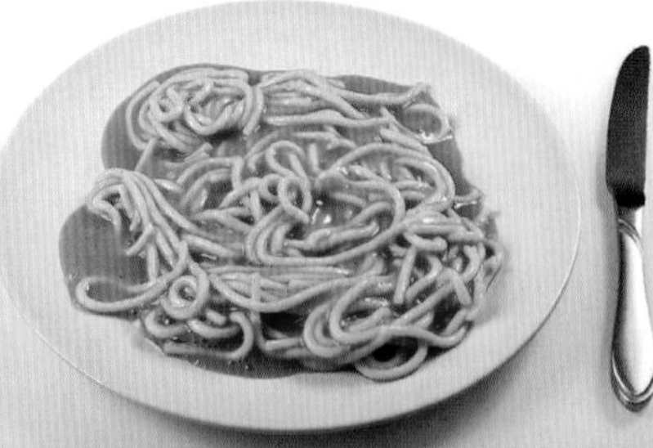

FIBRE		SAT FAT
4g	Weight: 425g (full tin)	0g

Spaghetti Hoops (tinned)

CARBS	CALS	PROTEIN	FAT
8g	40	1g	0g

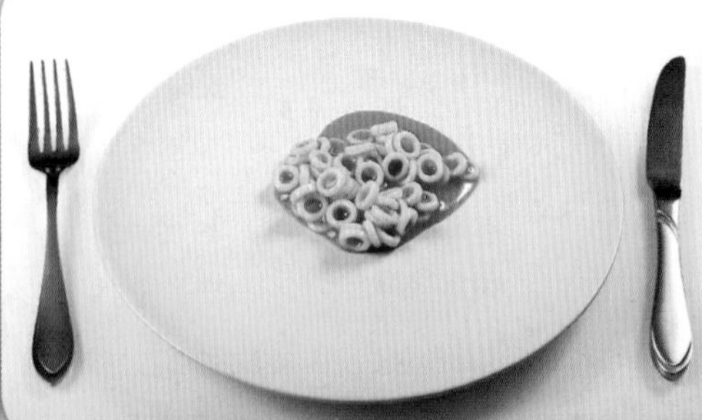

FIBRE		SAT FAT
0g	Weight: 70g	0g

CARBS	CALS	PROTEIN	FAT
25g	120	3g	0g

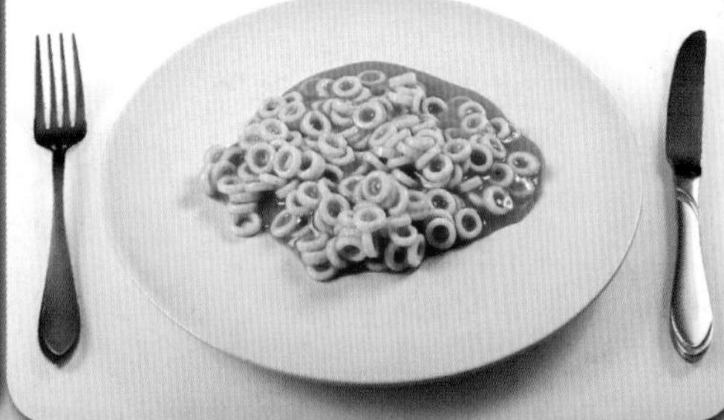

FIBRE		SAT FAT
1g	Weight: 210g (half tin)	0g

CARBS	CALS	PROTEIN	FAT
50g	239	7g	0g

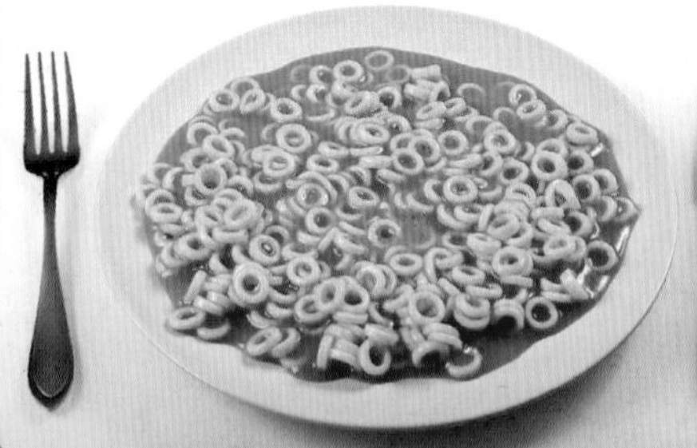

FIBRE		SAT FAT
1g	Weight: 420g (full tin)	0g

Noodles (egg)

20g CARBS	114 CALS	3g PROTEIN	2g FAT

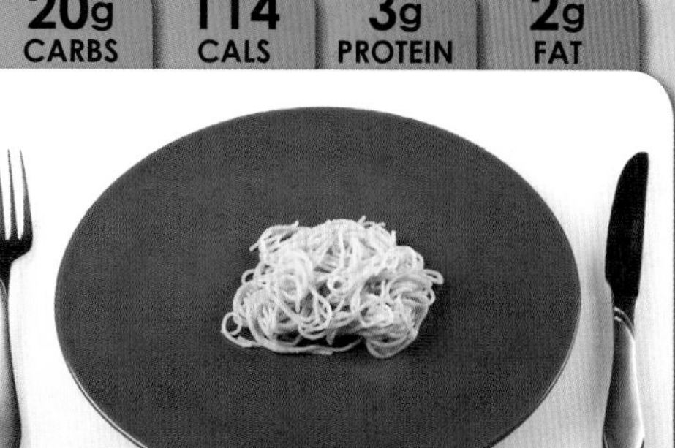

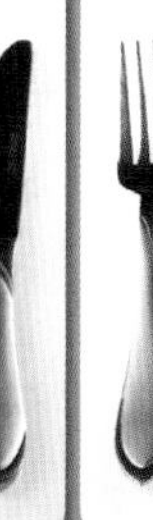

0g FIBRE	Weight: 58g	0g SAT FAT

40g CARBS	225 CALS	6g PROTEIN	4g FAT

1g FIBRE	Weight: 115g	0g SAT FAT

60g CARBS	333 CALS	10g PROTEIN	6g FAT

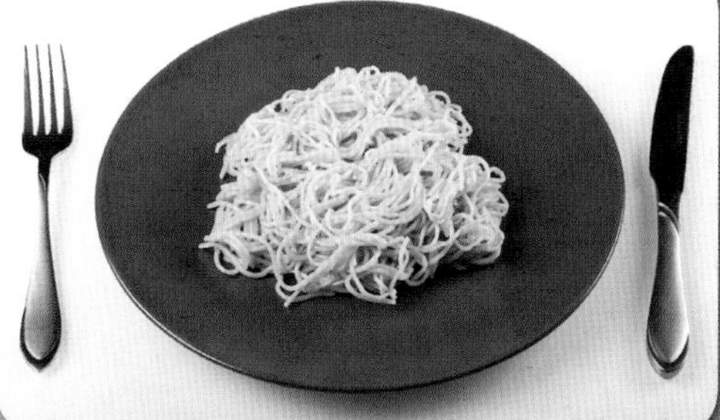

1g FIBRE	Weight: 170g	0g SAT FAT

80g CARBS	447 CALS	13g PROTEIN	9g FAT

2g FIBRE	Weight: 228g	0g SAT FAT

100g CARBS	559 CALS	16g PROTEIN	11g FAT

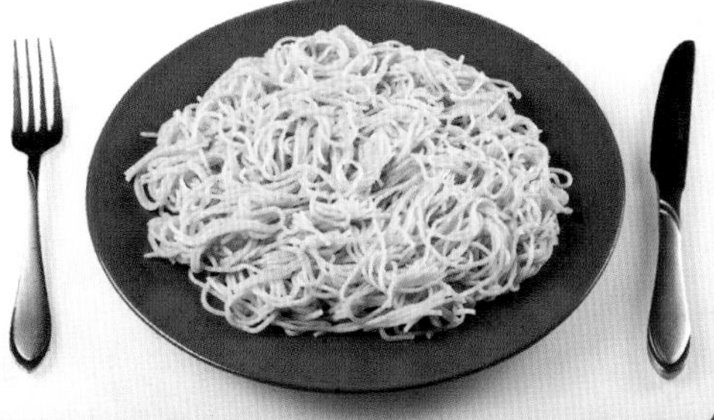

2g FIBRE	Weight: 285g	0g SAT FAT

120g CARBS	670 CALS	19g PROTEIN	13g FAT

3g FIBRE	Weight: 342g	1g SAT FAT

Noodles (rice)

CARBS	CALS	PROTEIN	FAT
20g	86	1g	0g

FIBRE	Weight	SAT FAT
1g	Weight: 70g	0g

CARBS	CALS	PROTEIN	FAT
40g	175	2g	0g

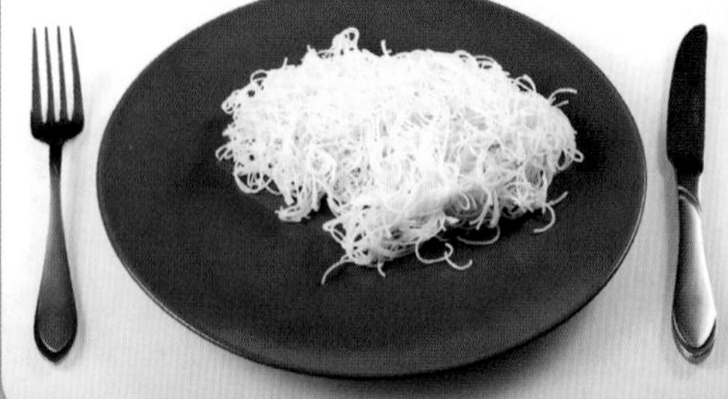

FIBRE	Weight	SAT FAT
1g	Weight: 142g	0g

CARBS	CALS	PROTEIN	FAT
60g	265	4g	0g

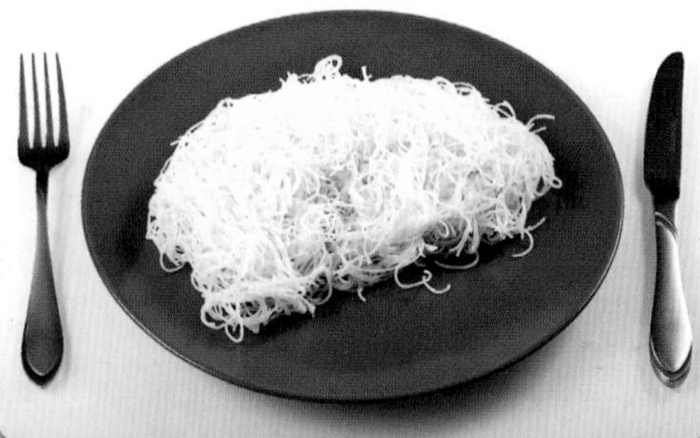

FIBRE	Weight	SAT FAT
2g	Weight: 215g	1g

CARBS	CALS	PROTEIN	FAT
80g	351	5g	0g

FIBRE	Weight	SAT FAT
2g	Weight: 285g	1g

CARBS	CALS	PROTEIN	FAT
100g	440	6g	0g

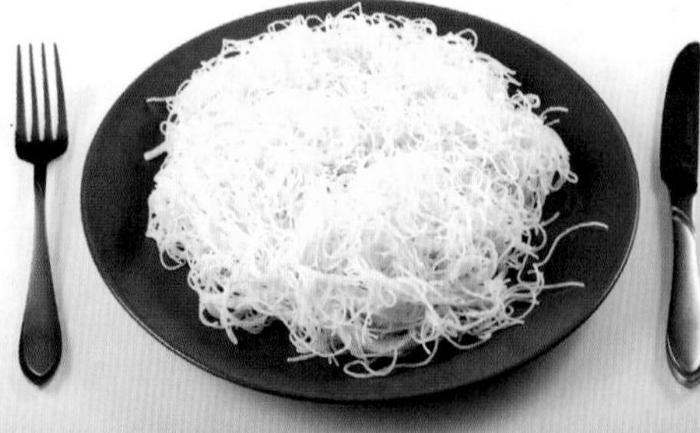

FIBRE	Weight	SAT FAT
3g	Weight: 358g	1g

CARBS	CALS	PROTEIN	FAT
120g	529	7g	0g

FIBRE	Weight	SAT FAT
3g	Weight: 430g	1g

Chips (deep fried)

CARBS	CALS	PROTEIN	FAT	FIBRE	SAT FAT	Weight
12g	90	1g	5g	1g	1g	33g
24g	180	3g	9g	2g	2g	66g
36g	273	4g	14g	3g	3g	100g
61g	459	7g	23g	5g	4g	168g
85g	642	10g	32g	8g	6g	235g
109g	827	12g	41g	10g	8g	303g

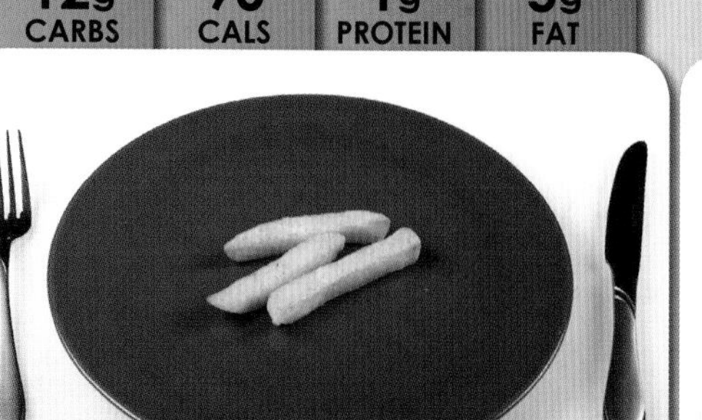

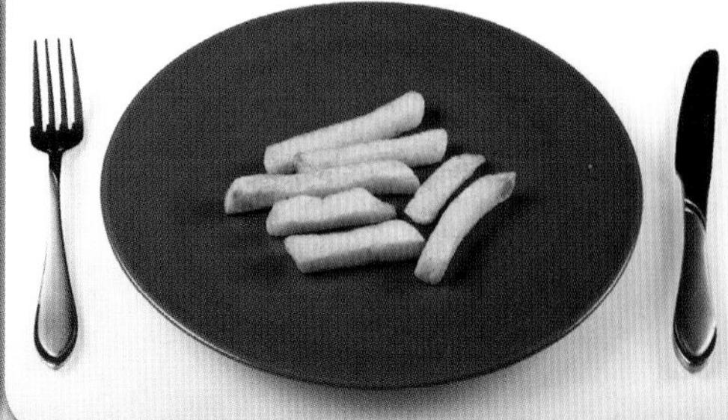

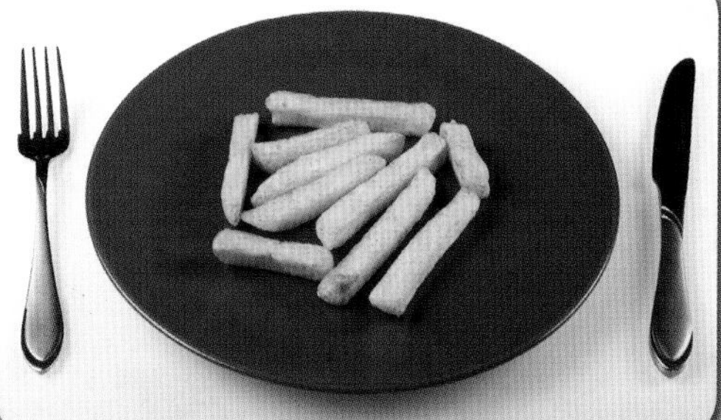

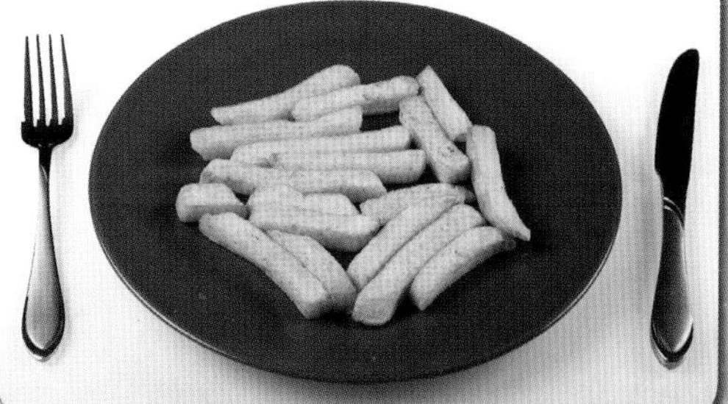

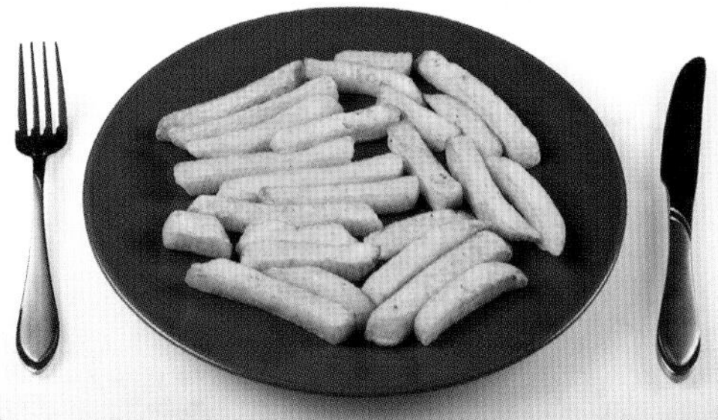

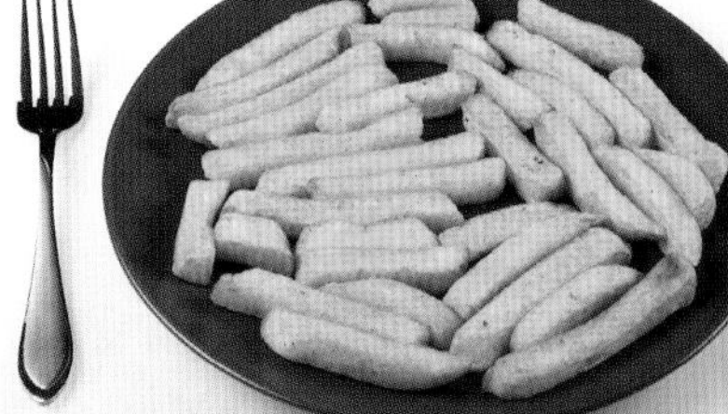

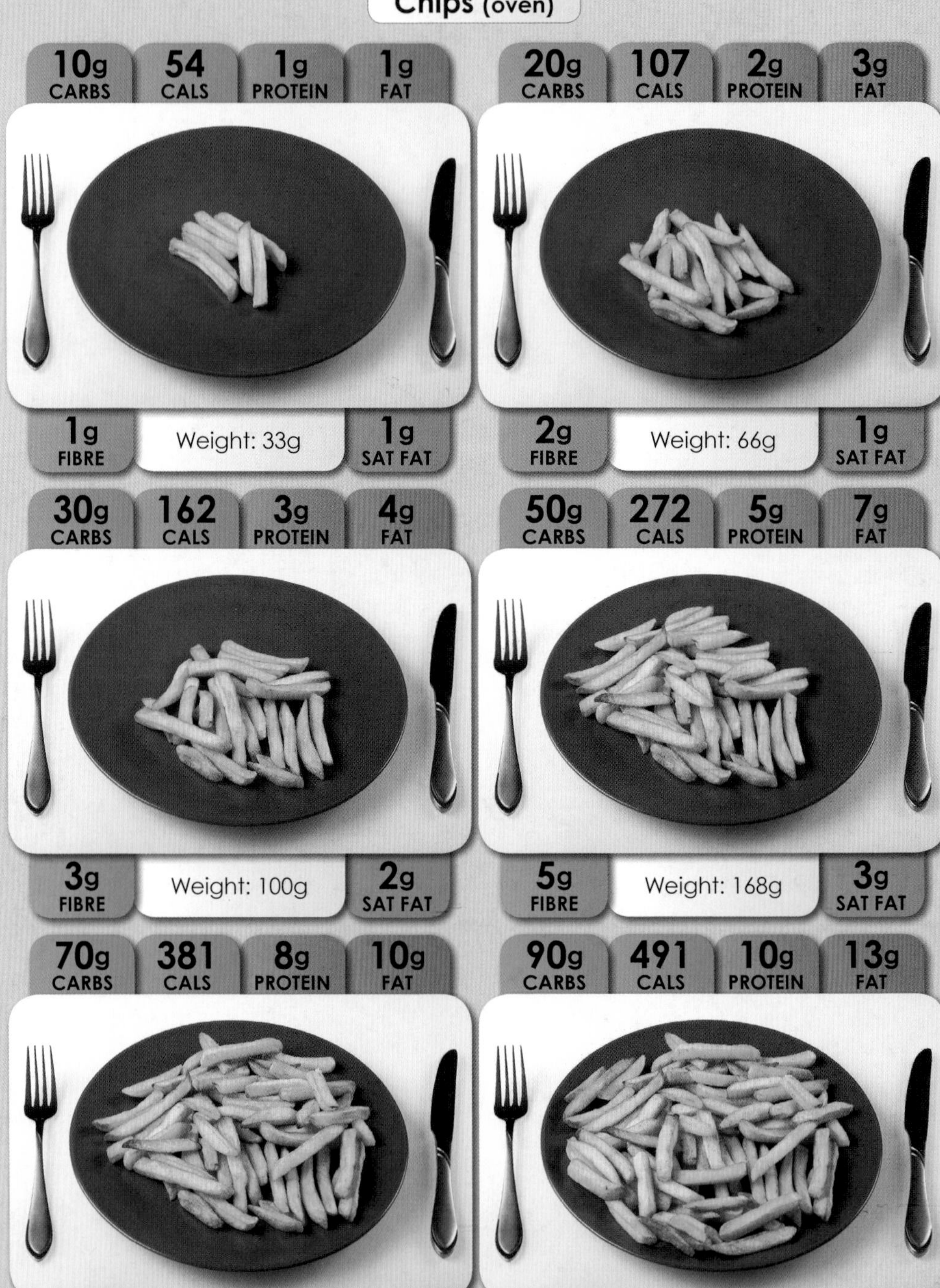
Chips (oven)
10g CARBS
54 CALS
1g PROTEIN
1g FAT
1g FIBRE
Weight: 33g
1g SAT FAT
20g CARBS
107 CALS
2g PROTEIN
3g FAT
2g FIBRE
Weight: 66g
1g SAT FAT
30g CARBS
162 CALS
3g PROTEIN
4g FAT
3g FIBRE
Weight: 100g
2g SAT FAT
50g CARBS
272 CALS
5g PROTEIN
7g FAT
5g FIBRE
Weight: 168g
3g SAT FAT
70g CARBS
381 CALS
8g PROTEIN
10g FAT
6g FIBRE
Weight: 235g
4g SAT FAT
90g CARBS
491 CALS
10g PROTEIN
13g FAT
8g FIBRE
Weight: 303g
6g SAT FAT

Dauphinoise Potatoes

10g CARBS	178 CALS	2g PROTEIN	15g FAT

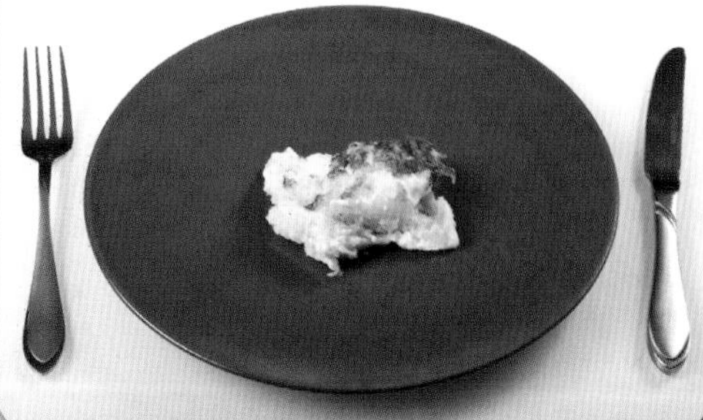

1g FIBRE	Weight: 72g	9g SAT FAT

30g CARBS	548 CALS	5g PROTEIN	46g FAT

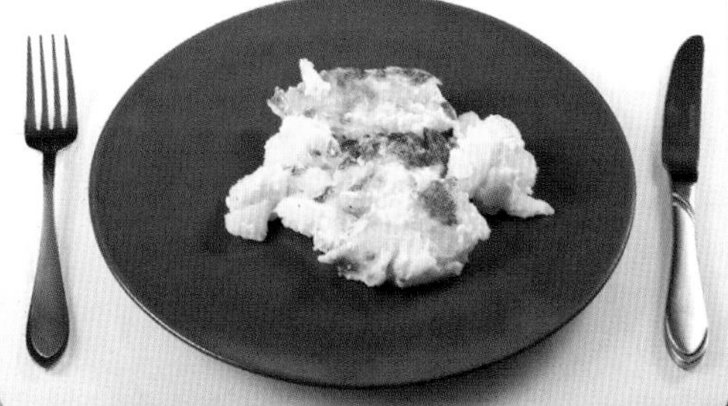

3g FIBRE	Weight: 222g	28g SAT FAT

50g CARBS	921 CALS	9g PROTEIN	78g FAT

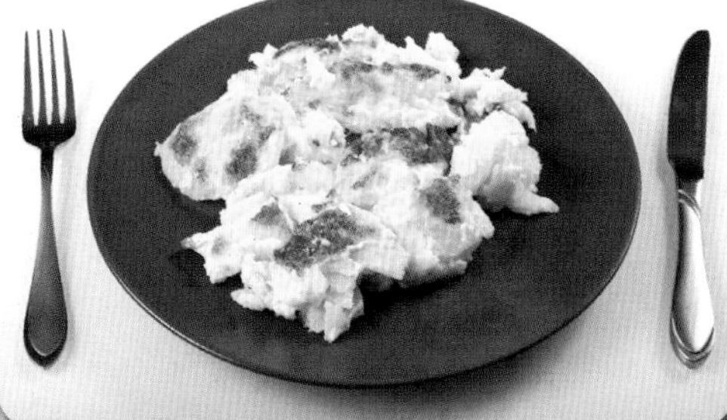

5g FIBRE	Weight: 373g	48g SAT FAT

Gnocchi

26g CARBS	120 CALS	3g PROTEIN	0g FAT

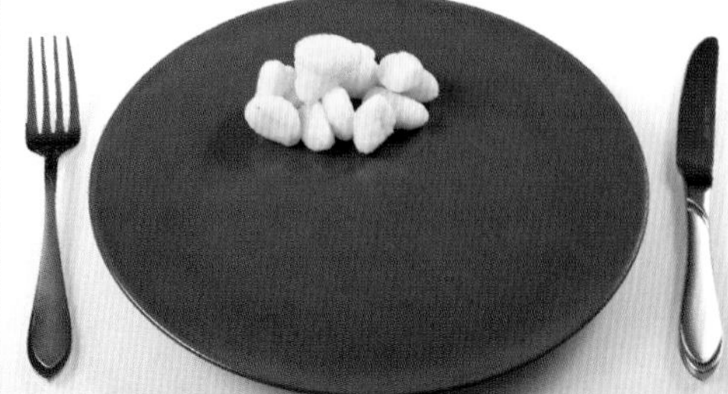

1g FIBRE	Weight: 80g	0g SAT FAT

77g CARBS	359 CALS	9g PROTEIN	1g FAT

3g FIBRE	Weight: 240g	0g SAT FAT

129g CARBS	601 CALS	14g PROTEIN	2g FAT

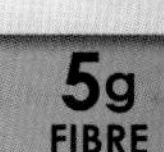

5g FIBRE	Weight: 402g	1g SAT FAT

26cm Dinner Plate

Jacket Potato (baked)

New Potatoes (boiled)

Jacket Potato (baked)

20g CARBS | 90 CALS | 3g PROTEIN | 0g FAT

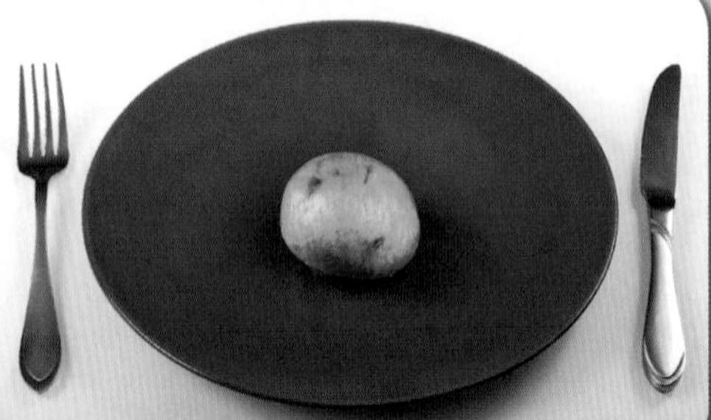

2g FIBRE | Weight: 95g | 0g SAT FAT

New Potatoes (boiled)

10g CARBS | 43 CALS | 1g PROTEIN | 0g FAT

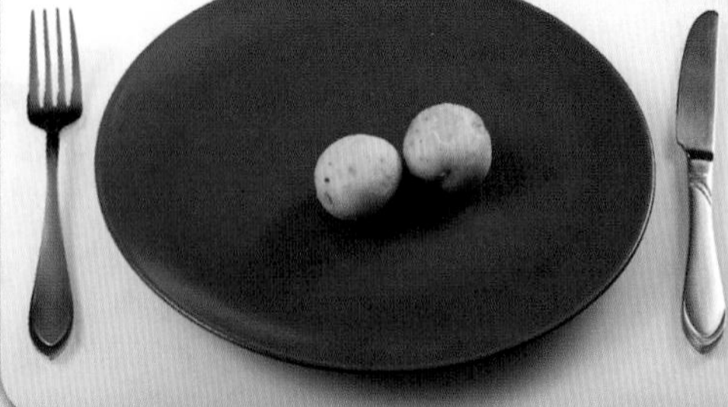

1g FIBRE | Weight: 65g | 0g SAT FAT

Jacket Potato (baked)

45g CARBS | 200 CALS | 6g PROTEIN | 1g FAT

New Potatoes (boiled)

30g CARBS | 129 CALS | 3g PROTEIN | 1g FAT

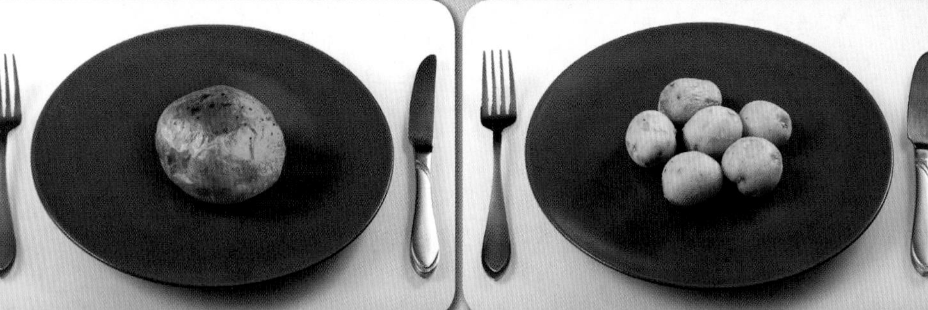

Jacket Potato (baked)

5g FIBRE | Weight: 220g | 0g SAT FAT

New Potatoes (boiled)

4g FIBRE | Weight: 195g | 0g SAT FAT

Jacket Potato (baked)

75g CARBS | 333 CALS | 9g PROTEIN | 1g FAT

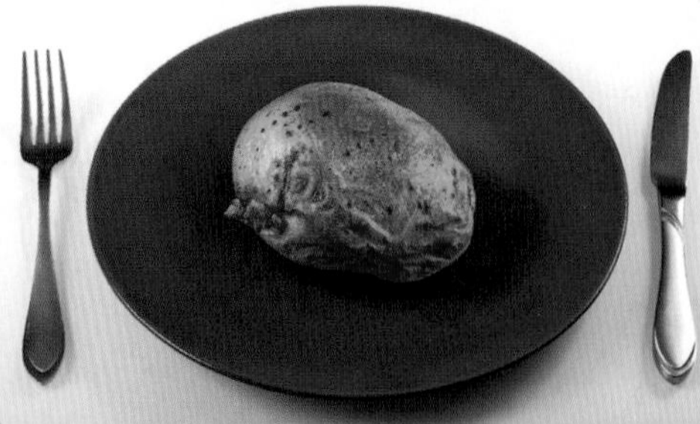

8g FIBRE | Weight: 348g | 0g SAT FAT

New Potatoes (boiled)

60g CARBS | 257 CALS | 6g PROTEIN | 1g FAT

8g FIBRE | Weight: 390g | 0g SAT FAT

Mashed Potato (with butter)

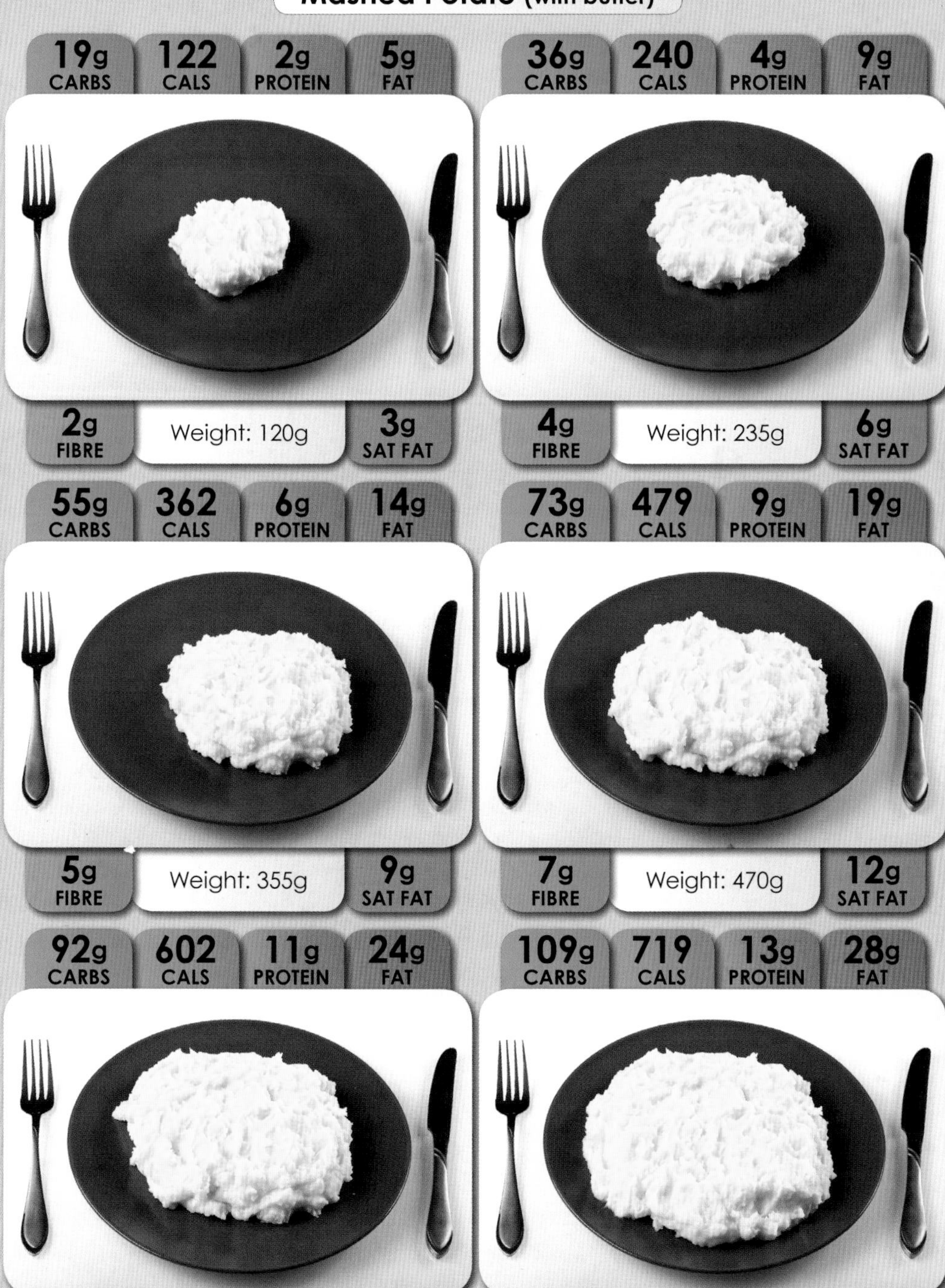

Mashed Potato (with semi-skimmed milk)

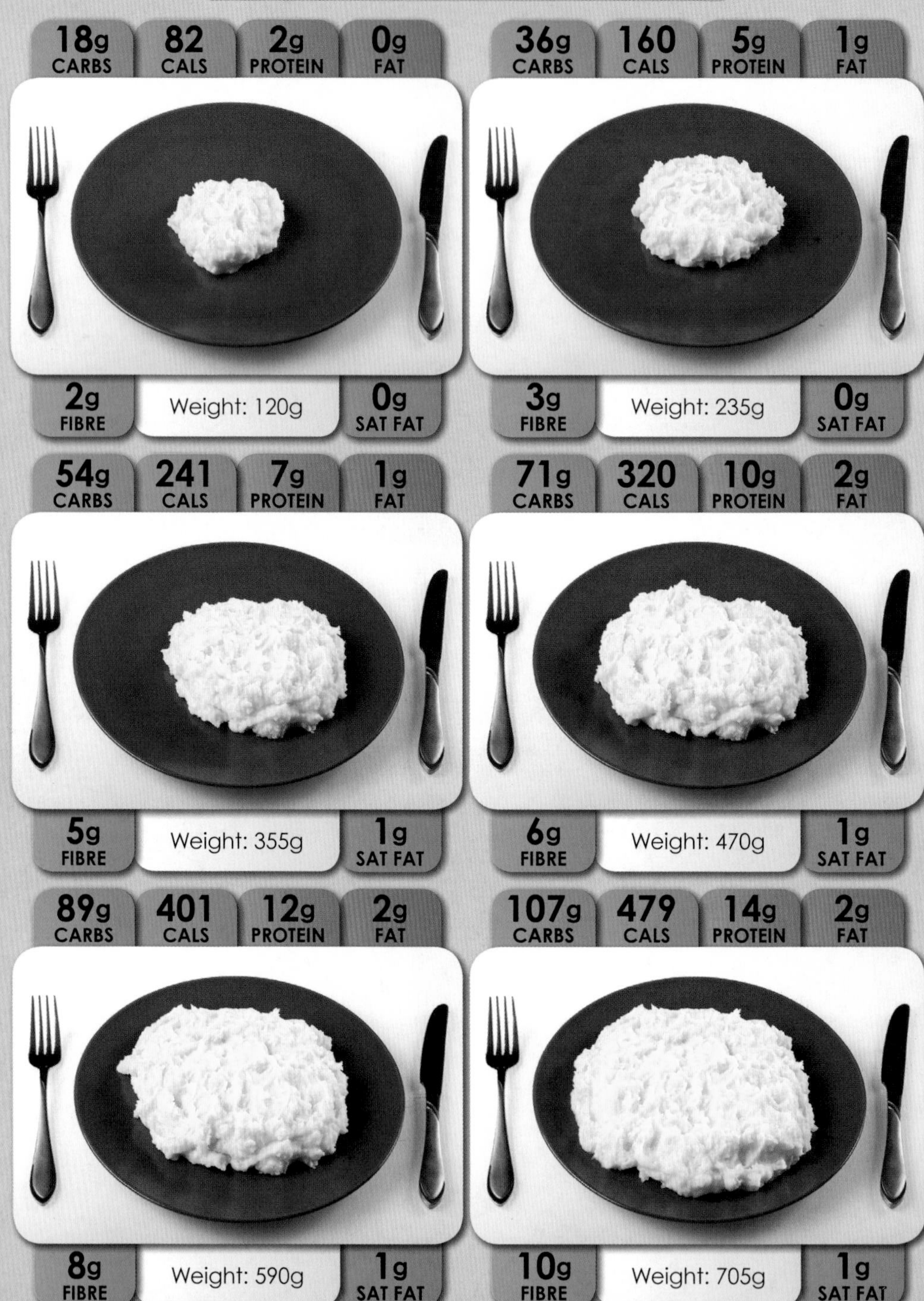

Potato Slices (baked)

8g CARBS	52 CALS	1g PROTEIN	2g FAT

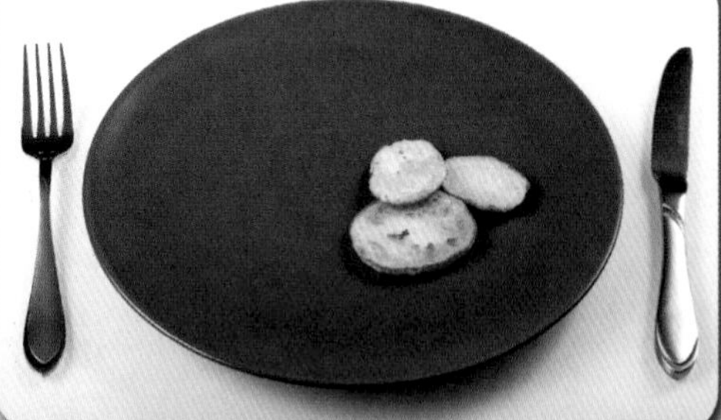

1g FIBRE	Weight: 28g	0g SAT FAT

23g CARBS	148 CALS	2g PROTEIN	5g FAT

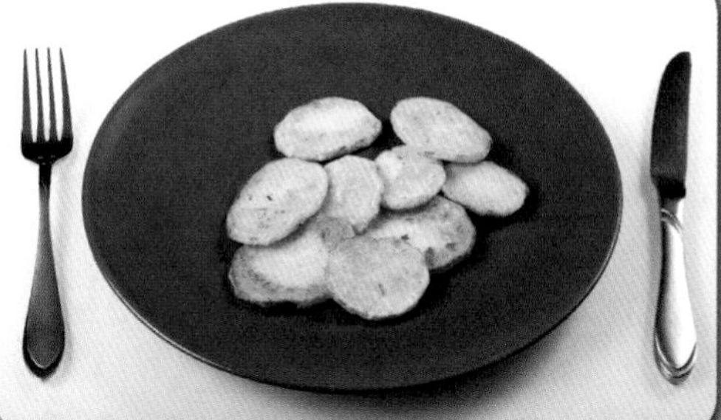

2g FIBRE	Weight: 80g	1g SAT FAT

39g CARBS	250 CALS	4g PROTEIN	9g FAT

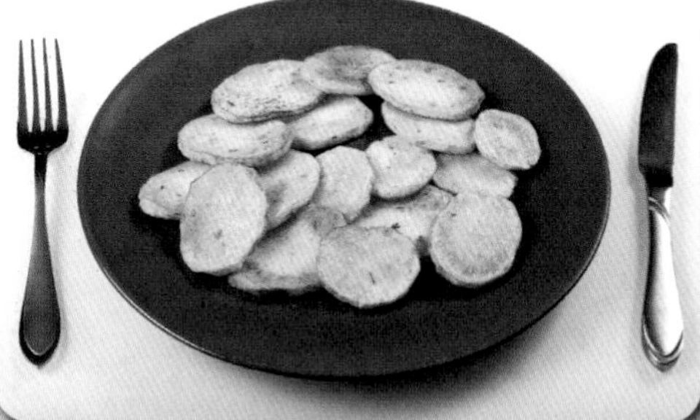

3g FIBRE	Weight: 135g	1g SAT FAT

Roast Potatoes

10g CARBS	57 CALS	1g PROTEIN	2g FAT

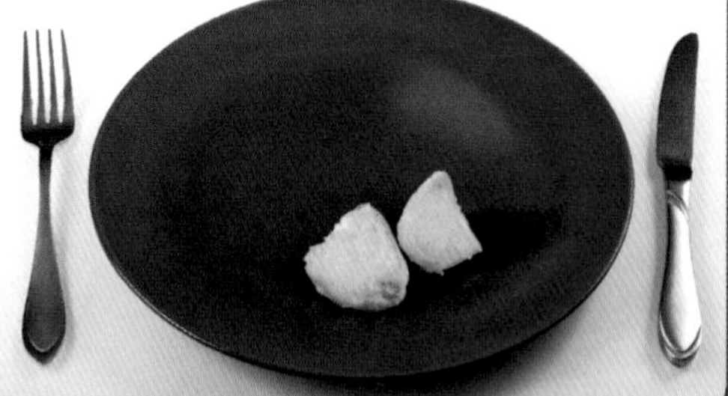

1g FIBRE	Weight: 38g	1g SAT FAT

40g CARBS	231 CALS	4g PROTEIN	7g FAT

4g FIBRE	Weight: 155g	3g SAT FAT

70g CARBS	402 CALS	8g PROTEIN	12g FAT

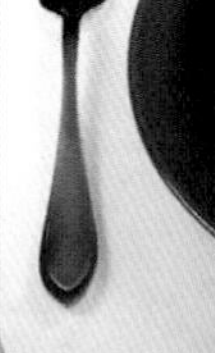

6g FIBRE	Weight: 270g	5g SAT FAT

26cm Dinner Plate

Sweet Potatoes (baked)

CARBS	CALS	PROTEIN	FAT
15g	63	1g	0g

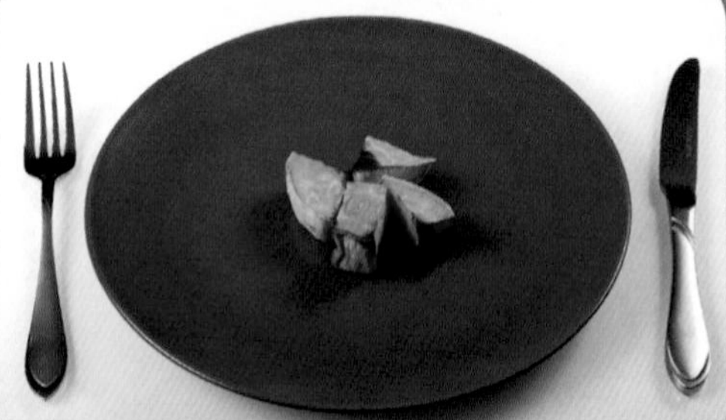

FIBRE	Weight	SAT FAT
2g	Weight: 55g	0g

CARBS	CALS	PROTEIN	FAT
45g	184	3g	1g

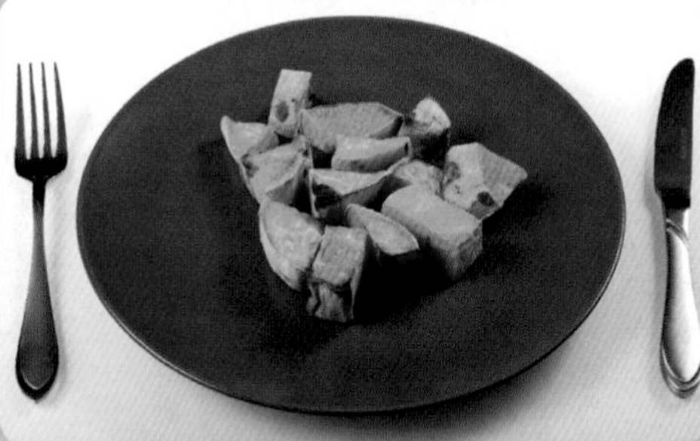

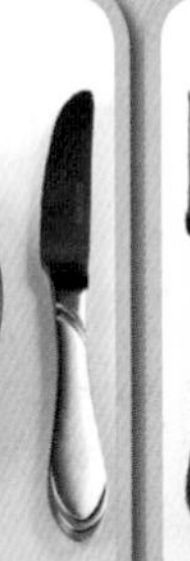

FIBRE	Weight	SAT FAT
7g	Weight: 160g	0g

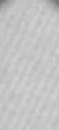

CARBS	CALS	PROTEIN	FAT
75g	311	4g	1g

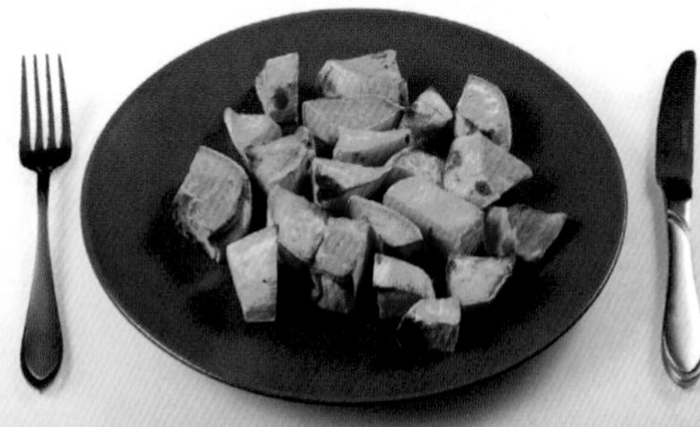

FIBRE	Weight	SAT FAT
12g	Weight: 270g	1g

Mashed Sweet Potato

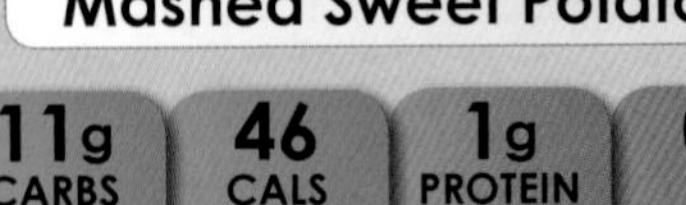

CARBS	CALS	PROTEIN	FAT
11g	46	1g	0g

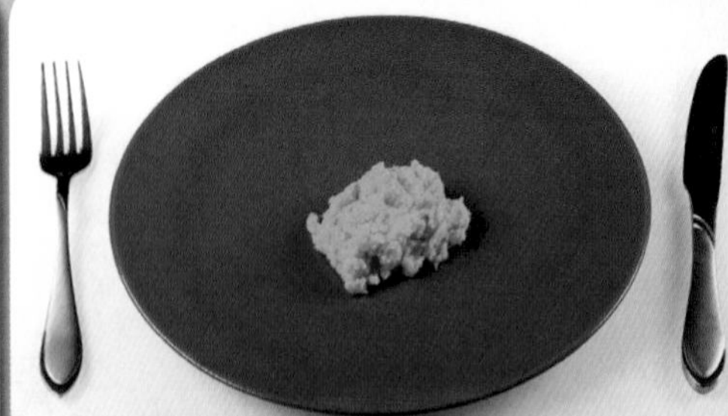

FIBRE	Weight	SAT FAT
2g	Weight: 55g	0g

CARBS	CALS	PROTEIN	FAT
33g	134	2g	0g

FIBRE	Weight	SAT FAT
5g	Weight: 160g	0g

CARBS	CALS	PROTEIN	FAT
55g	227	3g	1g

FIBRE	Weight	SAT FAT
8g	Weight: 270g	0g

Potato Salad (with mayonnaise)

Carbs	Cals	Protein	Fat
7g	172	1g	16g

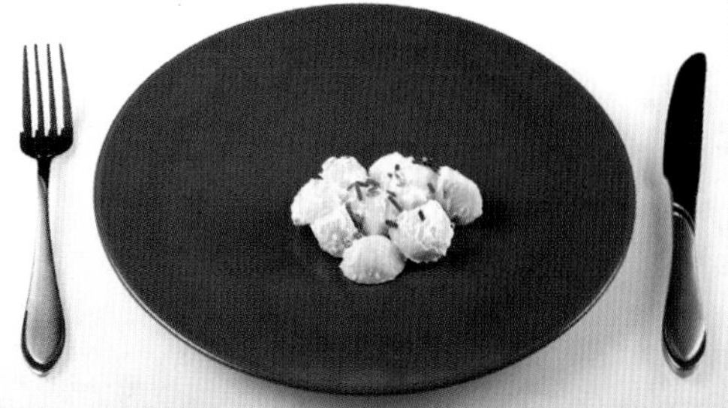

Fibre	Weight	Sat Fat
1g	Weight: 60g	2g

Carbs	Cals	Protein	Fat
14g	344	2g	32g

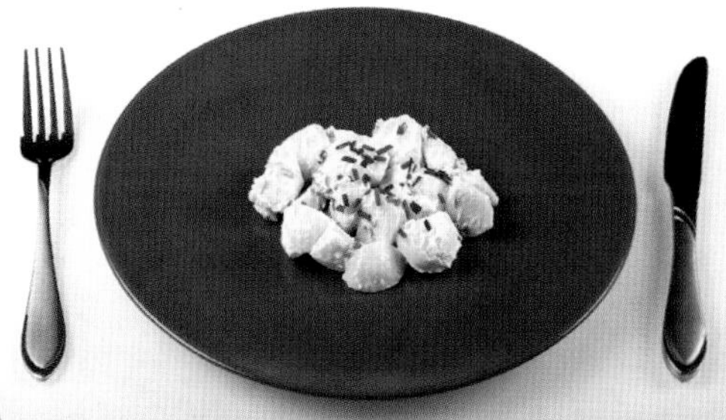

Fibre	Weight	Sat Fat
1g	Weight: 120g	5g

Carbs	Cals	Protein	Fat
21g	517	3g	48g

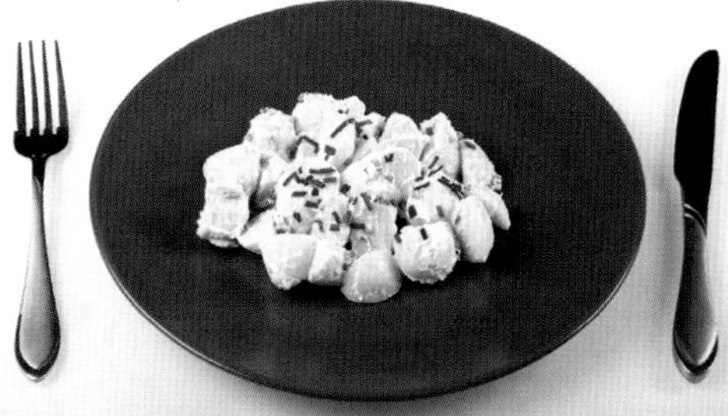

Fibre	Weight	Sat Fat
2g	Weight: 180g	7g

Wedges (baked)

Carbs	Cals	Protein	Fat
14g	89	2g	3g

Fibre	Weight	Sat Fat
2g	Weight: 55g	0g

Carbs	Cals	Protein	Fat
42g	267	5g	8g

Fibre	Weight	Sat Fat
5g	Weight: 165g	1g

Carbs	Cals	Protein	Fat
69g	437	8g	14g

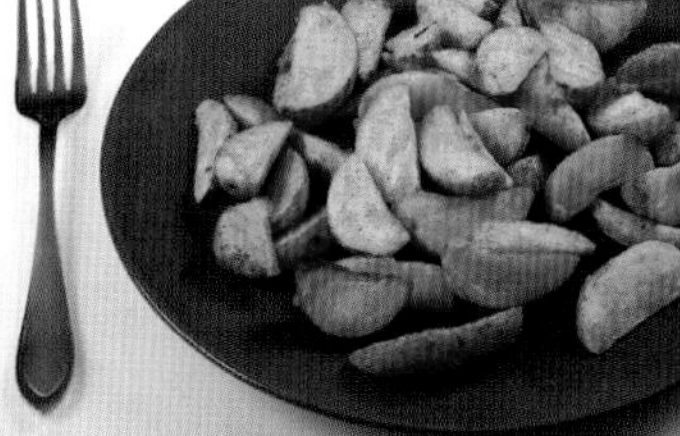

Fibre	Weight	Sat Fat
8g	Weight: 270g	2g

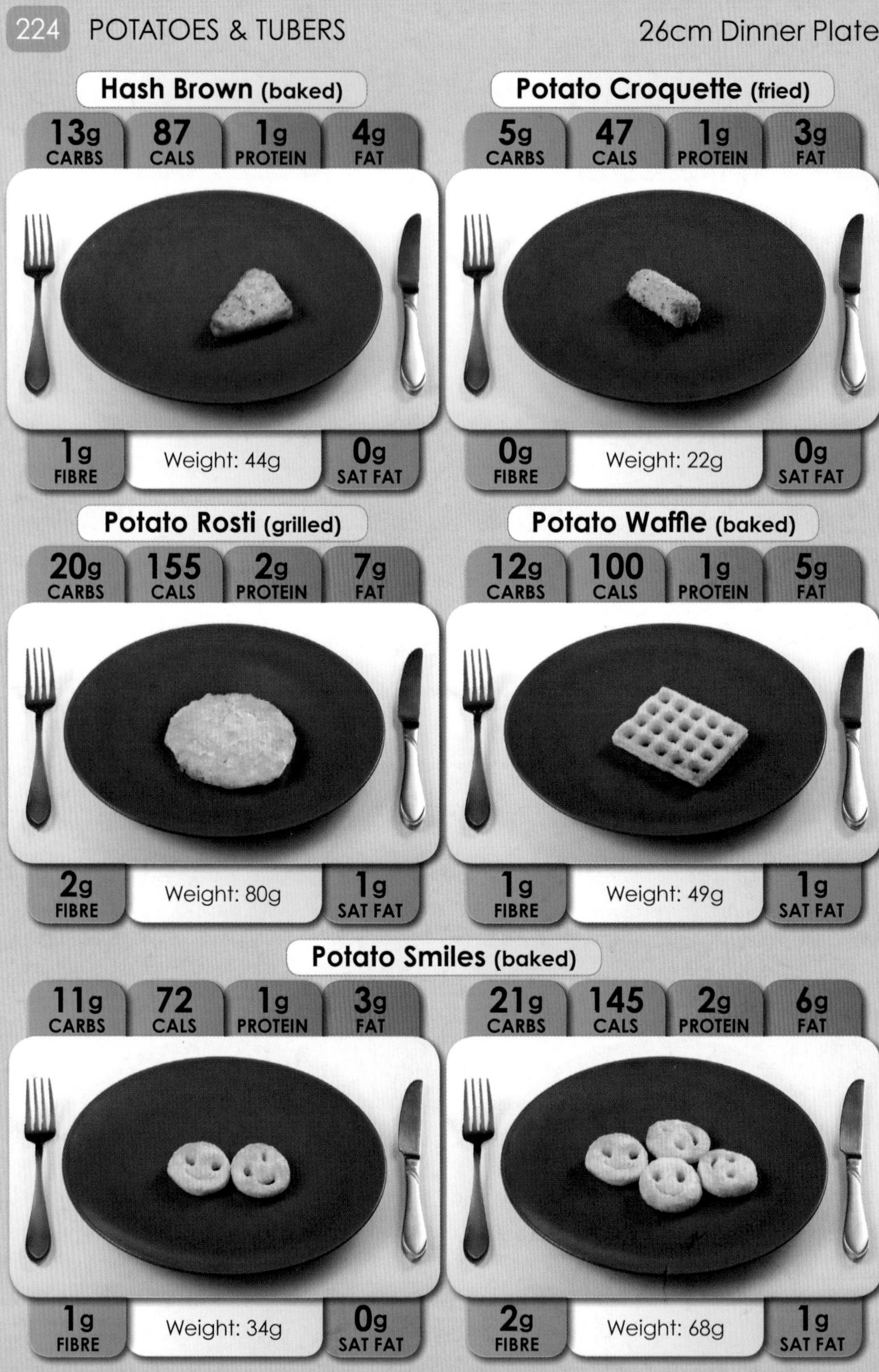

Hash Brown (baked)

Carbs	Cals	Protein	Fat	Fibre	Sat Fat	Weight
13g	87	1g	4g	1g	0g	44g

Potato Croquette (fried)

Carbs	Cals	Protein	Fat	Fibre	Sat Fat	Weight
5g	47	1g	3g	0g	0g	22g

Potato Rosti (grilled)

Carbs	Cals	Protein	Fat	Fibre	Sat Fat	Weight
20g	155	2g	7g	2g	1g	80g

Potato Waffle (baked)

Carbs	Cals	Protein	Fat	Fibre	Sat Fat	Weight
12g	100	1g	5g	1g	1g	49g

Potato Smiles (baked)

Carbs	Cals	Protein	Fat	Fibre	Sat Fat	Weight
11g	72	1g	3g	1g	0g	34g

Carbs	Cals	Protein	Fat	Fibre	Sat Fat	Weight
21g	145	2g	6g	2g	1g	68g

Cassava Chips (baked)

Carbs	Cals	Protein	Fat	Fibre	Weight	Sat Fat
23g	122	1g	3g	1g	45g	1g
71g	367	1g	8g	3g	136g	4g
119g	616	2g	14g	5g	228g	7g

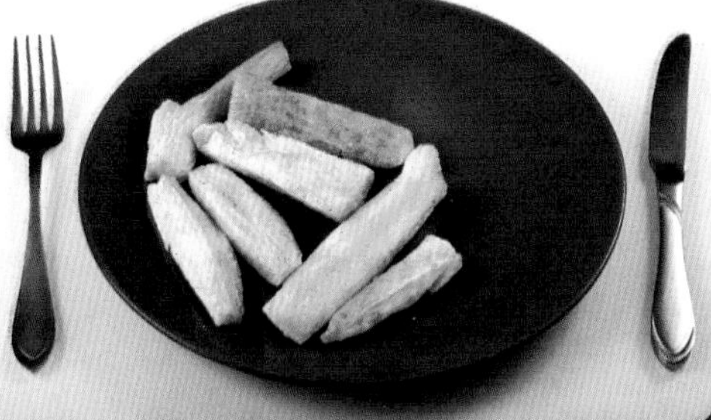

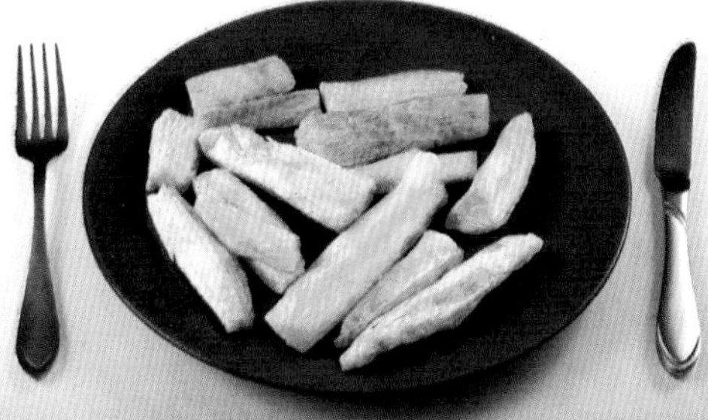

Eba / Gari

Carbs	Cals	Protein	Fat	Fibre	Weight	Sat Fat
45g	190	1g	1g	2g	130g	0g
91g	388	1g	1g	4g	265g	0g
129g	548	2g	2g	5g	375g	0g

Fufu (yam)

Carbs	Cals	Protein	Fat	Fibre	Weight	Sat Fat
49g	202	3g	0g	3g	130g	0g
99g	411	6g	1g	5g	265g	0g
140g	581	8g	1g	8g	375g	0g

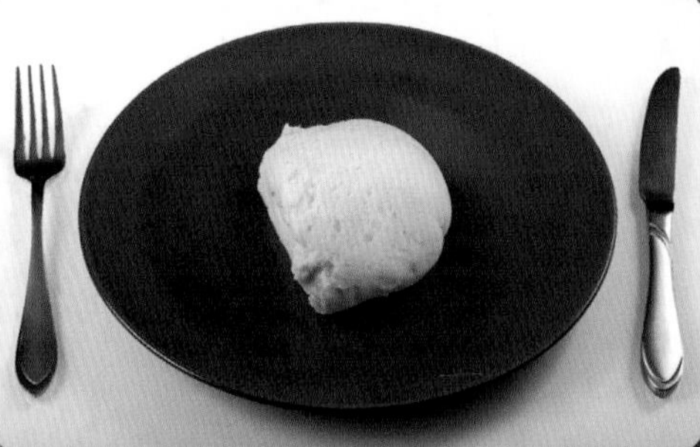

Yam (boiled)

Carbs	Cals	Protein	Fat	Fibre	Weight	Sat Fat
20g	80	1g	0g	1g	60g	0g
40g	160	2g	0g	2g	120g	0g
60g	242	3g	1g	4g	182g	0g

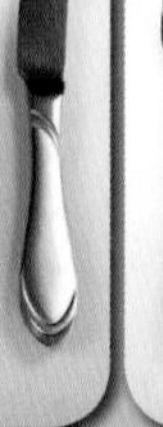

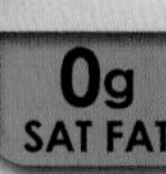

Basmati Rice

CARBS	CALS	PROTEIN	FAT	FIBRE	SAT FAT	Weight
10g	46	1g	0g	0g	0g	32g

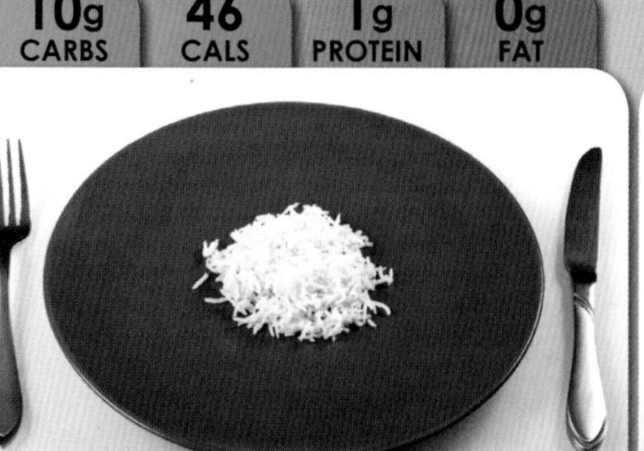

CARBS	CALS	PROTEIN	FAT	FIBRE	SAT FAT	Weight
30g	137	3g	1g	0g	0g	96g

CARBS	CALS	PROTEIN	FAT	FIBRE	SAT FAT	Weight
51g	233	5g	1g	0g	0g	163g

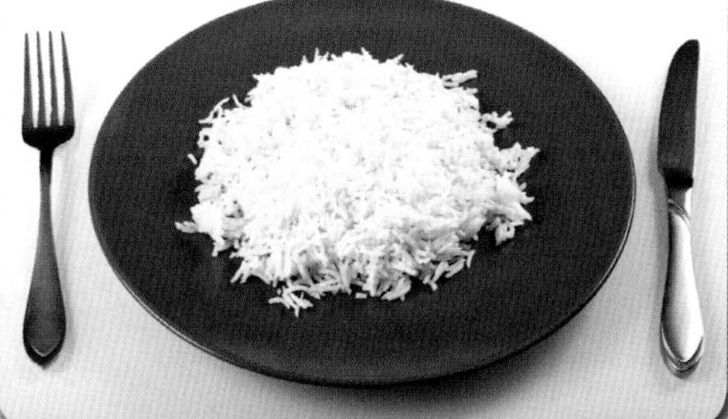

CARBS	CALS	PROTEIN	FAT	FIBRE	SAT FAT	Weight
71g	322	6g	2g	0g	0g	225g

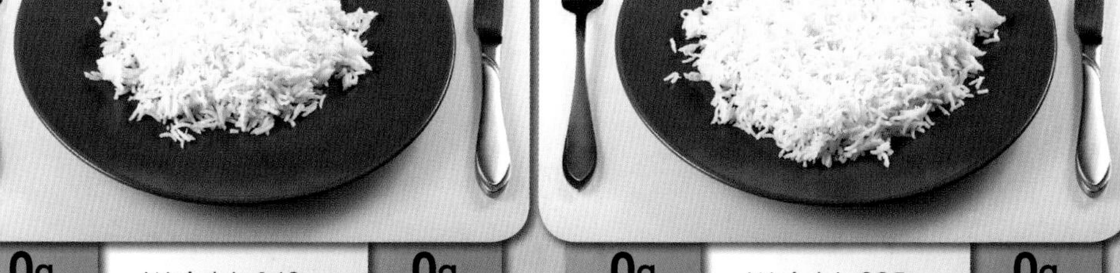

CARBS	CALS	PROTEIN	FAT	FIBRE	SAT FAT	Weight
91g	414	8g	2g	0g	1g	290g

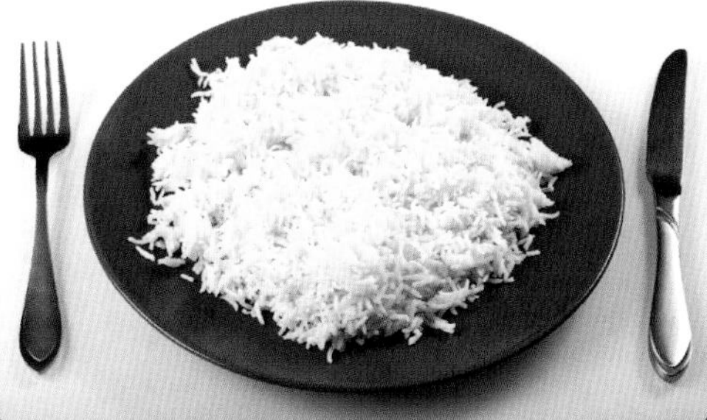

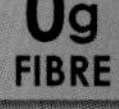

CARBS	CALS	PROTEIN	FAT	FIBRE	SAT FAT	Weight
112g	507	10g	3g	0g	1g	355g

Brown Rice (long grain)

10g CARBS | 42 CALS | 1g PROTEIN | 0g FAT

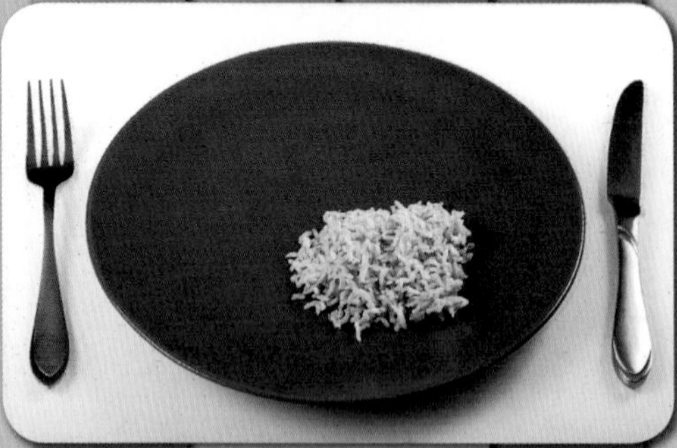

0g FIBRE | Weight: 30g | 0g SAT FAT

31g CARBS | 134 CALS | 3g PROTEIN | 1g FAT

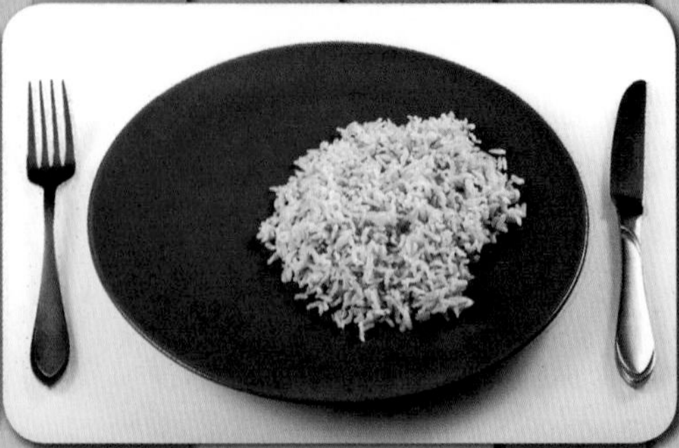

1g FIBRE | Weight: 95g | 0g SAT FAT

50g CARBS | 219 CALS | 4g PROTEIN | 2g FAT

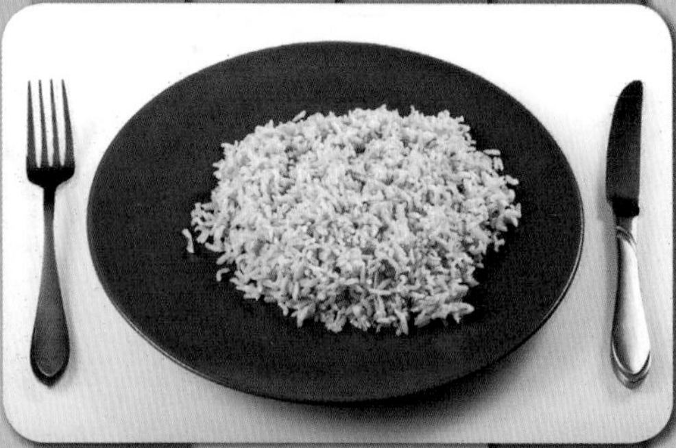

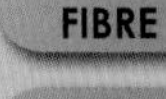

2g FIBRE | Weight: 155g | 1g SAT FAT

70g CARBS | 307 CALS | 6g PROTEIN | 2g FAT

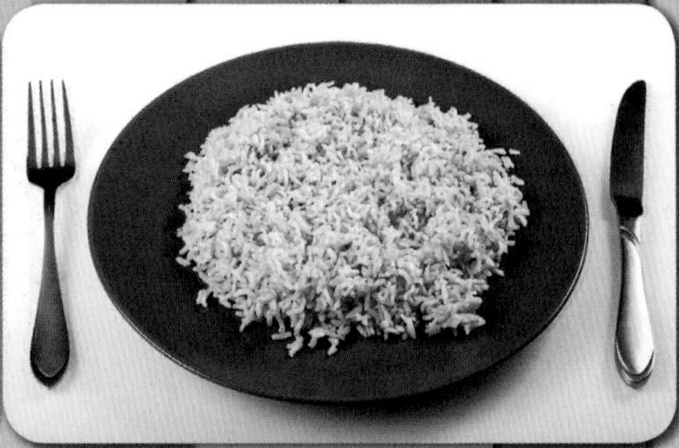

2g FIBRE | Weight: 218g | 1g SAT FAT

90g CARBS | 395 CALS | 7g PROTEIN | 3g FAT

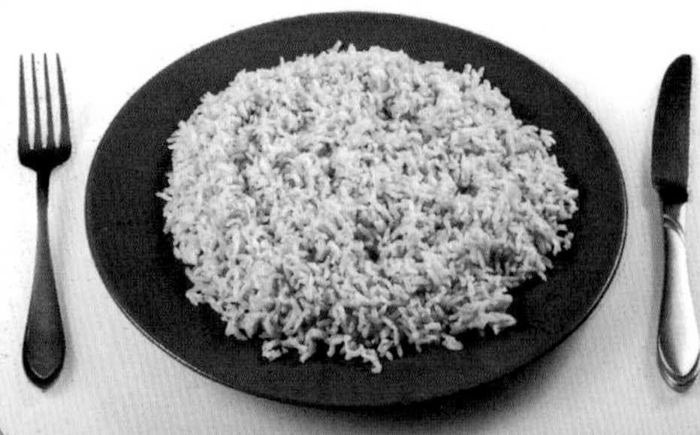

3g FIBRE | Weight: 280g | 1g SAT FAT

110g CARBS | 484 CALS | 9g PROTEIN | 4g FAT

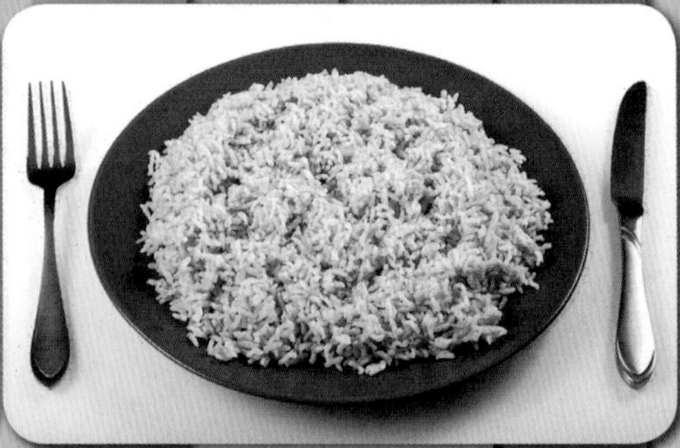

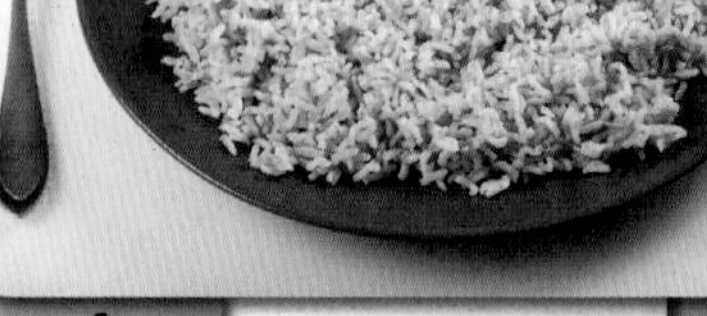

4g FIBRE | Weight: 343g | 1g SAT FAT

White Rice (long grain)

10g CARBS | 44 CALS | 1g PROTEIN | 0g FAT

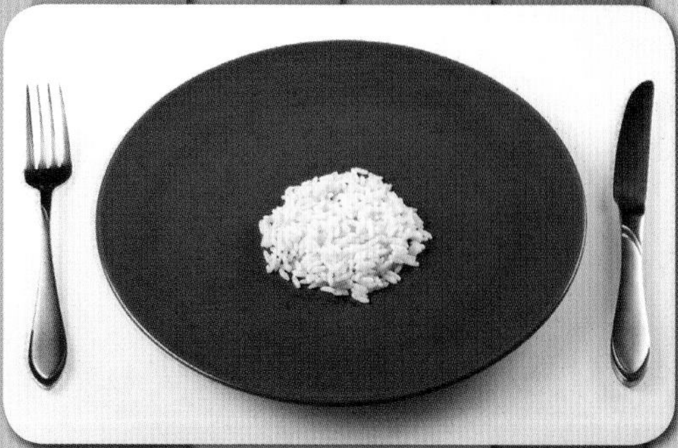

0g FIBRE | Weight: 32g | 0g SAT FAT

30g CARBS | 133 CALS | 3g PROTEIN | 1g FAT

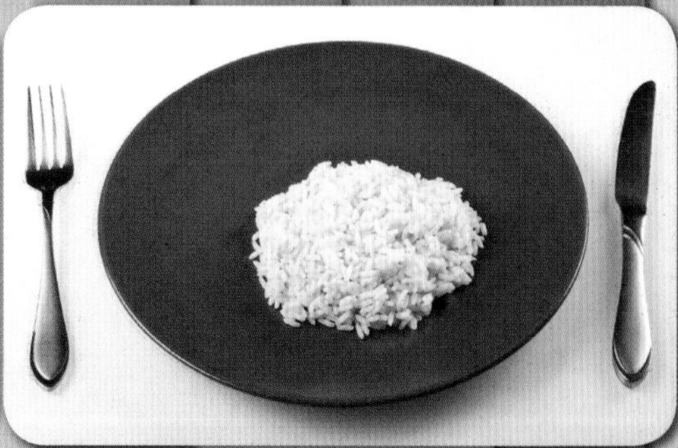

0g FIBRE | Weight: 96g | 0g SAT FAT

50g CARBS | 225 CALS | 4g PROTEIN | 2g FAT

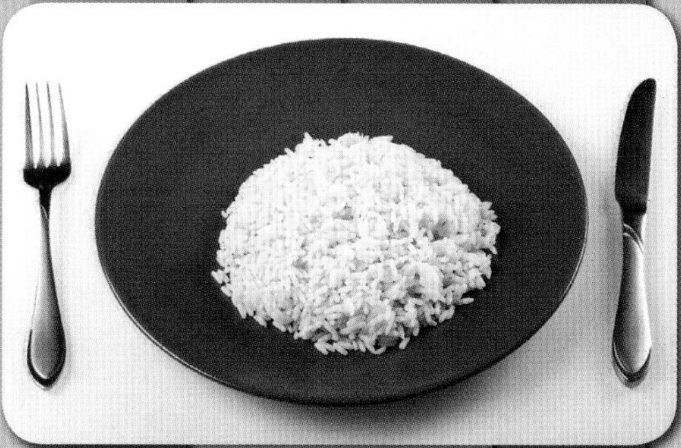

0g FIBRE | Weight: 163g | 1g SAT FAT

70g CARBS | 311 CALS | 6g PROTEIN | 3g FAT

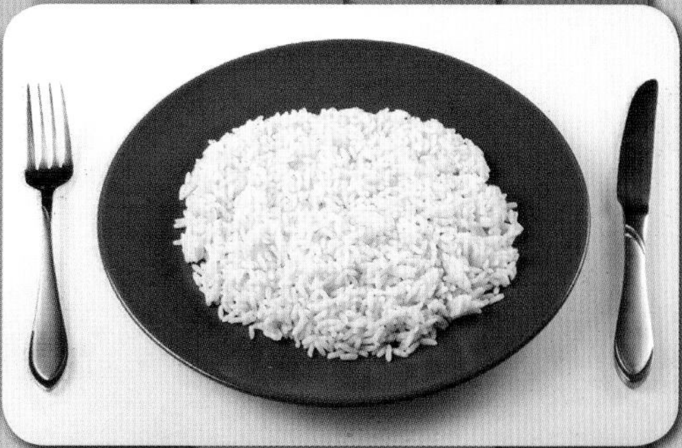

0g FIBRE | Weight: 225g | 1g SAT FAT

90g CARBS | 400 CALS | 8g PROTEIN | 4g FAT

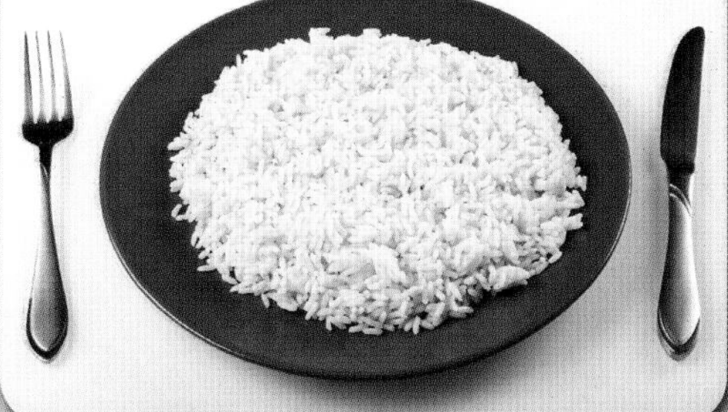

0g FIBRE | Weight: 290g | 1g SAT FAT

110g CARBS | 490 CALS | 9g PROTEIN | 5g FAT

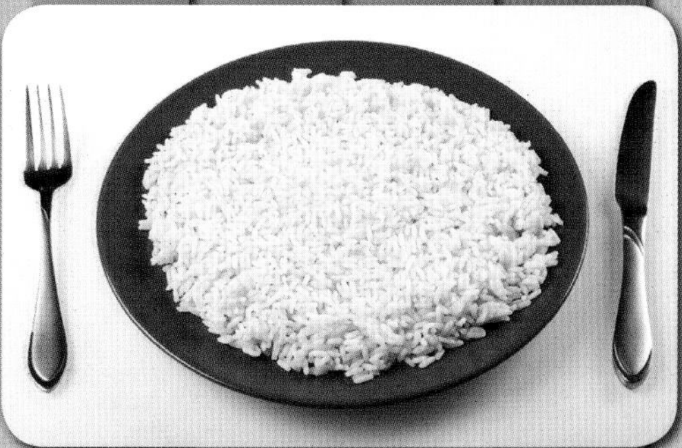

0g FIBRE | Weight: 355g | 1g SAT FAT

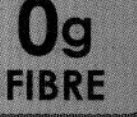

Egg Fried Rice

18g CARBS	102 CALS	2g PROTEIN	3g FAT

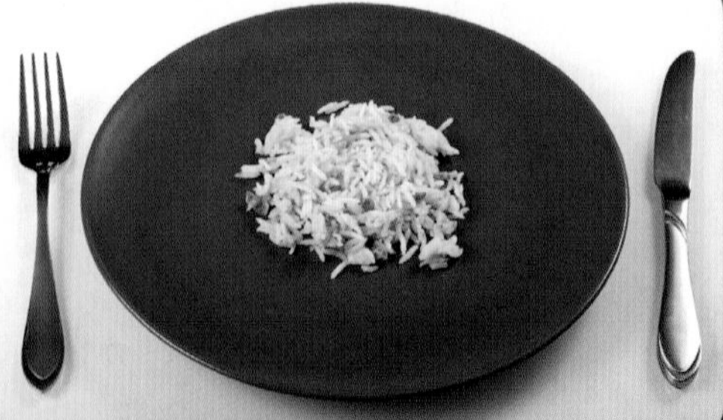

1g FIBRE	Weight: 55g	0g SAT FAT

57g CARBS	316 CALS	7g PROTEIN	8g FAT

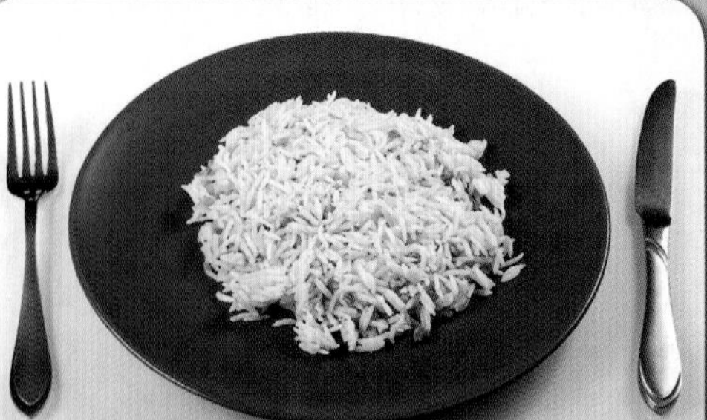

2g FIBRE	Weight: 170g	1g SAT FAT

93g CARBS	521 CALS	12g PROTEIN	14g FAT

3g FIBRE	Weight: 280g	2g SAT FAT

Jollof Rice

12g CARBS	71 CALS	1g PROTEIN	2g FAT

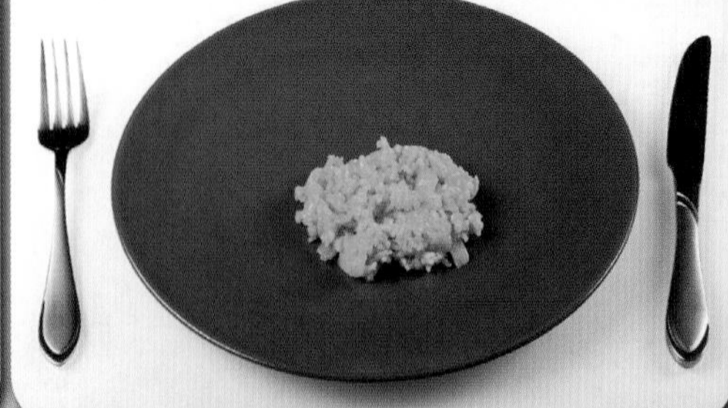

0g FIBRE	Weight: 55g	0g SAT FAT

36g CARBS	221 CALS	4g PROTEIN	7g FAT

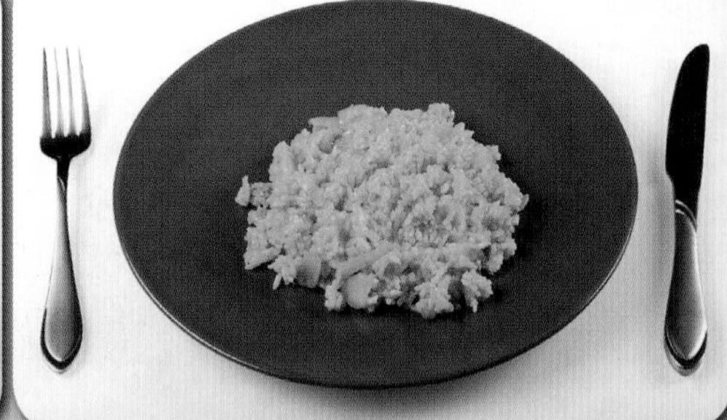

1g FIBRE	Weight: 170g	1g SAT FAT

59g CARBS	364 CALS	7g PROTEIN	11g FAT

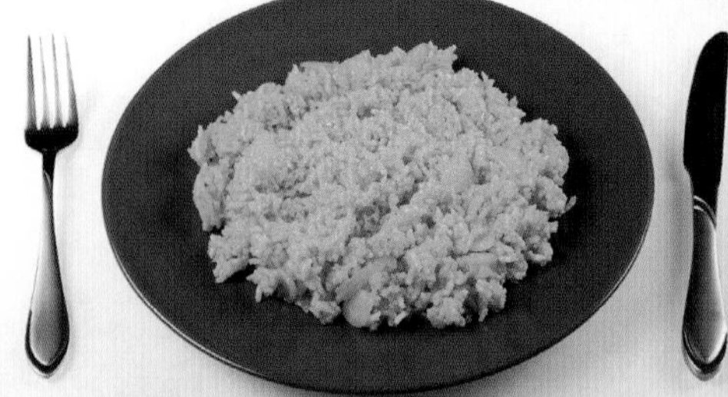

2g FIBRE	Weight: 280g	1g SAT FAT

Mexican Rice

17g CARBS | 86 CALS | 2g PROTEIN | 1g FAT

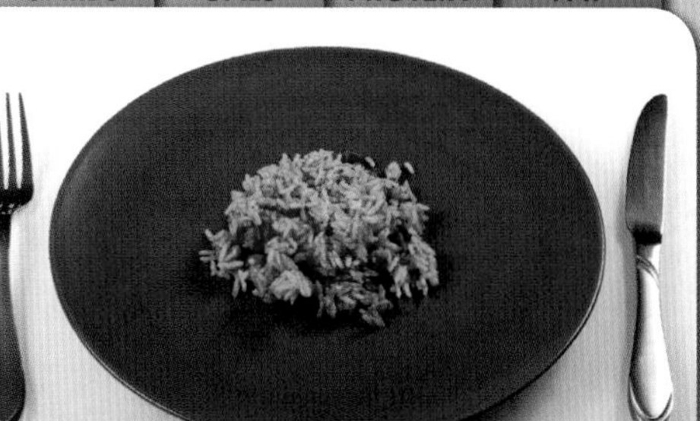

1g FIBRE | Weight: 55g | 0g SAT FAT

51g CARBS | 265 CALS | 6g PROTEIN | 4g FAT

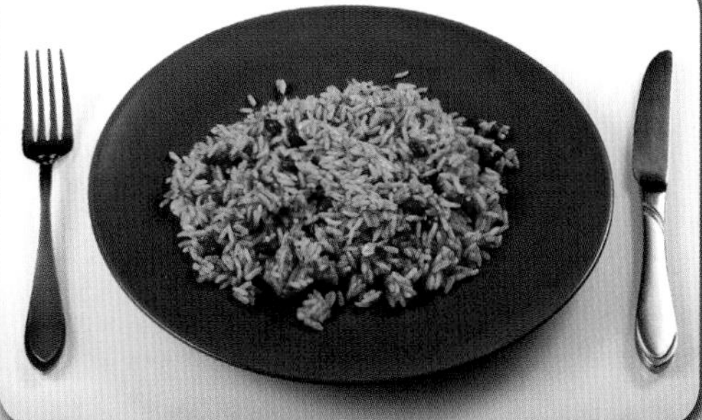

2g FIBRE | Weight: 170g | 0g SAT FAT

84g CARBS | 437 CALS | 10g PROTEIN | 6g FAT

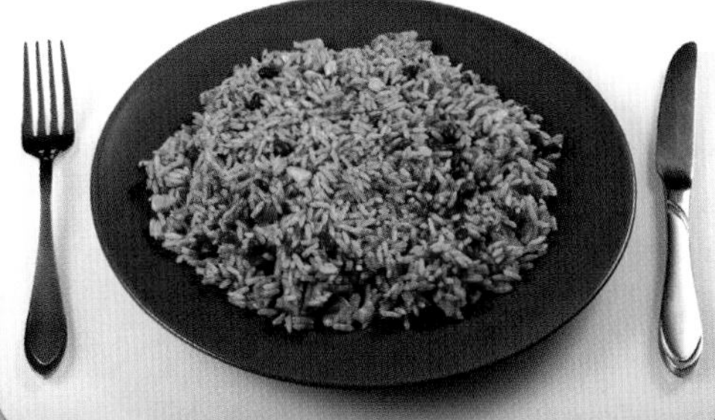

3g FIBRE | Weight: 280g | 1g SAT FAT

Pilau Rice

14g CARBS | 78 CALS | 1g PROTEIN | 3g FAT

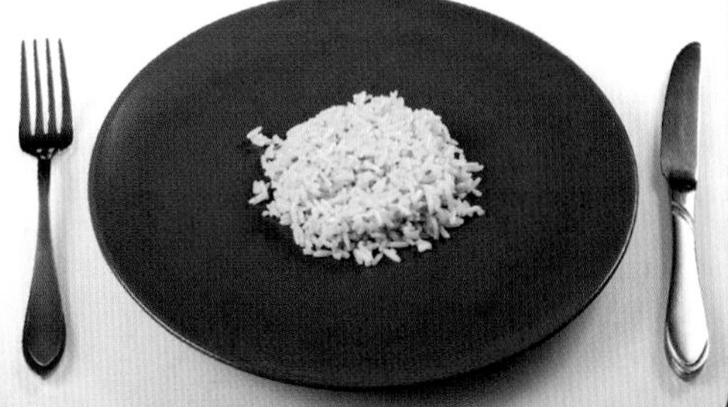

0g FIBRE | Weight: 55g | 1g SAT FAT

42g CARBS | 241 CALS | 4g PROTEIN | 8g FAT

1g FIBRE | Weight: 170g | 4g SAT FAT

69g CARBS | 398 CALS | 6g PROTEIN | 13g FAT

1g FIBRE | Weight: 280g | 7g SAT FAT

Rice & Peas

CARBS	CALS	PROTEIN	FAT
17g	88	3g	2g

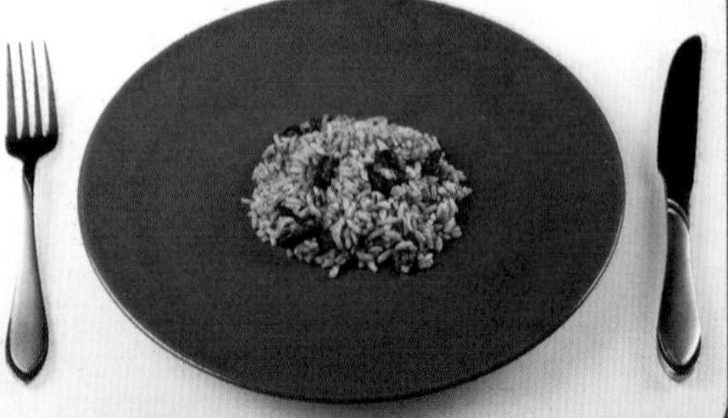

FIBRE	Weight	SAT FAT
2g	Weight: 55g	1g

CARBS	CALS	PROTEIN	FAT
52g	272	9g	5g

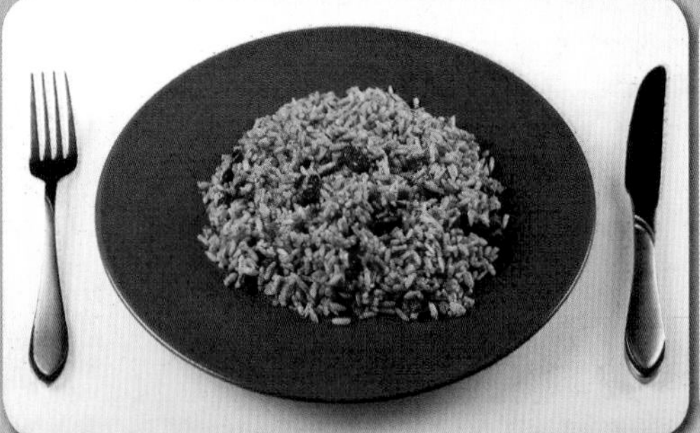

FIBRE	Weight	SAT FAT
5g	Weight: 170g	2g

CARBS	CALS	PROTEIN	FAT
85g	448	15g	8g

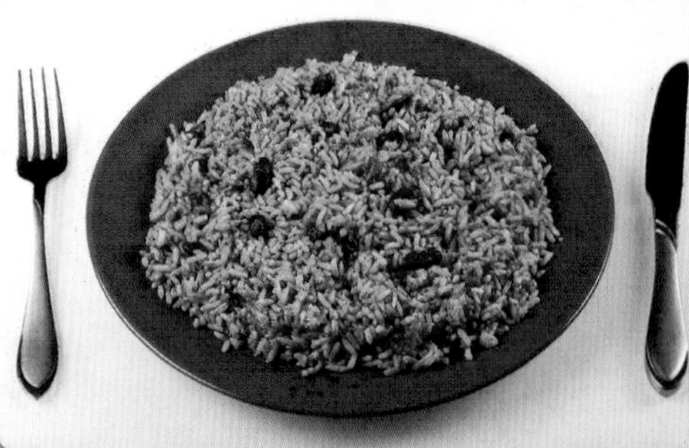

FIBRE	Weight	SAT FAT
9g	Weight: 280g	3g

Special Fried Rice

CARBS	CALS	PROTEIN	FAT
15g	87	2g	2g

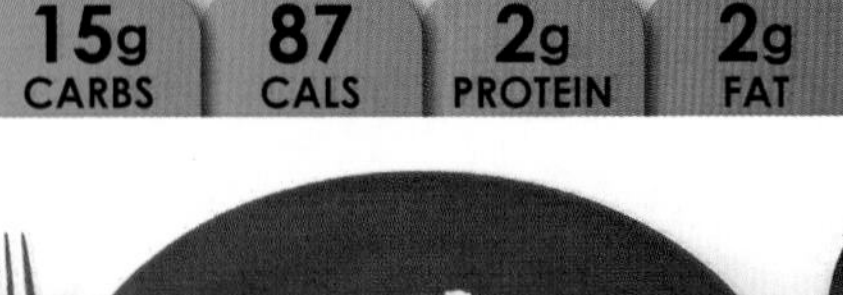

FIBRE	Weight	SAT FAT
0g	Weight: 55g	0g

CARBS	CALS	PROTEIN	FAT
46g	269	7g	6g

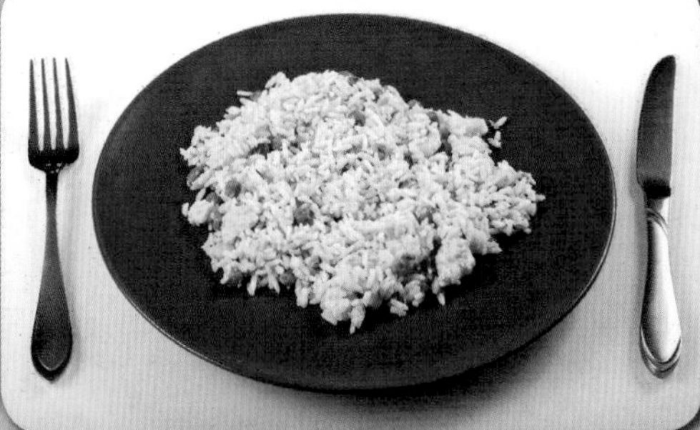

FIBRE	Weight	SAT FAT
1g	Weight: 170g	1g

CARBS	CALS	PROTEIN	FAT
76g	444	12g	10g

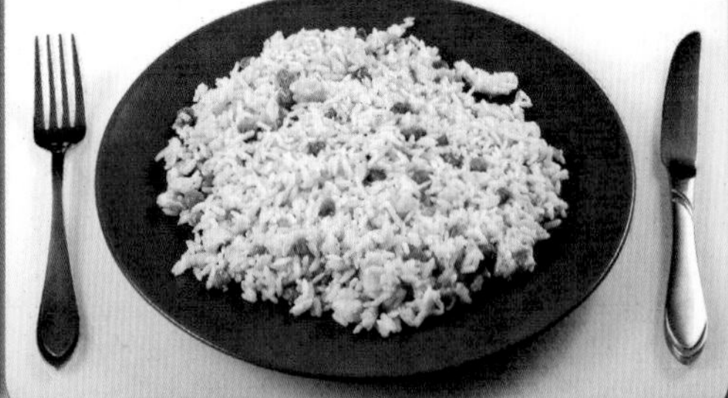

FIBRE	Weight	SAT FAT
2g	Weight: 280g	1g

Sticky White Rice

19g CARBS	100 CALS	2g PROTEIN	2g FAT

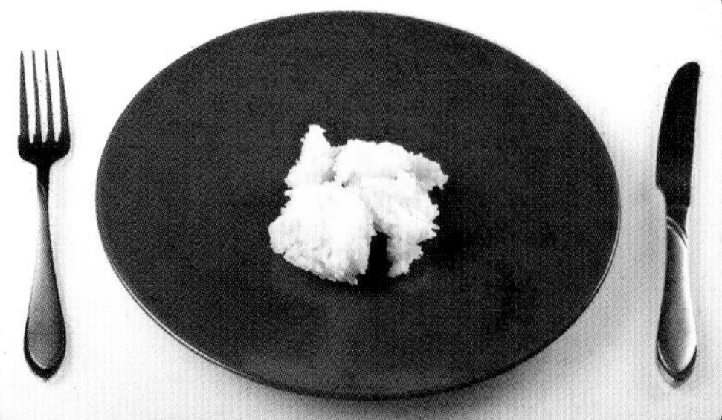

0g FIBRE	Weight: 70g	0g SAT FAT

39g CARBS	200 CALS	4g PROTEIN	4g FAT

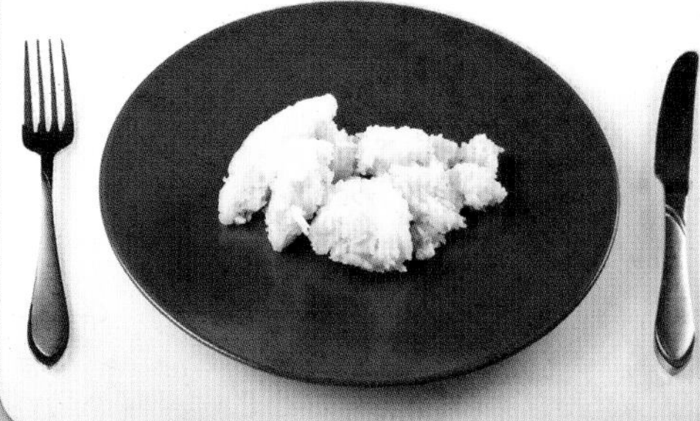

1g FIBRE	Weight: 140g	0g SAT FAT

77g CARBS	400 CALS	7g PROTEIN	7g FAT

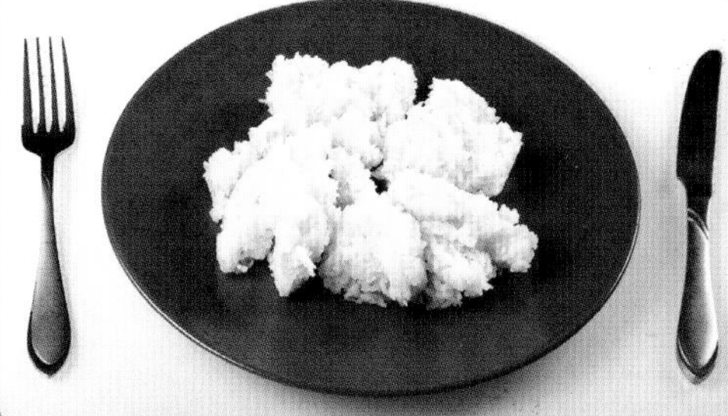

1g FIBRE	Weight: 280g	0g SAT FAT

Wild Rice

17g CARBS	81 CALS	2g PROTEIN	1g FAT

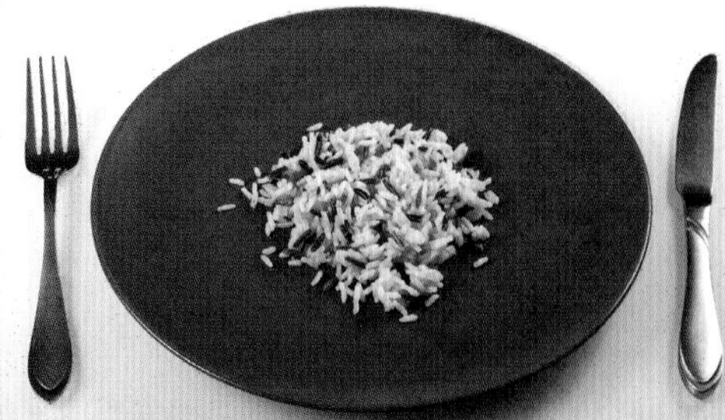

0g FIBRE	Weight: 55g	0g SAT FAT

52g CARBS	252 CALS	5g PROTEIN	2g FAT

1g FIBRE	Weight: 170g	0g SAT FAT

86g CARBS	414 CALS	9g PROTEIN	4g FAT

1g FIBRE	Weight: 280g	0g SAT FAT

26cm Dinner Plate

Bulgur Wheat

CARBS	CALS	PROTEIN	FAT	FIBRE	SAT FAT	Weight
20g	94	3g	0g	9g	0g	100g
40g	188	5g	1g	18g	0g	200g
60g	277	7g	1g	27g	0g	295g

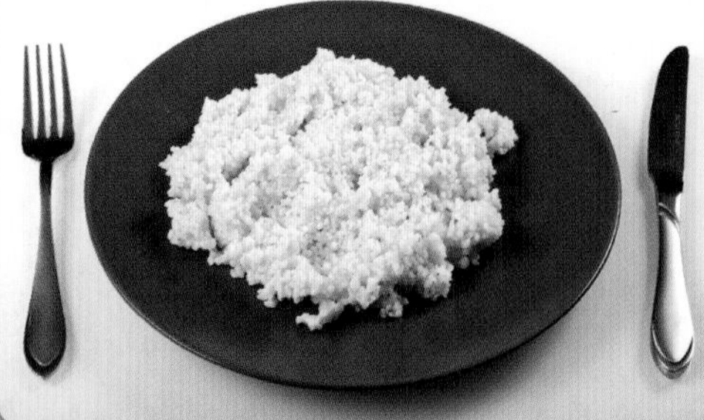

Quinoa

CARBS	CALS	PROTEIN	FAT	FIBRE	SAT FAT	Weight
20g	109	5g	2g	4g	0g	85g
40g	220	10g	4g	8g	0g	172g
60g	333	15g	6g	11g	0g	260g

Couscous

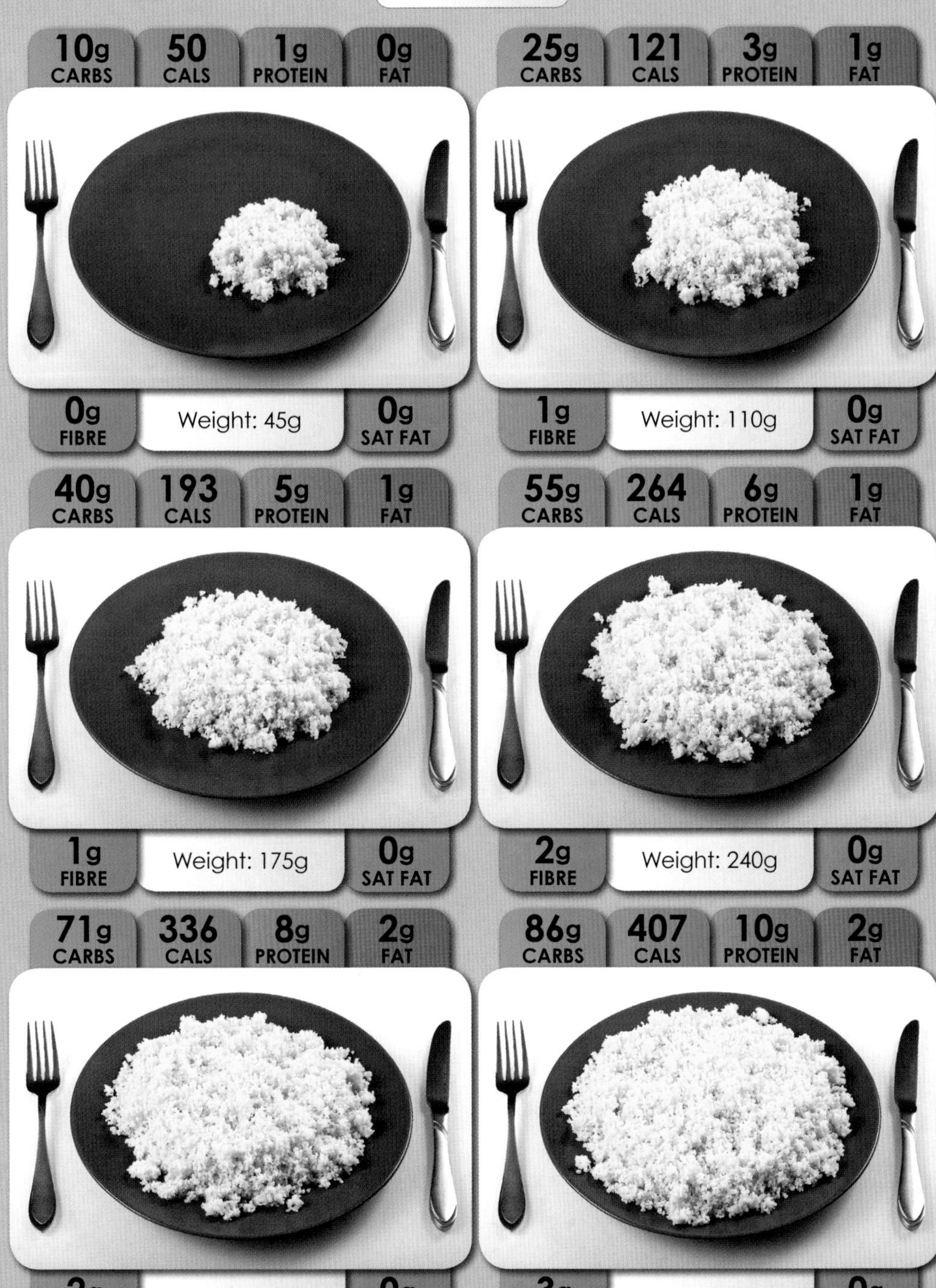
10g CARBS
50 CALS
1g PROTEIN
0g FAT
0g FIBRE
Weight: 45g
0g SAT FAT
25g CARBS
121 CALS
3g PROTEIN
1g FAT
1g FIBRE
Weight: 110g
0g SAT FAT
40g CARBS
193 CALS
5g PROTEIN
1g FAT
1g FIBRE
Weight: 175g
0g SAT FAT
55g CARBS
264 CALS
6g PROTEIN
1g FAT
2g FIBRE
Weight: 240g
0g SAT FAT
71g CARBS
336 CALS
8g PROTEIN
2g FAT
2g FIBRE
Weight: 305g
0g SAT FAT
86g CARBS
407 CALS
10g PROTEIN
2g FAT
3g FIBRE
Weight: 370g
0g SAT FAT

26cm Dinner Plate

Polenta

CARBS	CALS	PROTEIN	FAT
10g	47	1g	0g

FIBRE	Weight	SAT FAT
0g	Weight: 65g	0g

CARBS	CALS	PROTEIN	FAT
31g	140	3g	1g

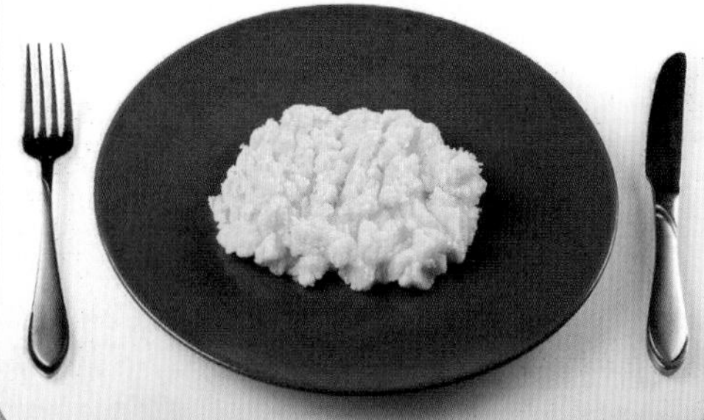

FIBRE	Weight	SAT FAT
1g	Weight: 195g	0g

CARBS	CALS	PROTEIN	FAT
51g	234	5g	1g

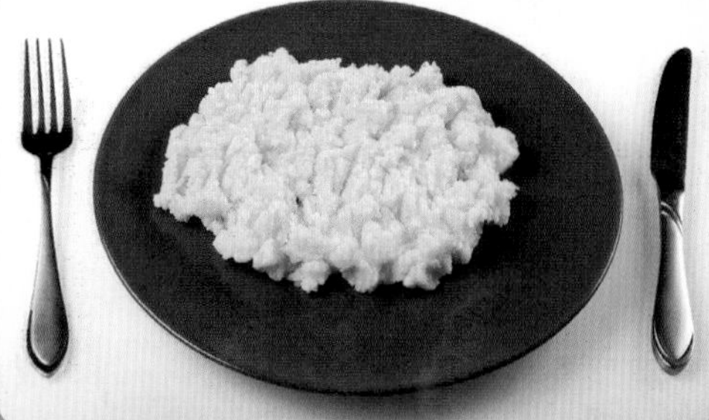

FIBRE	Weight	SAT FAT
2g	Weight: 325g	0g

Polenta (sliced)

CARBS	CALS	PROTEIN	FAT
10g	47	1g	0g

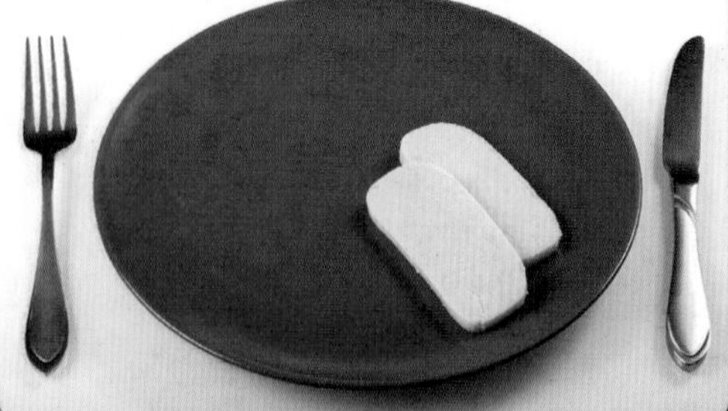

FIBRE	Weight	SAT FAT
0g	Weight: 65g	0g

CARBS	CALS	PROTEIN	FAT
20g	94	2g	0g

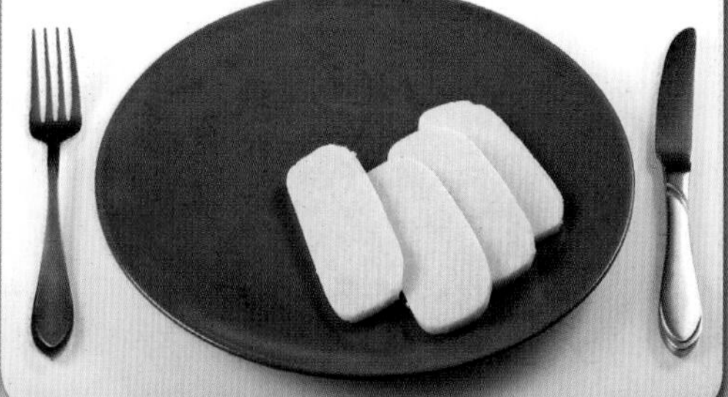

FIBRE	Weight	SAT FAT
1g	Weight: 130g	0g

CARBS	CALS	PROTEIN	FAT
30g	137	3g	1g

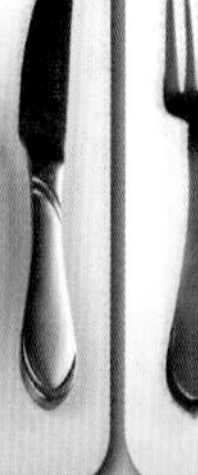

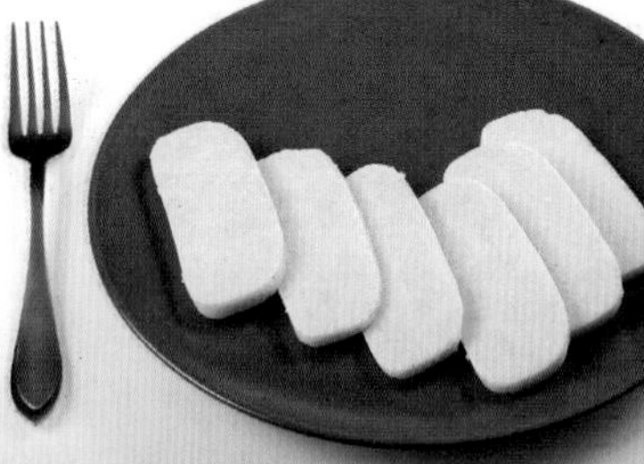

FIBRE	Weight	SAT FAT
1g	Weight: 190g	0g

BLT

	Small	Large
CARBS	21g	41g
CALS	200	400
PROTEIN	7g	14g
FAT	11g	21g
FIBRE	1g	2g
SAT FAT	2g	5g
Weight	85g	170g

Cheese & Pickle

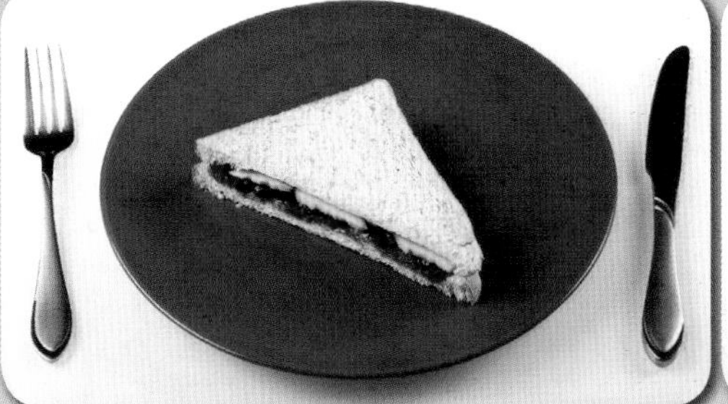

	Small	Large
CARBS	23g	46g
CALS	232	464
PROTEIN	10g	19g
FAT	12g	24g
FIBRE	1g	2g
SAT FAT	6g	12g
Weight	80g	160g

Chicken Salad

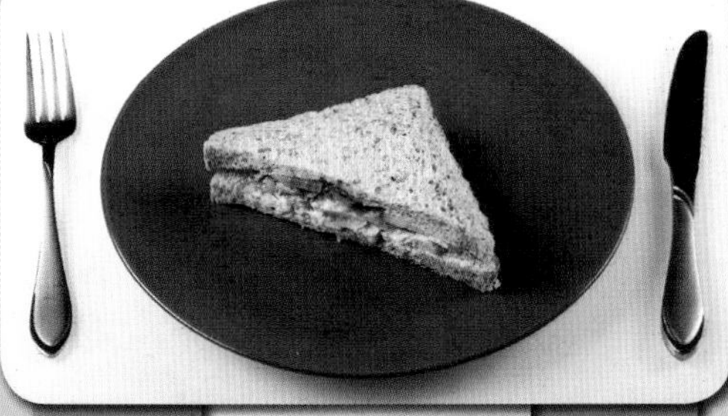

	Small	Large
CARBS	22g	43g
CALS	166	333
PROTEIN	10g	20g
FAT	5g	10g
FIBRE	1g	2g
SAT FAT	1g	2g
Weight	95g	190g

26cm Dinner Plate

Coronation Chicken

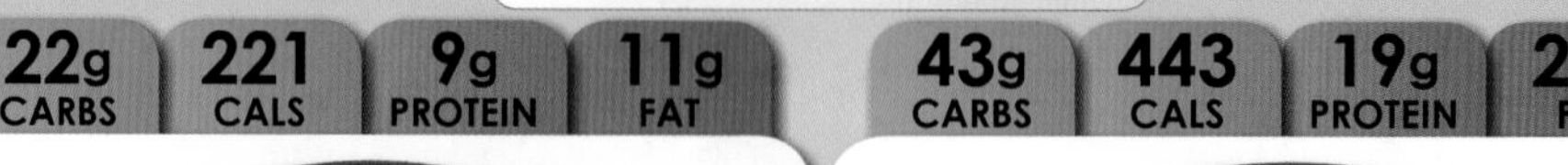

CARBS	CALS	PROTEIN	FAT	FIBRE	Weight	SAT FAT
22g	221	9g	11g	2g	90g	1g
43g	443	19g	22g	3g	180g	2g

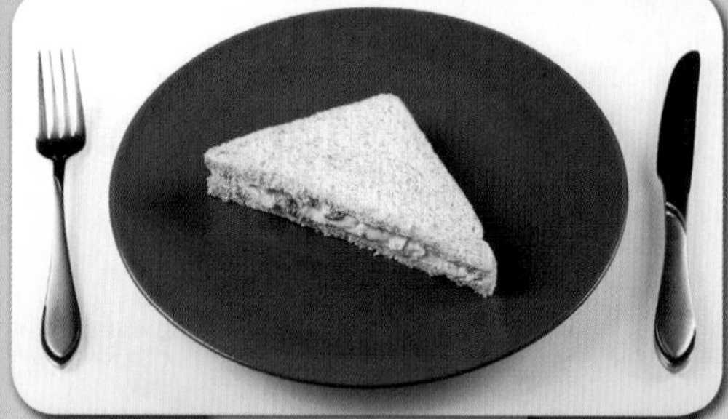

Egg Mayo

CARBS	CALS	PROTEIN	FAT	FIBRE	Weight	SAT FAT
17g	149	5g	7g	1g	60g	1g
34g	299	10g	14g	2g	120g	3g

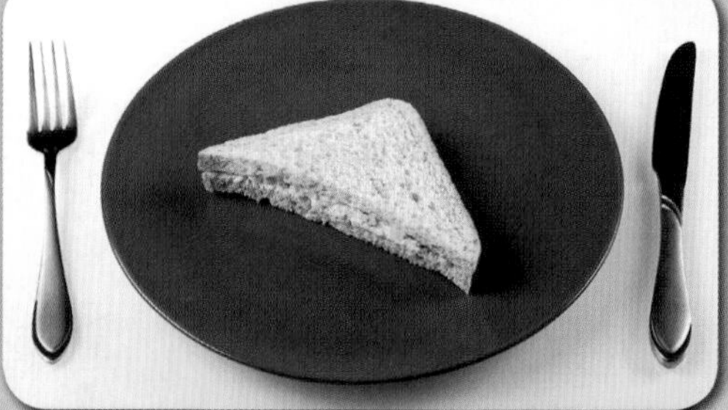

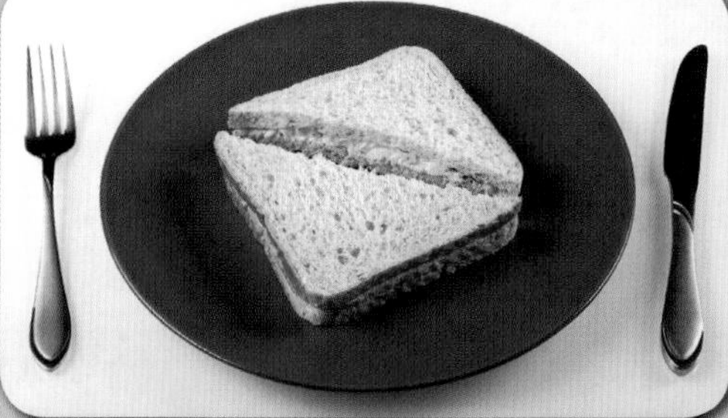

Grilled Cheese

CARBS	CALS	PROTEIN	FAT	FIBRE	Weight	SAT FAT
15g	197	10g	11g	1g	63g	7g
30g	394	20g	22g	2g	126g	13g

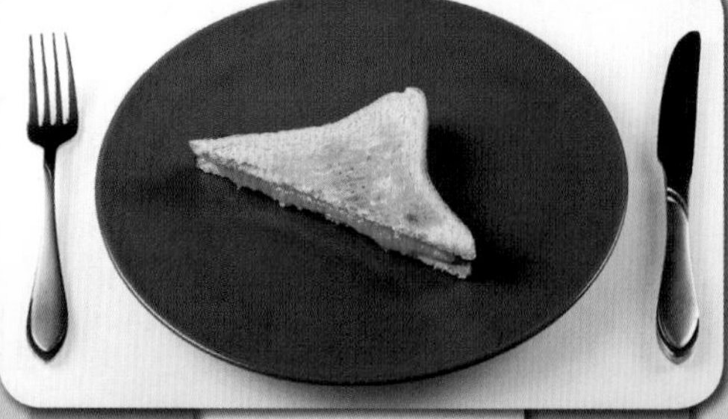

Ham Salad

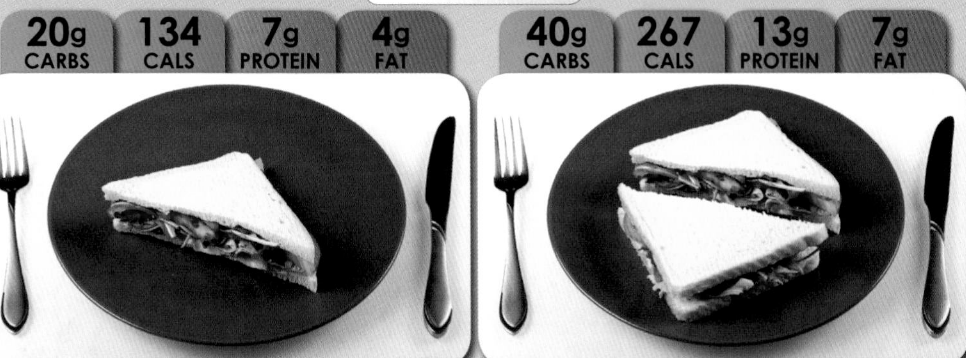

Carbs	Cals	Protein	Fat	Fibre	Weight	Sat Fat
20g	134	7g	4g	1g	80g	1g
40g	267	13g	7g	2g	160g	1g

Prawn Mayo

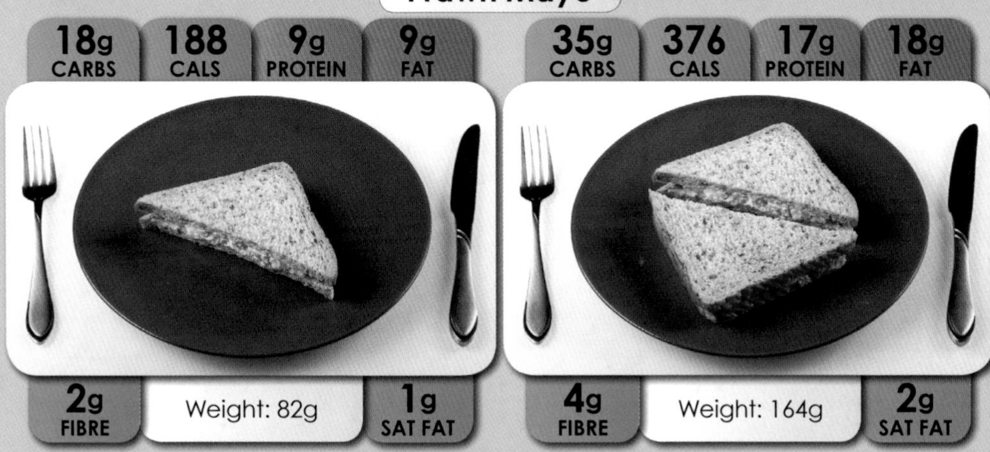

Carbs	Cals	Protein	Fat	Fibre	Weight	Sat Fat
18g	188	9g	9g	2g	82g	1g
35g	376	17g	18g	4g	164g	2g

Tuna Mayo & Sweetcorn

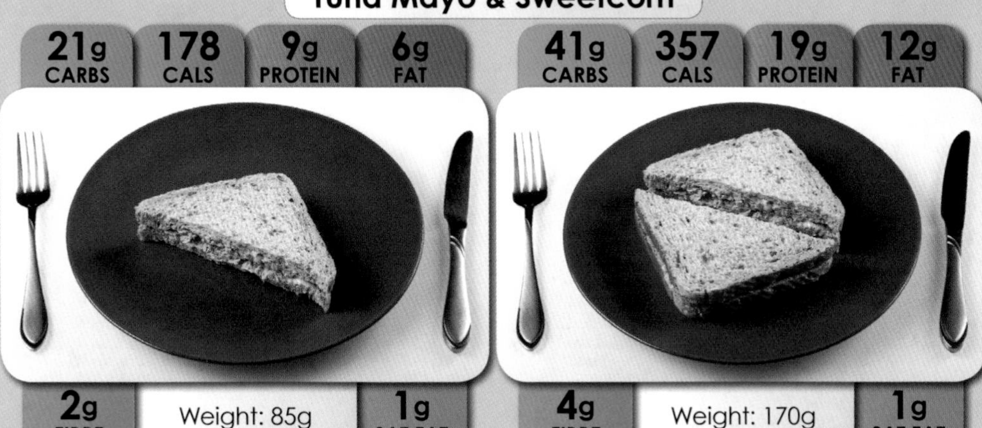

Carbs	Cals	Protein	Fat	Fibre	Weight	Sat Fat
21g	178	9g	6g	2g	85g	1g
41g	357	19g	12g	4g	170g	1g

14cm / 22cm Bowl

Bombay Mix

CARBS	CALS	PROTEIN	FAT	FIBRE	Weight	SAT FAT
10g	141	5g	9g	2g	28g	1g
20g	282	11g	18g	5g	56g	2g
30g	428	16g	28g	7g	85g	3g

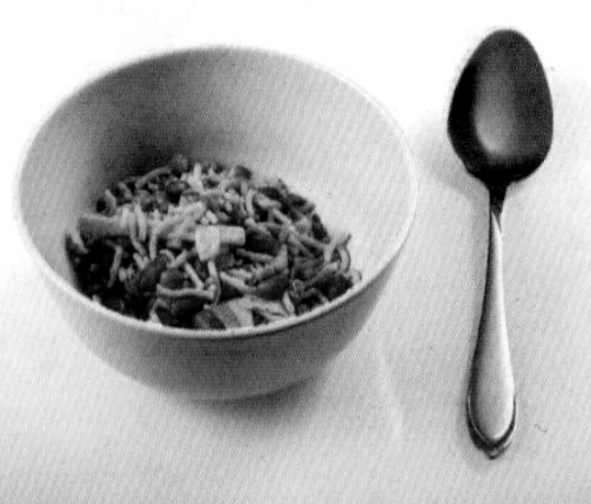

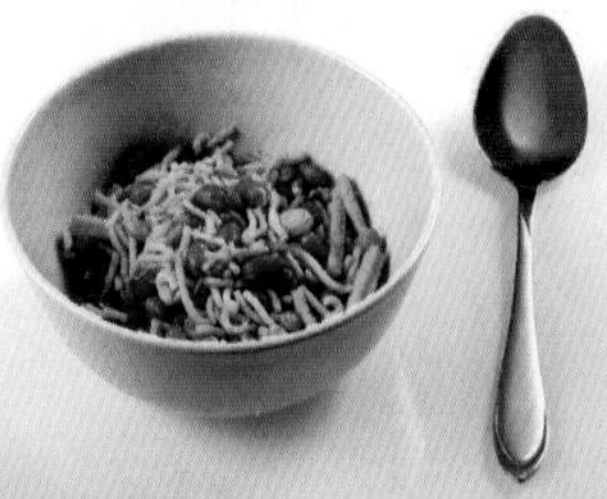

Crisps

CARBS	CALS	PROTEIN	FAT	FIBRE	Weight	SAT FAT
10g	95	1g	6g	1g	18g	3g
30g	297	3g	19g	4g	56g	8g
50g	498	5g	32g	7g	94g	13g

Popcorn (with butter)

CARBS	CALS	PROTEIN	FAT
5g	59	1g	4g

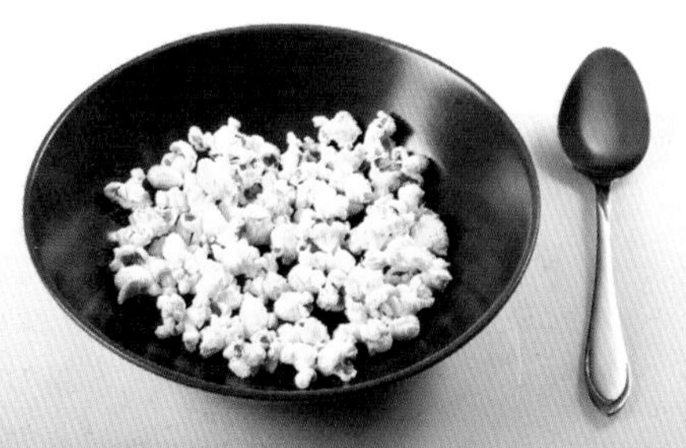

FIBRE	Weight	SAT FAT
1g	Weight: 10g	0g

CARBS	CALS	PROTEIN	FAT
10g	119	1g	9g

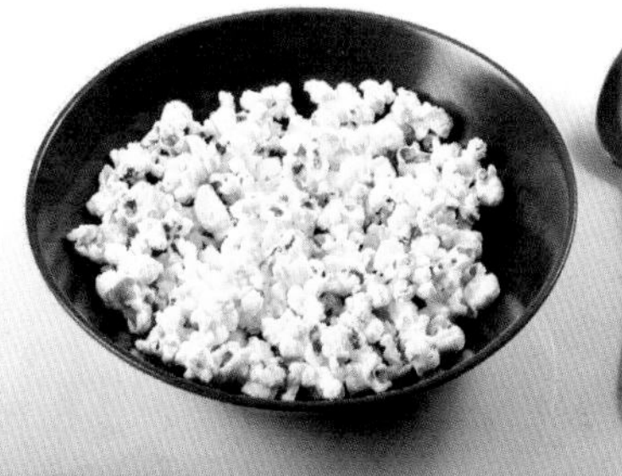

FIBRE	Weight	SAT FAT
1g	Weight: 20g	1g

CARBS	CALS	PROTEIN	FAT
20g	243	3g	18g

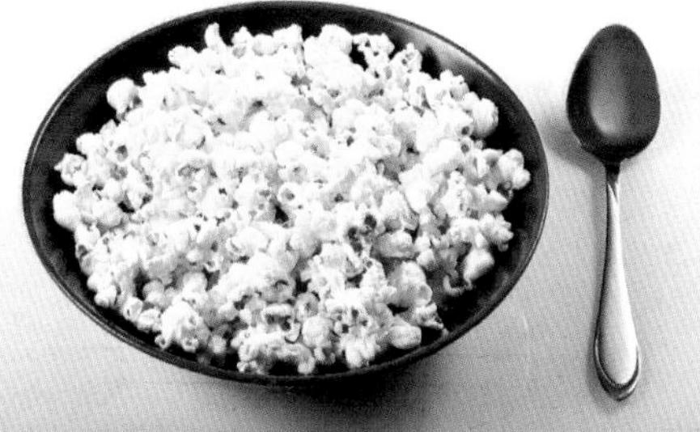

FIBRE	Weight	SAT FAT
3g	Weight: 41g	2g

Popcorn (sweet)

CARBS	CALS	PROTEIN	FAT
17g	106	1g	4g

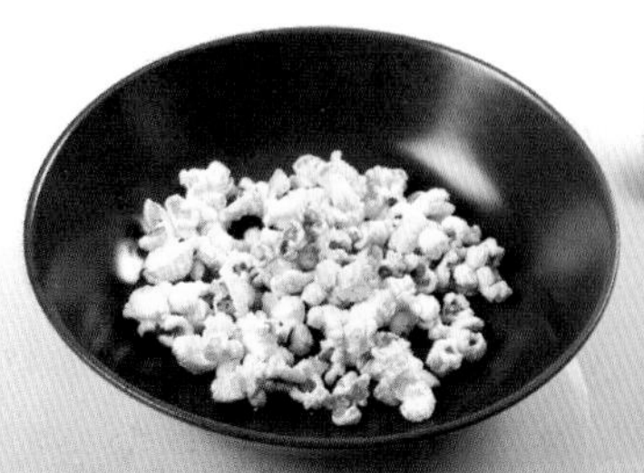

FIBRE	Weight	SAT FAT
1g	Weight: 22g	0g

CARBS	CALS	PROTEIN	FAT
53g	326	1g	14g

FIBRE	Weight	SAT FAT
4g	Weight: 68g	1g

CARBS	CALS	PROTEIN	FAT
88g	542	2g	23g

FIBRE	Weight	SAT FAT
7g	Weight: 113g	2g

Pretzels

CARBS	CALS	PROTEIN	FAT
10g	50	1g	1g

FIBRE	Weight	SAT FAT
0g	Weight: 13g	0g

CARBS	CALS	PROTEIN	FAT
21g	99	2g	1g

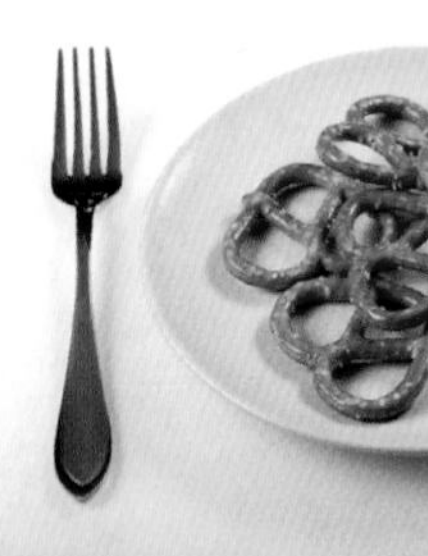
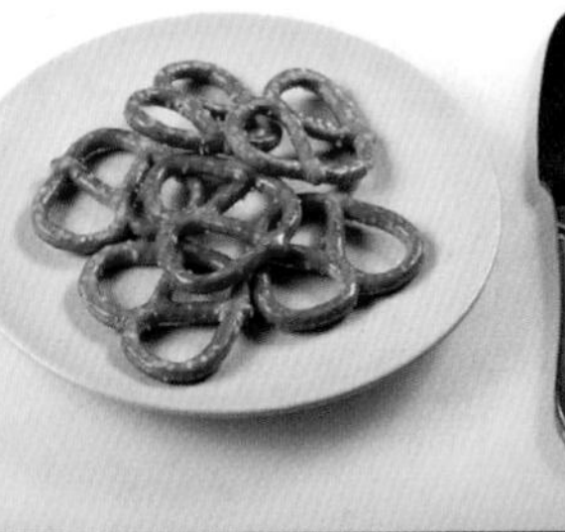
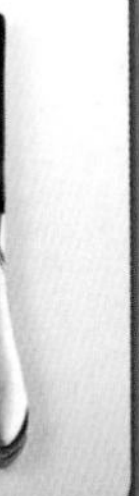

FIBRE	Weight	SAT FAT
1g	Weight: 26g	0g

CARBS	CALS	PROTEIN	FAT
32g	152	4g	1g

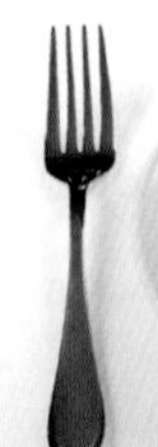
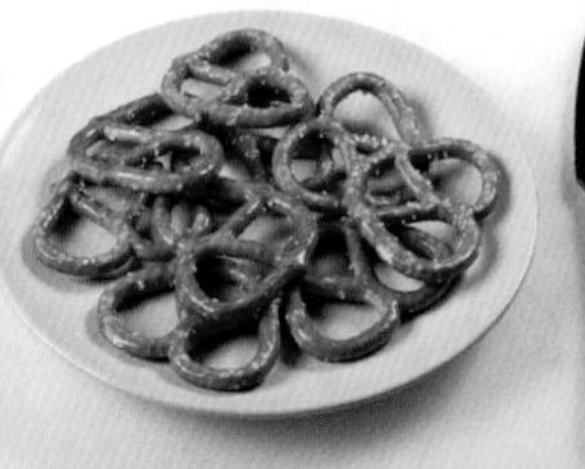
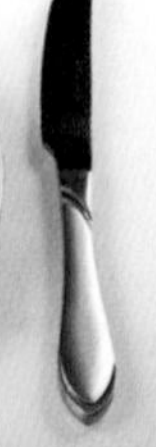

FIBRE	Weight	SAT FAT
1g	Weight: 40g	0g

Tortilla Chips

CARBS	CALS	PROTEIN	FAT
10g	73	1g	4g

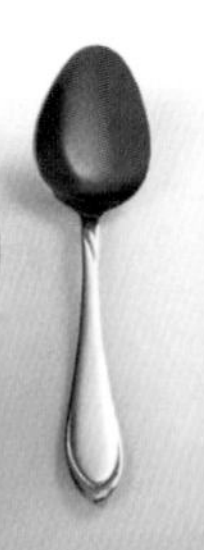

FIBRE	Weight	SAT FAT
1g	Weight: 16g	1g

CARBS	CALS	PROTEIN	FAT
30g	230	4g	11g

FIBRE	Weight	SAT FAT
4g	Weight: 50g	2g

CARBS	CALS	PROTEIN	FAT
60g	459	8g	23g

FIBRE	Weight	SAT FAT
8g	Weight: 100g	4g

Fudge

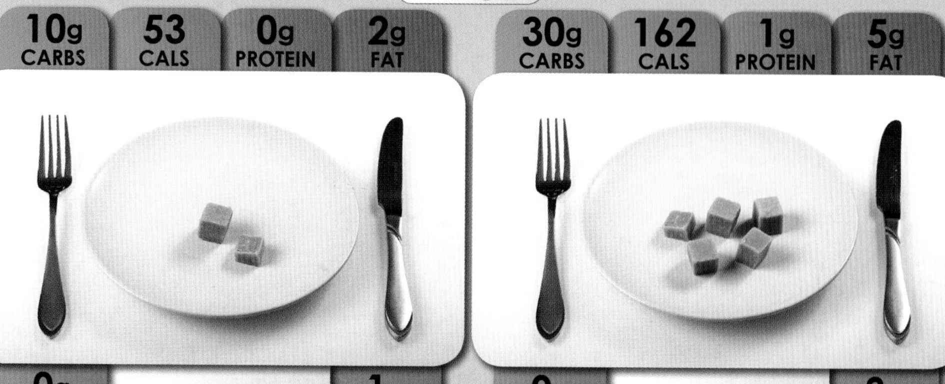

	Portion 1	Portion 2
CARBS	10g	30g
CALS	53	162
PROTEIN	0g	1g
FAT	2g	5g
FIBRE	0g	0g
Weight	12g	37g
SAT FAT	1g	3g

Marshmallows (small)

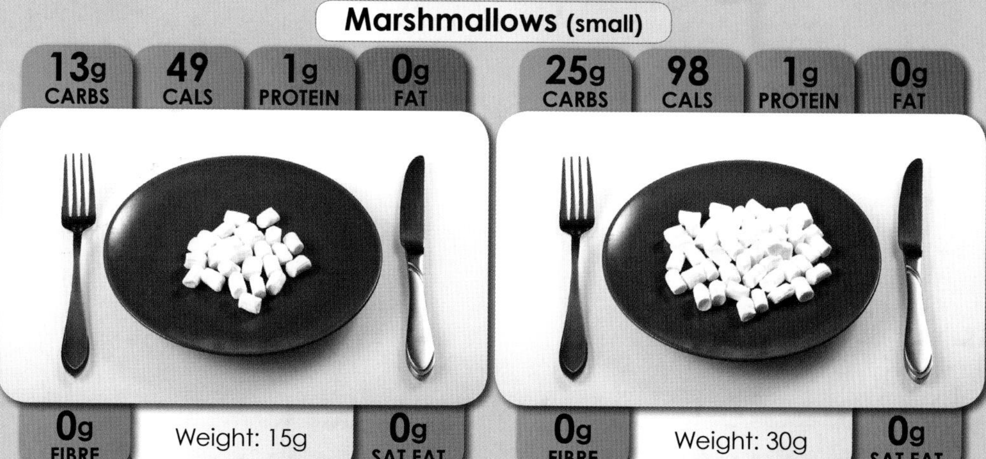

	Portion 1	Portion 2
CARBS	13g	25g
CALS	49	98
PROTEIN	1g	1g
FAT	0g	0g
FIBRE	0g	0g
Weight	15g	30g
SAT FAT	0g	0g

Marshmallows (large)

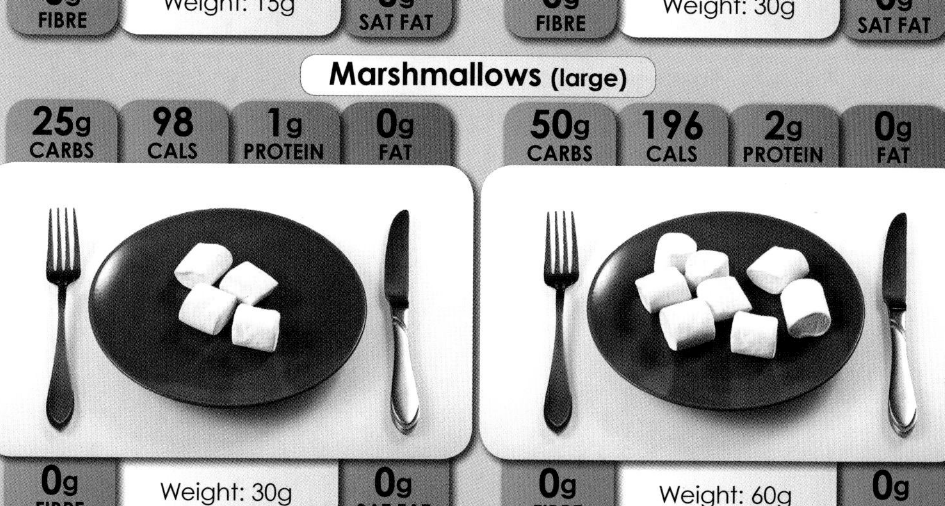

	Portion 1	Portion 2
CARBS	25g	50g
CALS	98	196
PROTEIN	1g	2g
FAT	0g	0g
FIBRE	0g	0g
Weight	30g	60g
SAT FAT	0g	0g

Chocolate (milk)

CARBS	CALS	PROTEIN	FAT
9g	83	1g	5g

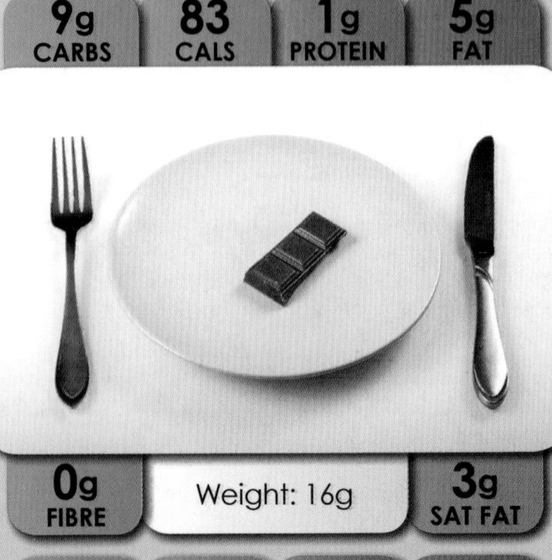

FIBRE	Weight	SAT FAT
0g	Weight: 16g	3g

CARBS	CALS	PROTEIN	FAT
29g	260	4g	15g

FIBRE	Weight	SAT FAT
1g	Weight: 50g	9g

CARBS	CALS	PROTEIN	FAT
58g	525	8g	31g

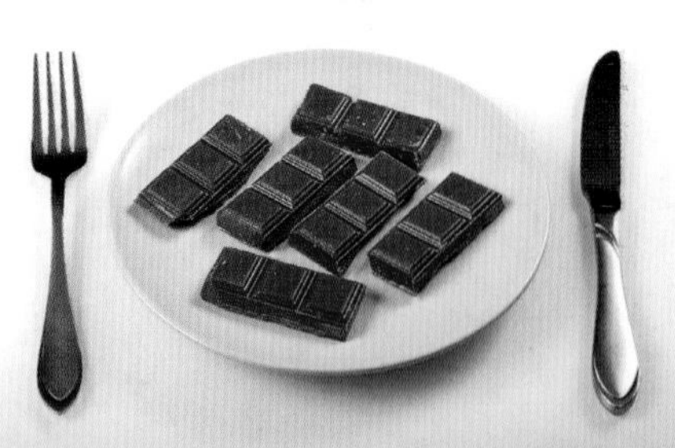

FIBRE	Weight	SAT FAT
1g	Weight: 101g	19g

Chocolate (dark)

CARBS	CALS	PROTEIN	FAT
10g	82	1g	5g

FIBRE	Weight	SAT FAT
1g	Weight: 16g	3g

CARBS	CALS	PROTEIN	FAT
31g	245	2g	13g

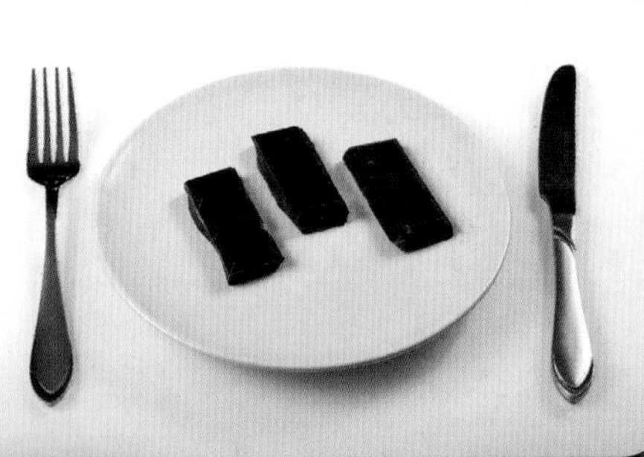

FIBRE	Weight	SAT FAT
2g	Weight: 48g	8g

CARBS	CALS	PROTEIN	FAT
60g	479	5g	26g

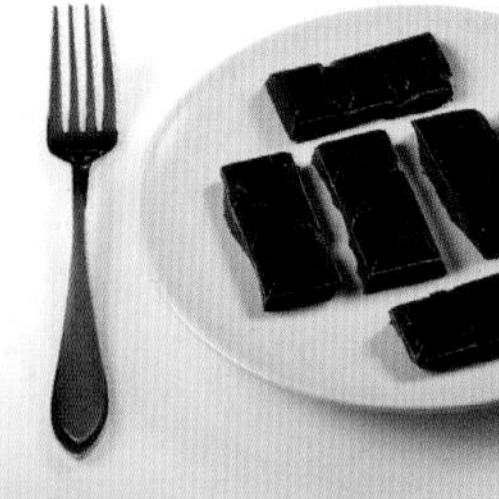

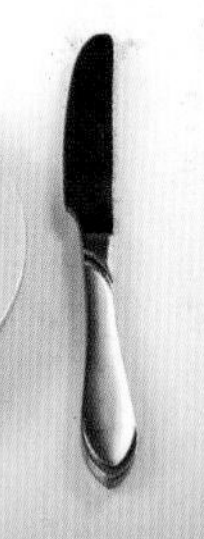

FIBRE	Weight	SAT FAT
3g	Weight: 94g	16g

Chocolate (white)

12g CARBS	111 CALS	2g PROTEIN	6g FAT

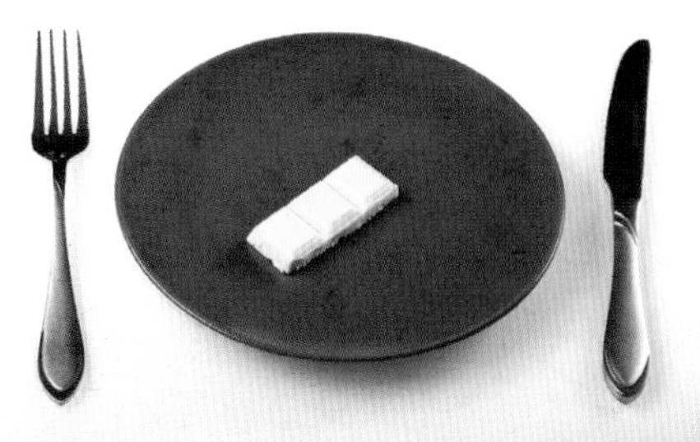

0g FIBRE	Weight: 21g	4g SAT FAT

37g CARBS	333 CALS	5g PROTEIN	19g FAT

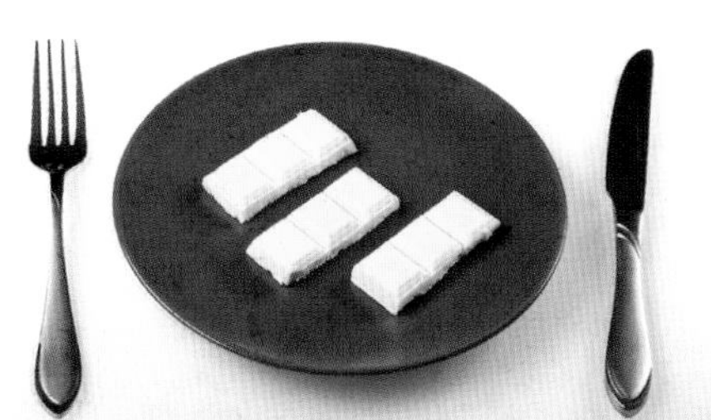

0g FIBRE	Weight: 63g	12g SAT FAT

73g CARBS	667 CALS	10g PROTEIN	39g FAT

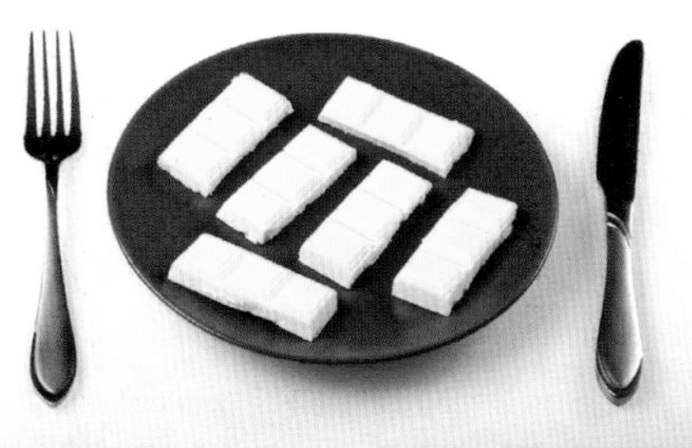

1g FIBRE	Weight: 126g	23g SAT FAT

Chocolate (milk, with hazelnuts)

12g CARBS	140 CALS	2g PROTEIN	9g FAT

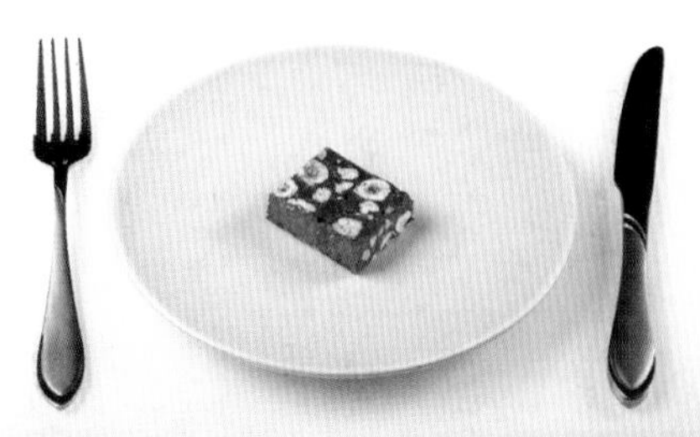

1g FIBRE	Weight: 25g	4g SAT FAT

24g CARBS	280 CALS	4g PROTEIN	18g FAT

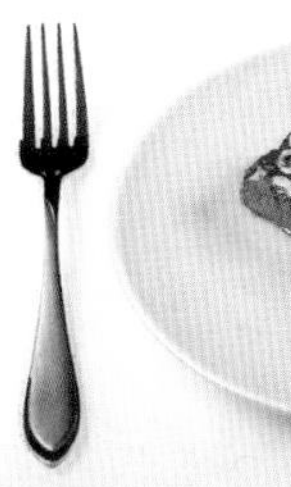

1g FIBRE	Weight: 50g	9g SAT FAT

49g CARBS	560 CALS	9g PROTEIN	36g FAT

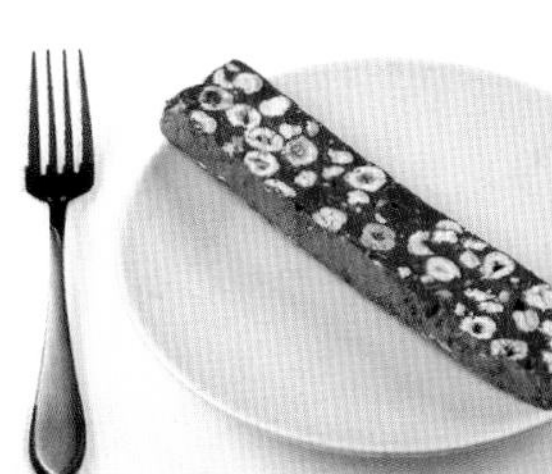

2g FIBRE	Weight: 100g	17g SAT FAT

Chocolate Honeycomb Balls

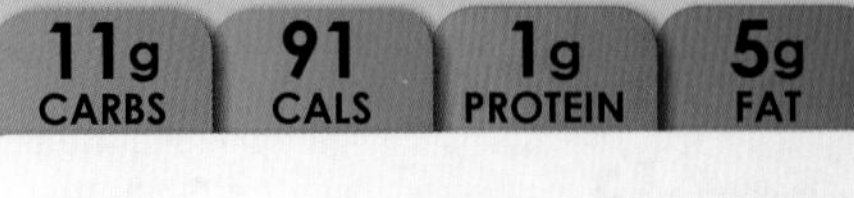

11g CARBS	91 CALS	1g PROTEIN	5g FAT

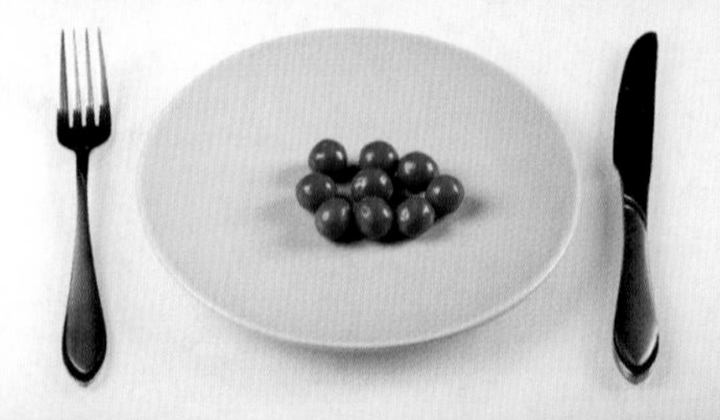

0g FIBRE	Weight: 18g	3g SAT FAT

23g CARBS	187 CALS	3g PROTEIN	9g FAT

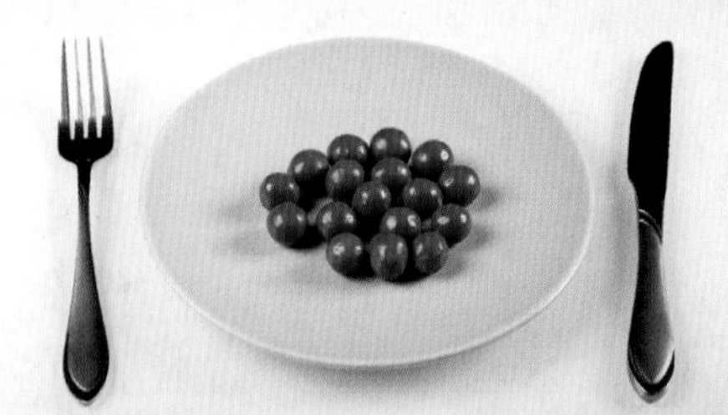

0g FIBRE	Weight: 37g	6g SAT FAT

Chocolate Mint

10g CARBS	67 CALS	1g PROTEIN	3g FAT

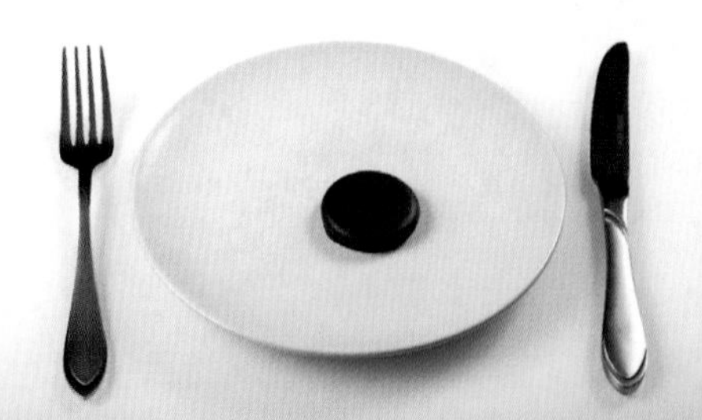

1g FIBRE	Weight: 15g	2g SAT FAT

Individual Chocolate

7g CARBS	53 CALS	0g PROTEIN	3g FAT

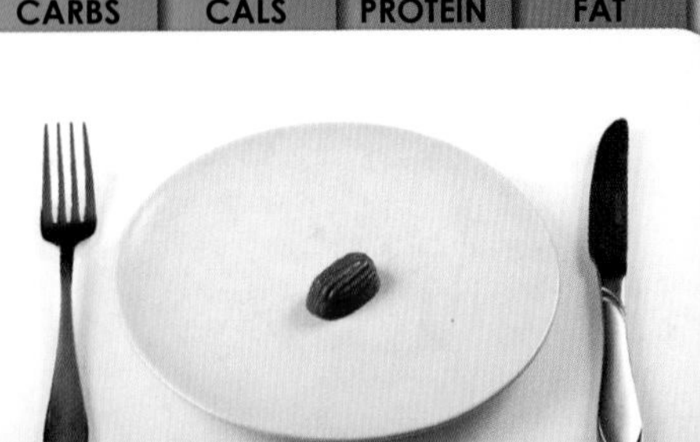

0g FIBRE	Weight: 11g	2g SAT FAT

7g CARBS	76 CALS	1g PROTEIN	5g FAT

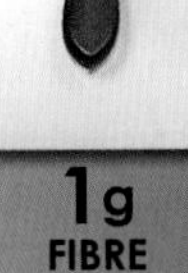

1g FIBRE	Weight: 14g	3g SAT FAT

6g CARBS	78 CALS	1g PROTEIN	6g FAT

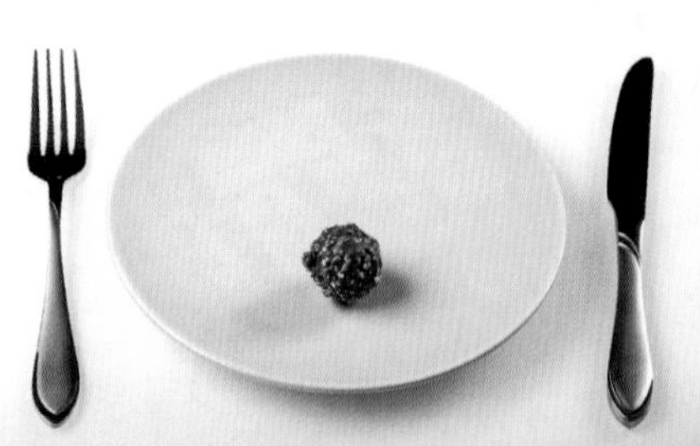

1g FIBRE	Weight: 13g	2g SAT FAT

Cola Bottles

20g CARBS	88 CALS	2g PROTEIN	0g FAT
0g FIBRE	Weight: 27g	0g SAT FAT	

Dextrose Tablets

20g CARBS	81 CALS	0g PROTEIN	0g FAT
0g FIBRE	Weight: 20g	0g SAT FAT	

Jelly Babies

20g CARBS	84 CALS	1g PROTEIN	0g FAT

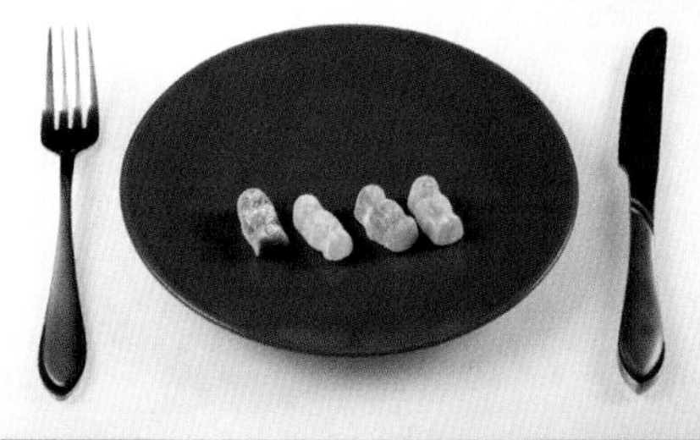

0g FIBRE	Weight: 25g	0g SAT FAT

Jelly Beans

20g CARBS	80 CALS	0g PROTEIN	0g FAT
0g FIBRE	Weight: 22g	0g SAT FAT	

Licorice Allsorts

20g CARBS	91 CALS	1g PROTEIN	1g FAT

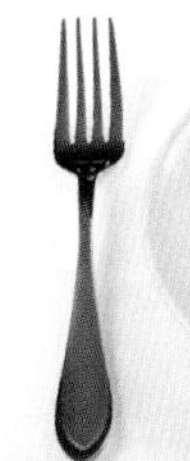

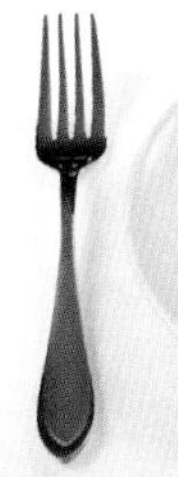

1g FIBRE	Weight: 26g	1g SAT FAT

Wine Gums

20g CARBS	87 CALS	1g PROTEIN	0g FAT

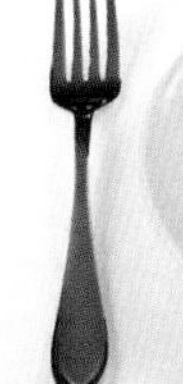

0g FIBRE	Weight: 27g	0g SAT FAT

Broccoli & Stilton Soup

CARBS	CALS	PROTEIN	FAT
4g	67	3g	4g

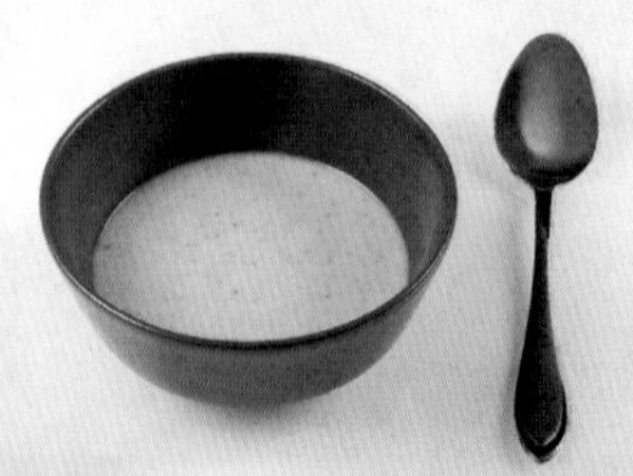

FIBRE	Weight	SAT FAT
1g	Weight: 130g	2g

CARBS	CALS	PROTEIN	FAT
8g	134	5g	9g

FIBRE	Weight	SAT FAT
3g	Weight: 260g	5g

CARBS	CALS	PROTEIN	FAT
12g	206	8g	13g

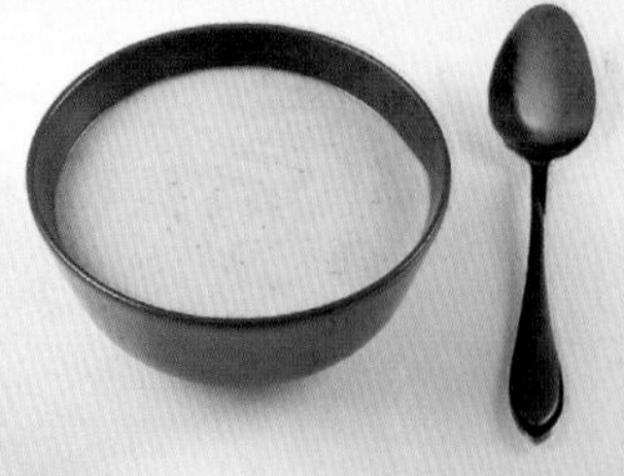

FIBRE	Weight	SAT FAT
4g	Weight: 400g	8g

Chicken Noodle Soup

CARBS	CALS	PROTEIN	FAT
4g	25	1g	0g

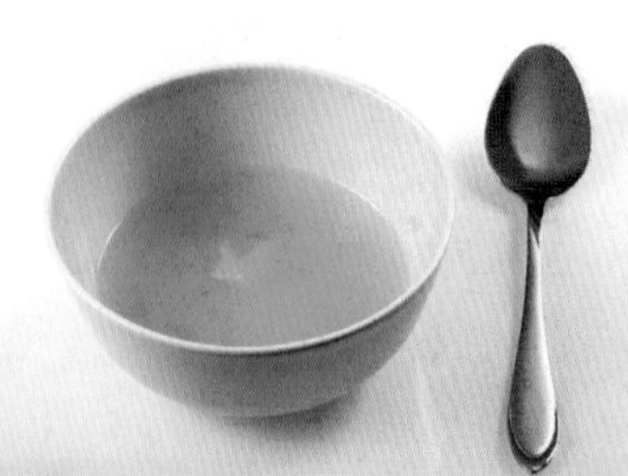

FIBRE	Weight	SAT FAT
0g	Weight: 130g	0g

CARBS	CALS	PROTEIN	FAT
8g	49	3g	1g

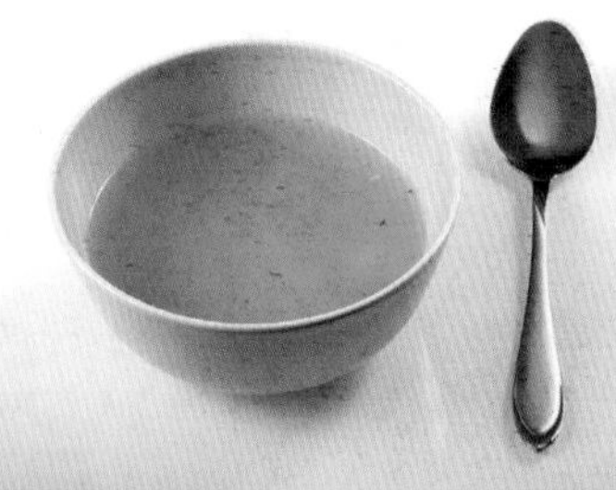

FIBRE	Weight	SAT FAT
1g	Weight: 260g	0g

CARBS	CALS	PROTEIN	FAT
13g	76	4g	1g

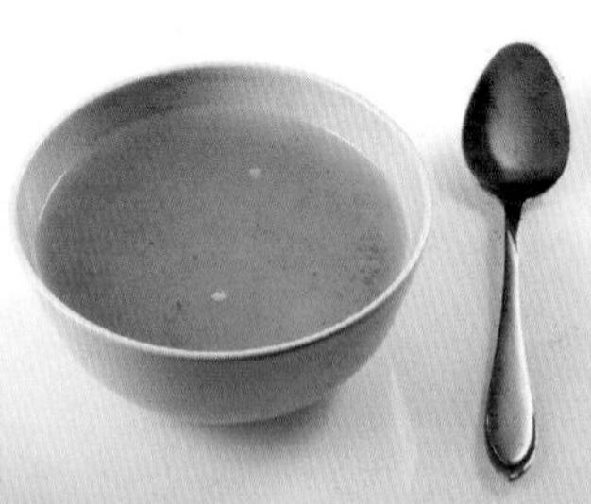

FIBRE	Weight	SAT FAT
1g	Weight: 400g	0g

Chunky Veg Soup

Weight	Carbs	Cals	Protein	Fat	Fibre	Sat Fat
130g	11g	58	2g	1g	2g	0g
260g	21g	115	4g	2g	4g	0g
400g	32g	177	6g	2g	6g	0g

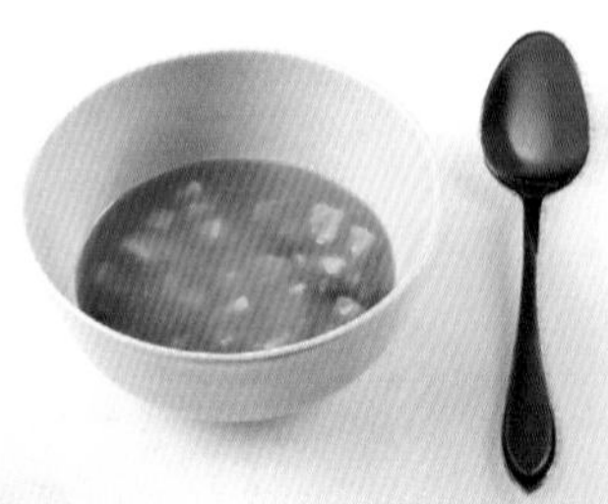

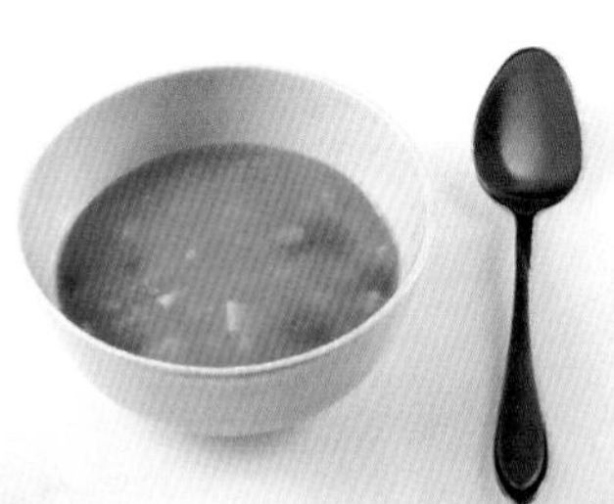

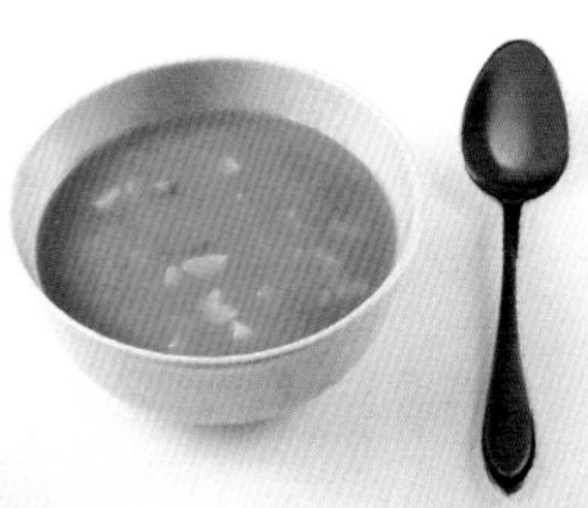

Mushroom Soup

Weight	Carbs	Cals	Protein	Fat	Fibre	Sat Fat
130g	5g	60	1g	4g	0g	1g
260g	10g	120	3g	8g	0g	1g
400g	16g	184	4g	12g	0g	2g

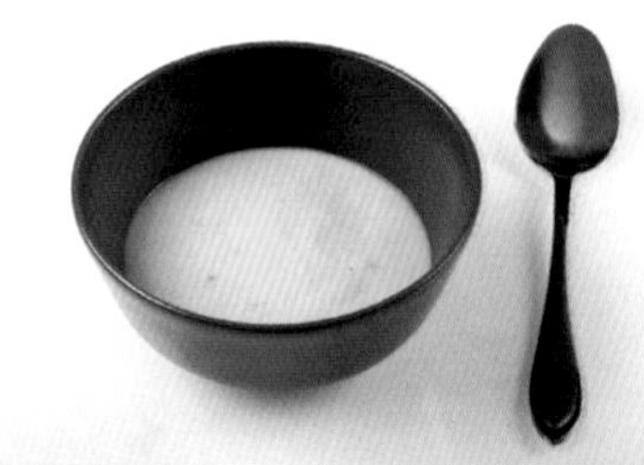

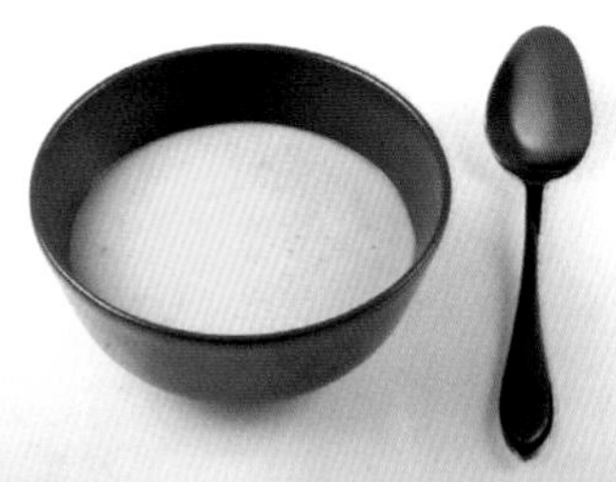

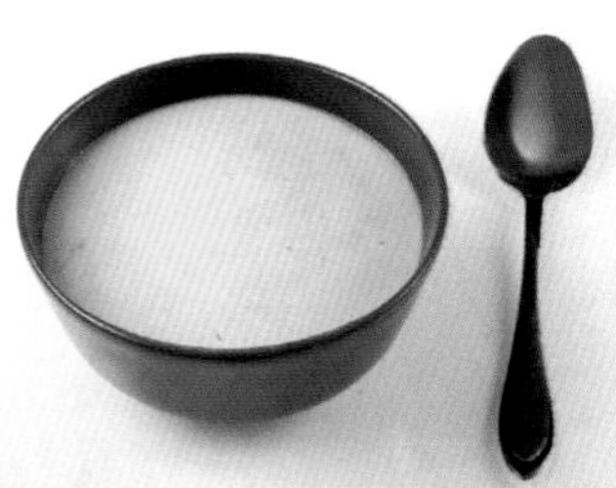

Onion Soup

CARBS	CALS	PROTEIN	FAT
7g	53	1g	3g

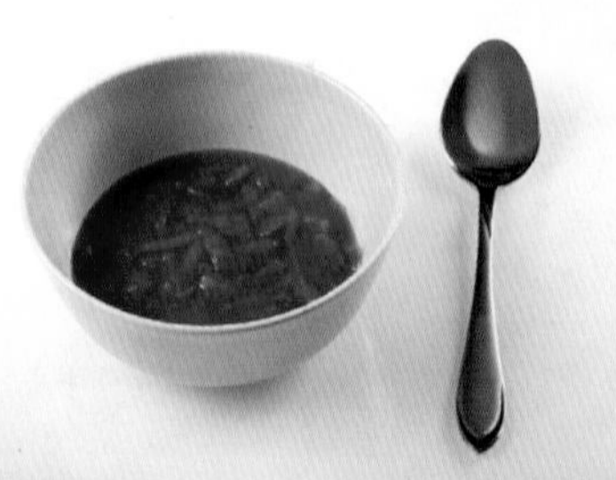

FIBRE	Weight	SAT FAT
2g	Weight: 130g	0g

CARBS	CALS	PROTEIN	FAT
13g	107	3g	6g

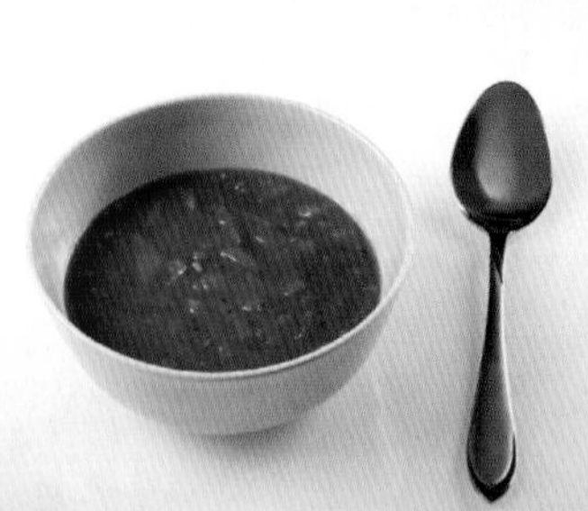

FIBRE	Weight	SAT FAT
3g	Weight: 260g	1g

CARBS	CALS	PROTEIN	FAT
20g	164	4g	9g

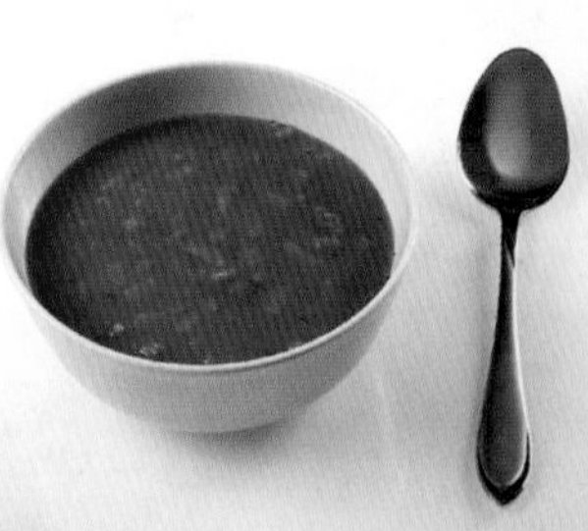

FIBRE	Weight	SAT FAT
5g	Weight: 400g	1g

Tomato Soup

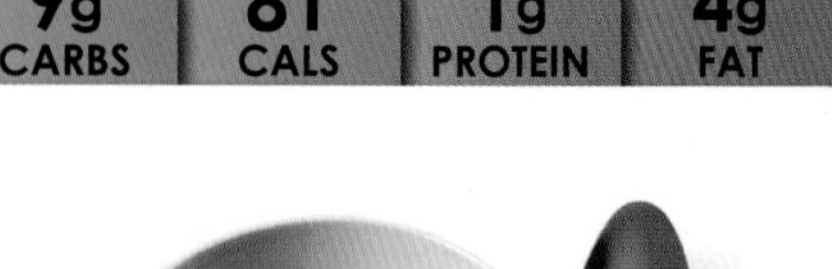

CARBS	CALS	PROTEIN	FAT
9g	81	1g	4g

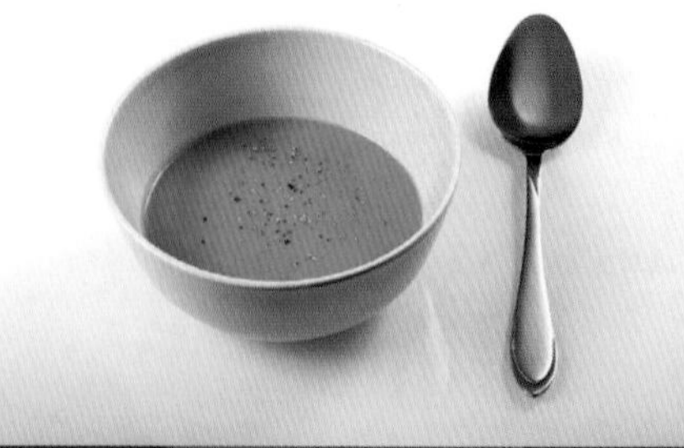

FIBRE	Weight	SAT FAT
1g	Weight: 130g	1g

CARBS	CALS	PROTEIN	FAT
19g	161	2g	9g

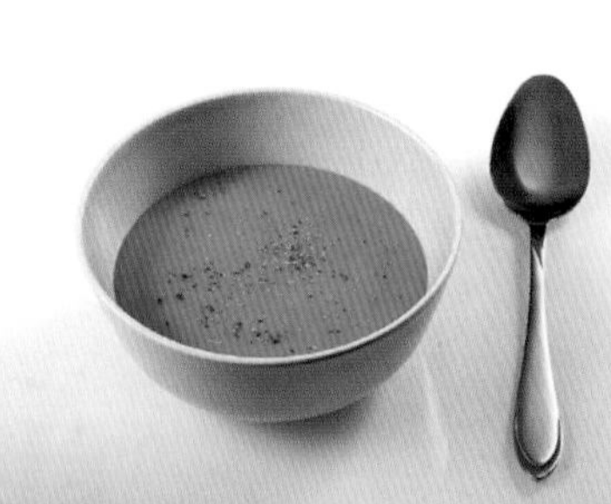

FIBRE	Weight	SAT FAT
2g	Weight: 260g	1g

CARBS	CALS	PROTEIN	FAT
29g	248	4g	14g

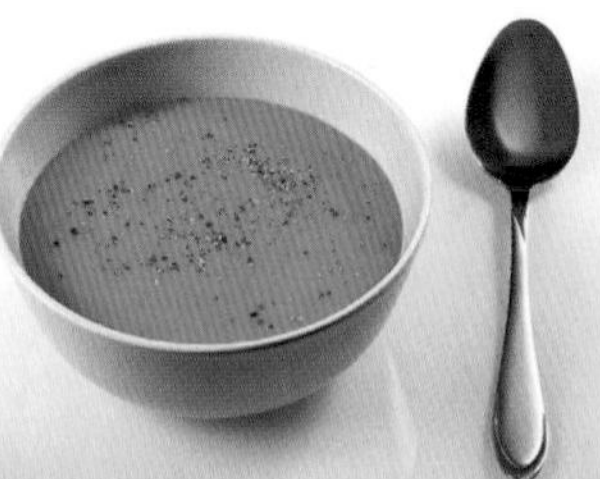

FIBRE	Weight	SAT FAT
3g	Weight: 400g	2g

Butter

CARBS	CALS	PROTEIN	FAT	FIBRE	Weight	SAT FAT
0g	37	0g	4g	0g	Weight: 5g (teaspoon)	3g
0g	112	0g	12g	0g	Weight: 15g (tablespoon)	8g

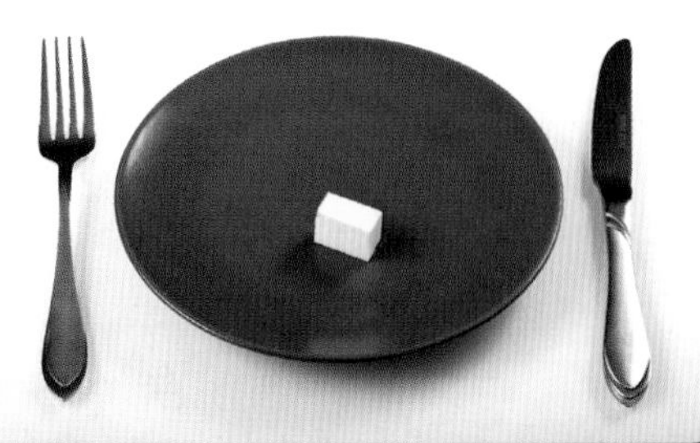

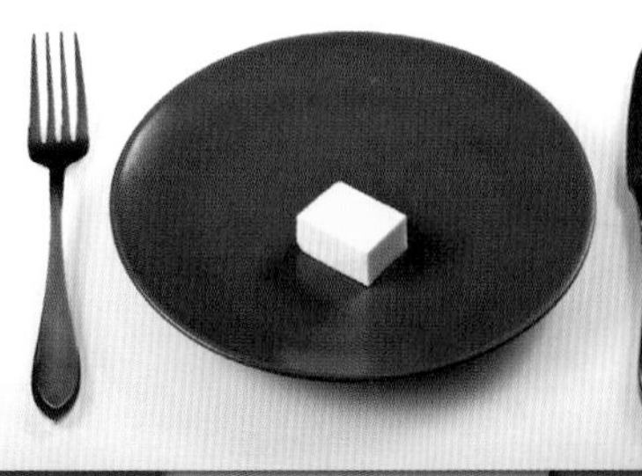

Margarine

CARBS	CALS	PROTEIN	FAT	FIBRE	Weight	SAT FAT
0g	37	0g	4g	0g	Weight: 5g (teaspoon)	1g
0g	112	0g	12g	0g	Weight: 15g (tablespoon)	3g

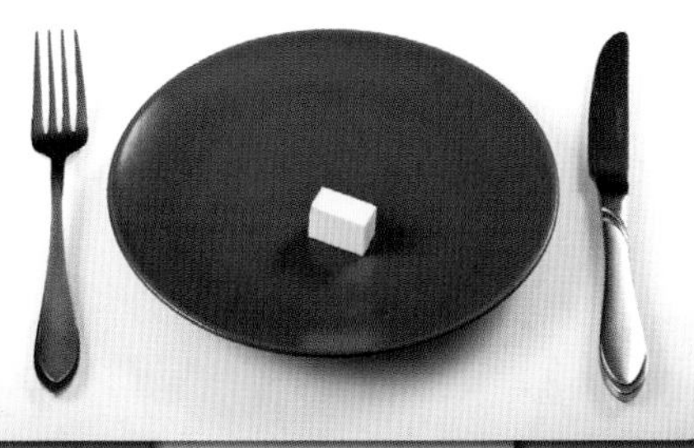

Margarine (light)

CARBS	CALS	PROTEIN	FAT	FIBRE	Weight	SAT FAT
0g	14	0g	2g	0g	Weight: 5g (teaspoon)	0g
1g	42	0g	5g	0g	Weight: 15g (tablespoon)	1g

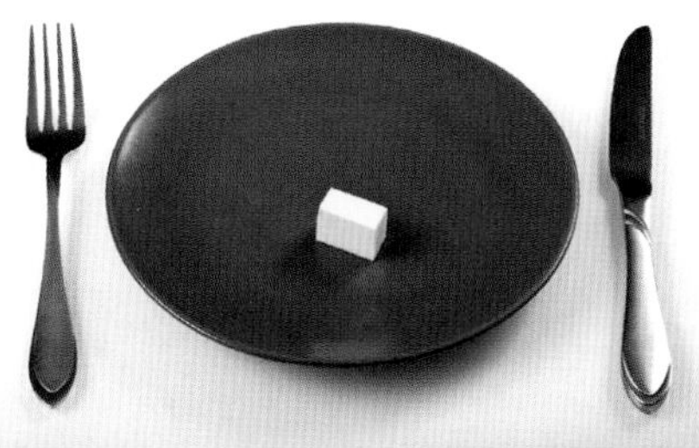

Olive Oil Spread

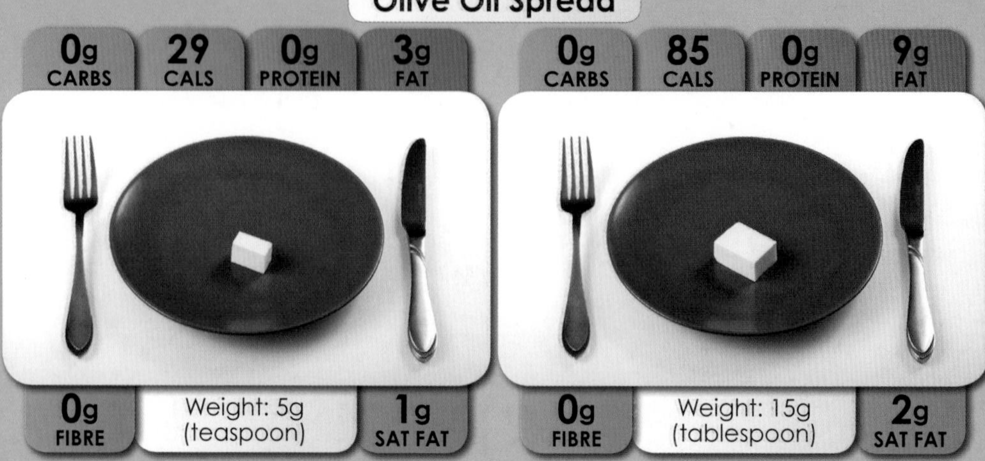

Weight	Carbs	Cals	Protein	Fat	Fibre	Sat Fat
5g (teaspoon)	0g	29	0g	3g	0g	1g
15g (tablespoon)	0g	85	0g	9g	0g	2g

Lard

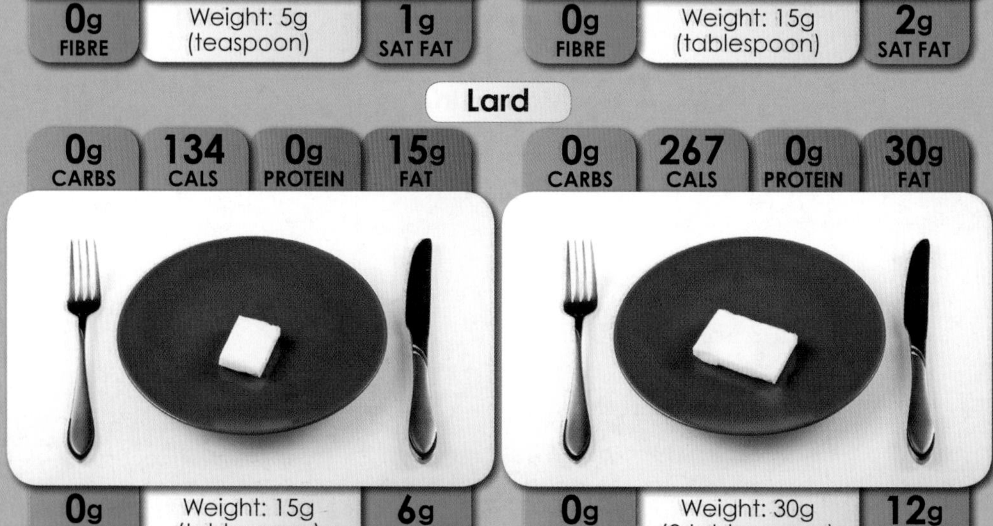

Weight	Carbs	Cals	Protein	Fat	Fibre	Sat Fat
15g (tablespoon)	0g	134	0g	15g	0g	6g
30g (2 tablespoons)	0g	267	0g	30g	0g	12g

Ghee

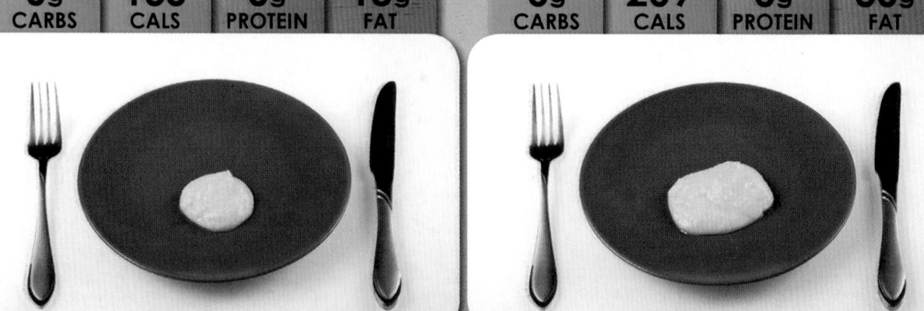

Weight	Carbs	Cals	Protein	Fat	Fibre	Sat Fat
15g (tablespoon)	0g	135	0g	15g	0g	10g
30g (2 tablespoons)	0g	269	0g	30g	0g	20g

Olive / Vegetable / Sesame Oil

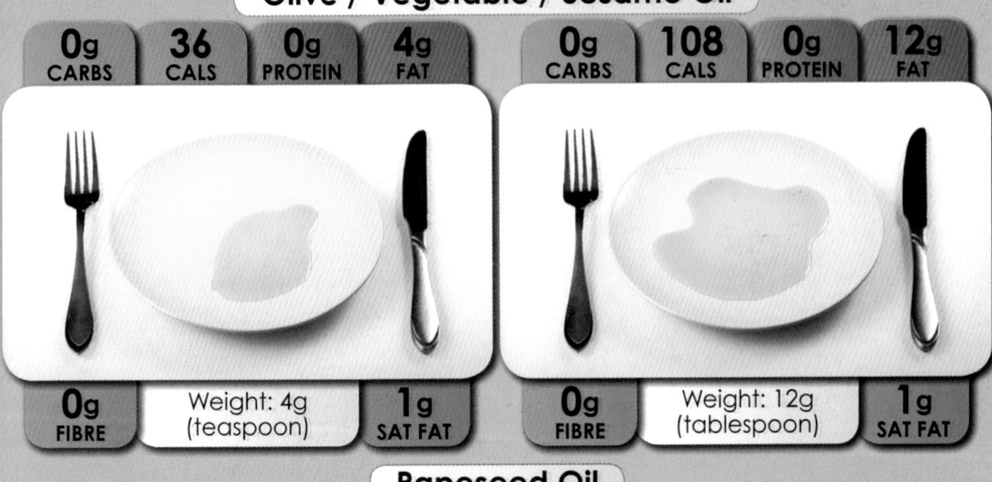

Rapeseed Oil

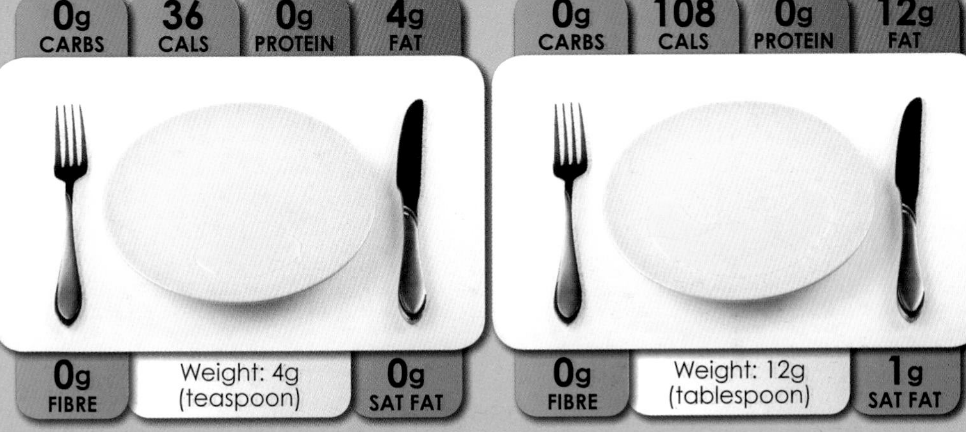

Palm Oil

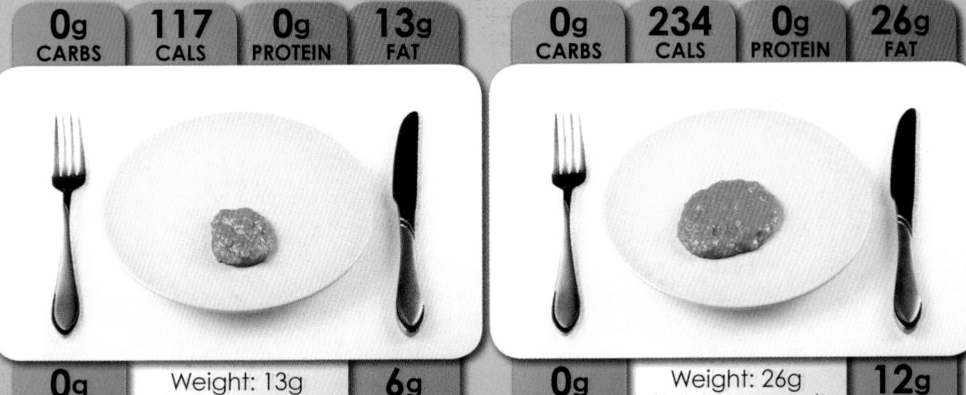

20cm Side Plate

Chocolate Nut Spread

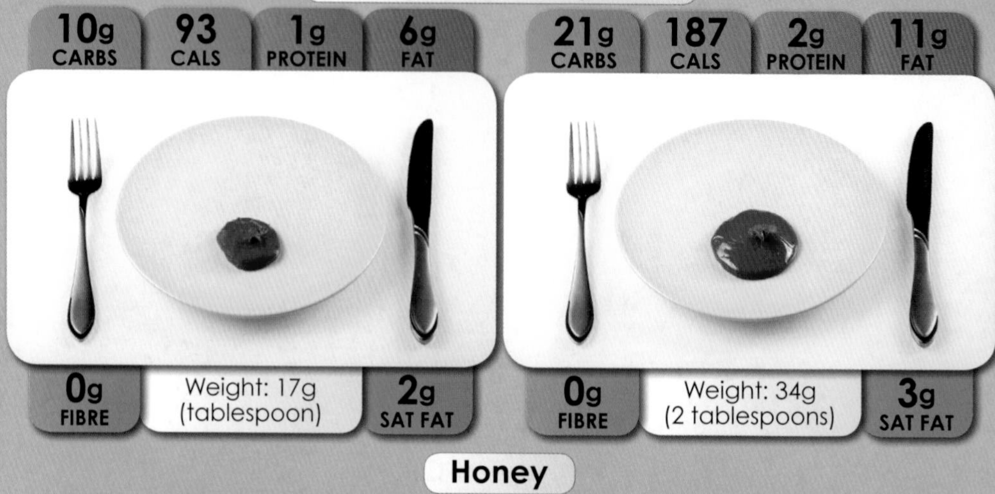

Weight	Carbs	Cals	Protein	Fat	Fibre	Sat Fat
Weight: 17g (tablespoon)	10g	93	1g	6g	0g	2g
Weight: 34g (2 tablespoons)	21g	187	2g	11g	0g	3g

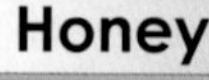

Honey

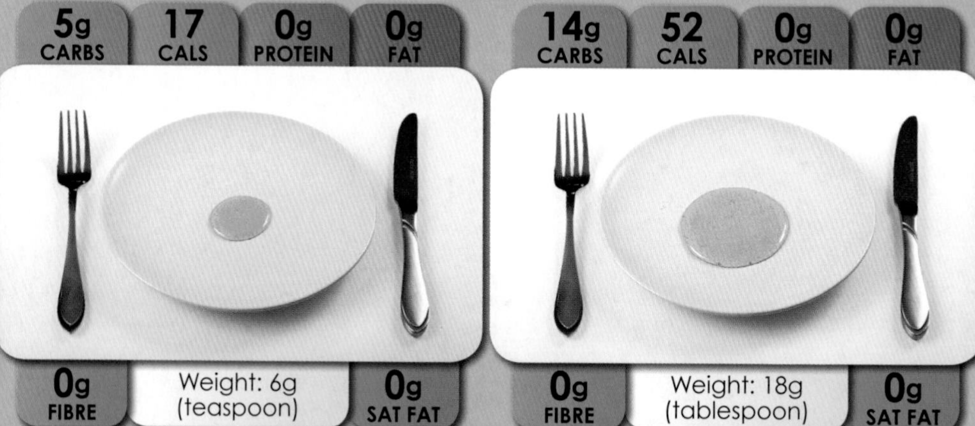

Weight	Carbs	Cals	Protein	Fat	Fibre	Sat Fat
Weight: 6g (teaspoon)	5g	17	0g	0g	0g	0g
Weight: 18g (tablespoon)	14g	52	0g	0g	0g	0g

Jam

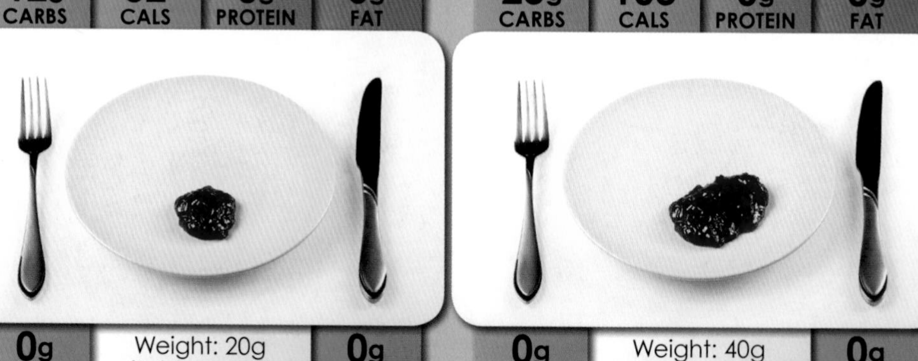

Weight	Carbs	Cals	Protein	Fat	Fibre	Sat Fat
Weight: 20g (tablespoon)	12g	52	0g	0g	0g	0g
Weight: 40g (2 tablespoons)	25g	103	0g	0g	0g	0g

Lemon Curd

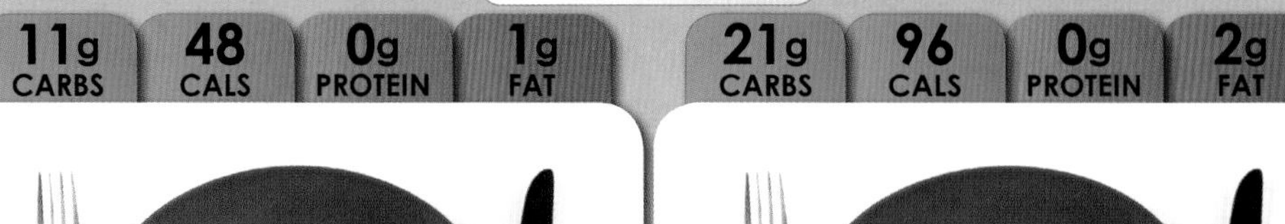

11g CARBS	48 CALS	0g PROTEIN	1g FAT

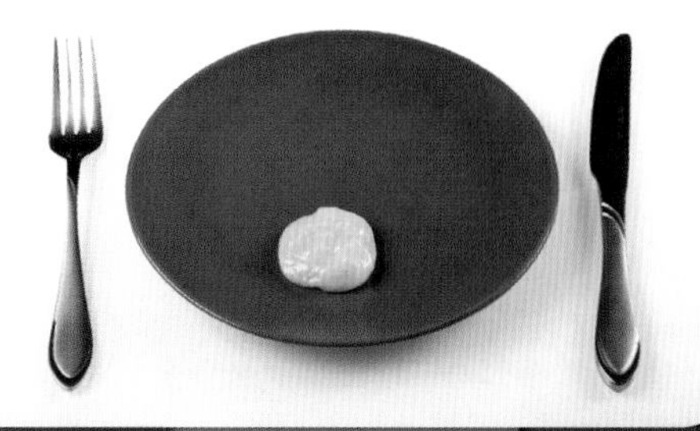

0g FIBRE	Weight: 17g (tablespoon)	0g SAT FAT

21g CARBS	96 CALS	0g PROTEIN	2g FAT

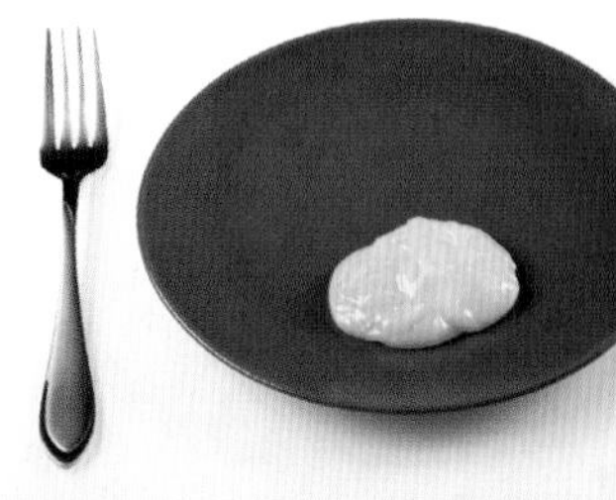

0g FIBRE	Weight: 34g (2 tablespoons)	1g SAT FAT

Maple Syrup

11g CARBS	45 CALS	0g PROTEIN	0g FAT

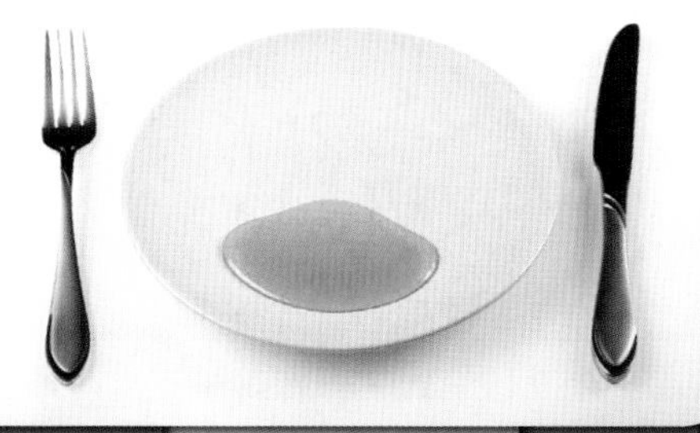

0g FIBRE	Weight: 17g (tablespoon)	0g SAT FAT

23g CARBS	89 CALS	0g PROTEIN	0g FAT

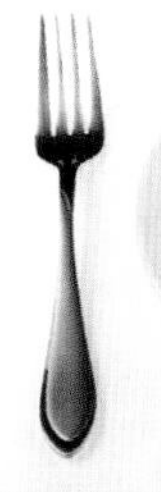

0g FIBRE	Weight: 34g (2 tablespoons)	0g SAT FAT

Marmalade

14g CARBS	52 CALS	0g PROTEIN	0g FAT

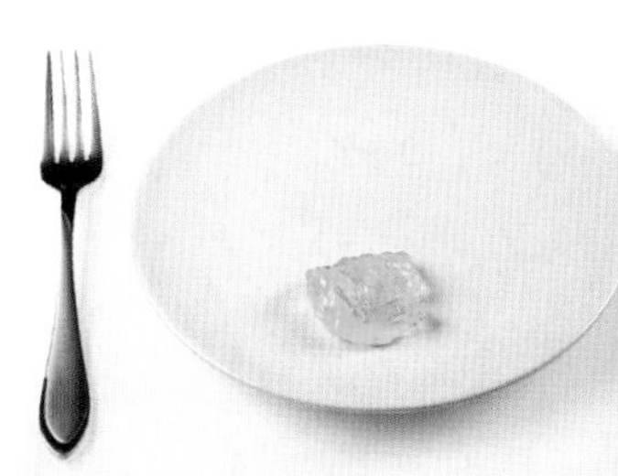

0g FIBRE	Weight: 20g (tablespoon)	0g SAT FAT

28g CARBS	104 CALS	0g PROTEIN	0g FAT

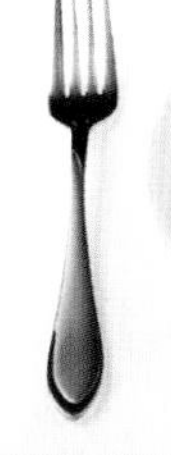

0g FIBRE	Weight: 40g (2 tablespoons)	0g SAT FAT

Marmite

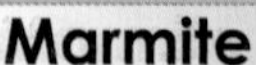

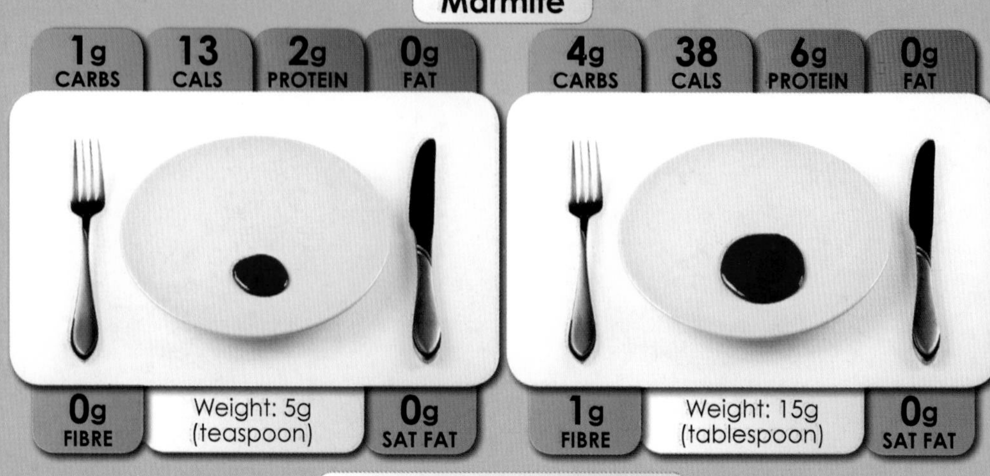

Peanut Butter (crunchy)

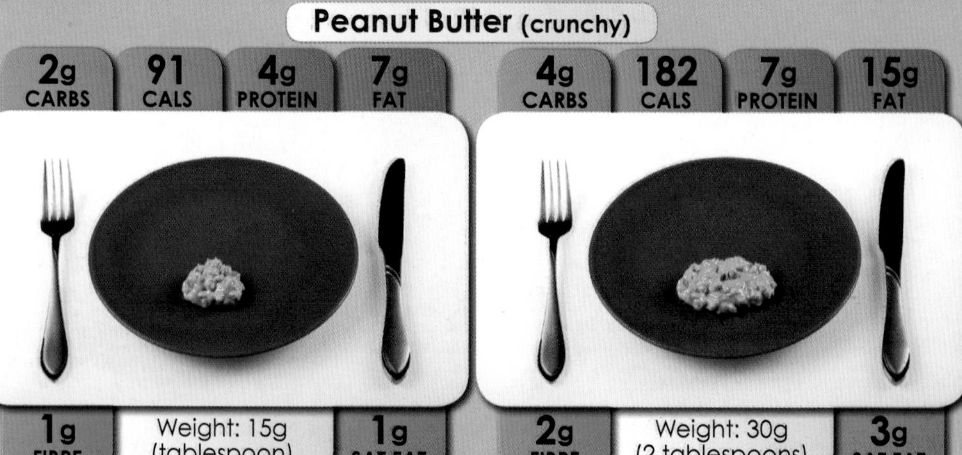

Peanut Butter (smooth)

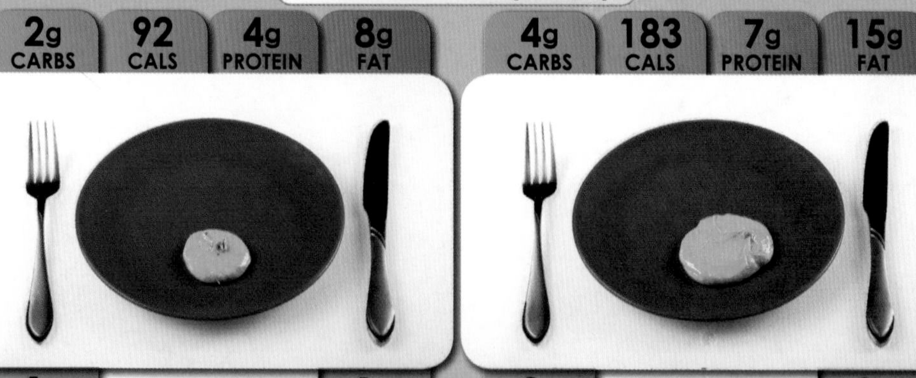

Sugar (white)

	Carbs	Cals	Protein	Fat	Fibre	Sat Fat	Weight
Teaspoon	5g	20	0g	0g	0g	0g	5g (teaspoon)
Tablespoon	16g	59	0g	0g	0g	0g	15g (tablespoon)

Sugar (brown)

	Carbs	Cals	Protein	Fat	Fibre	Sat Fat	Weight
Teaspoon	5g	18	0g	0g	0g	0g	5g (teaspoon)
Tablespoon	15g	54	0g	0g	0g	0g	15g (tablespoon)

Sweetener

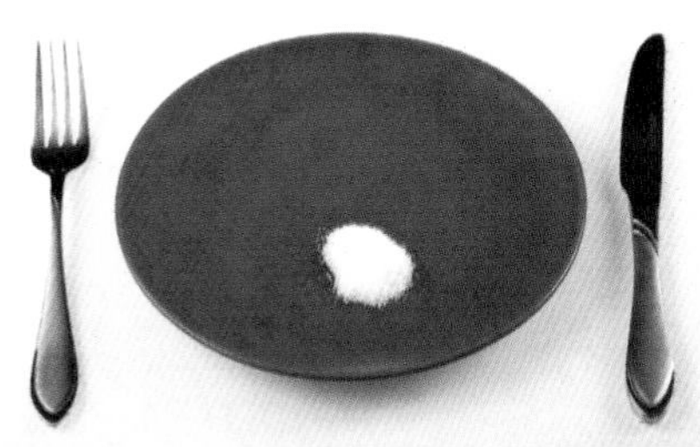

	Carbs	Cals	Protein	Fat	Fibre	Sat Fat	Weight
Teaspoon	0g	2	0g	0g	0g	0g	0.5g (teaspoon)
Tablespoon	1g	6	0g	0g	0g	0g	1.5g (tablespoon)

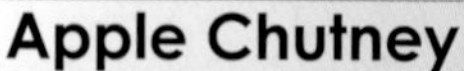

Apple Chutney

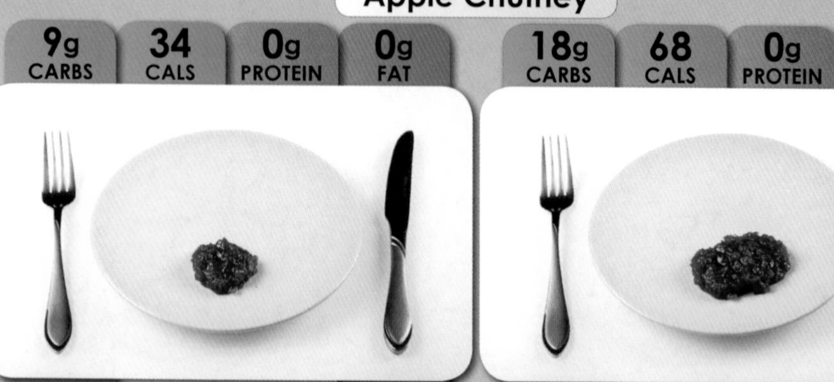

	Tablespoon	2 tablespoons
Carbs	9g	18g
Cals	34	68
Protein	0g	0g
Fat	0g	0g
Fibre	0g	1g
Weight	18g (tablespoon)	36g (2 tablespoons)
Sat fat	0g	0g

BBQ Sauce

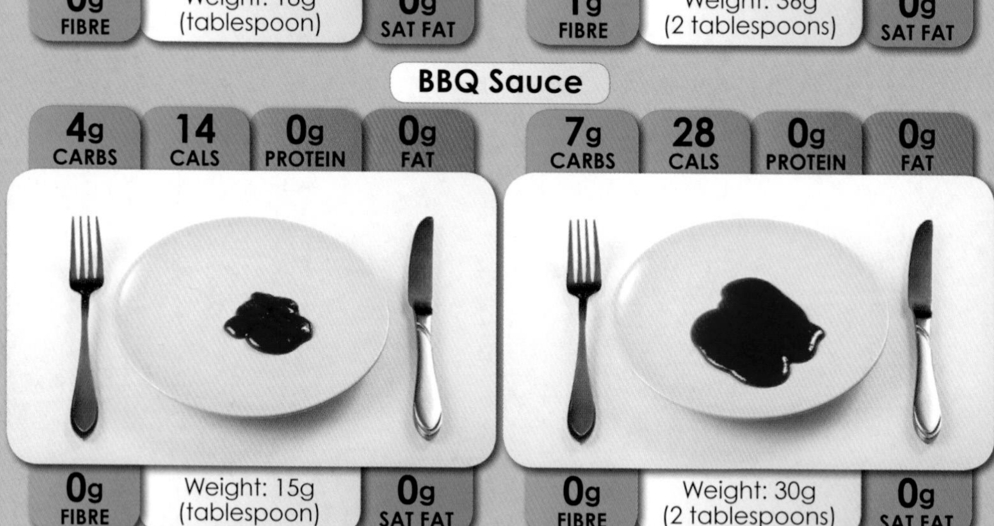

	Tablespoon	2 tablespoons
Carbs	4g	7g
Cals	14	28
Protein	0g	0g
Fat	0g	0g
Fibre	0g	0g
Weight	15g (tablespoon)	30g (2 tablespoons)
Sat fat	0g	0g

Béarnaise Sauce

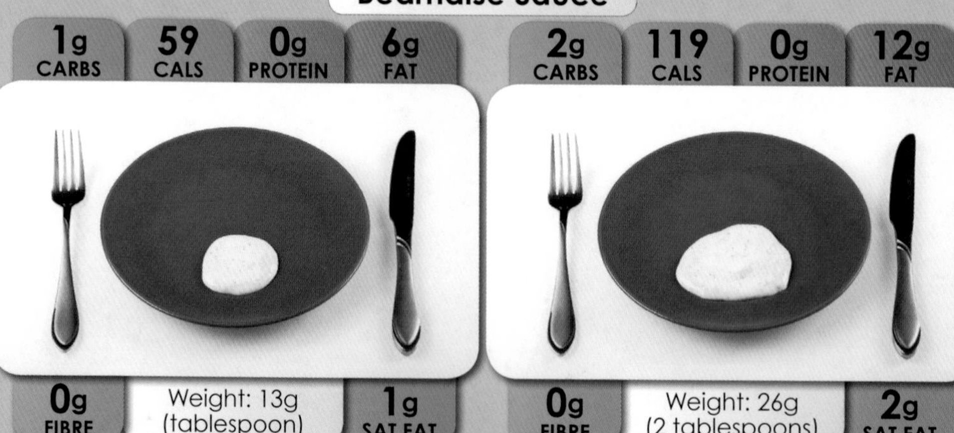

	Tablespoon	2 tablespoons
Carbs	1g	2g
Cals	59	119
Protein	0g	0g
Fat	6g	12g
Fibre	0g	0g
Weight	13g (tablespoon)	26g (2 tablespoons)
Sat fat	1g	2g

Brown Sauce

CARBS	CALS	PROTEIN	FAT	FIBRE	Weight	SAT FAT
4g	17	0g	0g	0g	Weight: 17g (tablespoon)	0g
8g	33	0g	0g	0g	Weight: 34g (2 tablespoons)	0g

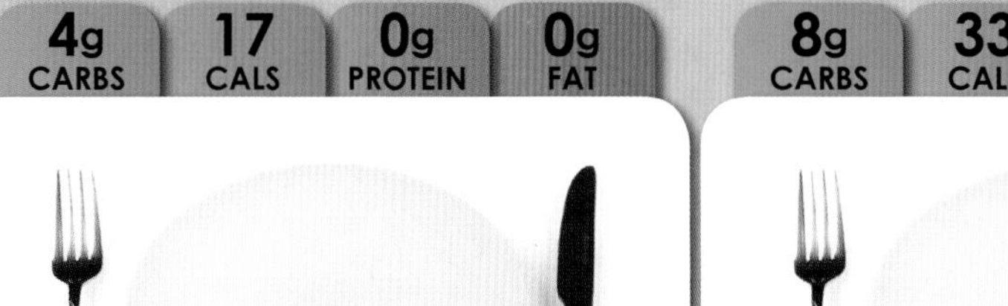
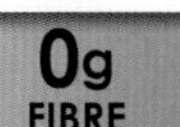
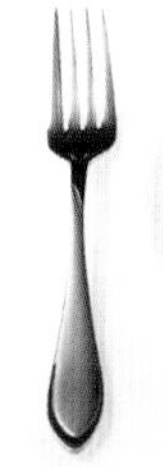

Caesar Dressing

CARBS	CALS	PROTEIN	FAT	FIBRE	Weight	SAT FAT
1g	70	0g	7g	0g	Weight: 15g (tablespoon)	1g
2g	140	1g	14g	0g	Weight: 30g (2 tablespoons)	1g

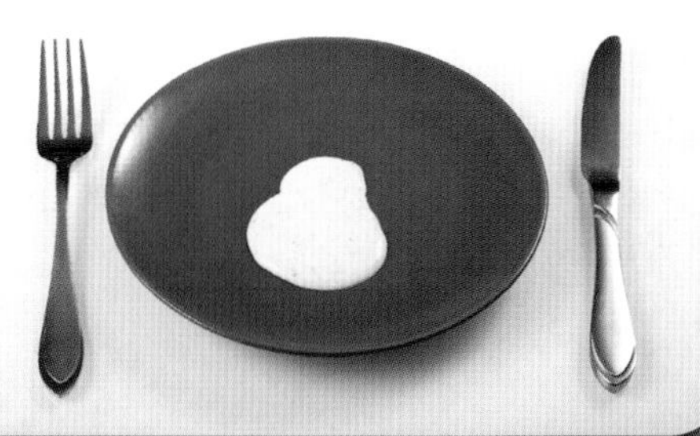
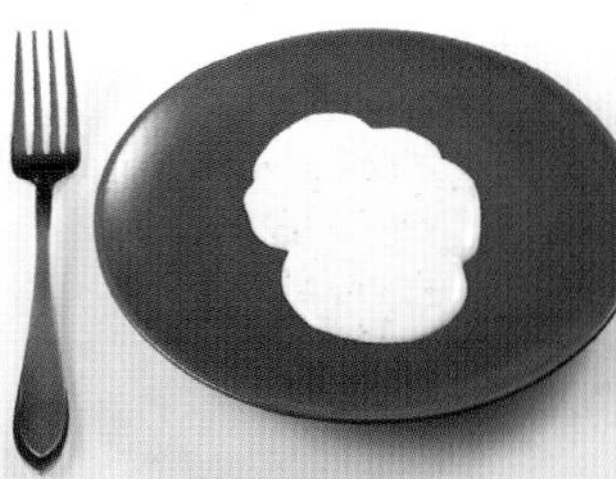

Chilli Sauce

CARBS	CALS	PROTEIN	FAT	FIBRE	Weight	SAT FAT
4g	16	0g	0g	0g	Weight: 20g (tablespoon)	0g
7g	32	1g	0g	1g	Weight: 40g (2 tablespoons)	0g

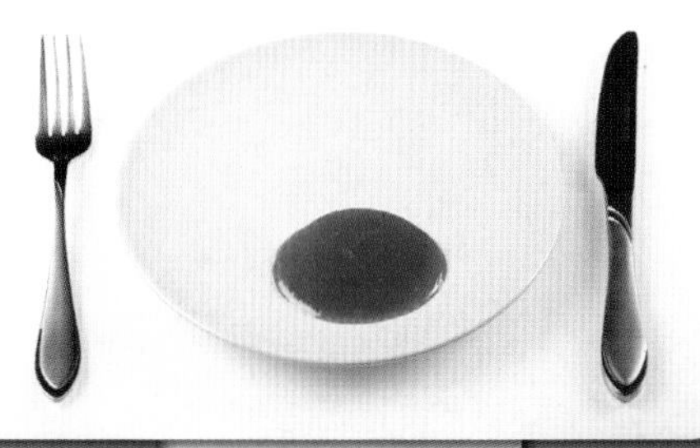
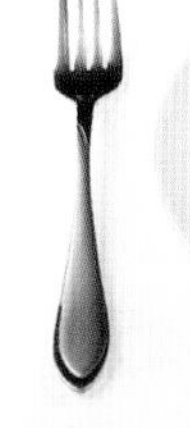

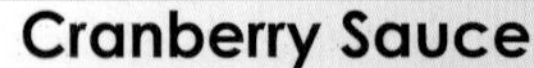

Cranberry Sauce

	Side plate	Dinner plate
CARBS	8g	16g
CALS	30	60
PROTEIN	0g	0g
FAT	0g	0g
FIBRE	0g	1g
Weight	20g (tablespoon)	40g (2 tablespoons)
SAT FAT	0g	0g

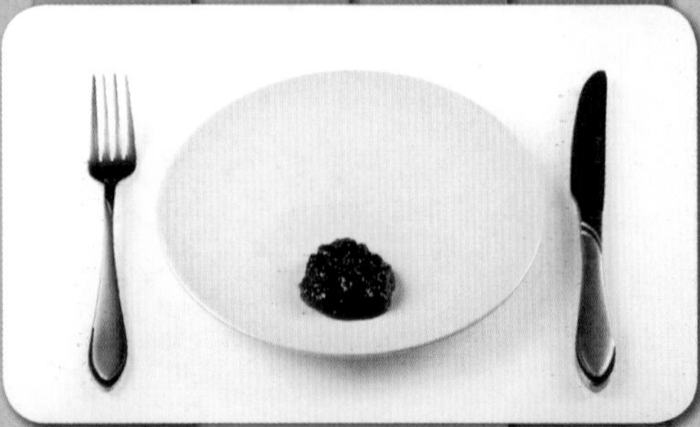

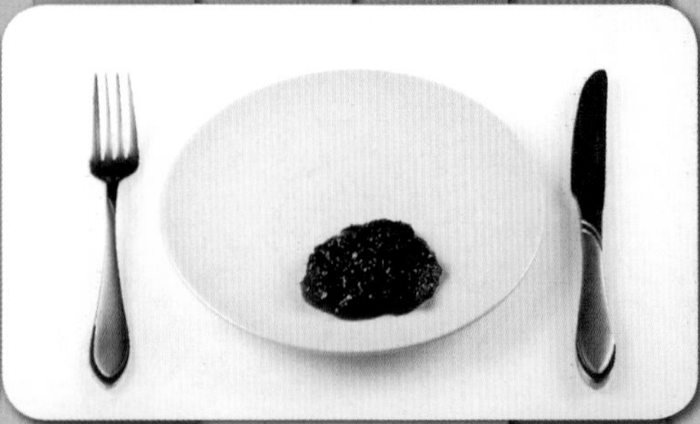

Gravy

	Side plate	Dinner plate
CARBS	4g	7g
CALS	39	78
PROTEIN	0g	1g
FAT	3g	6g
FIBRE	0g	0g
Weight	115g	230g
SAT FAT	1g	2g

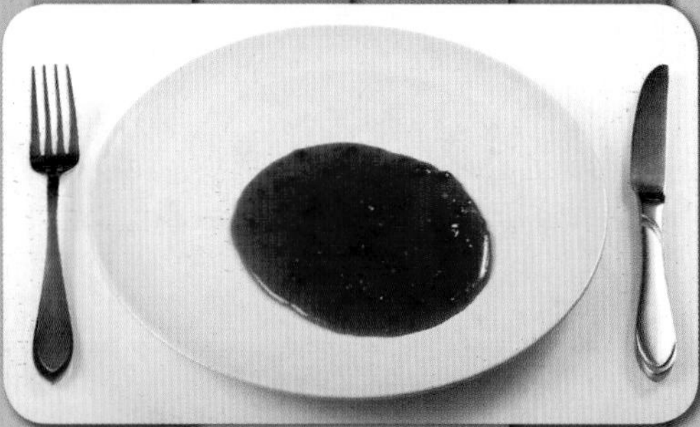

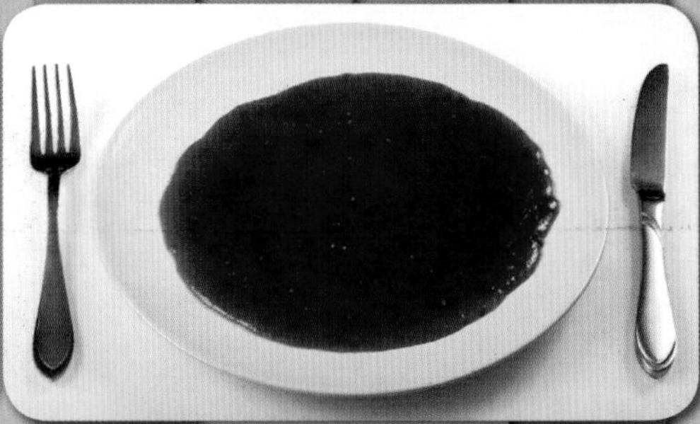

Guacamole

	Side plate	Dinner plate
CARBS	1g	1g
CALS	38	77
PROTEIN	0g	1g
FAT	4g	8g
FIBRE	1g	2g
Weight	30g (2 tablespoons)	60g (4 tablespoons)
SAT FAT	1g	2g

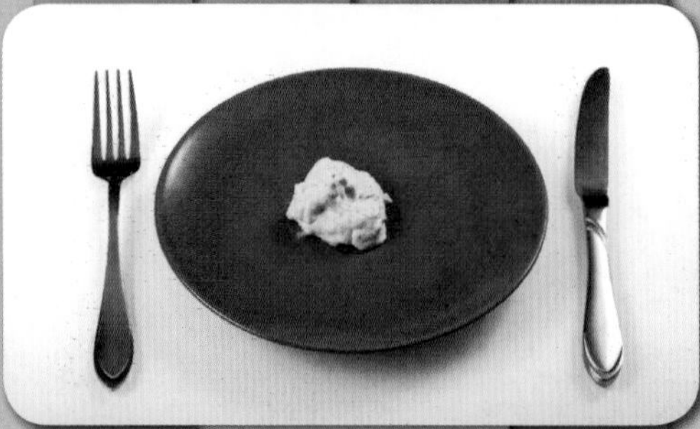

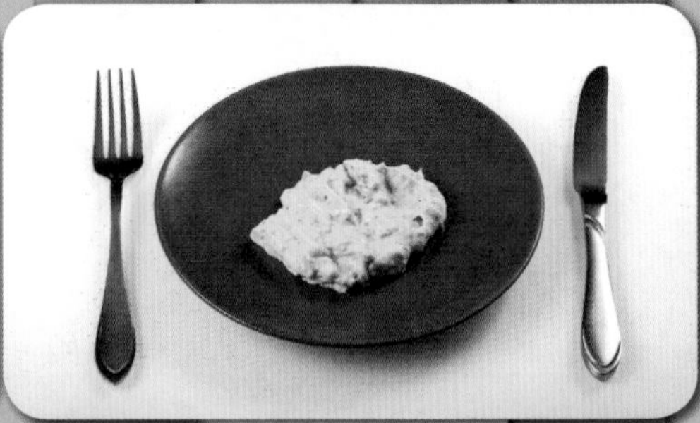

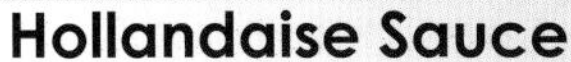

Hollandaise Sauce

Weight	Carbs	Cals	Protein	Fat	Fibre	Sat Fat
13g (tablespoon)	0g	93	1g	10g	0g	6g
26g (2 tablespoons)	0g	186	1g	20g	0g	12g

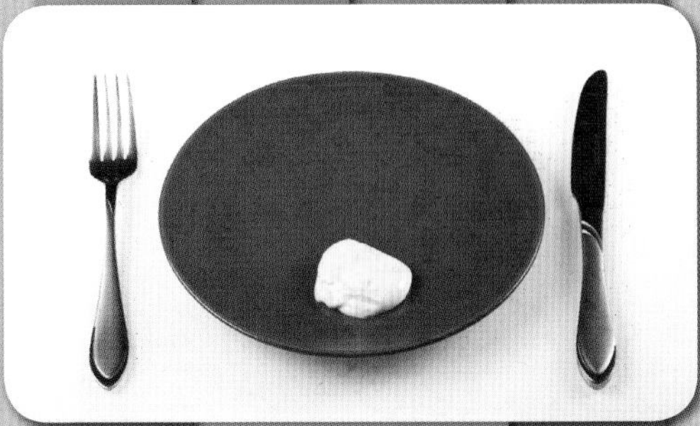

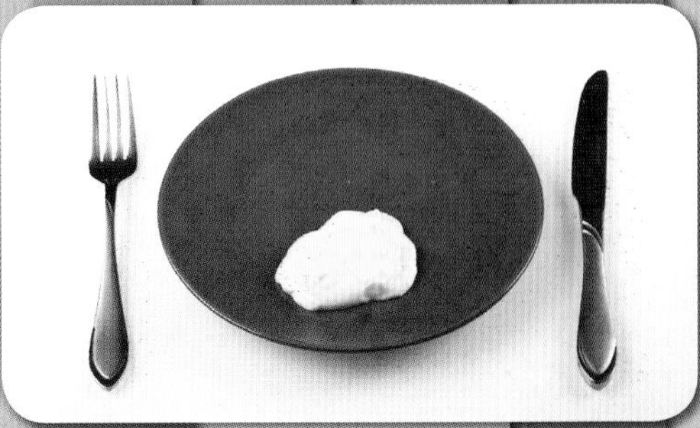

Horseradish Sauce

Weight	Carbs	Cals	Protein	Fat	Fibre	Sat Fat
13g (tablespoon)	2g	20	0g	1g	0g	0g
26g (2 tablespoons)	5g	40	1g	2g	1g	0g

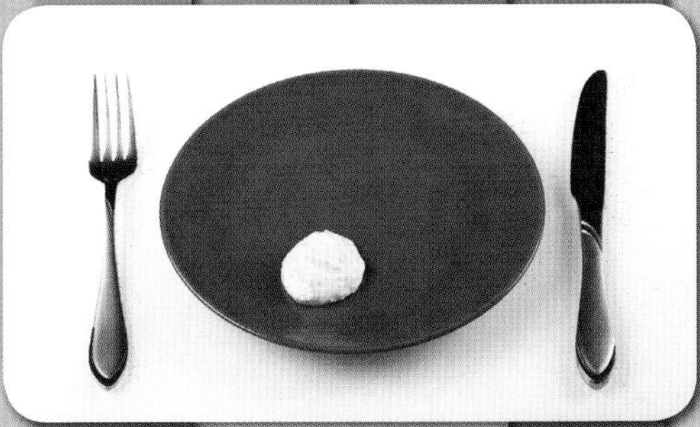

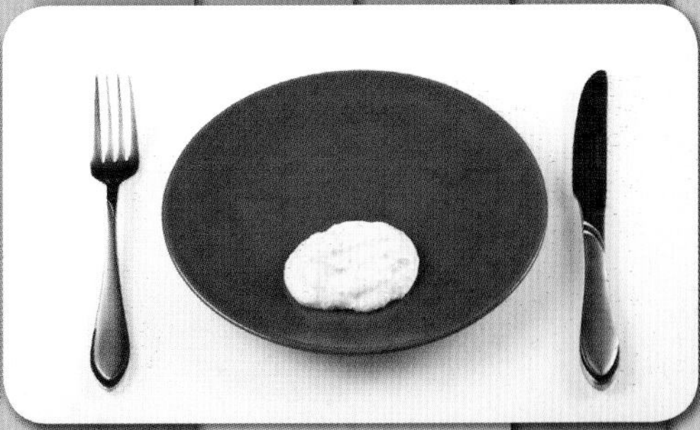

Houmous

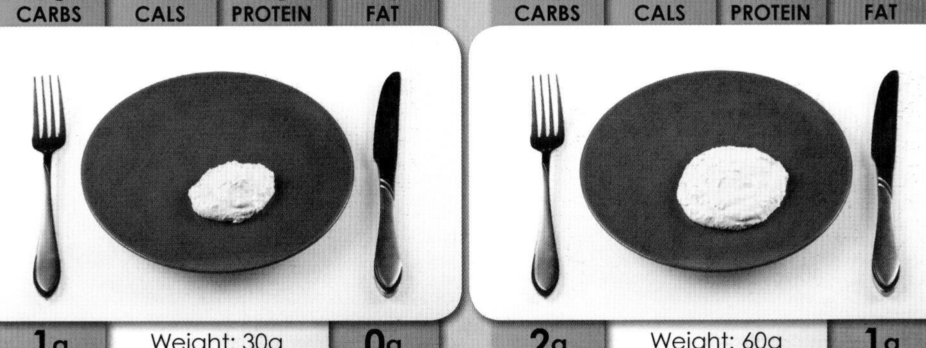

Weight	Carbs	Cals	Protein	Fat	Fibre	Sat Fat
30g (2 tablespoons)	3g	56	2g	4g	1g	0g
60g (4 tablespoons)	7g	112	5g	8g	2g	1g

20cm Side Plate

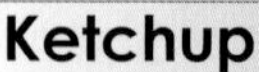

Ketchup

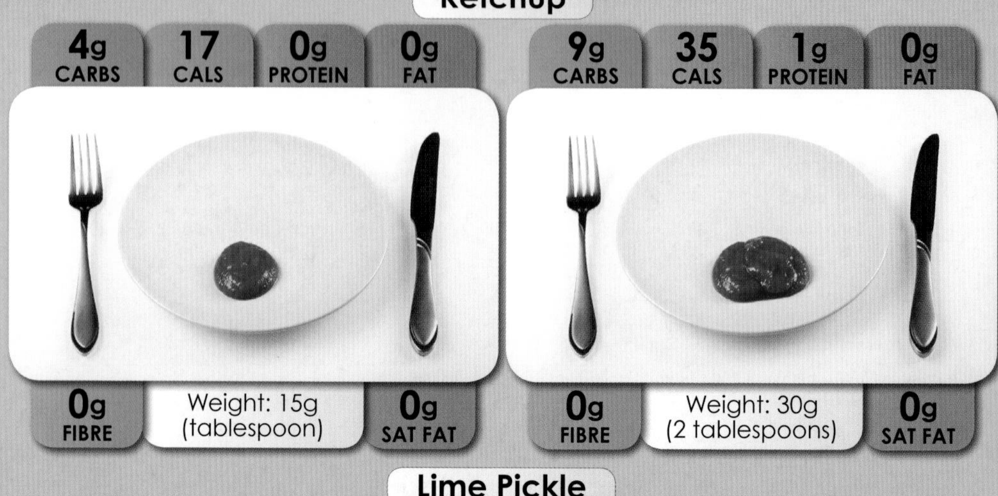

	Carbs	Cals	Protein	Fat	Fibre	Sat Fat	Weight
Tablespoon	4g	17	0g	0g	0g	0g	15g (tablespoon)
2 tablespoons	9g	35	1g	0g	0g	0g	30g (2 tablespoons)

Lime Pickle

	Carbs	Cals	Protein	Fat	Fibre	Sat Fat	Weight
Tablespoon	1g	29	0g	3g	1g	0g	16g (tablespoon)
2 tablespoons	2g	59	1g	5g	1g	1g	32g (2 tablespoons)

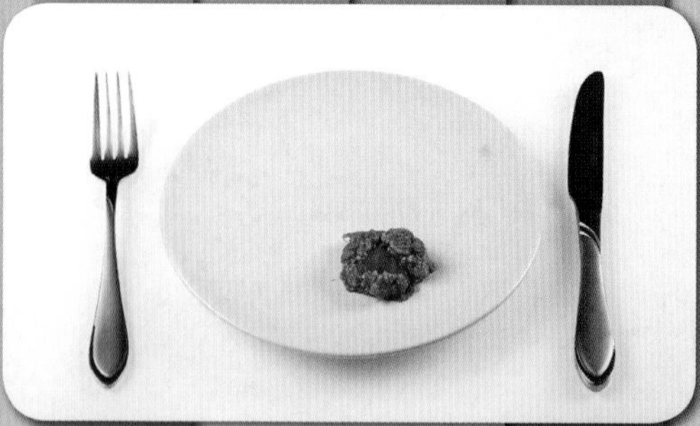

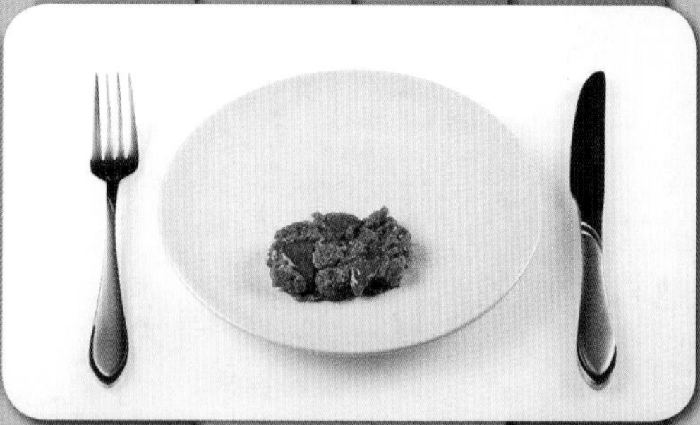

Mango Chutney

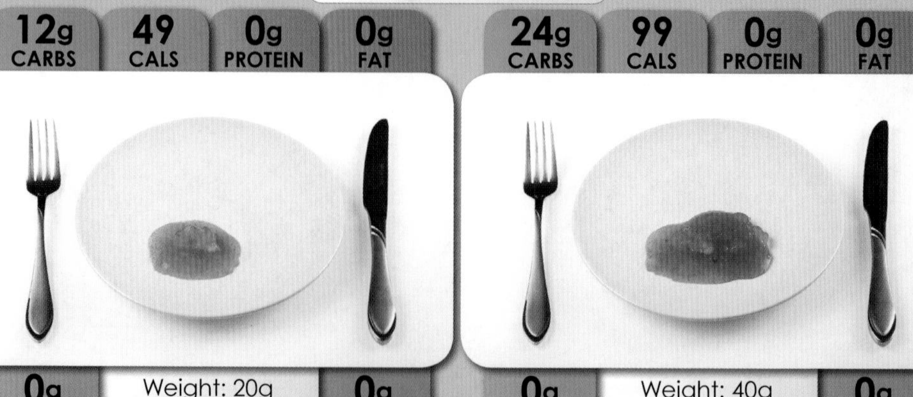

	Carbs	Cals	Protein	Fat	Fibre	Sat Fat	Weight
Tablespoon	12g	49	0g	0g	0g	0g	20g (tablespoon)
2 tablespoons	24g	99	0g	0g	0g	0g	40g (2 tablespoons)

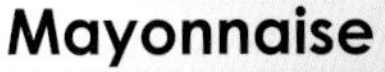

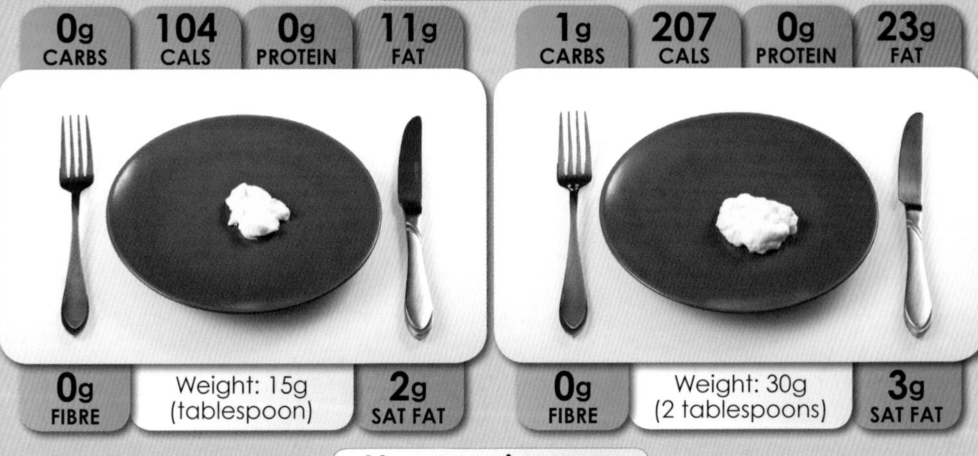

Mayonnaise (light)

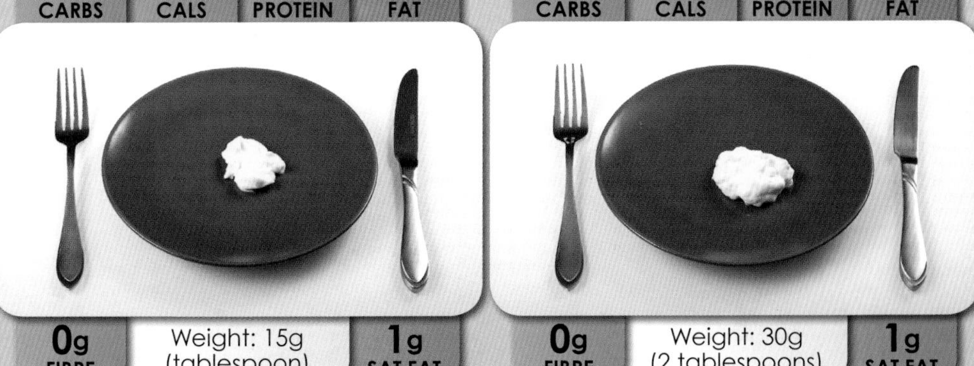

Mint Sauce

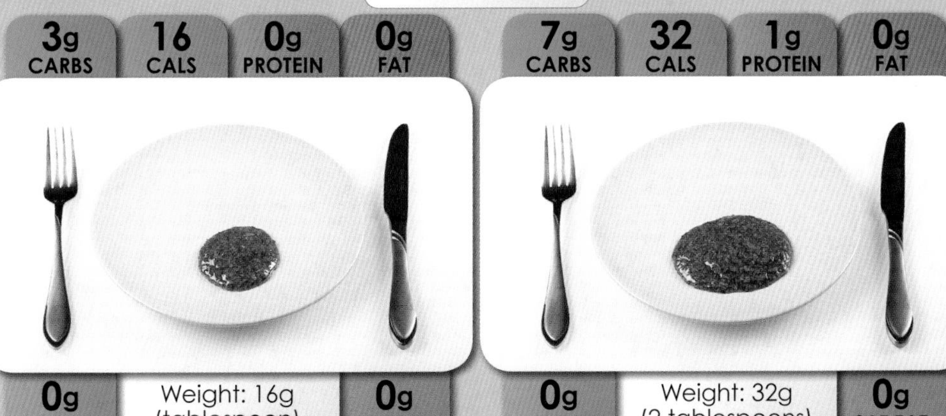

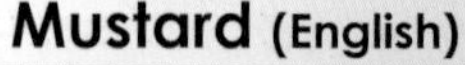

Mustard (English)

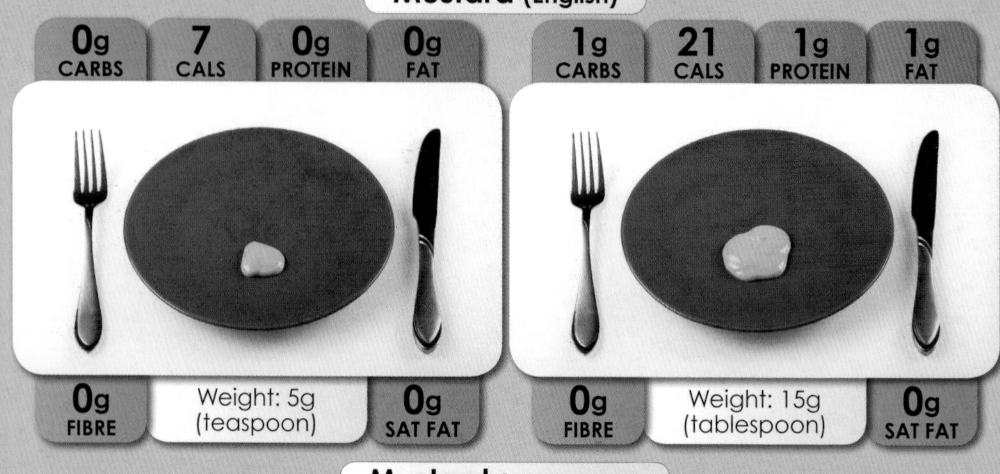

	Carbs	Cals	Protein	Fat	Fibre	Sat Fat	Weight
Left	0g	7	0g	0g	0g	0g	5g (teaspoon)
Right	1g	21	1g	1g	0g	0g	15g (tablespoon)

Mustard (wholegrain)

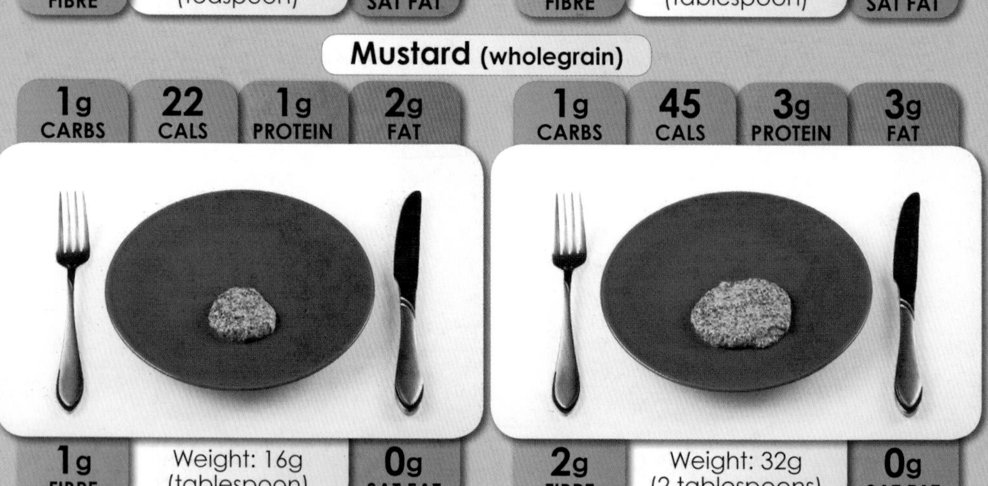

	Carbs	Cals	Protein	Fat	Fibre	Sat Fat	Weight
Left	1g	22	1g	2g	1g	0g	16g (tablespoon)
Right	1g	45	3g	3g	2g	0g	32g (2 tablespoons)

Parsley Sauce

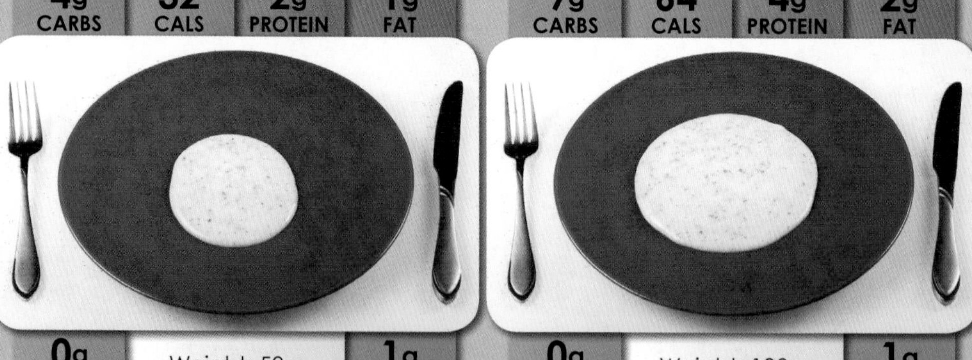

	Carbs	Cals	Protein	Fat	Fibre	Sat Fat	Weight
Left	4g	32	2g	1g	0g	1g	50g
Right	9g	64	4g	2g	0g	1g	100g

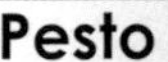

Pesto

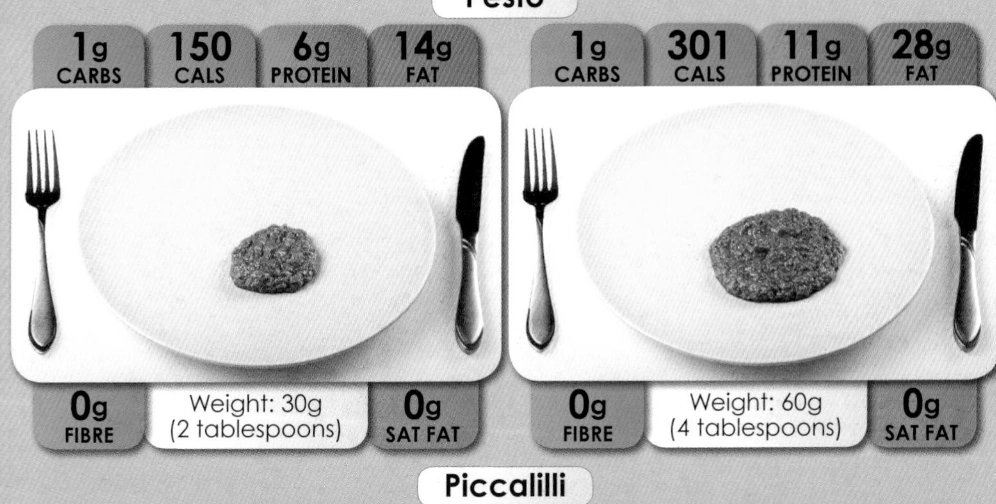

Weight	Carbs	Cals	Protein	Fat	Fibre	Sat Fat
Weight: 30g (2 tablespoons)	1g	150	6g	14g	0g	0g
Weight: 60g (4 tablespoons)	1g	301	11g	28g	0g	0g

Piccalilli

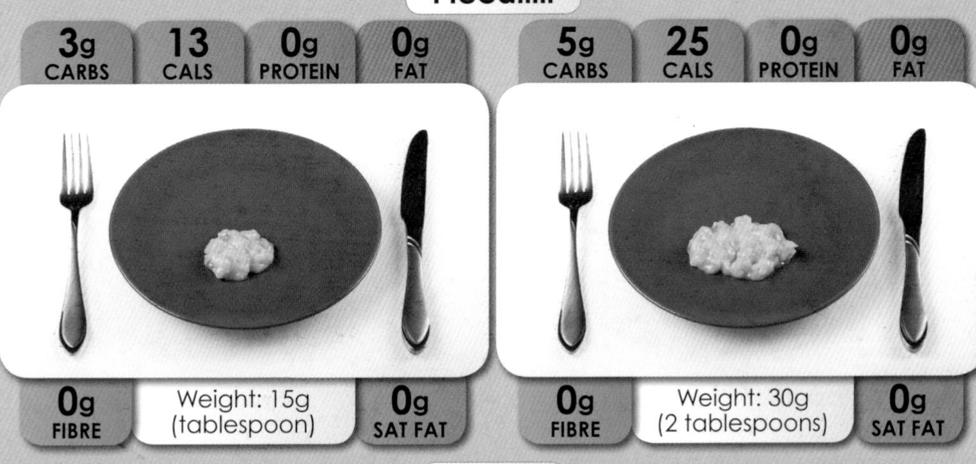

Weight	Carbs	Cals	Protein	Fat	Fibre	Sat Fat
Weight: 15g (tablespoon)	3g	13	0g	0g	0g	0g
Weight: 30g (2 tablespoons)	5g	25	0g	0g	0g	0g

Pickle

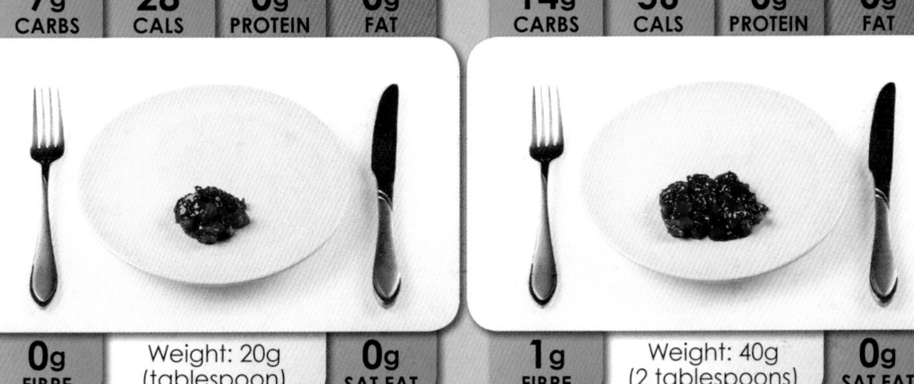

Weight	Carbs	Cals	Protein	Fat	Fibre	Sat Fat
Weight: 20g (tablespoon)	7g	28	0g	0g	0g	0g
Weight: 40g (2 tablespoons)	14g	56	0g	0g	1g	0g

Raita

1g CARBS	15 CALS	0g PROTEIN	1g FAT

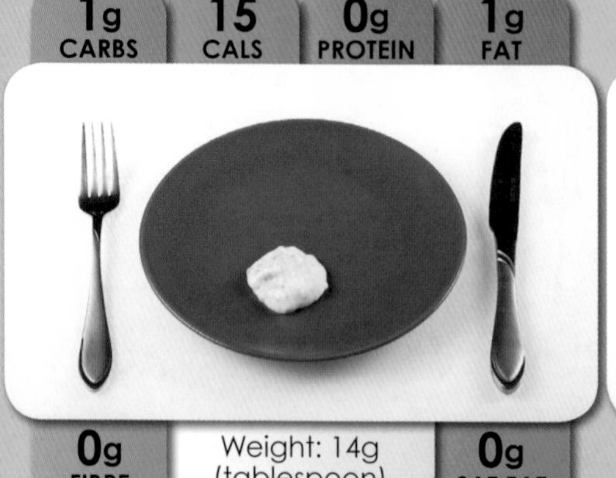

0g FIBRE	Weight: 14g (tablespoon)	0g SAT FAT

2g CARBS	30 CALS	1g PROTEIN	2g FAT

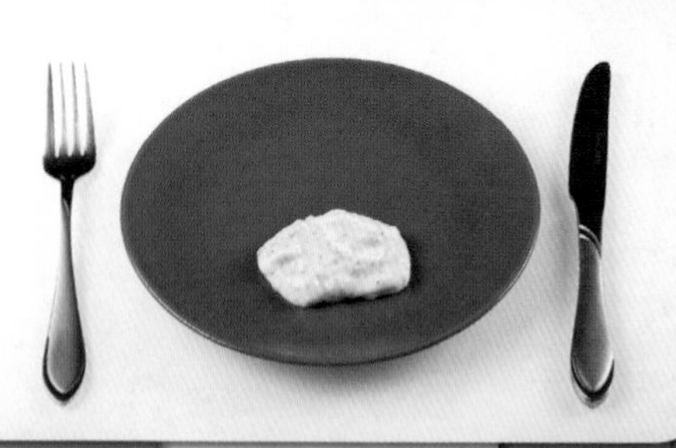

0g FIBRE	Weight: 28g (2 tablespoons)	0g SAT FAT

Salad Cream

3g CARBS	52 CALS	0g PROTEIN	5g FAT

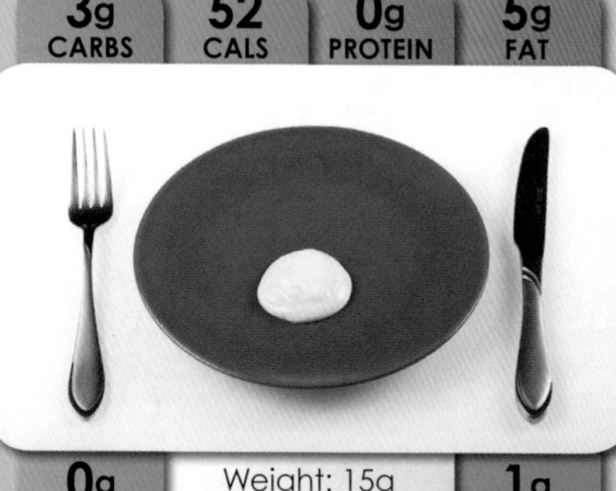

0g FIBRE	Weight: 15g (tablespoon)	1g SAT FAT

5g CARBS	104 CALS	1g PROTEIN	9g FAT

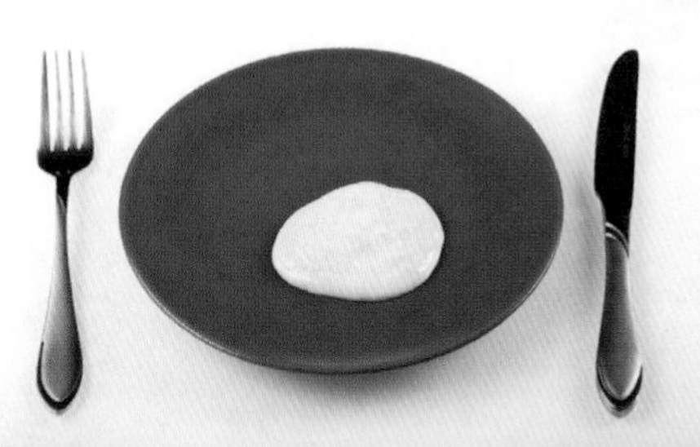

0g FIBRE	Weight: 30g (2 tablespoons)	1g SAT FAT

Soy Sauce

1g CARBS	7 CALS	1g PROTEIN	0g FAT

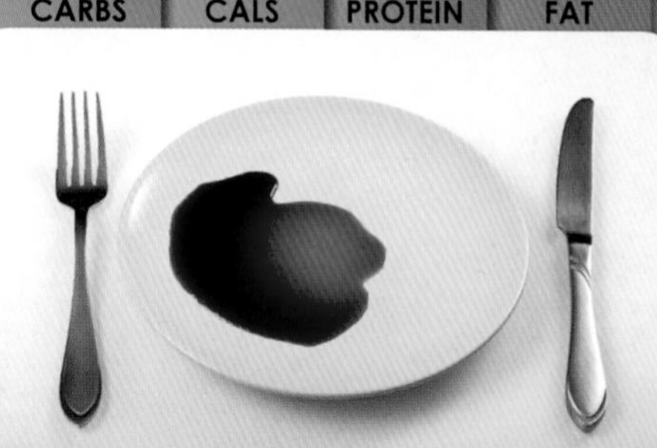

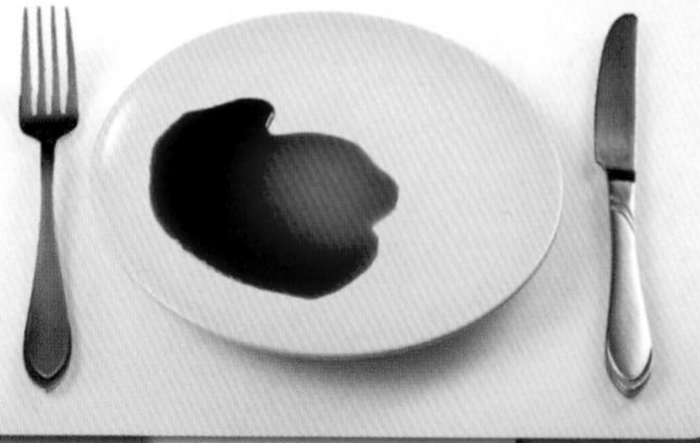

0g FIBRE	Weight: 15g (tablespoon)	0g SAT FAT

3g CARBS	13 CALS	1g PROTEIN	0g FAT

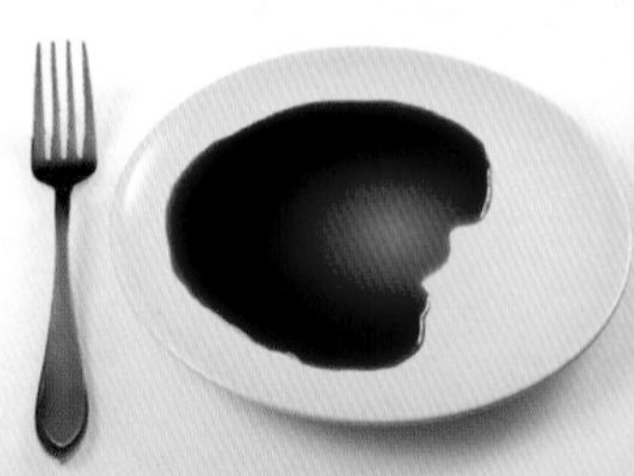

0g FIBRE	Weight: 30g (2 tablespoons)	0g SAT FAT

Sweet Chilli Sauce

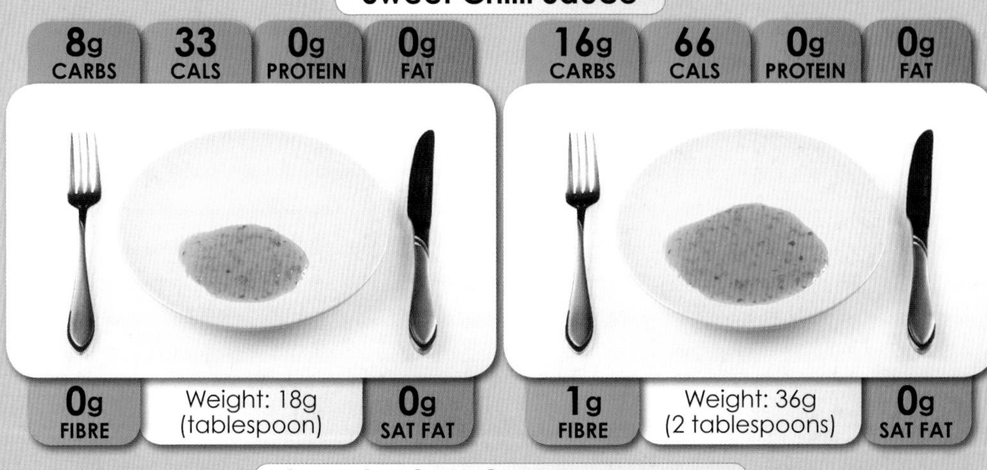

	Carbs	Cals	Protein	Fat	Fibre	Sat Fat	Weight
1 tablespoon	8g	33	0g	0g	0g	0g	18g
2 tablespoons	16g	66	0g	0g	1g	0g	36g

Sweet & Sour Sauce (takeaway)

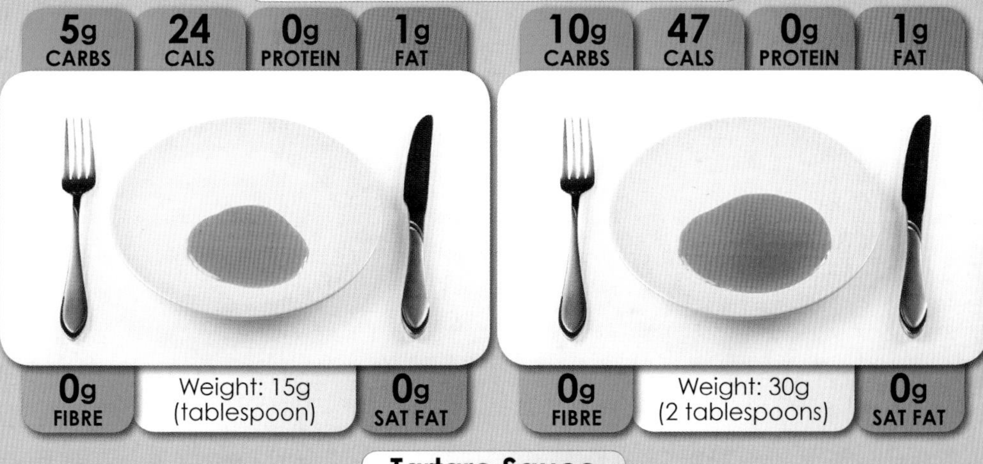

	Carbs	Cals	Protein	Fat	Fibre	Sat Fat	Weight
1 tablespoon	5g	24	0g	1g	0g	0g	15g
2 tablespoons	10g	47	0g	1g	0g	0g	30g

Tartare Sauce

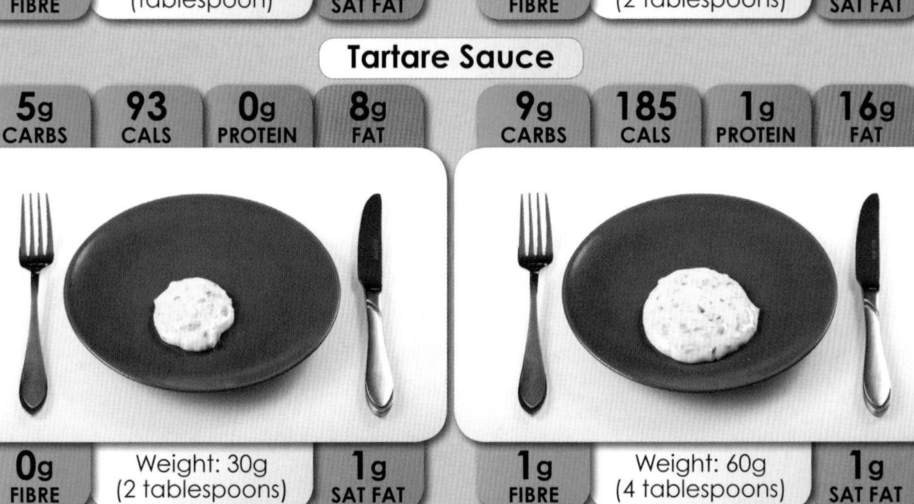

	Carbs	Cals	Protein	Fat	Fibre	Sat Fat	Weight
2 tablespoons	5g	93	0g	8g	0g	1g	30g
4 tablespoons	9g	185	1g	16g	1g	1g	60g

Thousand Island Dressing

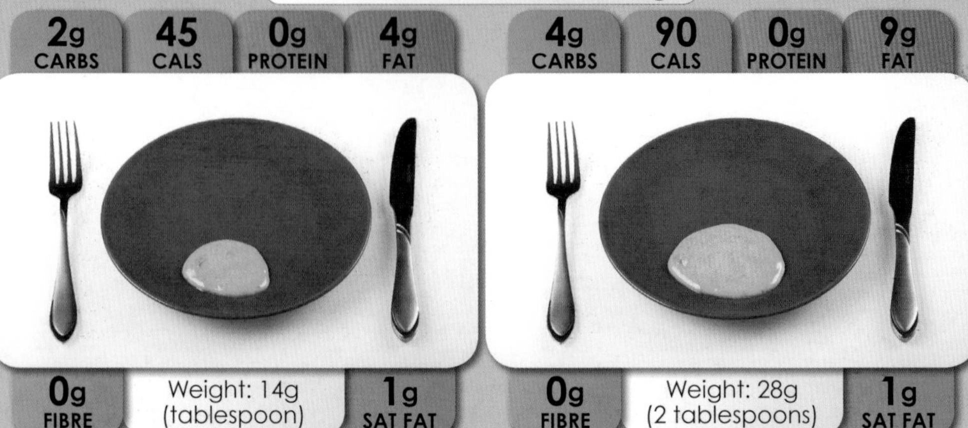

	Carbs	Cals	Protein	Fat	Fibre	Sat Fat	Weight
Side	2g	45	0g	4g	0g	1g	14g (tablespoon)
Dinner	4g	90	0g	9g	0g	1g	28g (2 tablespoons)

White Sauce (made with whole milk)

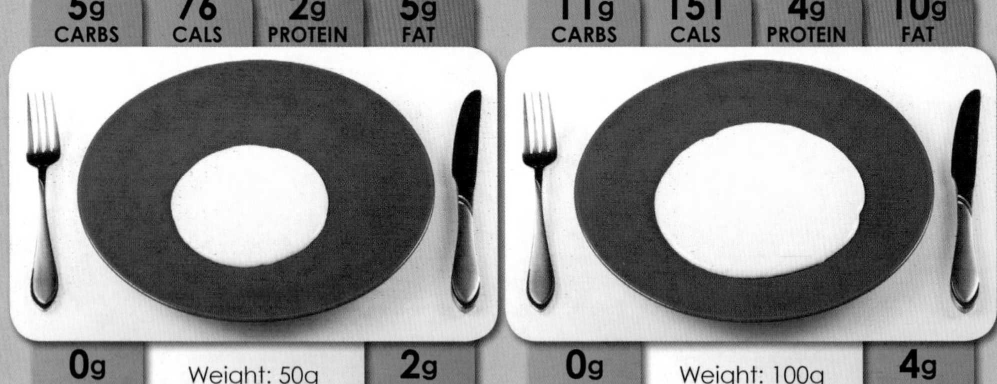

	Carbs	Cals	Protein	Fat	Fibre	Sat Fat	Weight
Side	5g	76	2g	5g	0g	2g	50g
Dinner	11g	151	4g	10g	0g	4g	100g

Worcestershire Sauce

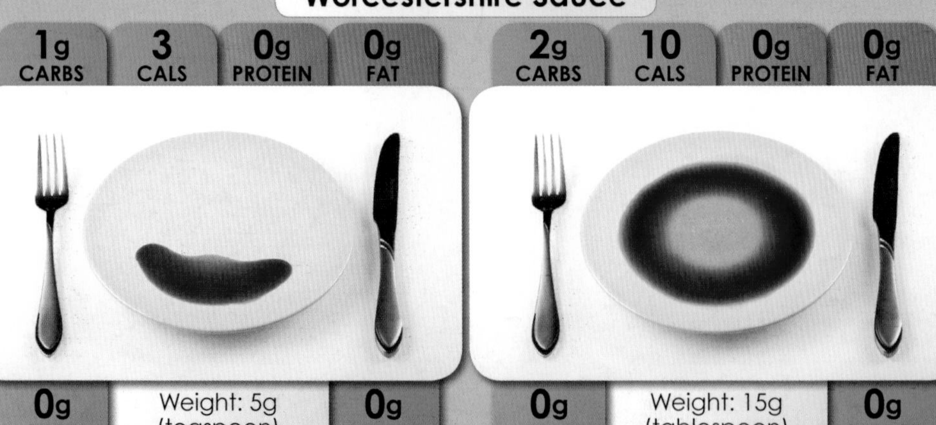

	Carbs	Cals	Protein	Fat	Fibre	Sat Fat	Weight
Side	1g	3	0g	0g	0g	0g	5g (teaspoon)
Dinner	2g	10	0g	0g	0g	0g	15g (tablespoon)

Doner Kebab

	Carbs	Cals	Protein	Fat	Fibre	Weight	Sat Fat
Left	49g	580	28g	31g	3g	250g	14g
Right	80g	1053	53g	60g	5g	415g	27g

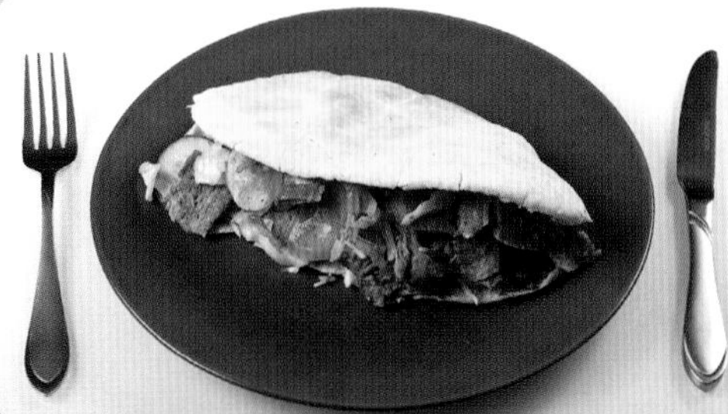

Shish Kebab

	Carbs	Cals	Protein	Fat	Fibre	Weight	Sat Fat
Left	49g	434	33g	13g	3g	250g	4g
Right	80g	762	63g	23g	5g	415g	8g

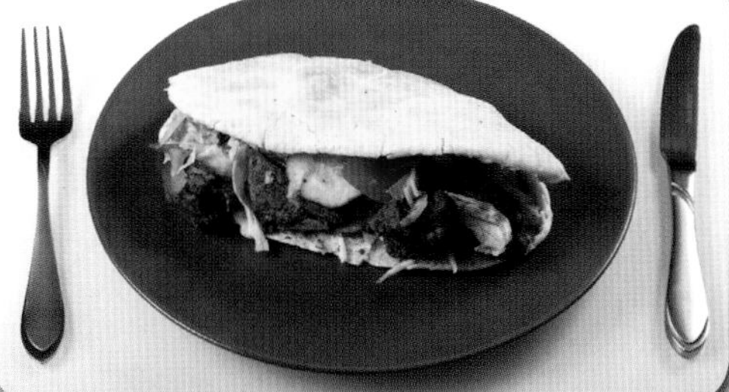

Falafel in Pitta

	Carbs	Cals	Protein	Fat	Fibre	Weight	Sat Fat
Left	59g	371	13g	11g	6g	200g	1g
Right	101g	648	22g	21g	11g	350g	3g

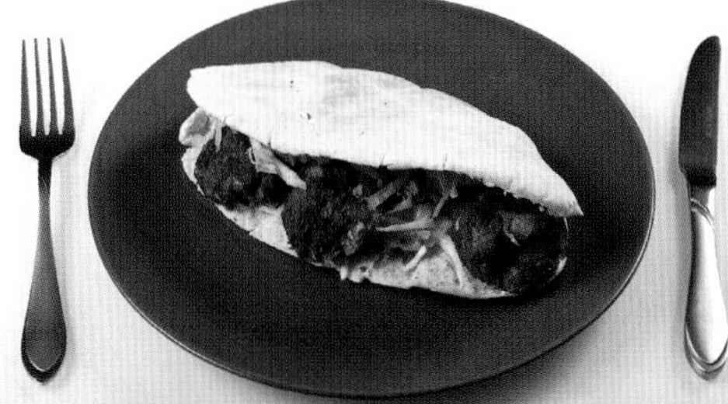

26cm Dinner Plate

Fish

14g CARBS	313 CALS	23g PROTEIN	19g FAT

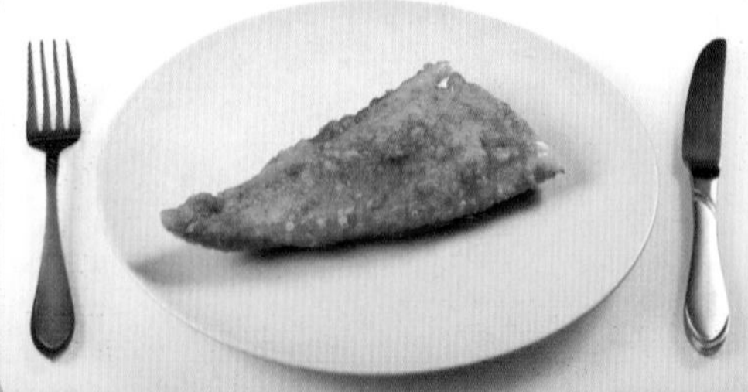

1g FIBRE	Weight: 135g	5g SAT FAT

33g CARBS	766 CALS	56g PROTEIN	46g FAT

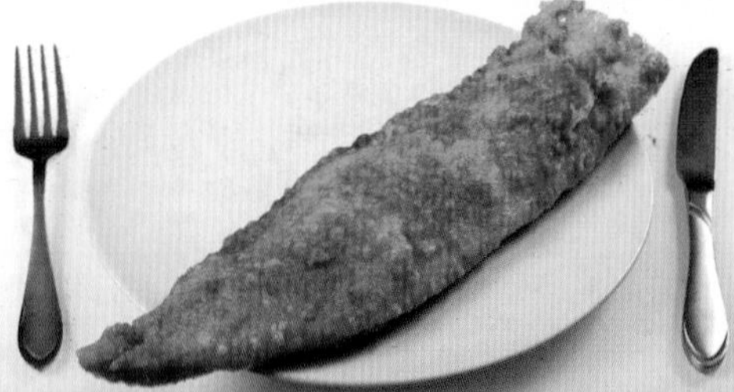

2g FIBRE	Weight: 330g	12g SAT FAT

Battered Sausage

25g CARBS	421 CALS	16g PROTEIN	29g FAT

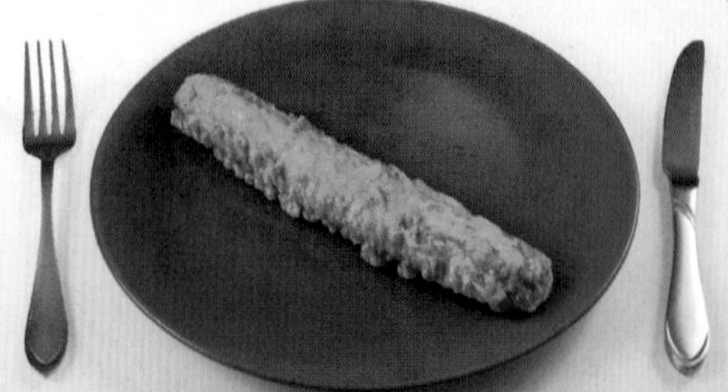

0g FIBRE	Weight: 137g	13g SAT FAT

Chips

40g CARBS	311 CALS	4g PROTEIN	16g FAT

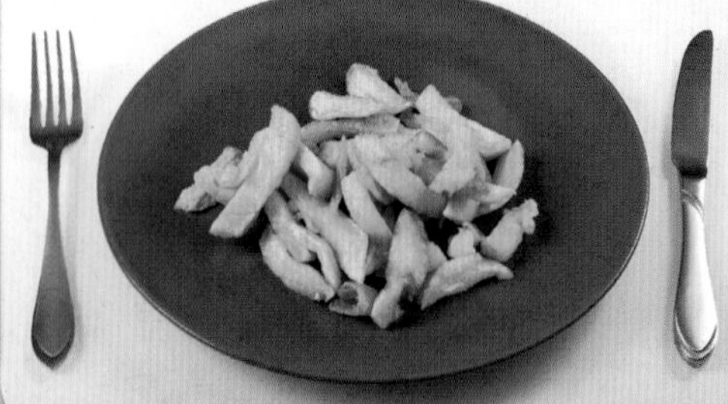

4g FIBRE	Weight: 130g	1g SAT FAT

80g CARBS	626 CALS	8g PROTEIN	33g FAT

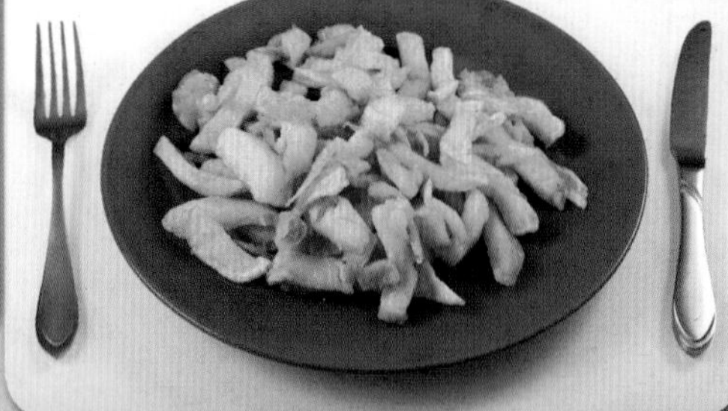

8g FIBRE	Weight: 262g	3g SAT FAT

121g CARBS	944 CALS	13g PROTEIN	49g FAT

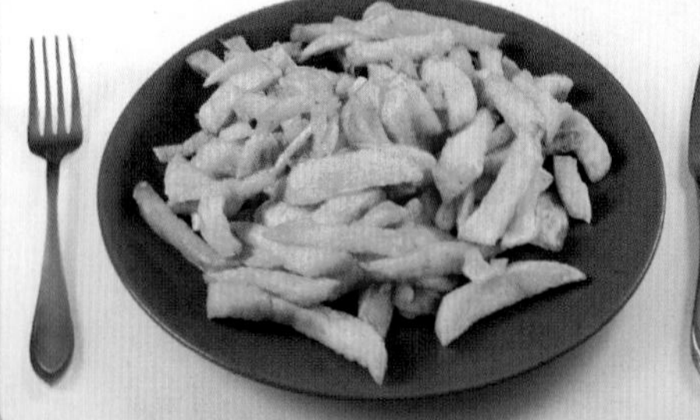

12g FIBRE	Weight: 395g	4g SAT FAT

Margherita Pizza (thin crust)

CARBS	CALS	PROTEIN	FAT	FIBRE	Weight	SAT FAT
17g	156	7g	6g	1g	Weight: 40g	3g
30g	273	12g	11g	2g	Weight: 70g	5g

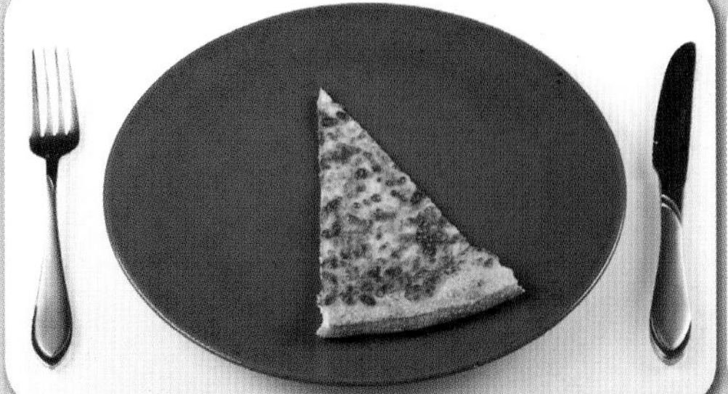

Pepperoni Pizza (thin crust)

CARBS	CALS	PROTEIN	FAT	FIBRE	Weight	SAT FAT
17g	199	9g	10g	1g	Weight: 55g	4g
36g	416	19g	21g	3g	Weight: 115g	8g

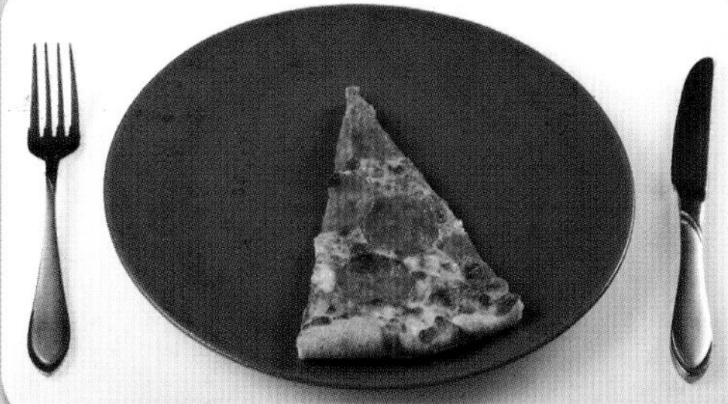

Vegetable Pizza (thin crust)

CARBS	CALS	PROTEIN	FAT	FIBRE	Weight	SAT FAT
18g	140	6g	5g	1g	Weight: 55g	2g
38g	293	12g	10g	3g	Weight: 115g	4g

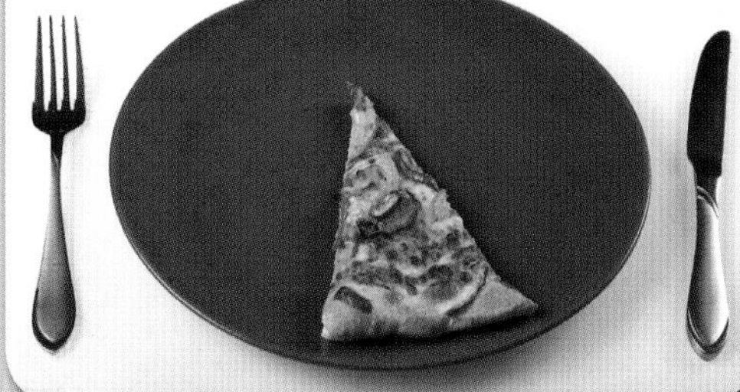

Margherita Pizza (deep pan)

24g CARBS	216 CALS	10g PROTEIN	9g FAT

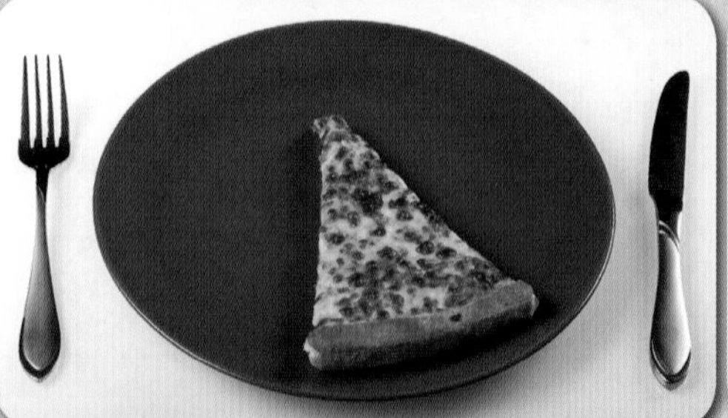

2g FIBRE	Weight: 85g	4g SAT FAT

47g CARBS	432 CALS	19g PROTEIN	18g FAT

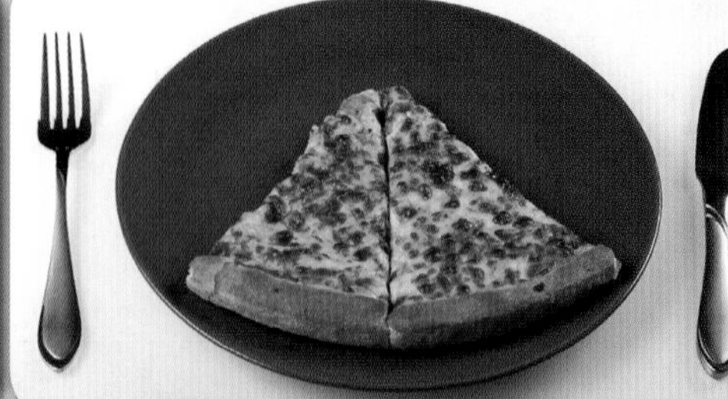

4g FIBRE	Weight: 170g	8g SAT FAT

Pepperoni Pizza (deep pan)

24g CARBS	259 CALS	12g PROTEIN	13g FAT

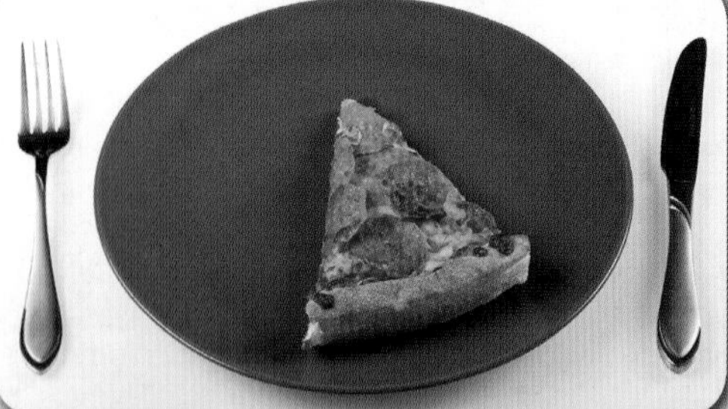

2g FIBRE	Weight: 85g	5g SAT FAT

39g CARBS	427 CALS	19g PROTEIN	21g FAT

3g FIBRE	Weight: 140g	8g SAT FAT

Vegetable Pizza (deep pan)

25g CARBS	197 CALS	8g PROTEIN	7g FAT

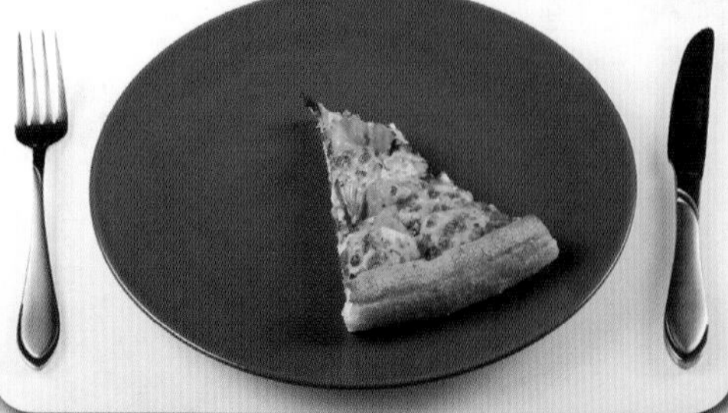

2g FIBRE	Weight: 70g	3g SAT FAT

46g CARBS	366 CALS	15g PROTEIN	14g FAT

3g FIBRE	Weight: 130g	5g SAT FAT

Margherita Pizza (stuffed crust)

30g	274	12g	12g
CARBS	CALS	PROTEIN	FAT

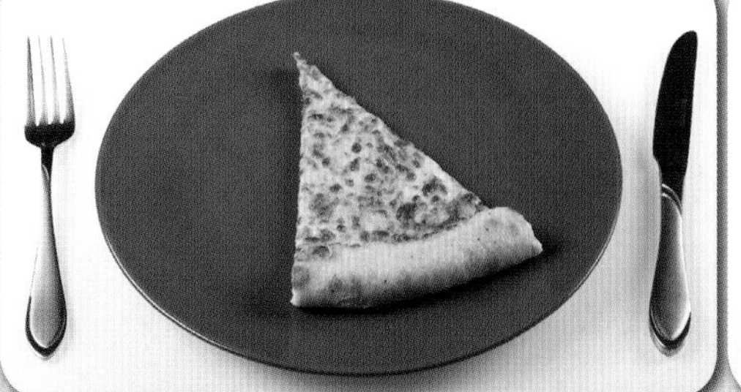

2g FIBRE	Weight: 90g	6g SAT FAT

54g	502	22g	21g
CARBS	CALS	PROTEIN	FAT

4g FIBRE	Weight: 165g	10g SAT FAT

Pepperoni Pizza (stuffed crust)

30g	317	14g	15g
CARBS	CALS	PROTEIN	FAT

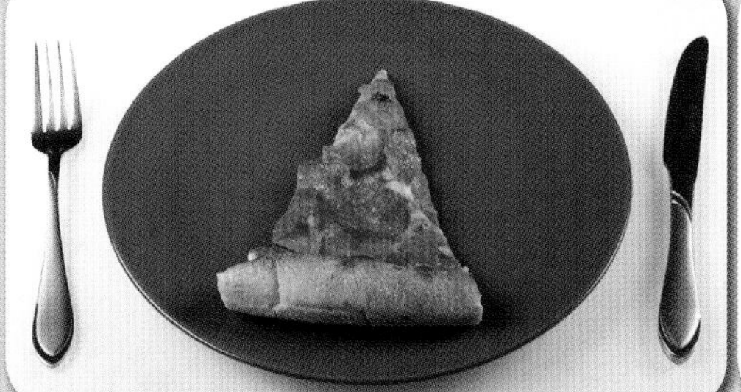

2g FIBRE	Weight: 110g	7g SAT FAT

50g	533	23g	26g
CARBS	CALS	PROTEIN	FAT

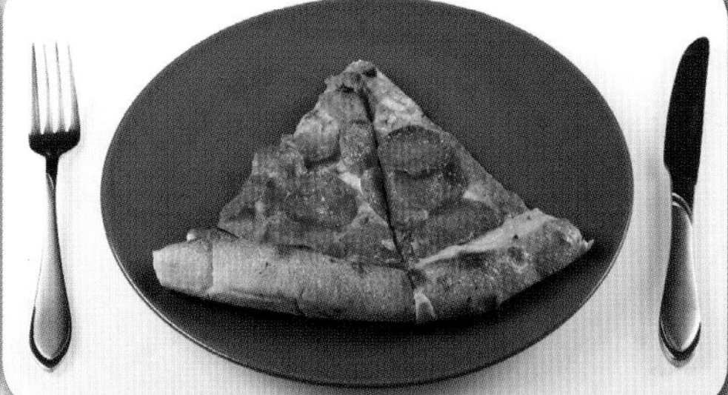

4g FIBRE	Weight: 185g	11g SAT FAT

Vegetable Pizza (stuffed crust)

30g	253	11g	10g
CARBS	CALS	PROTEIN	FAT

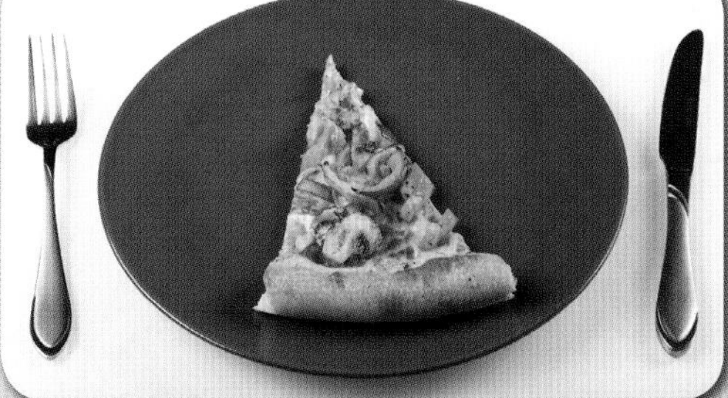

2g FIBRE	Weight: 100g	5g SAT FAT

52g	430	18g	17g
CARBS	CALS	PROTEIN	FAT

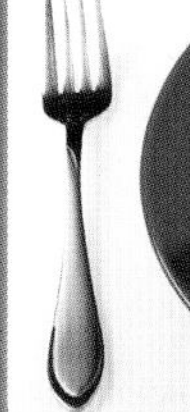

4g FIBRE	Weight: 170g	8g SAT FAT

26cm Dinner Plate / 22cm Large Bowl

Chicken Balls

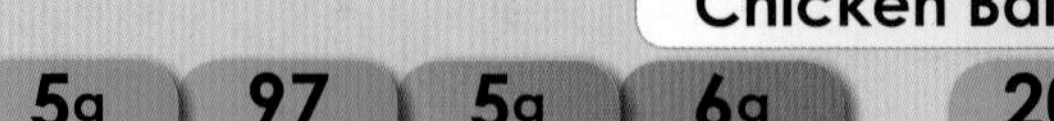

CARBS	CALS	PROTEIN	FAT	FIBRE	Weight	SAT FAT
5g	97	5g	6g	0g	38g	2g
20g	357	17g	20g	1g	140g	6g

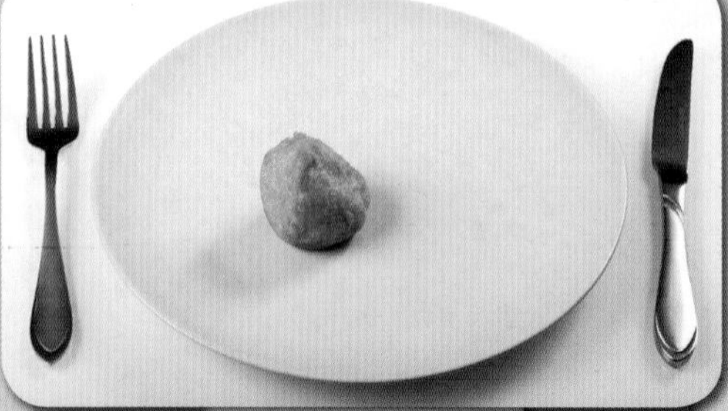

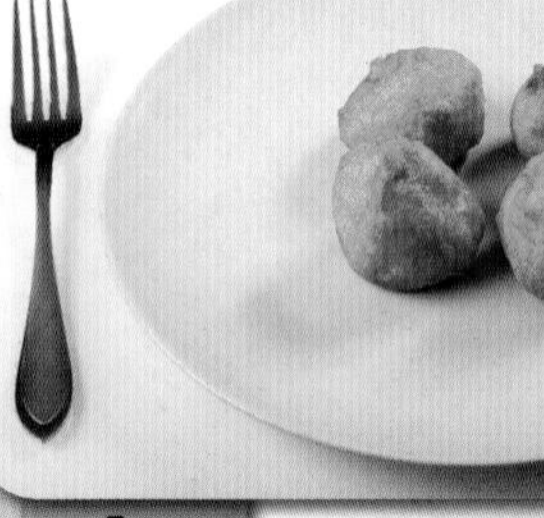

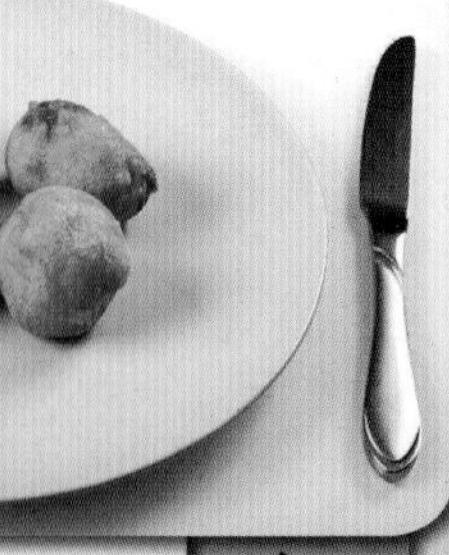

Duck Pancake

CARBS	CALS	PROTEIN	FAT	FIBRE	Weight	SAT FAT
14g	125	7g	5g	1g	50g	1g
14g	125	7g	5g	1g	50g	1g

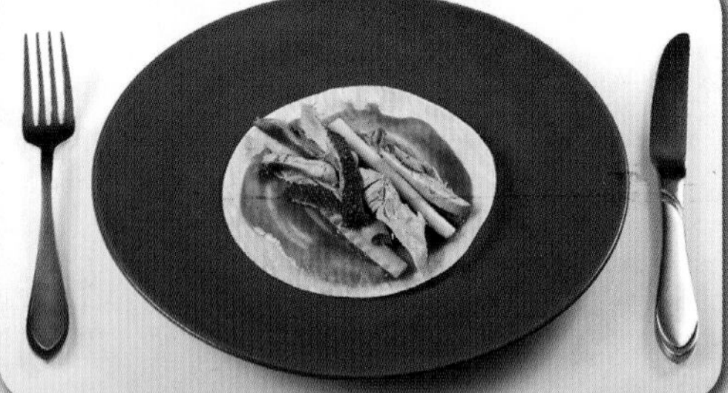

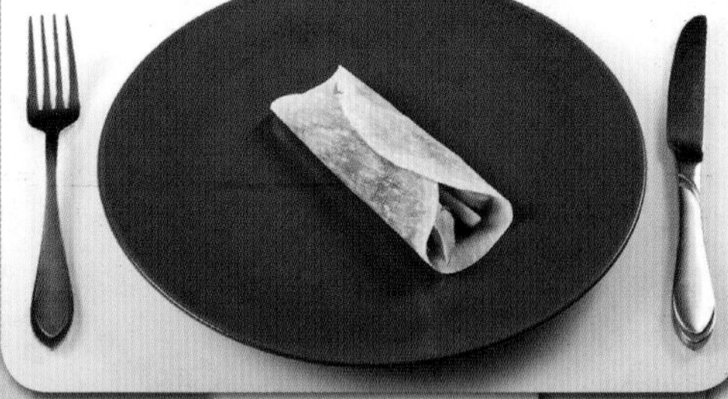

Prawn Crackers

CARBS	CALS	PROTEIN	FAT	FIBRE	Weight	SAT FAT
5g	51	0g	4g	0g	9g	0g
20g	200	0g	14g	0g	35g	1g

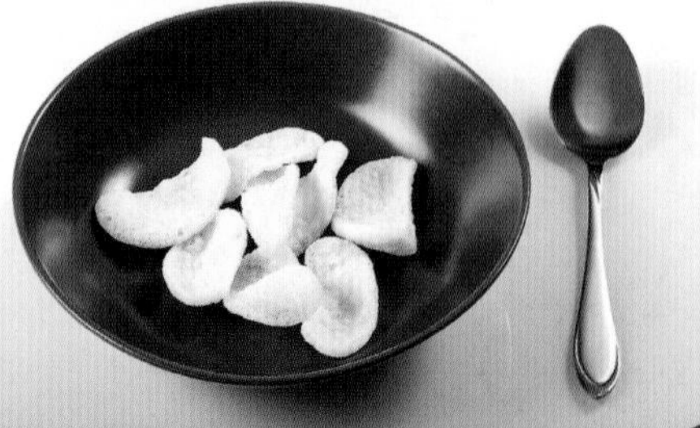

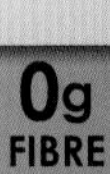

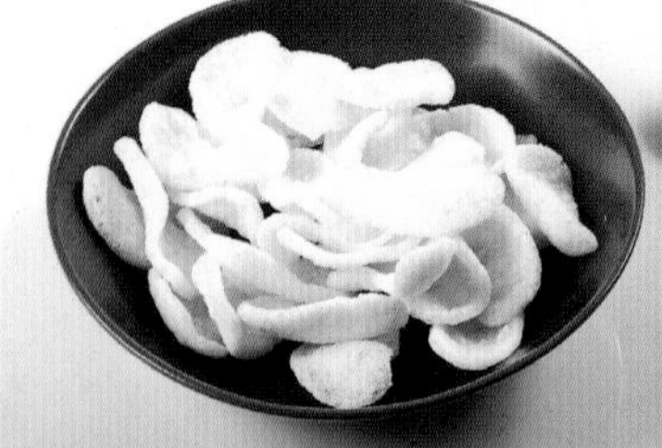

Prawn Toast

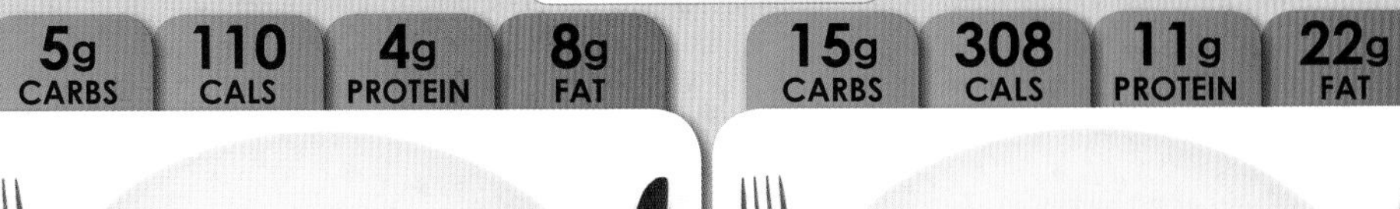

CARBS	CALS	PROTEIN	FAT	FIBRE	Weight	SAT FAT
5g	110	4g	8g	1g	Weight: 32g	3g
15g	308	11g	22g	3g	Weight: 90g	7g

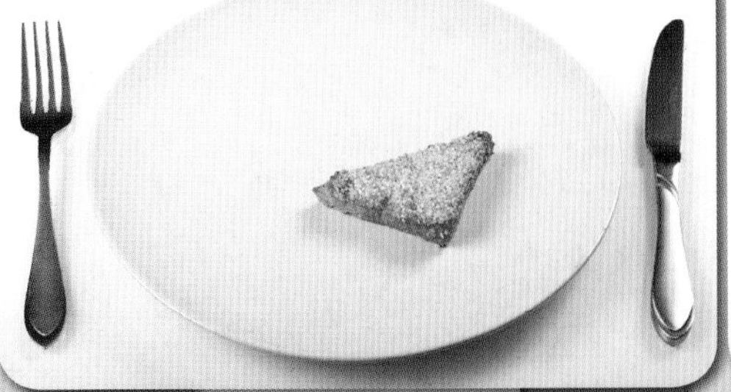

Spare Ribs

CARBS	CALS	PROTEIN	FAT	FIBRE	Weight	SAT FAT
18g	326	24g	17g	2g	Weight: 150g	6g
36g	662	49g	35g	5g	Weight: 305g	13g

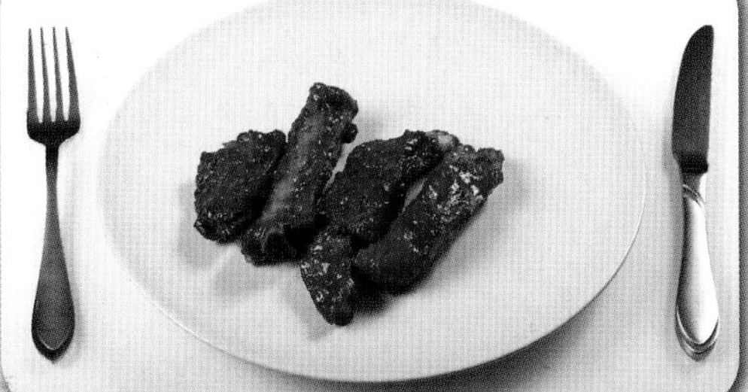

Spring Roll (meat)

CARBS	CALS	PROTEIN	FAT	FIBRE	Weight	SAT FAT
4g	58	2g	4g	0g	Weight: 24g	1g
13g	169	5g	12g	1g	Weight: 70g	3g

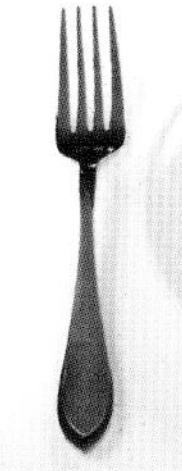
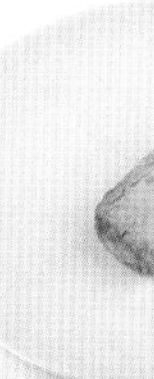
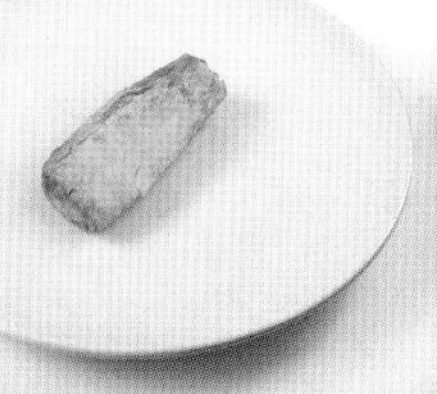
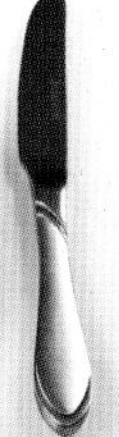
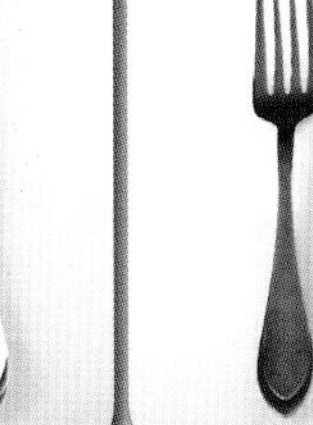
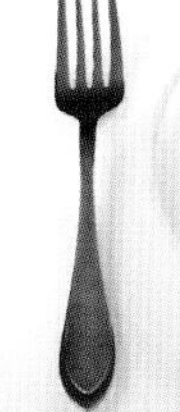
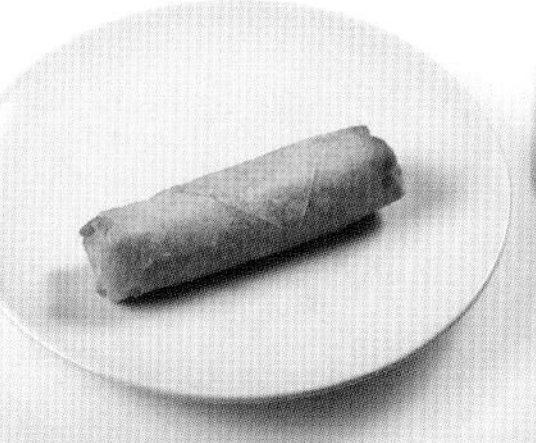
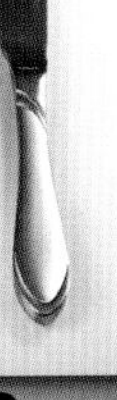

26cm Dinner Plate

Beef Chow Mein

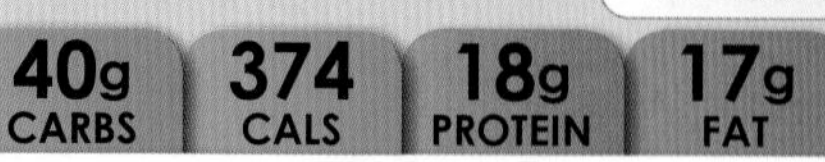

CARBS	CALS	PROTEIN	FAT	FIBRE	Weight	SAT FAT
40g	374	18g	17g	7g	275g	4g
80g	741	37g	33g	13g	545g	7g

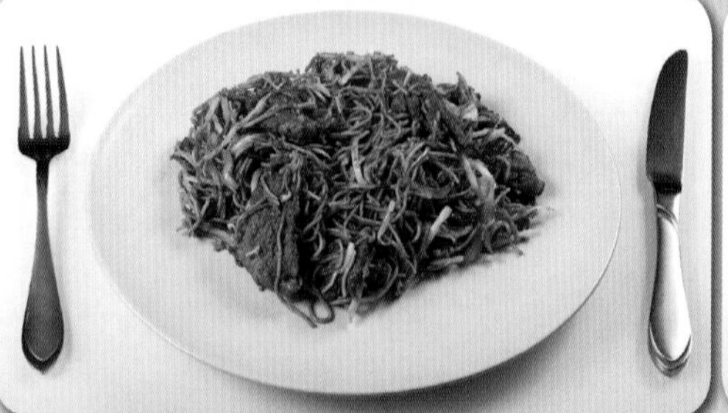

Beef in Black Bean Sauce

CARBS	CALS	PROTEIN	FAT	FIBRE	Weight	SAT FAT
15g	206	19g	7g	4g	225g	2g
29g	412	38g	14g	7g	450g	3g

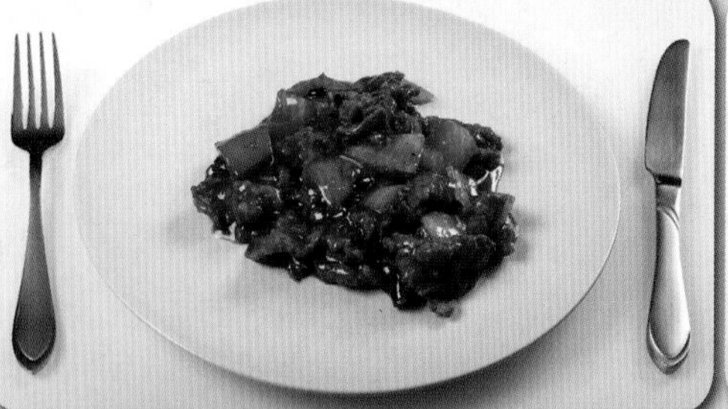

Chicken Curry

CARBS	CALS	PROTEIN	FAT	FIBRE	Weight	SAT FAT
5g	276	22g	19g	4g	190g	6g
10g	551	45g	37g	8g	380g	11g

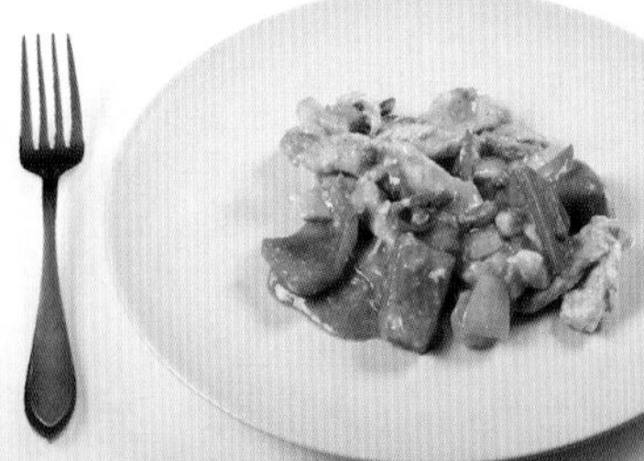

Crispy Shredded Beef

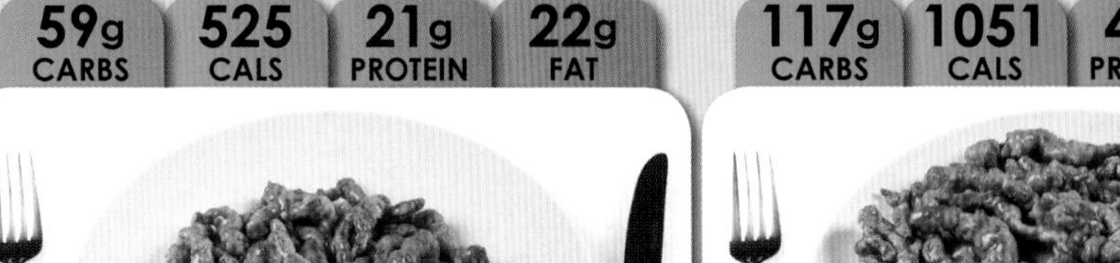

Weight	Carbs	Cals	Protein	Fat	Fibre	Sat Fat
170g	59g	525	21g	22g	2g	2g
340g	117g	1051	42g	44g	4g	4g

Lemon Chicken

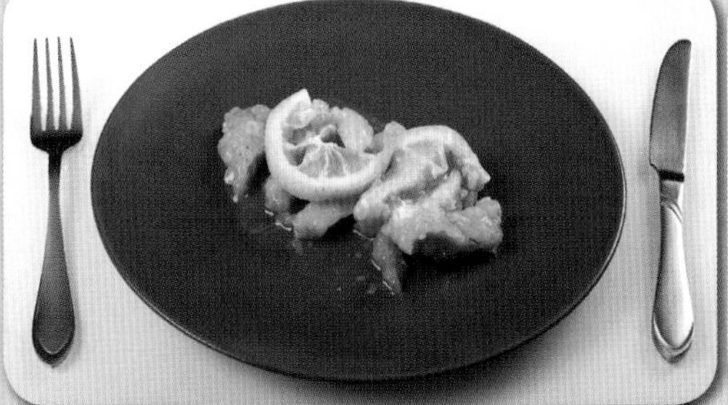

Weight	Carbs	Cals	Protein	Fat	Fibre	Sat Fat
170g	12g	253	28g	11g	0g	1g
340g	24g	507	57g	21g	0g	3g

Roast Peking Duck

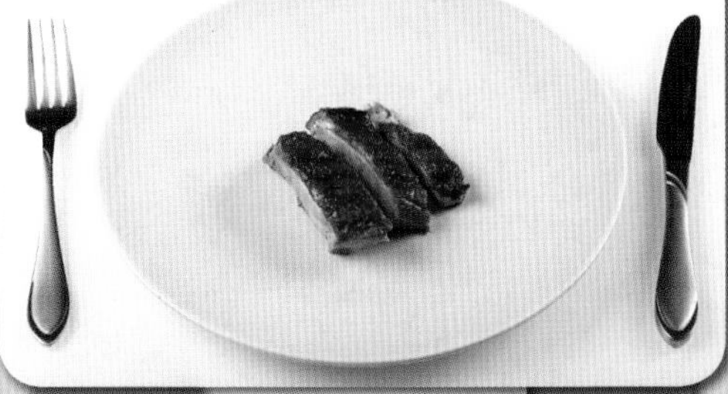

Weight	Carbs	Cals	Protein	Fat	Fibre	Sat Fat
75g	0g	317	15g	29g	0g	9g
115g	0g	486	23g	44g	0g	13g

26cm Dinner Plate

Singapore Noodles

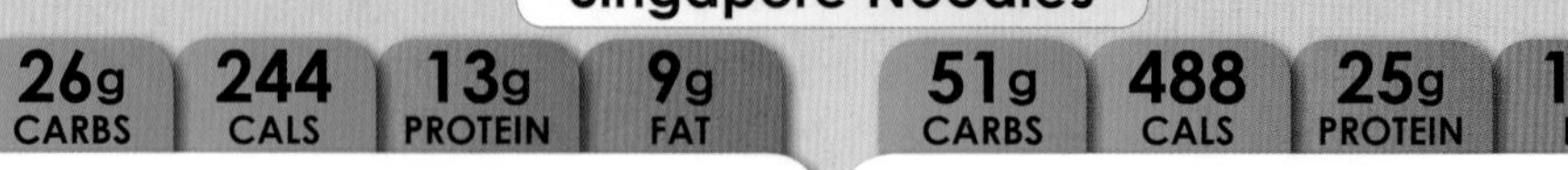

	Carbs	Cals	Protein	Fat	Fibre	Weight	Sat Fat
Small	26g	244	13g	9g	5g	205g	1g
Large	51g	488	25g	19g	10g	410g	2g

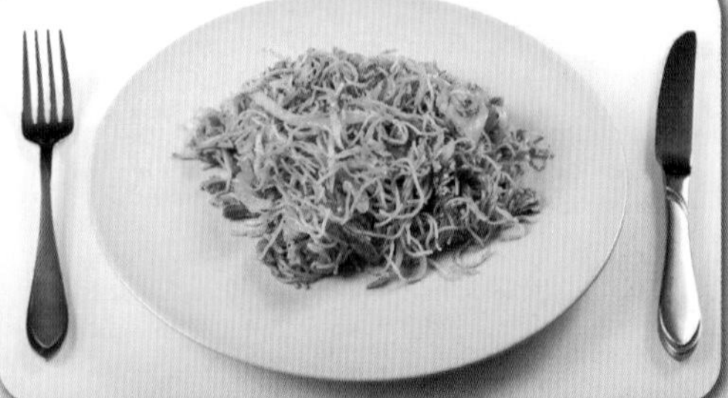

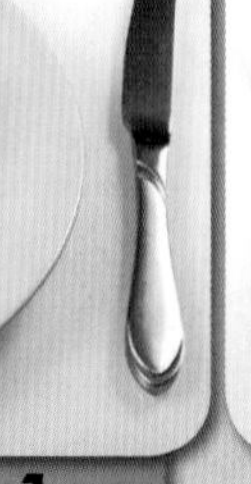

Sweet & Sour Pork

	Carbs	Cals	Protein	Fat	Fibre	Weight	Sat Fat
Small	28g	443	32g	22g	2g	250g	5g
Large	57g	885	64g	43g	4g	500g	10g

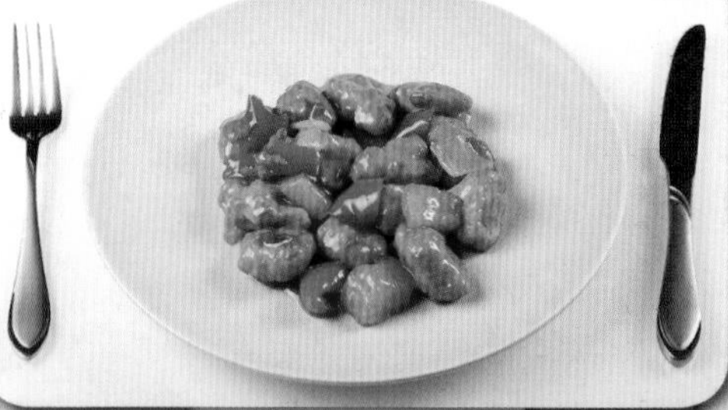

Szechuan Prawns

	Carbs	Cals	Protein	Fat	Fibre	Weight	Sat Fat
Small	4g	141	13g	8g	2g	170g	1g
Large	9g	282	27g	16g	4g	340g	2g

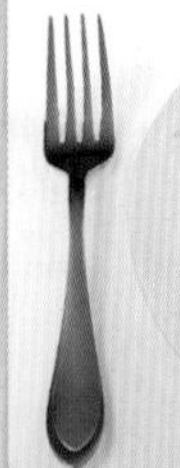

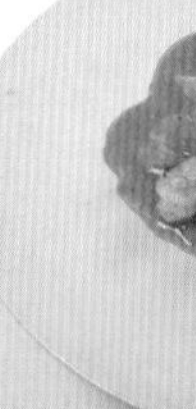

Miso Soup

CARBS	CALS	PROTEIN	FAT	FIBRE	Weight	SAT FAT
2g	28	1g	1g	1g	200g	0g
4g	56	2g	2g	2g	400g	0g

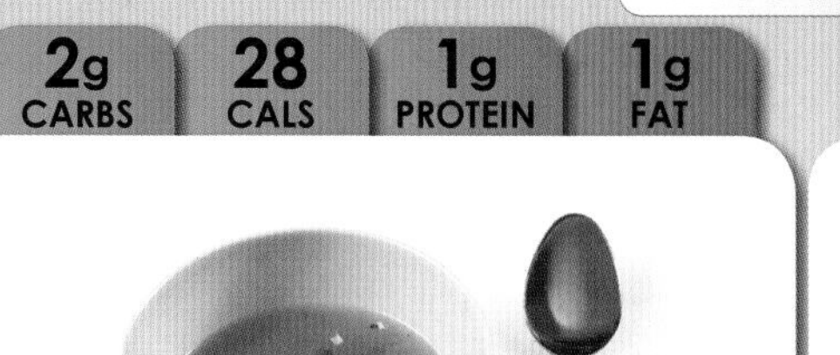

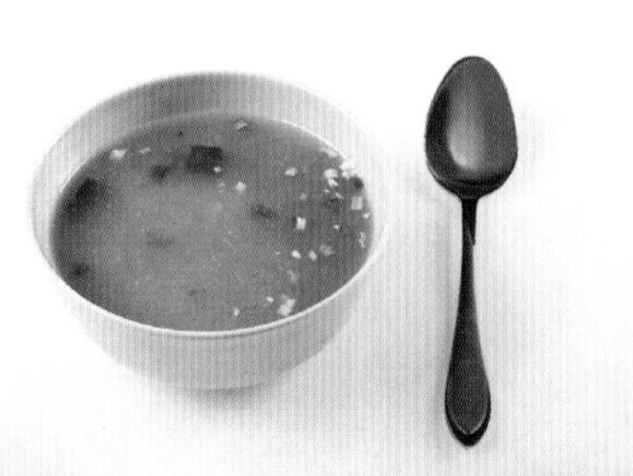

Pork Gyoza

CARBS	CALS	PROTEIN	FAT	FIBRE	Weight	SAT FAT
0g	37	2g	3g	0g	16g	1g
1g	111	5g	10g	0g	48g	3g

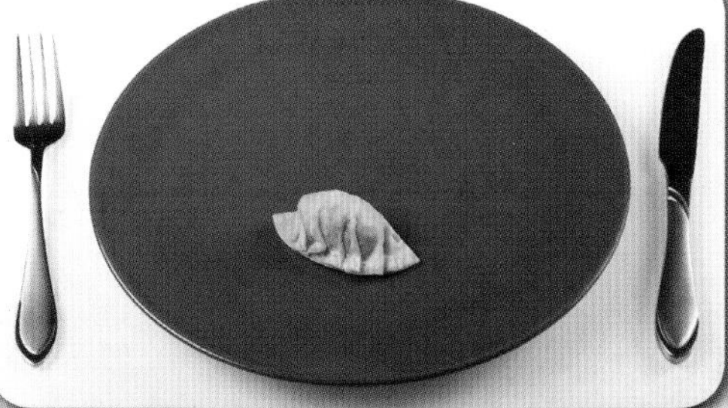

Prawn Tempura

CARBS	CALS	PROTEIN	FAT	FIBRE	Weight	SAT FAT
2g	38	2g	2g	0g	15g	1g
7g	114	5g	7g	0g	45g	3g

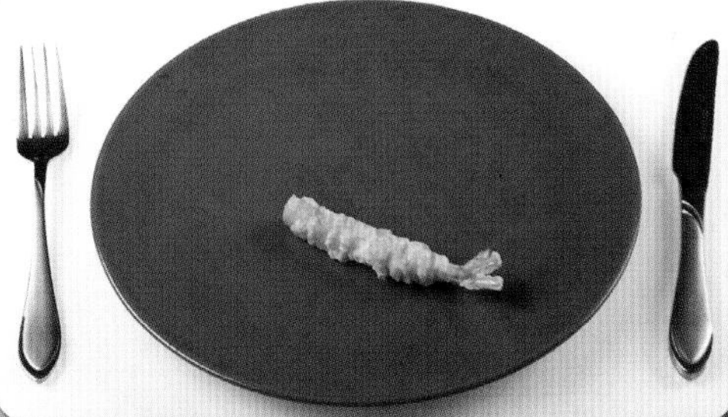

California Roll

CARBS	CALS	PROTEIN	FAT
6g	34	1g	1g

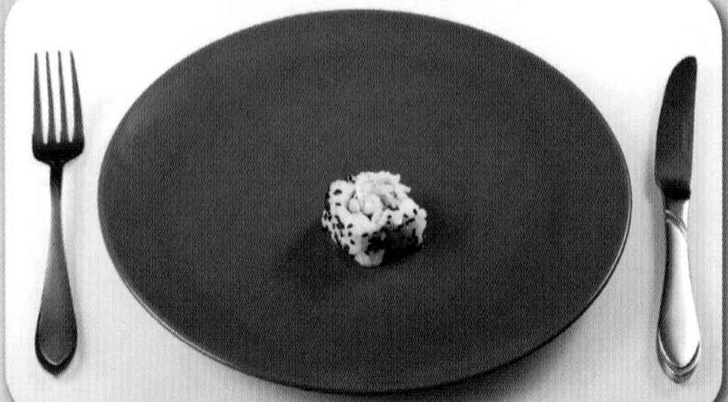

FIBRE	Weight	SAT FAT
0g	Weight: 24g	0g

CARBS	CALS	PROTEIN	FAT
9g	50	1g	1g

FIBRE	Weight	SAT FAT
0g	Weight: 35g	0g

Prawn Maki

CARBS	CALS	PROTEIN	FAT
7g	40	1g	1g

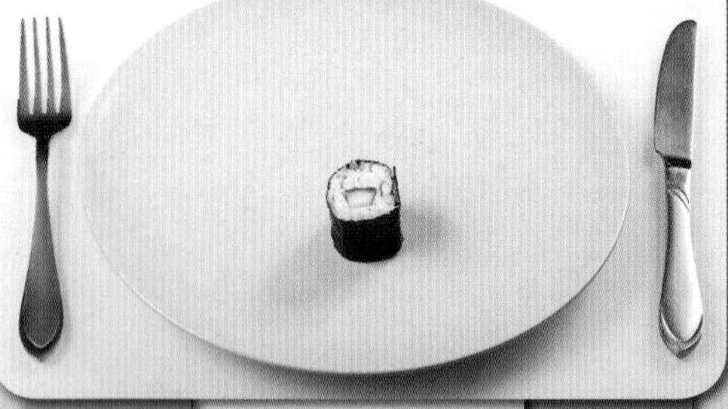

FIBRE	Weight	SAT FAT
0g	Weight: 24g	0g

Prawn Nigiri

CARBS	CALS	PROTEIN	FAT
9g	50	2g	1g

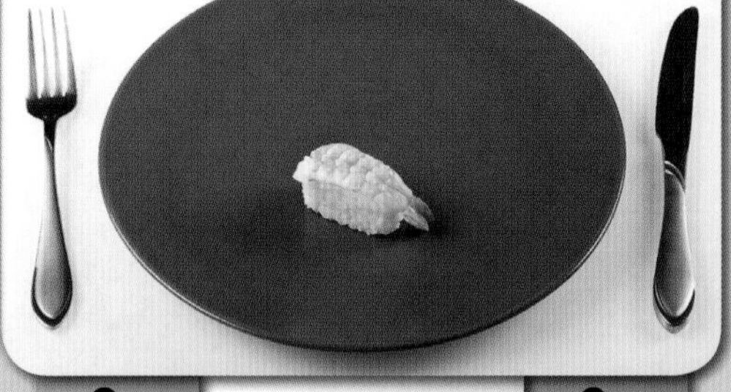

FIBRE	Weight	SAT FAT
0g	Weight: 30g	0g

Salmon Nigiri

CARBS	CALS	PROTEIN	FAT
8g	54	2g	2g

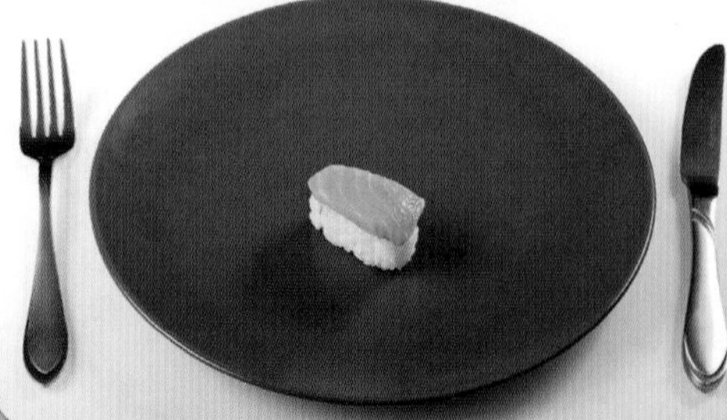

FIBRE	Weight	SAT FAT
0g	Weight: 34g	0g

Tuna Nigiri

CARBS	CALS	PROTEIN	FAT
7g	40	3g	0g

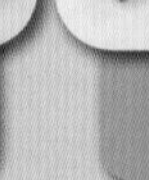

FIBRE	Weight	SAT FAT
0g	Weight: 28g	0g

Mackerel Sashimi

CARBS	CALS	PROTEIN	FAT
0g	33	3g	2g

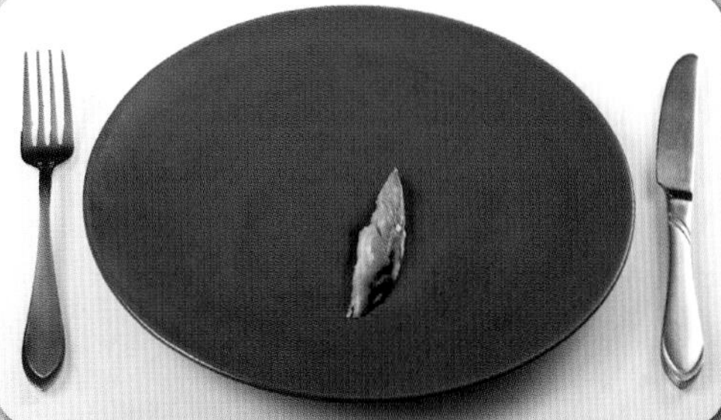

FIBRE	Weight	SAT FAT
0g	Weight: 15g	1g

Salmon Sashimi

CARBS	CALS	PROTEIN	FAT
0g	27	3g	2g

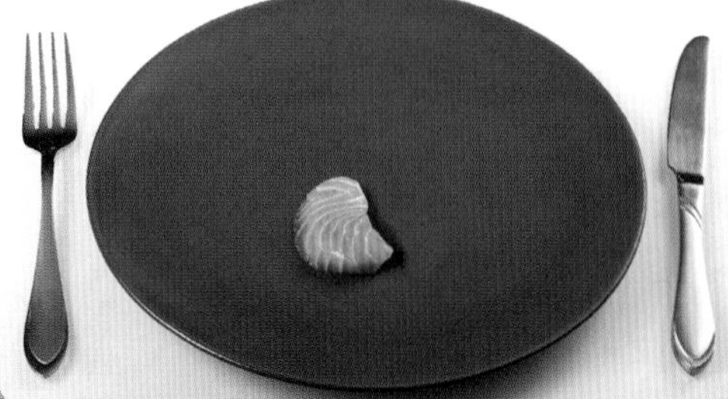

FIBRE	Weight	SAT FAT
0g	Weight: 15g	0g

Tuna Sashimi

CARBS	CALS	PROTEIN	FAT
0g	20	4g	0g

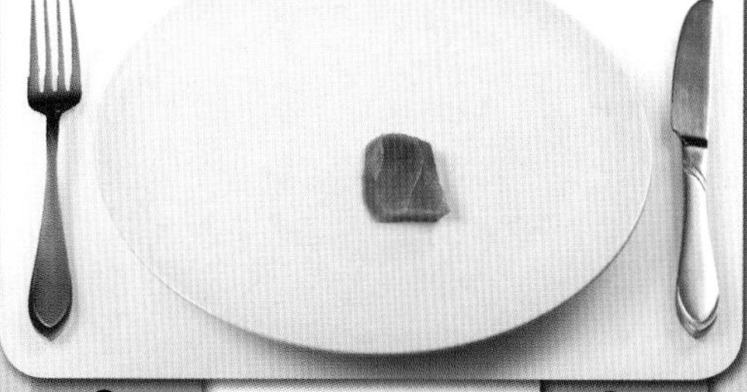

FIBRE	Weight	SAT FAT
0g	Weight: 15g	0g

Rice Ball

CARBS	CALS	PROTEIN	FAT
19g	96	2g	2g

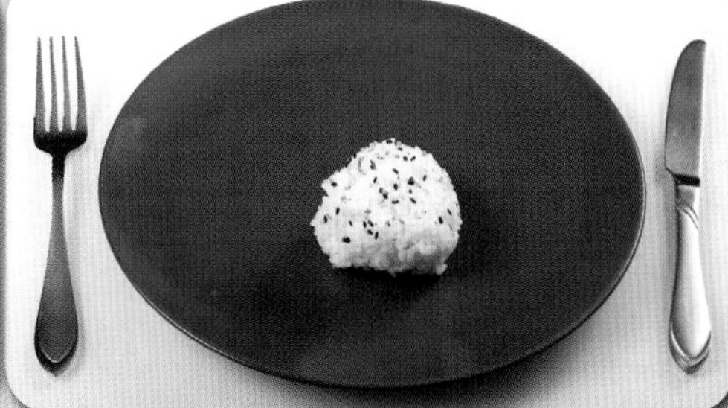

FIBRE	Weight	SAT FAT
1g	Weight: 70g	0g

Chicken Teriyaki

CARBS	CALS	PROTEIN	FAT
7g	261	50g	4g

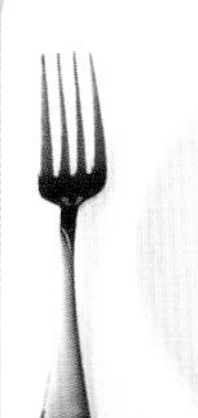
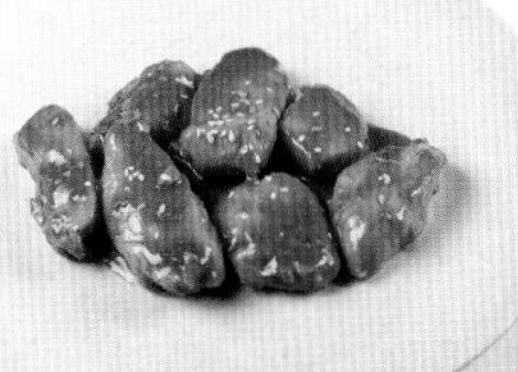
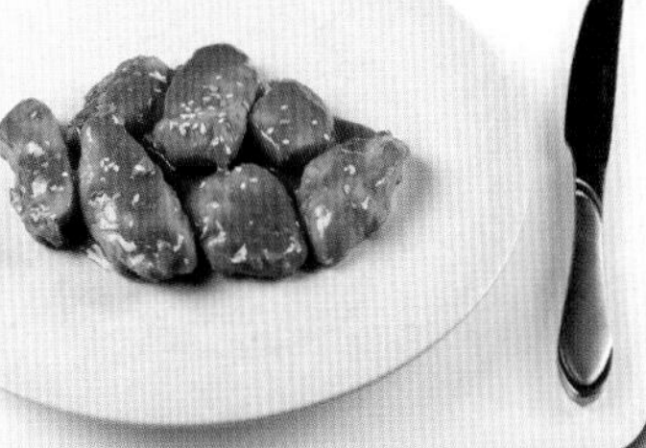
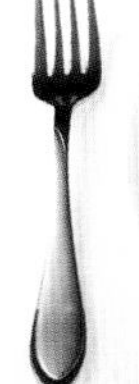

FIBRE	Weight	SAT FAT
0g	Weight: 185g	1g

CARBS	CALS	PROTEIN	FAT
13g	522	100g	8g

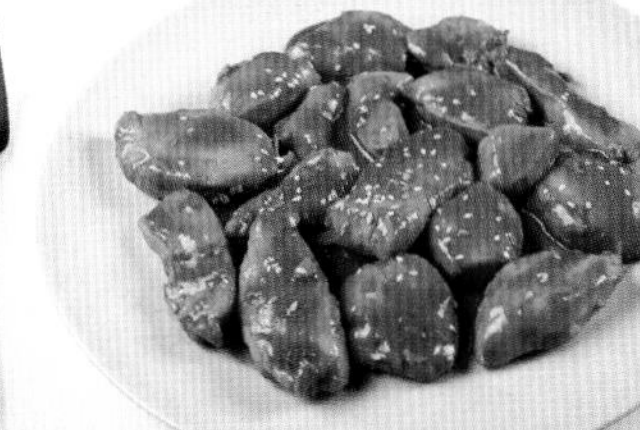

FIBRE	Weight	SAT FAT
0g	Weight: 370g	2g

Onion Bhaji

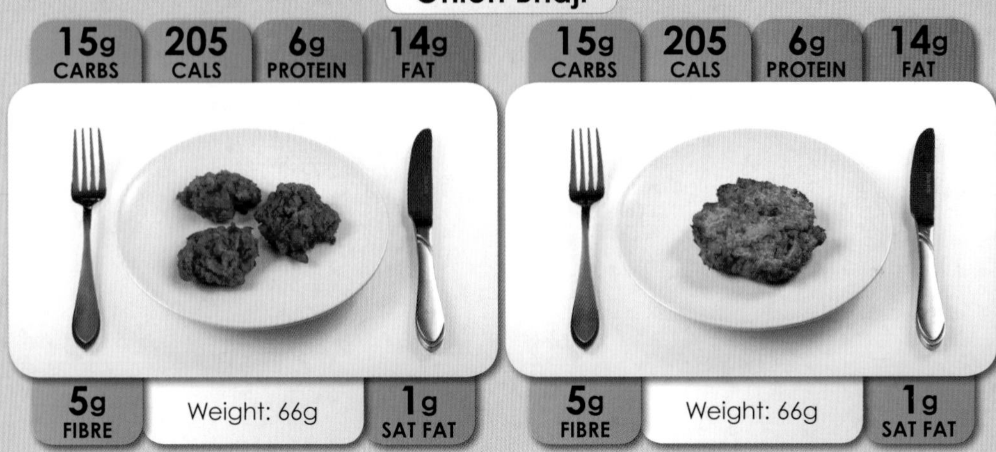

	Carbs	Cals	Protein	Fat	Fibre	Sat Fat	Weight
Left	15g	205	6g	14g	5g	1g	66g
Right	15g	205	6g	14g	5g	1g	66g

Lamb Samosa

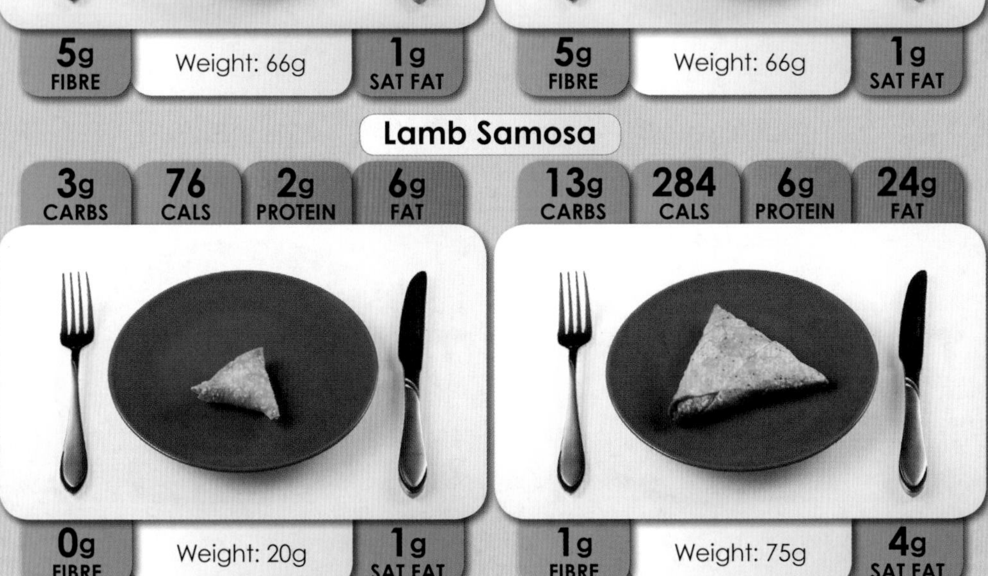

	Carbs	Cals	Protein	Fat	Fibre	Sat Fat	Weight
Left	3g	76	2g	6g	0g	1g	20g
Right	13g	284	6g	24g	1g	4g	75g

Vegetable Samosa

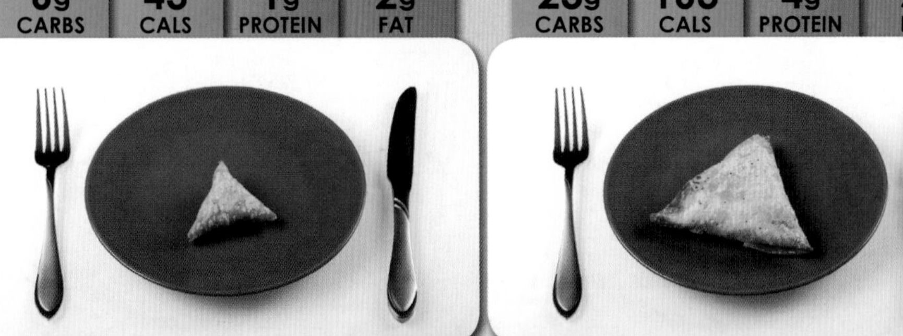

	Carbs	Cals	Protein	Fat	Fibre	Sat Fat	Weight
Left	6g	43	1g	2g	1g	0g	20g
Right	23g	163	4g	7g	3g	1g	75g

Vegetable Pakora

	CARBS	CALS	PROTEIN	FAT	FIBRE	Weight	SAT FAT
Side Plate	5g	52	1g	3g	1g	22g	0g
Dinner Plate	10g	106	3g	7g	2g	45g	1g

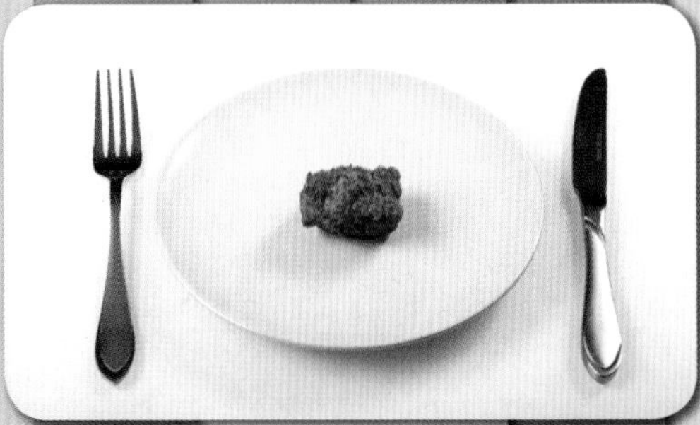

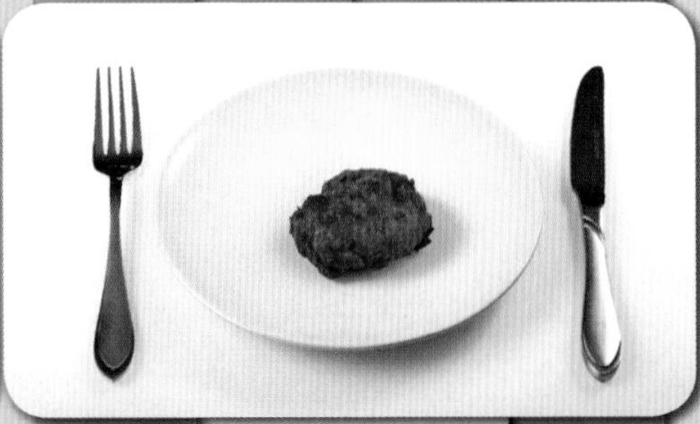

Bombay Potatoes

	CARBS	CALS	PROTEIN	FAT	FIBRE	Weight	SAT FAT
Side Plate	21g	177	3g	10g	2g	150g	1g
Dinner Plate	41g	354	6g	20g	5g	300g	2g

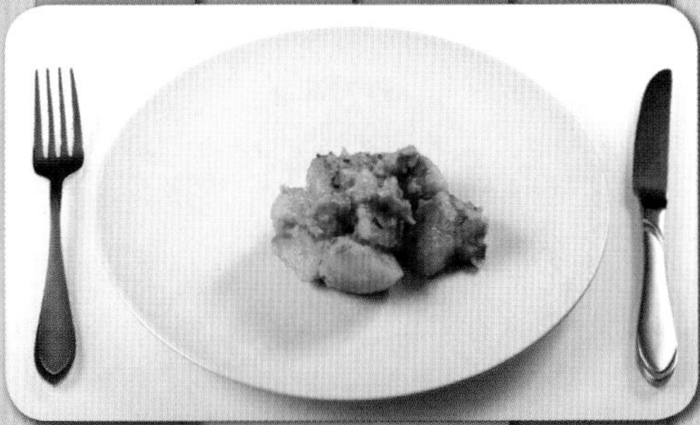

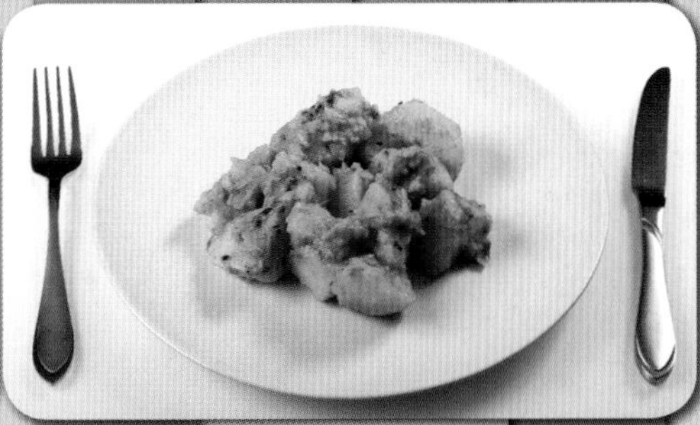

Sag Aloo Gobi

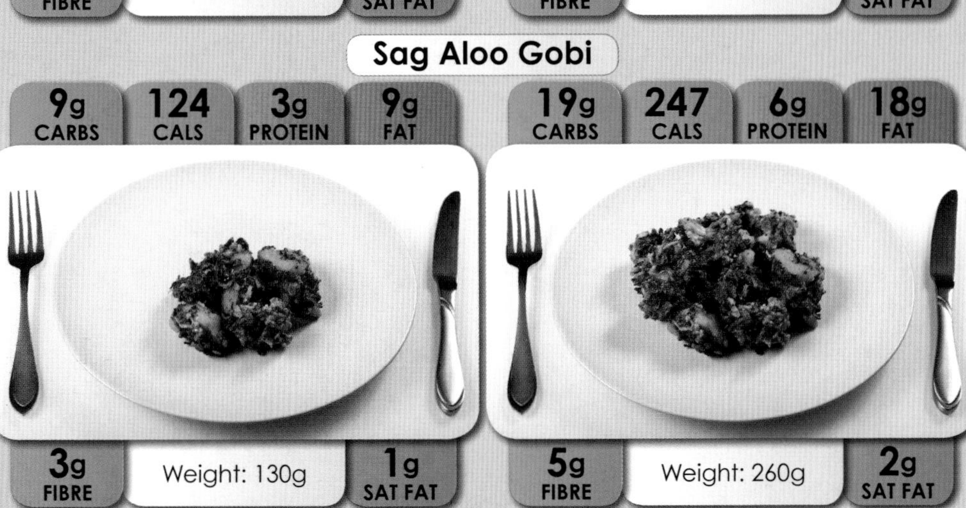

	CARBS	CALS	PROTEIN	FAT	FIBRE	Weight	SAT FAT
Side Plate	9g	124	3g	9g	3g	130g	1g
Dinner Plate	19g	247	6g	18g	5g	260g	2g

26cm Dinner Plate

Chicken Korma

	CARBS	CALS	PROTEIN	FAT	FIBRE	Weight	SAT FAT
Small	10g	286	33g	13g	1g	225g	4g
Large	21g	572	66g	27g	2g	450g	8g

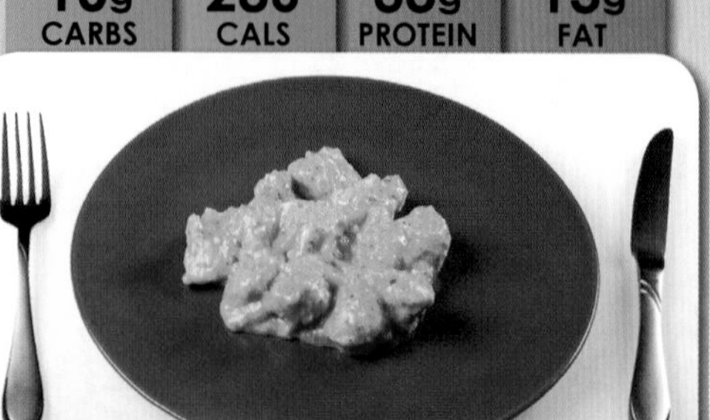

Chicken Tandoori

	CARBS	CALS	PROTEIN	FAT	FIBRE	Weight	SAT FAT
Small	9g	372	37g	21g	2g	175g	6g
Large	15g	648	64g	36g	3g	305g	11g

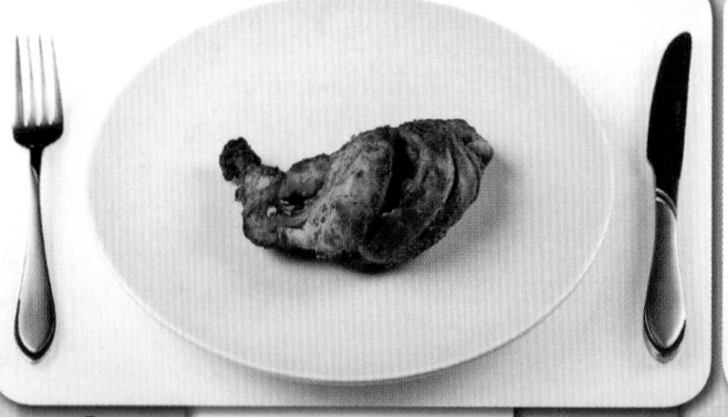

Chicken Tikka Masala

	CARBS	CALS	PROTEIN	FAT	FIBRE	Weight	SAT FAT
Small	5g	291	24g	20g	4g	185g	7g
Large	10g	581	48g	39g	9g	370g	13g

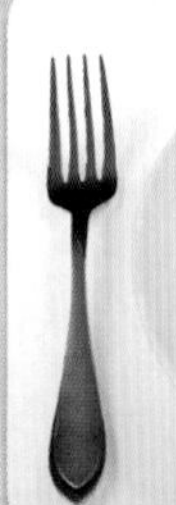

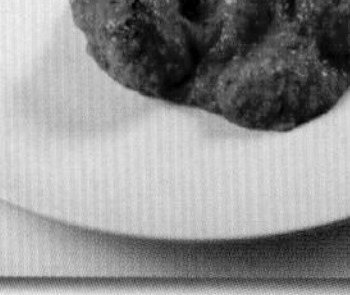

King Prawn Bhuna

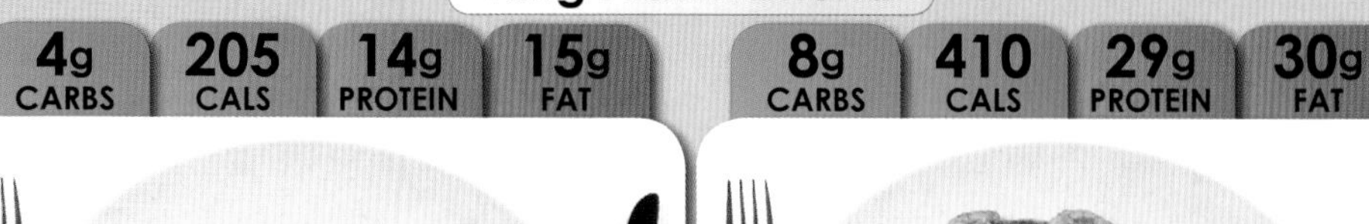

CARBS	CALS	PROTEIN	FAT	FIBRE	SAT FAT	Weight
4g	205	14g	15g	4g	3g	175g
8g	410	29g	30g	9g	5g	350g

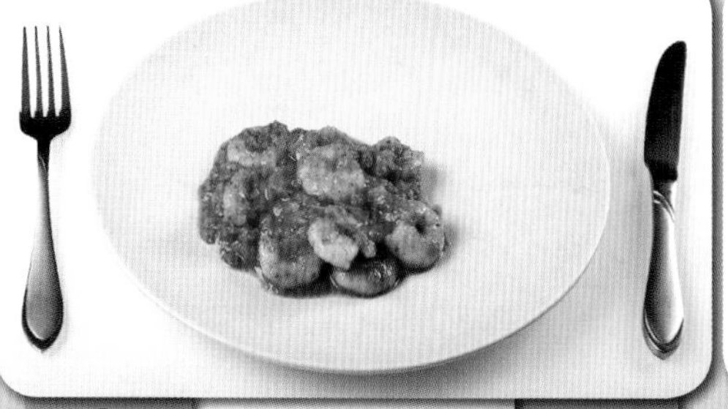

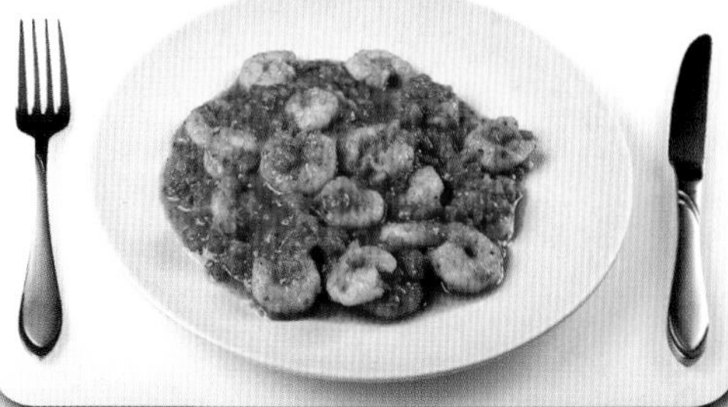

Lamb Biryani

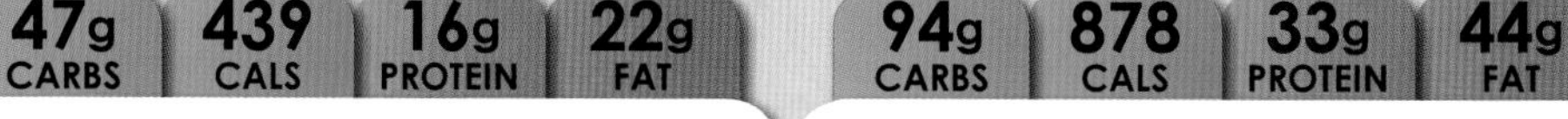

CARBS	CALS	PROTEIN	FAT	FIBRE	SAT FAT	Weight
47g	439	16g	22g	2g	5g	225g
94g	878	33g	44g	4g	10g	450g

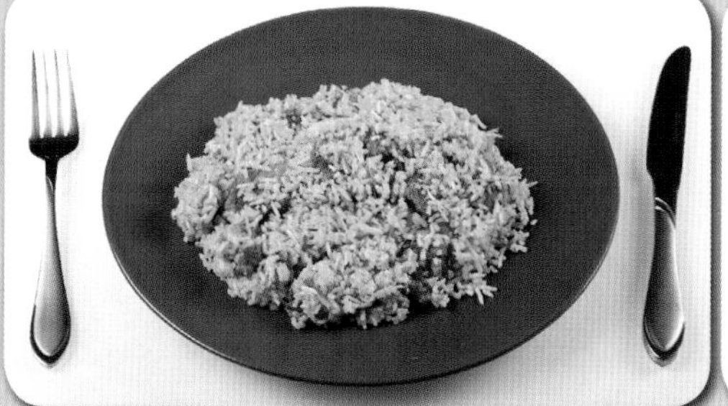

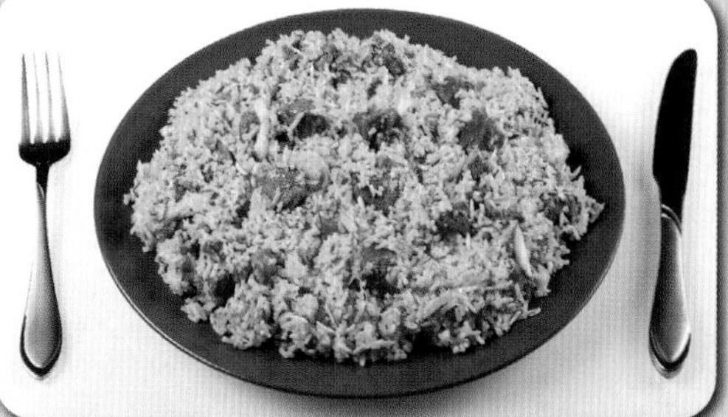

Lamb Rogan Josh

CARBS	CALS	PROTEIN	FAT	FIBRE	SAT FAT	Weight
7g	261	25g	16g	2g	6g	175g
14g	522	50g	32g	4g	13g	350g

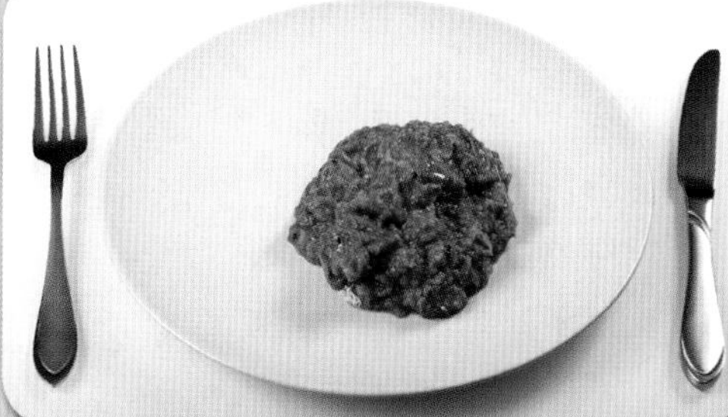

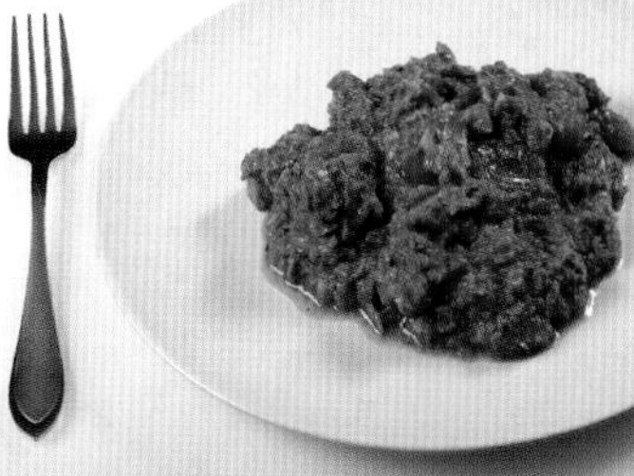

Burrito (bean)

CARBS	CALS	PROTEIN	FAT
60g	414	13g	14g

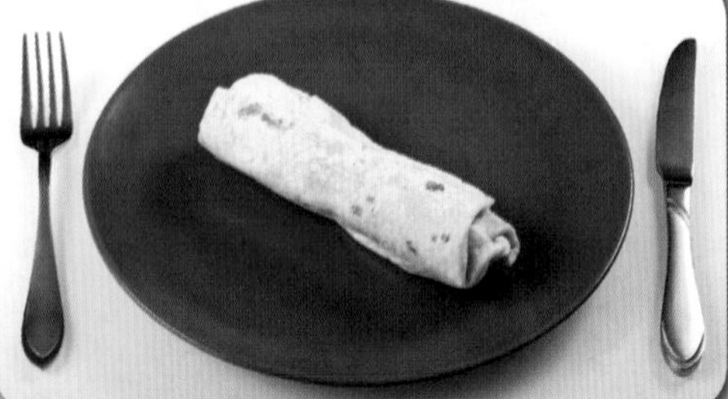

FIBRE	Weight	SAT FAT
6g	Weight: 200g	5g

Burrito (chicken)

CARBS	CALS	PROTEIN	FAT
48g	383	21g	10g

FIBRE	Weight	SAT FAT
5g	Weight: 225g	2g

Enchilada (chicken)

CARBS	CALS	PROTEIN	FAT
29g	324	24g	13g

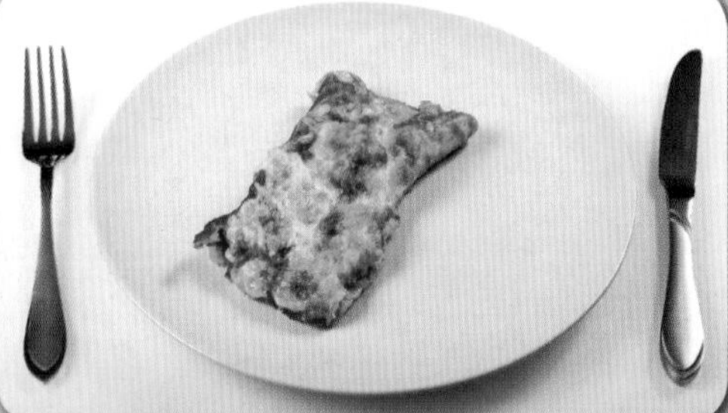

FIBRE	Weight	SAT FAT
2g	Weight: 146g	5g

Fajita (chicken)

CARBS	CALS	PROTEIN	FAT
30g	237	19g	5g

FIBRE	Weight	SAT FAT
2g	Weight: 160g	1g

Quesadilla (bean)

CARBS	CALS	PROTEIN	FAT
18g	162	5g	8g

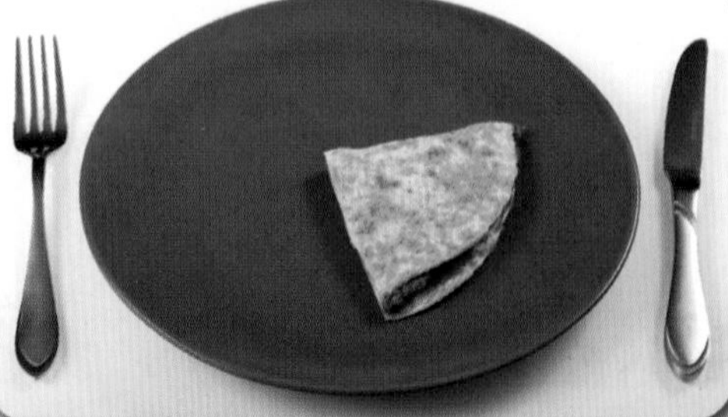

FIBRE	Weight	SAT FAT
2g	Weight: 74g	3g

Taco (beef)

CARBS	CALS	PROTEIN	FAT
10g	236	12g	16g

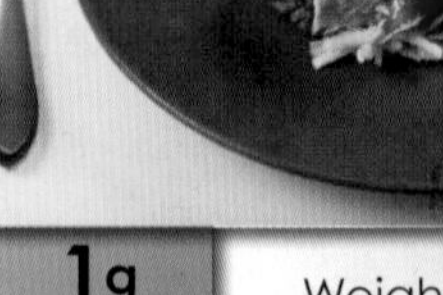

FIBRE	Weight	SAT FAT
1g	Weight: 80g	7g

Chicken Satay

CARBS	CALS	PROTEIN	FAT	FIBRE	Weight	SAT FAT
1g	76	9g	4g	1g	Weight: 40g	1g
2g	153	17g	8g	2g	Weight: 80g	2g

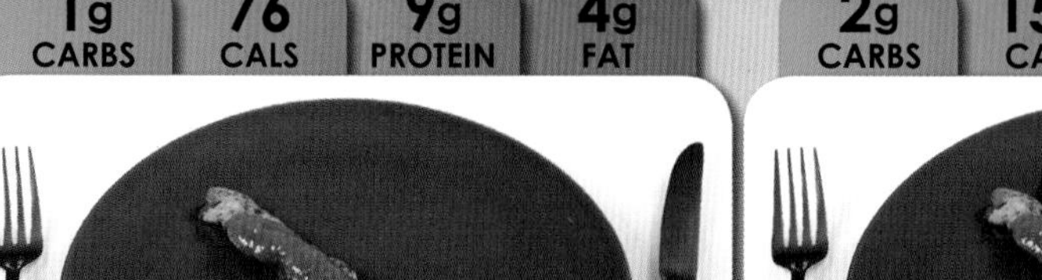

Tom Yum Soup (prawn)

CARBS	CALS	PROTEIN	FAT	FIBRE	Weight	SAT FAT
21g	142	5g	4g	3g	Weight: 200g	1g
42g	284	10g	8g	5g	Weight: 400g	2g

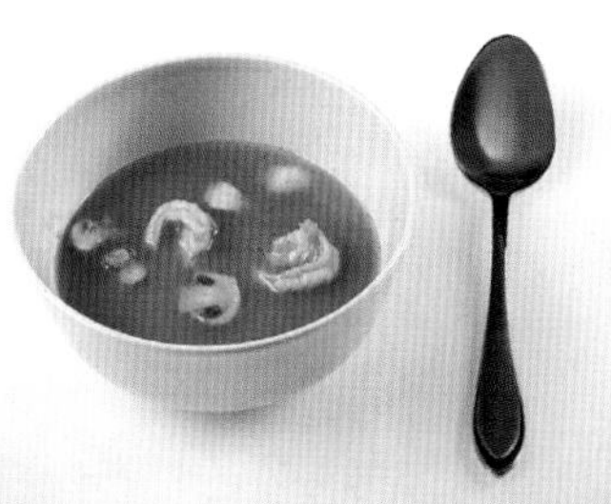

Chicken, Prawn & Pineapple Rice

CARBS	CALS	PROTEIN	FAT	FIBRE	Weight	SAT FAT
69g	481	15g	16g	2g	Weight: 250g	5g
139g	963	29g	32g	4g	Weight: 500g	10g

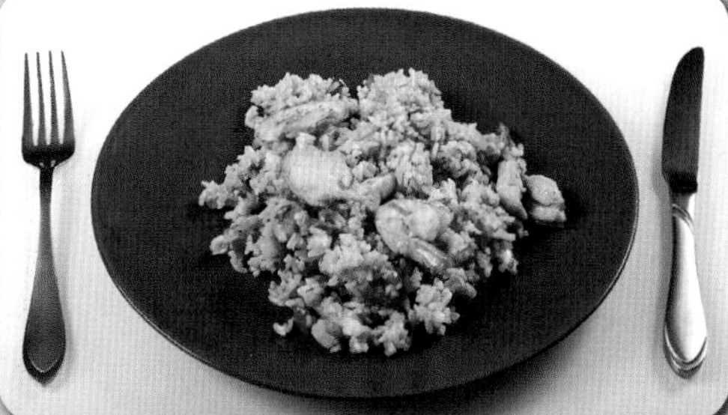

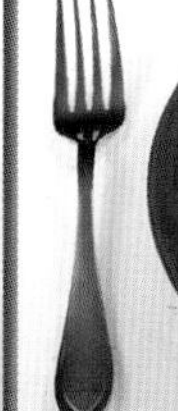

26cm Dinner Plate

Green Curry (chicken)

7g CARBS	271 CALS	29g PROTEIN	14g FAT

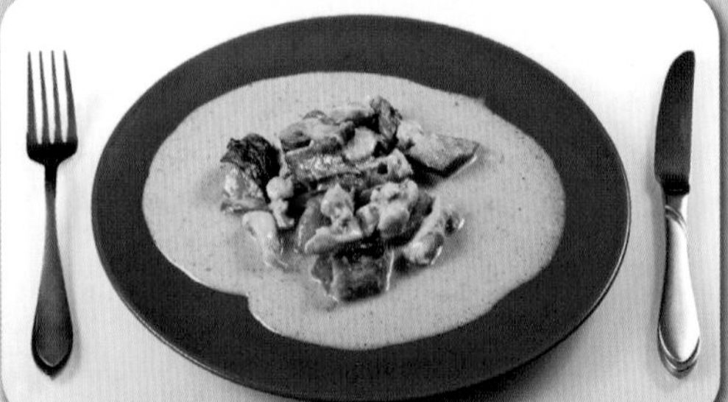

2g FIBRE	Weight: 195g	7g SAT FAT

13g CARBS	542 CALS	58g PROTEIN	29g FAT

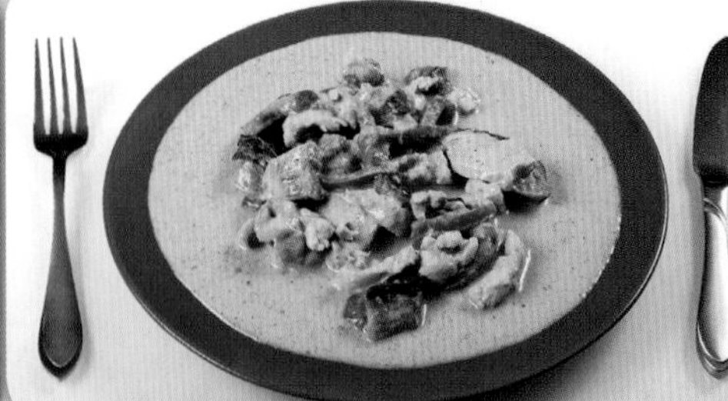

3g FIBRE	Weight: 390g	14g SAT FAT

Massaman Curry (beef)

14g CARBS	338 CALS	21g PROTEIN	21g FAT

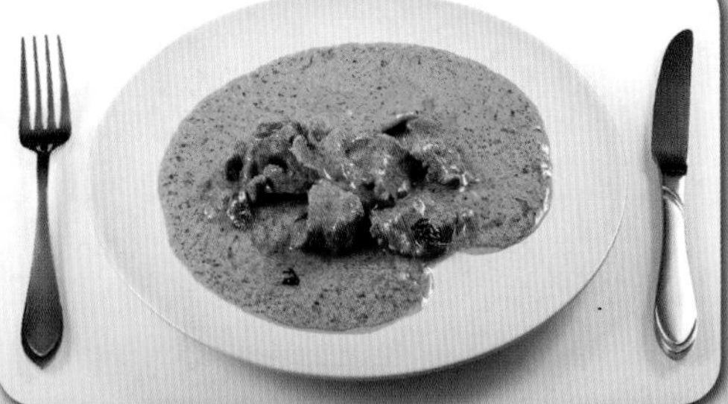

6g FIBRE	Weight: 200g	11g SAT FAT

27g CARBS	676 CALS	43g PROTEIN	42g FAT

12g FIBRE	Weight: 400g	22g SAT FAT

Pad Thai (chicken & prawn)

42g CARBS	307 CALS	15g PROTEIN	9g FAT

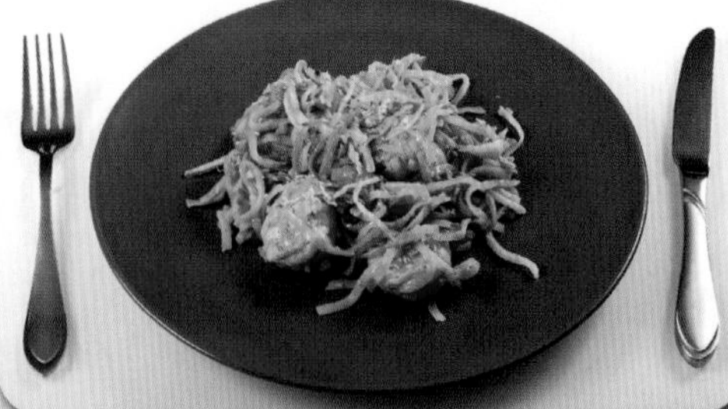

5g FIBRE	Weight: 200g	1g SAT FAT

84g CARBS	613 CALS	29g PROTEIN	17g FAT

9g FIBRE	Weight: 400g	2g SAT FAT

Ackee (tinned)

CARBS	CALS	PROTEIN	FAT
1g	61	1g	6g

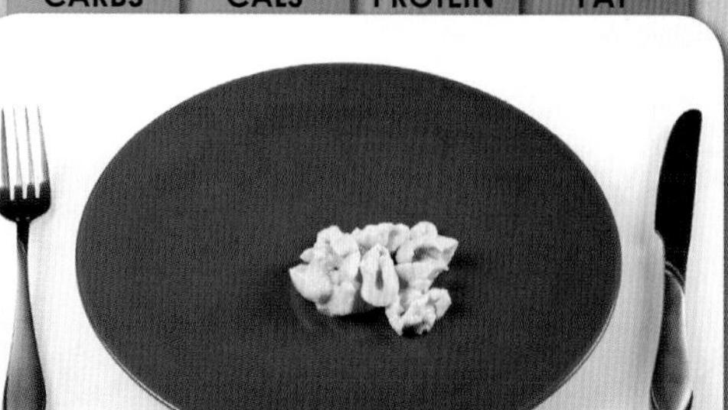

FIBRE	Weight	SAT FAT
1g	Weight: 40g	0g

CARBS	CALS	PROTEIN	FAT
1g	122	2g	11g

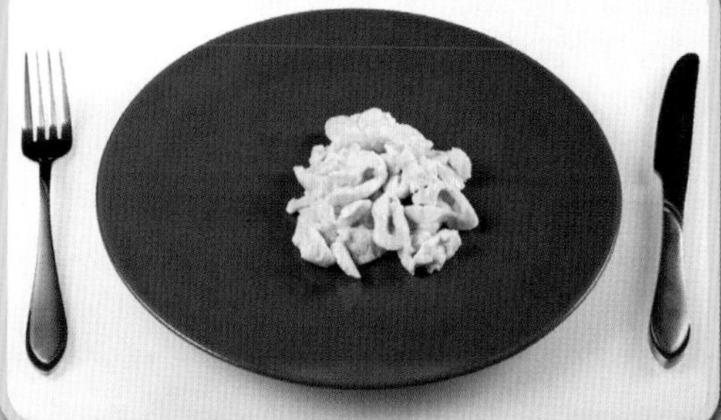

FIBRE	Weight	SAT FAT
2g	Weight: 80g	0g

CARBS	CALS	PROTEIN	FAT
2g	243	5g	22g

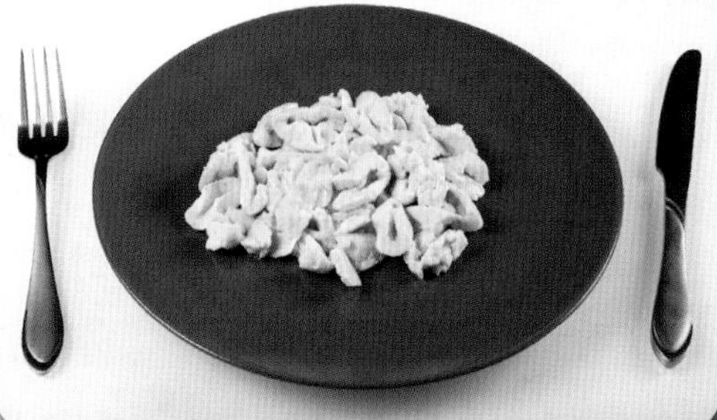

FIBRE	Weight	SAT FAT
4g	Weight: 160g	0g

Artichokes (tinned)

CARBS	CALS	PROTEIN	FAT
2g	11	1g	0g

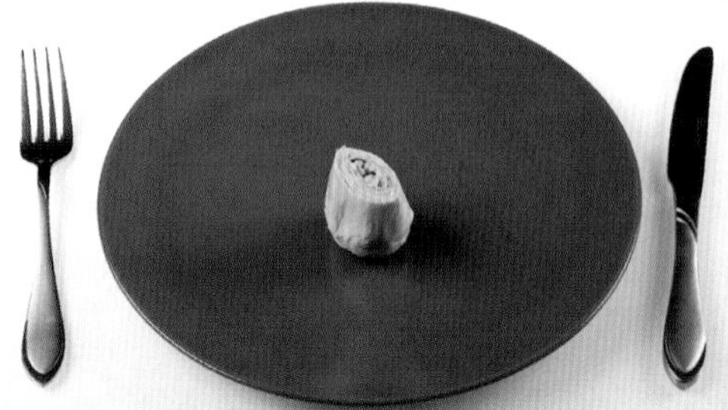

FIBRE	Weight	SAT FAT
1g	Weight: 40g	0g

CARBS	CALS	PROTEIN	FAT
4g	23	1g	0g

FIBRE	Weight	SAT FAT
1g	Weight: 80g	0g

CARBS	CALS	PROTEIN	FAT
8g	45	3g	0g

FIBRE	Weight	SAT FAT
3g	Weight: 160g	0g

Asparagus (boiled)

Weight	Carbs	Cals	Protein	Fat	Fibre	Sat Fat
40g	1g	10	1g	0g	1g	0g
80g	1g	21	3g	1g	2g	0g
120g	2g	31	4g	1g	2g	0g

Aubergine (fried in oil)

Weight	Carbs	Cals	Protein	Fat	Fibre	Sat Fat
30g	1g	91	0g	10g	1g	1g
60g	2g	181	1g	19g	2g	3g
90g	3g	272	1g	29g	3g	4g

Avocado

1g CARBS	76 CALS	1g PROTEIN	8g FAT

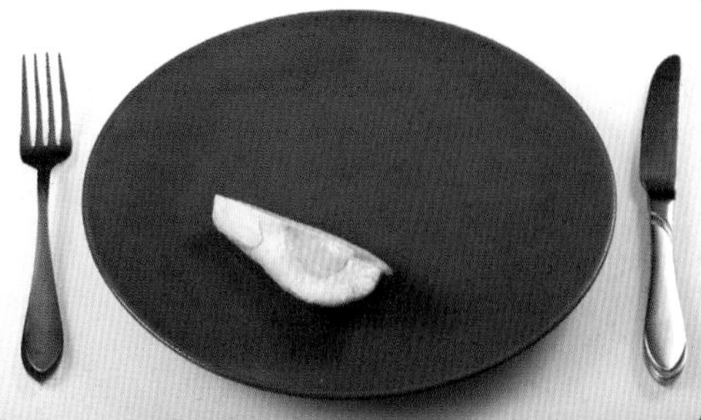

2g FIBRE	Weight: 40g	2g SAT FAT

2g CARBS	153 CALS	1g PROTEIN	16g FAT

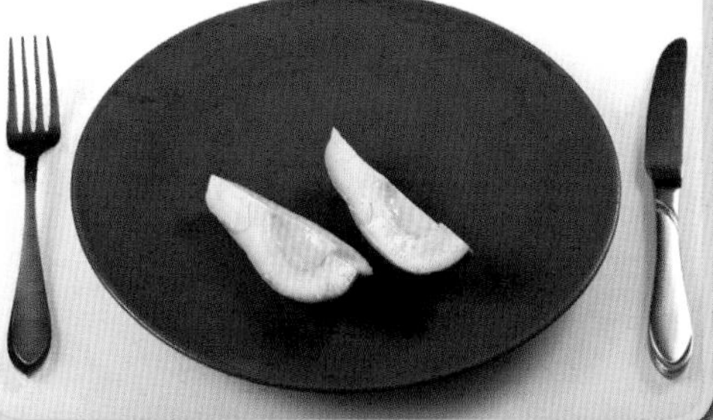

4g FIBRE	Weight: 80g (half)	4g SAT FAT

3g CARBS	287 CALS	2g PROTEIN	30g FAT

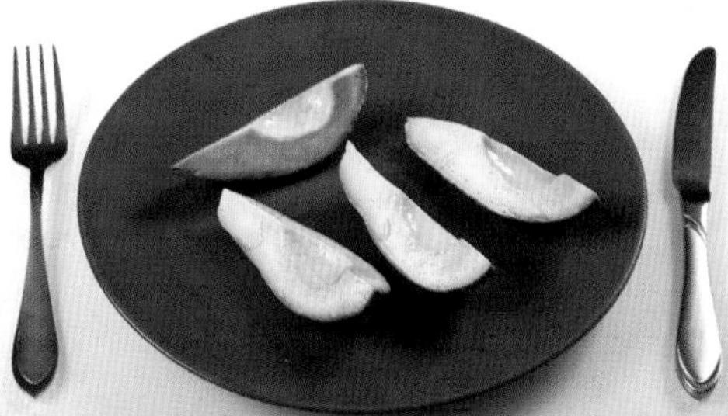

7g FIBRE	Weight: 150g (whole)	7g SAT FAT

Baked Beans (in tomato sauce)

12g CARBS	67 CALS	4g PROTEIN	0g FAT

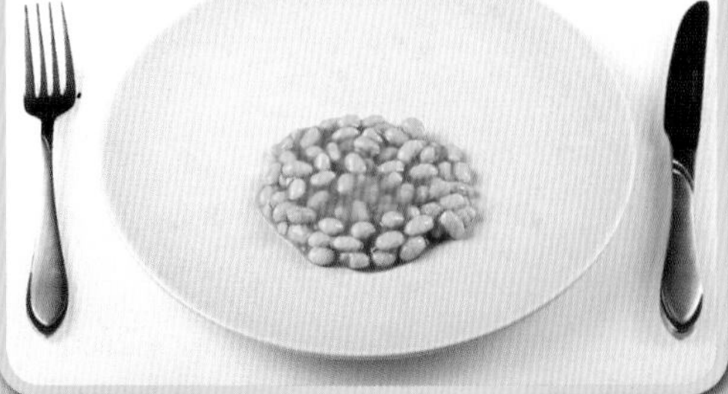

4g FIBRE	Weight: 80g	0g SAT FAT

31g CARBS	168 CALS	10g PROTEIN	1g FAT

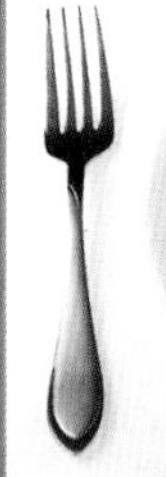

10g FIBRE	Weight: 200g	0g SAT FAT

61g CARBS	336 CALS	21g PROTEIN	2g FAT

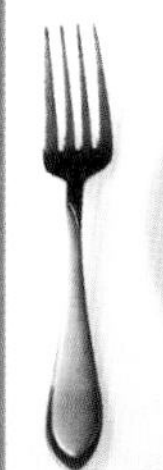

20g FIBRE	Weight: 400g	0g SAT FAT

Bamboo Shoots

0g CARBS	3 CALS	0g PROTEIN	0g FAT

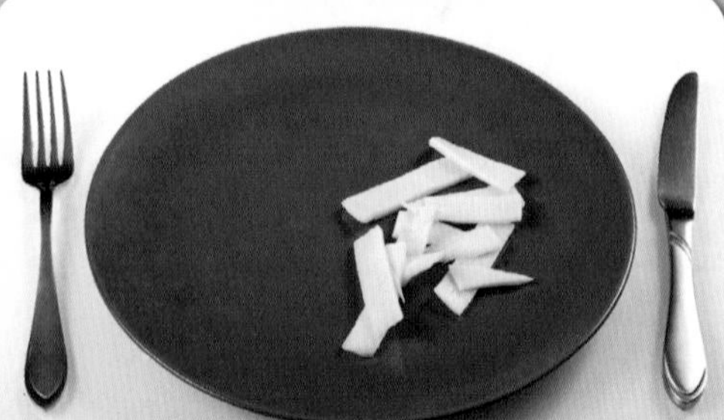

1g FIBRE	Weight: 30g	0g SAT FAT

0g CARBS	6 CALS	1g PROTEIN	0g FAT

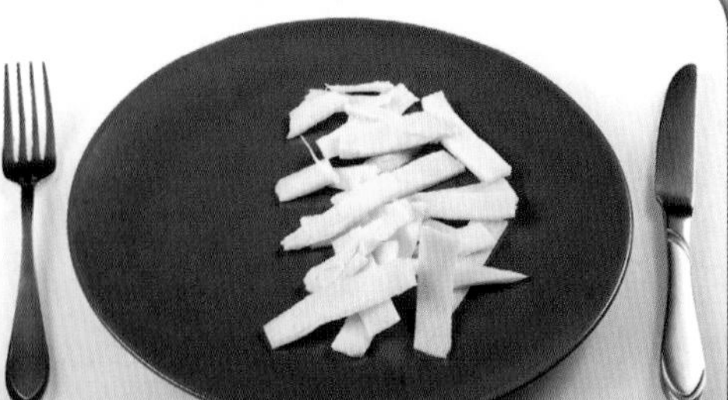

1g FIBRE	Weight: 55g	0g SAT FAT

1g CARBS	9 CALS	1g PROTEIN	0g FAT

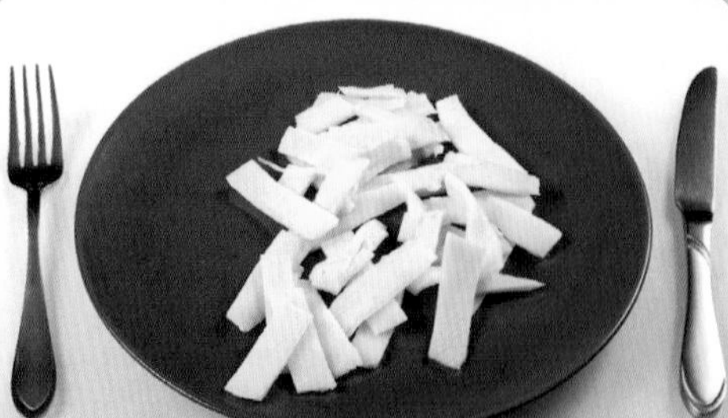

2g FIBRE	Weight: 80g	0g SAT FAT

Bean Sprouts

1g CARBS	9 CALS	1g PROTEIN	0g FAT

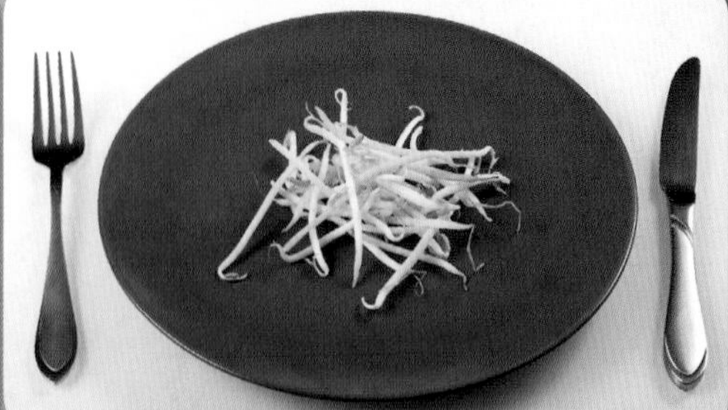

1g FIBRE	Weight: 30g	0g SAT FAT

3g CARBS	25 CALS	2g PROTEIN	0g FAT

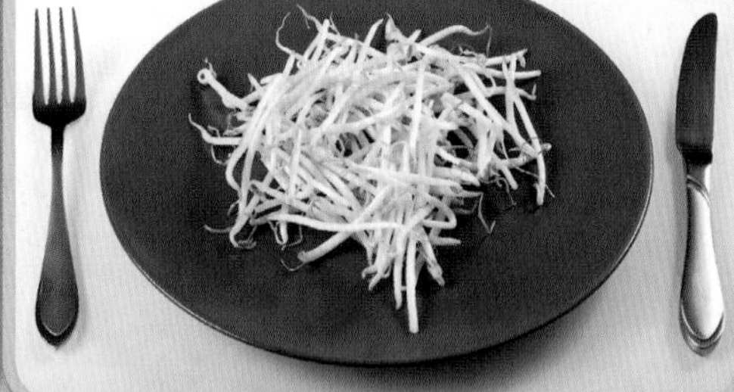

2g FIBRE	Weight: 80g	0g SAT FAT

7g CARBS	53 CALS	5g PROTEIN	1g FAT

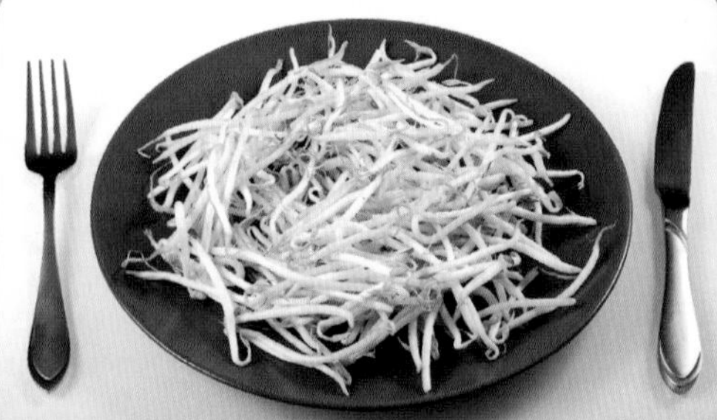

3g FIBRE	Weight: 170g	0g SAT FAT

Beetroot (boiled)

CARBS	CALS	PROTEIN	FAT
3g	14	1g	0g

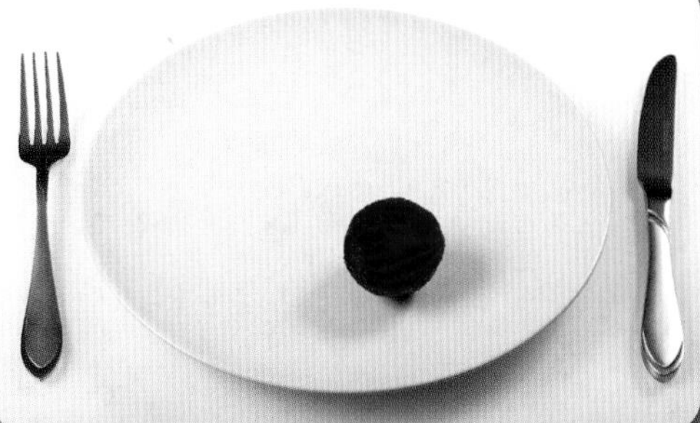

FIBRE	Weight	SAT FAT
1g	Weight: 30g	0g

CARBS	CALS	PROTEIN	FAT
8g	37	2g	0g

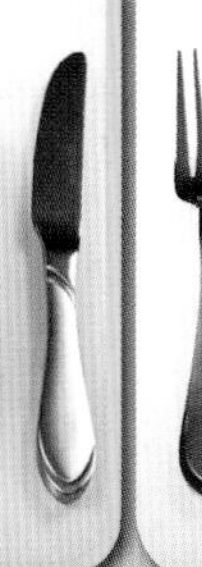

FIBRE	Weight	SAT FAT
2g	Weight: 80g	0g

CARBS	CALS	PROTEIN	FAT
13g	64	3g	0g

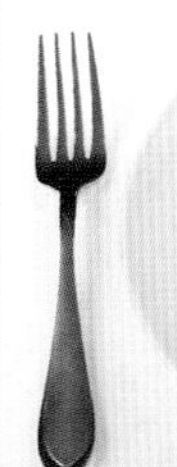

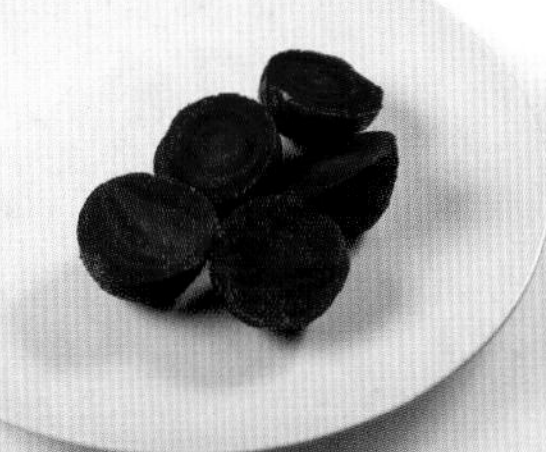

FIBRE	Weight	SAT FAT
4g	Weight: 140g	0g

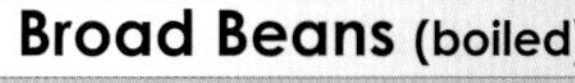

Broad Beans (boiled)

CARBS	CALS	PROTEIN	FAT
2g	14	2g	0g

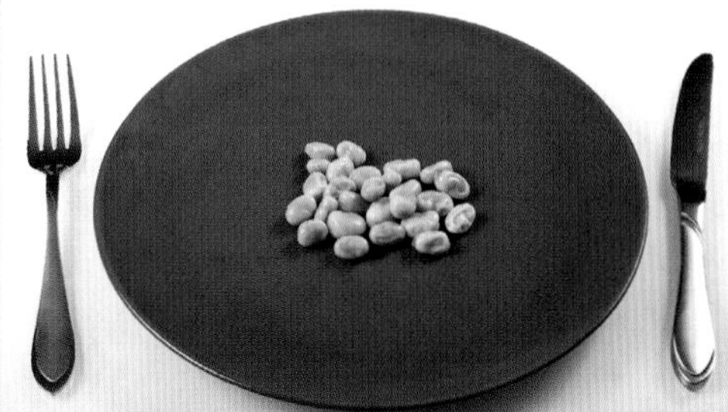

FIBRE	Weight	SAT FAT
2g	Weight: 30g	0g

CARBS	CALS	PROTEIN	FAT
3g	26	3g	0g

FIBRE	Weight	SAT FAT
4g	Weight: 55g	0g

CARBS	CALS	PROTEIN	FAT
4g	38	4g	1g

FIBRE	Weight	SAT FAT
6g	Weight: 80g	0g

Broccoli (boiled)

CARBS	CALS	PROTEIN	FAT	FIBRE	Weight	SAT FAT
0g	10	1g	0g	1g	40g	0g
1g	19	3g	1g	3g	80g	0g
1g	29	4g	1g	4g	120g	0g

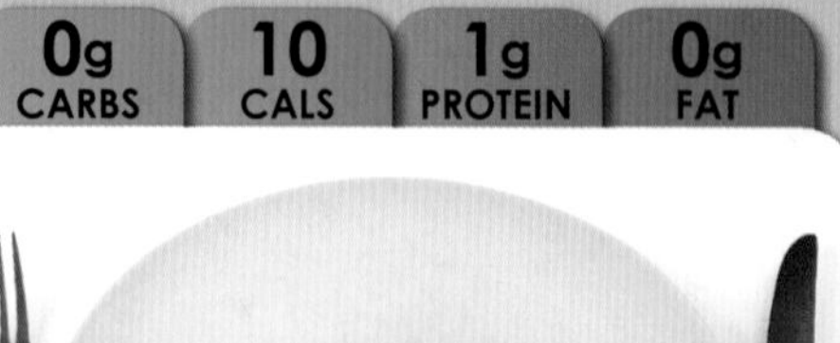
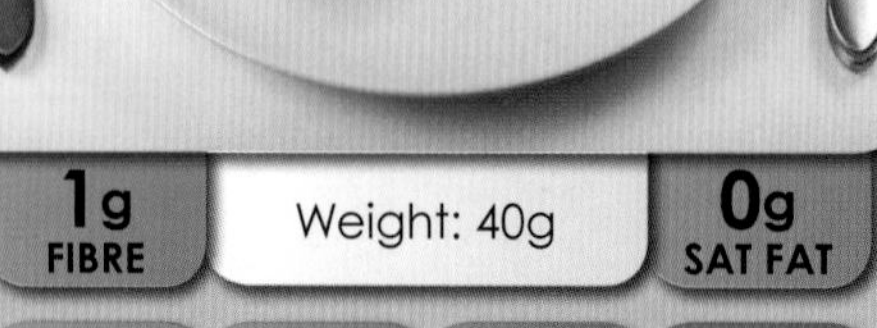
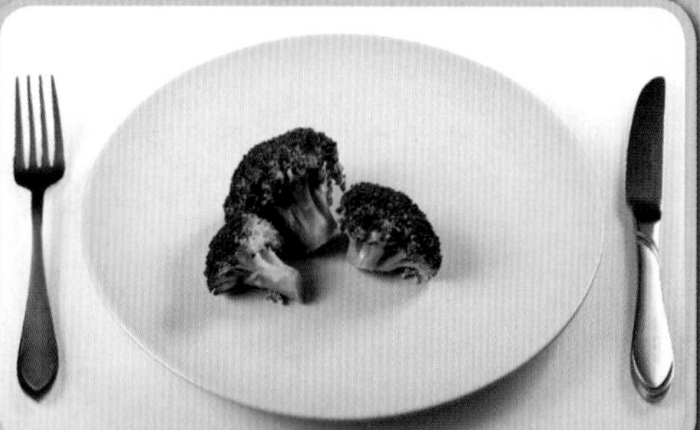
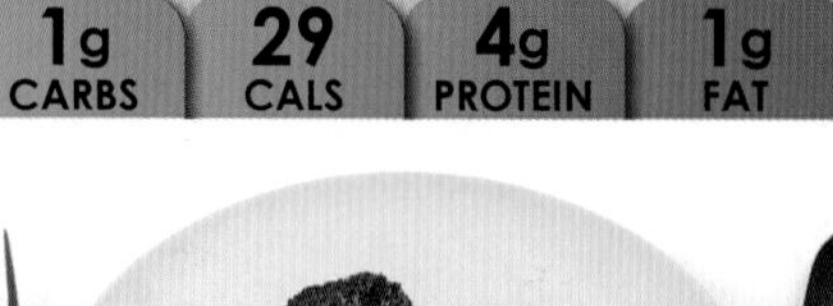
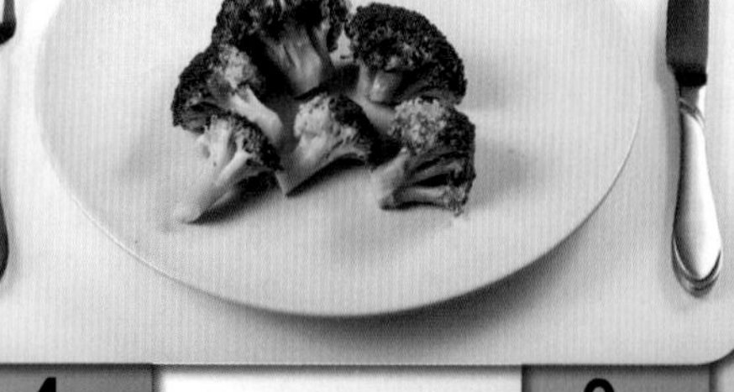

Brussels Sprouts (boiled)

CARBS	CALS	PROTEIN	FAT	FIBRE	Weight	SAT FAT
1g	14	1g	1g	2g	40g	0g
3g	28	2g	1g	3g	80g	0g
6g	56	5g	2g	7g	160g	0g

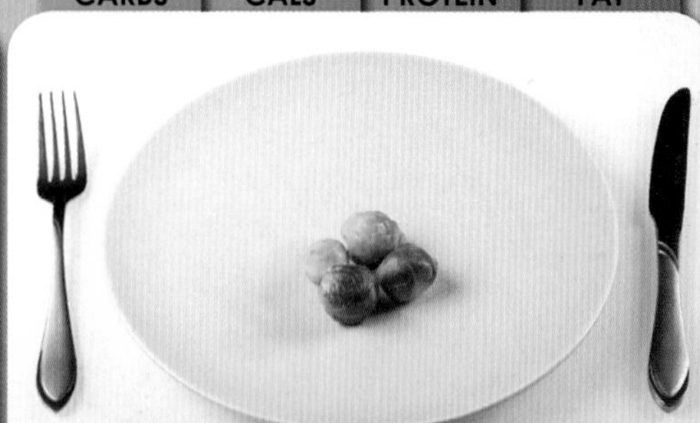
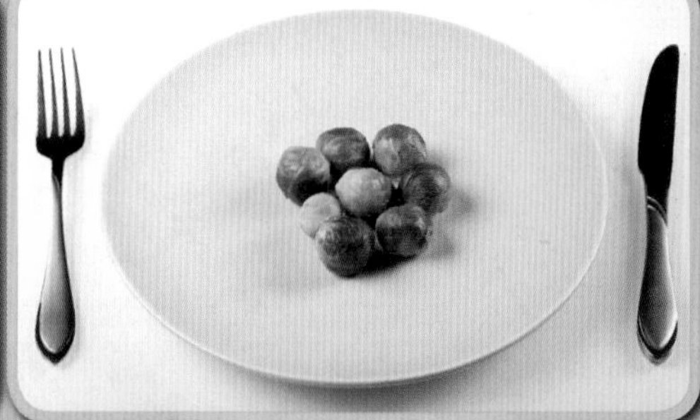
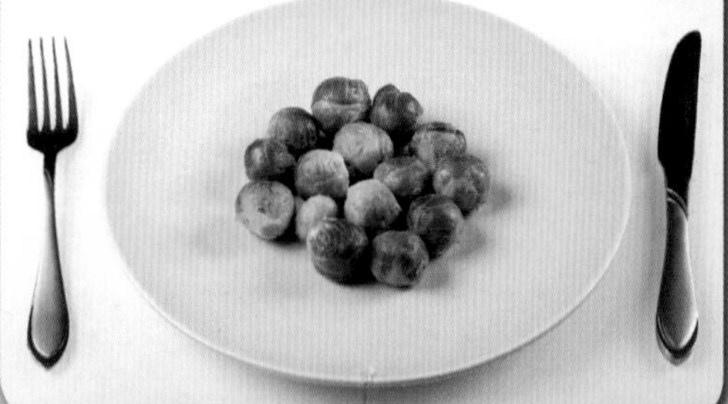

Butter Beans

CARBS	CALS	PROTEIN	FAT
5g	31	2g	0g

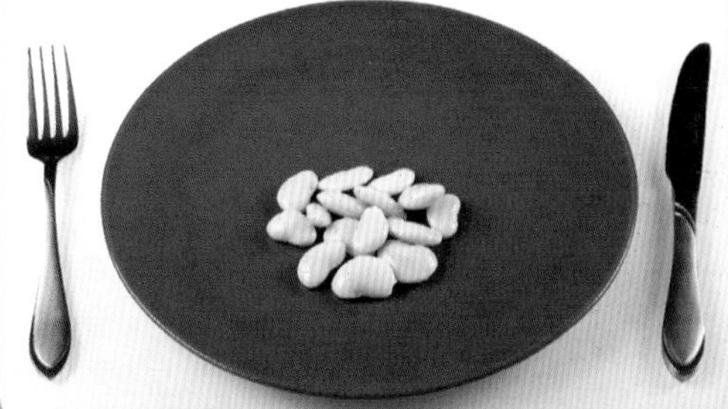

FIBRE	Weight	SAT FAT
2g	Weight: 40g	0g

CARBS	CALS	PROTEIN	FAT
10g	62	5g	0g

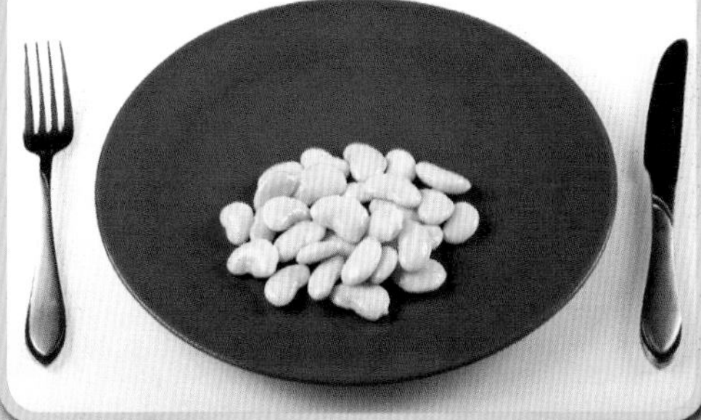

FIBRE	Weight	SAT FAT
5g	Weight: 80g	0g

CARBS	CALS	PROTEIN	FAT
21g	123	9g	1g

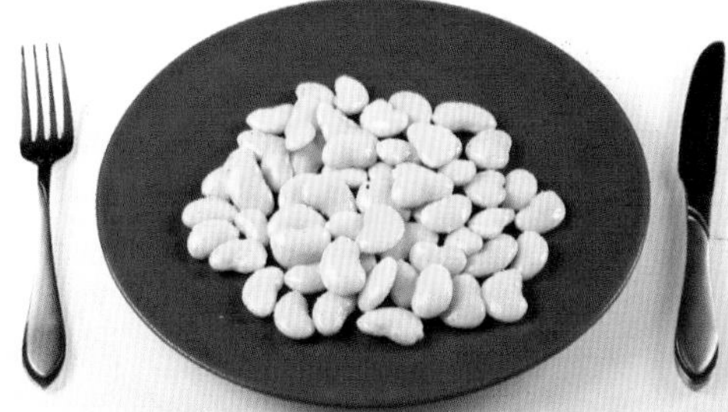

FIBRE	Weight	SAT FAT
10g	Weight: 160g	0g

Butternut Squash (baked)

CARBS	CALS	PROTEIN	FAT
10g	42	1g	0g

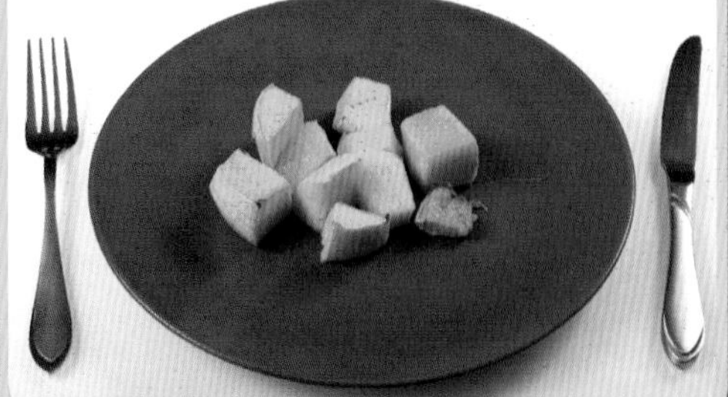

FIBRE	Weight	SAT FAT
3g	Weight: 130g	0g

CARBS	CALS	PROTEIN	FAT
20g	85	2g	0g

FIBRE	Weight	SAT FAT
5g	Weight: 265g	0g

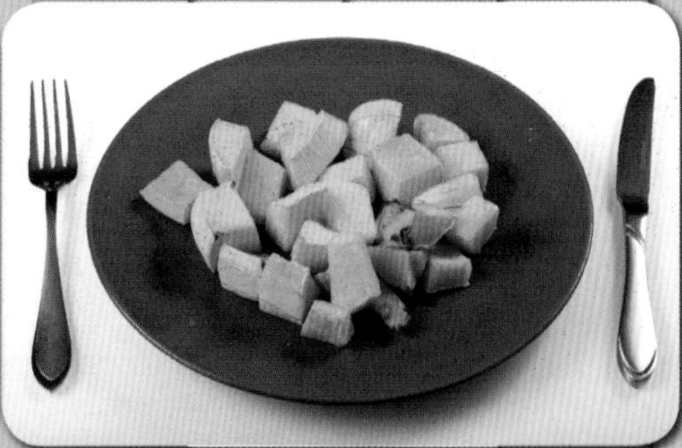

CARBS	CALS	PROTEIN	FAT
30g	128	4g	0g

FIBRE	Weight	SAT FAT
8g	Weight: 400g	0g

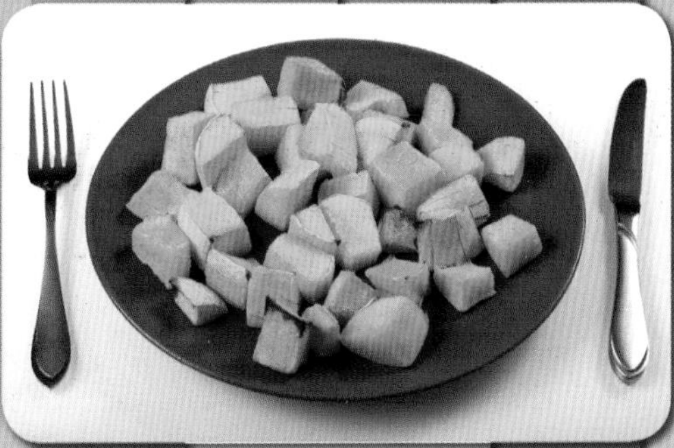

Cabbage (boiled)

CARBS	CALS	PROTEIN	FAT	FIBRE	SAT FAT	Weight
1g	6	0g	0g	1g	0g	40g
2g	13	1g	0g	2g	0g	80g
3g	19	1g	1g	3g	0g	120g

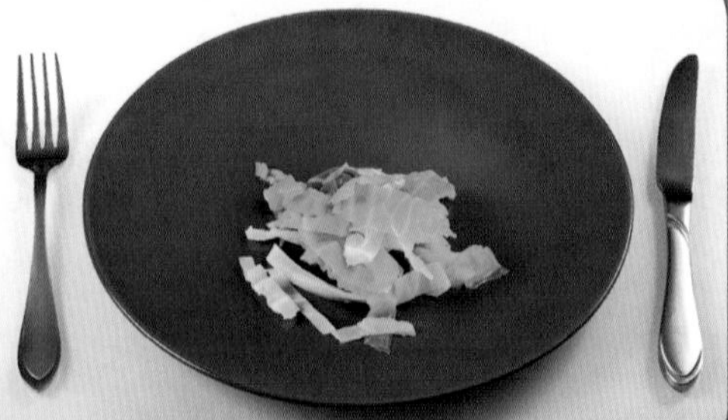

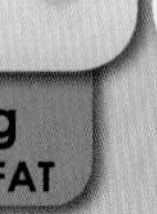

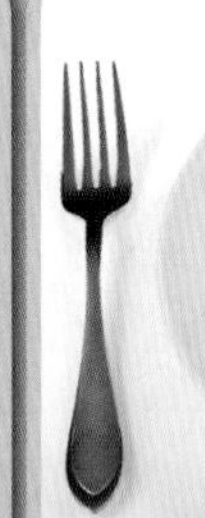

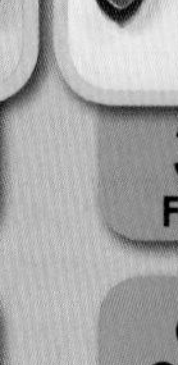

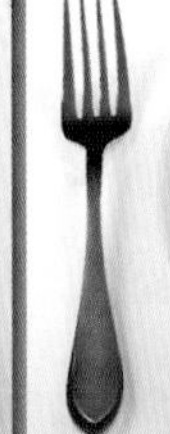

Carrots (boiled)

CARBS	CALS	PROTEIN	FAT	FIBRE	SAT FAT	Weight
2g	10	0g	0g	1g	0g	40g
4g	19	1g	0g	3g	0g	80g
6g	29	1g	1g	4g	0g	120g

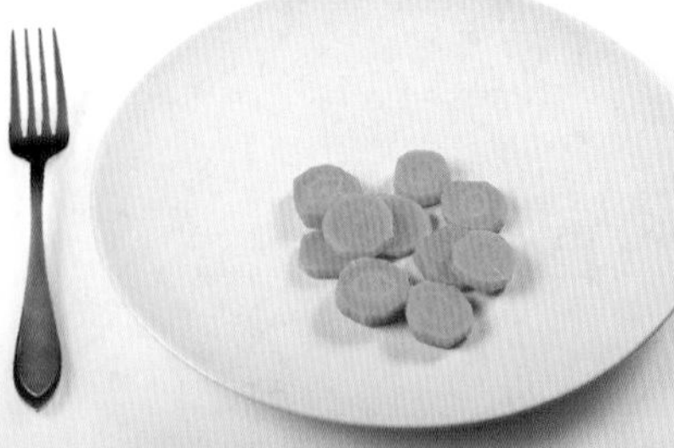

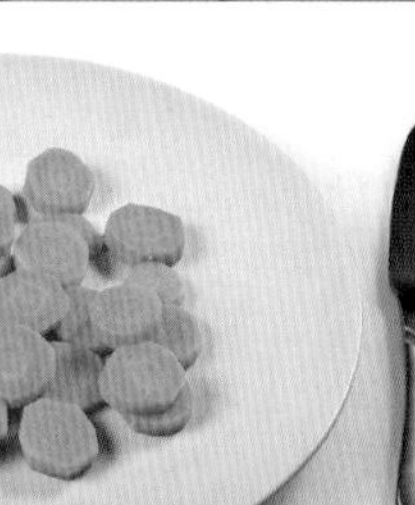

Cauliflower (boiled)

1g CARBS	11 CALS	1g PROTEIN	0g FAT

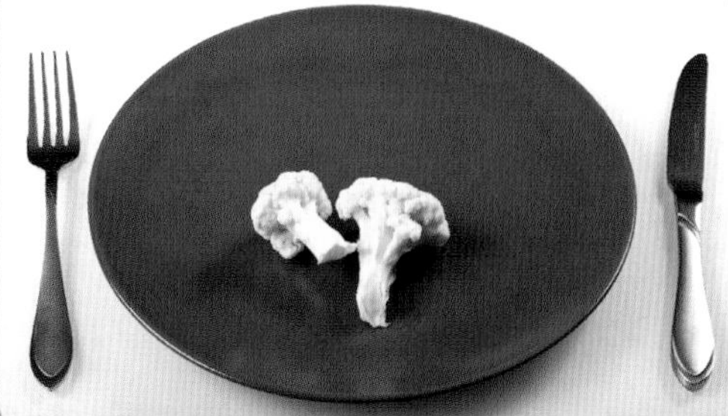

1g FIBRE	Weight: 40g	0g SAT FAT

2g CARBS	22 CALS	2g PROTEIN	1g FAT

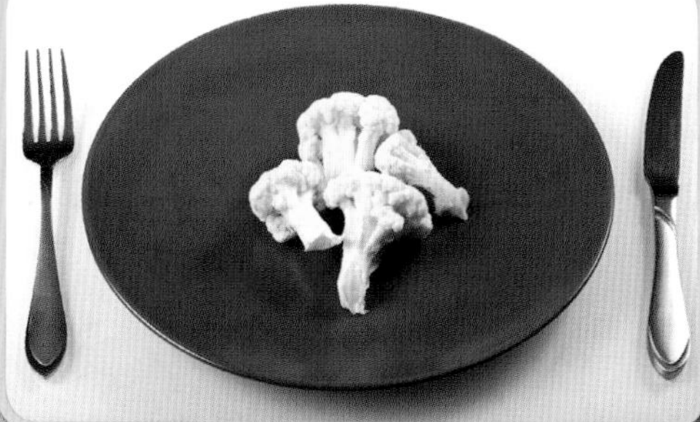

2g FIBRE	Weight: 80g	0g SAT FAT

3g CARBS	34 CALS	4g PROTEIN	1g FAT

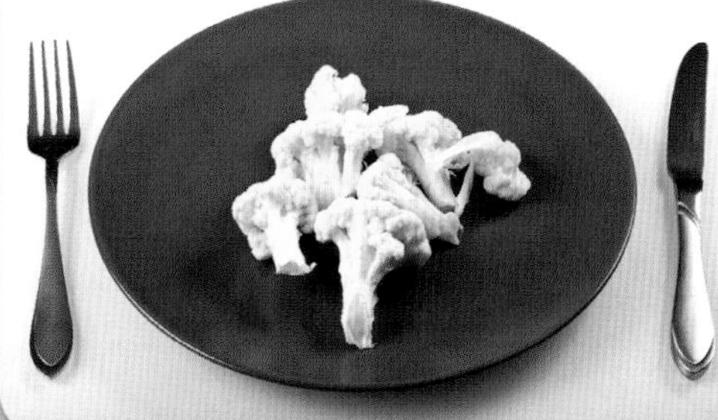

3g FIBRE	Weight: 120g	0g SAT FAT

Celery

0g CARBS	3 CALS	0g PROTEIN	0g FAT

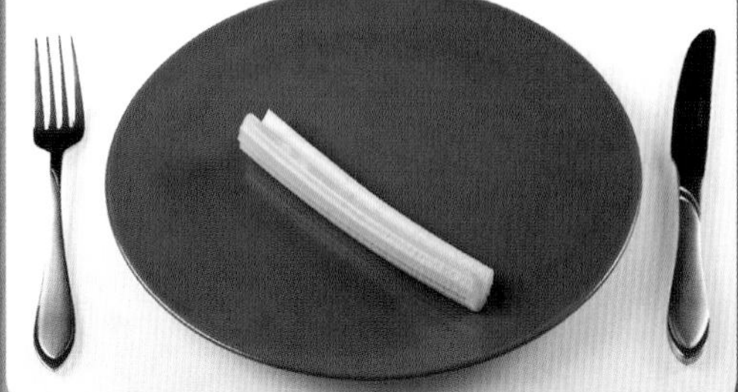

1g FIBRE	Weight: 40g	0g SAT FAT

1g CARBS	6 CALS	0g PROTEIN	0g FAT

1g FIBRE	Weight: 80g	0g SAT FAT

1g CARBS	6 CALS	0g PROTEIN	0g FAT

1g FIBRE	Weight: 80g	0g SAT FAT

Cherry Tomatoes

CARBS	CALS	PROTEIN	FAT
1g	7	0g	0g

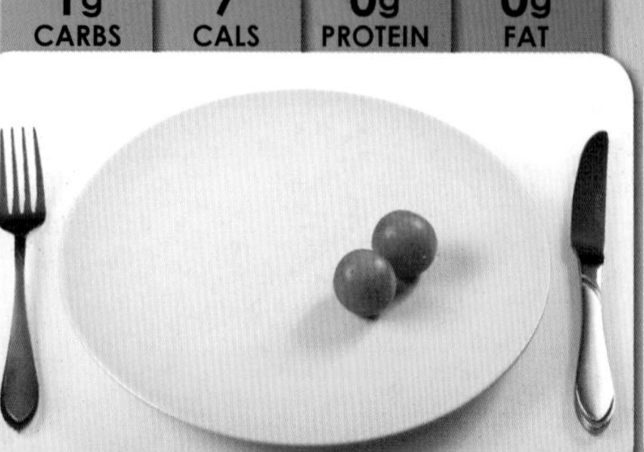

FIBRE	Weight	SAT FAT
1g	Weight: 40g	0g

CARBS	CALS	PROTEIN	FAT
2g	14	1g	0g

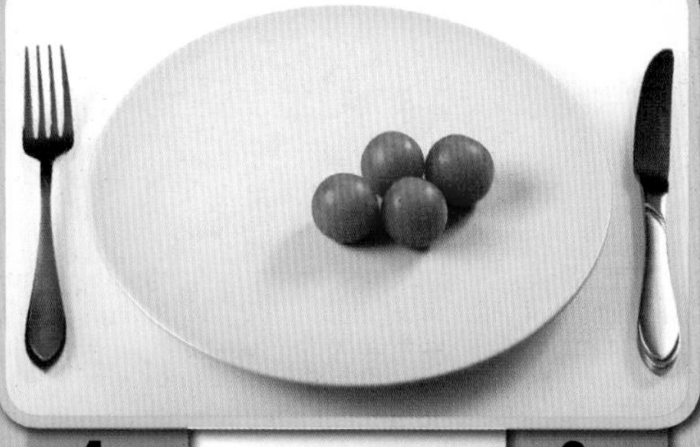

FIBRE	Weight	SAT FAT
1g	Weight: 80g	0g

CARBS	CALS	PROTEIN	FAT
4g	22	1g	1g

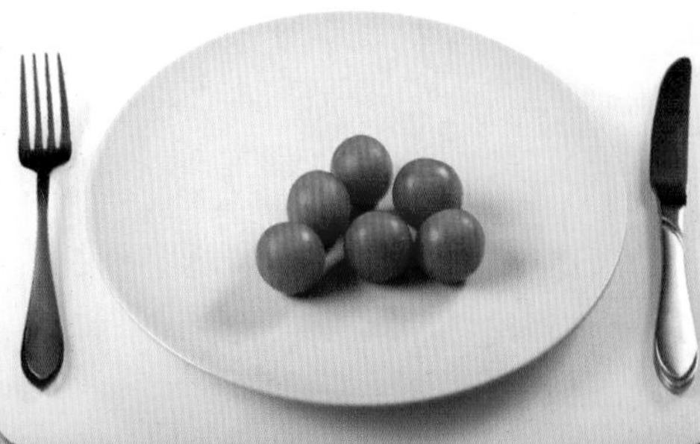

FIBRE	Weight	SAT FAT
2g	Weight: 120g	0g

Chick Peas (tinned)

CARBS	CALS	PROTEIN	FAT
6g	46	3g	1g

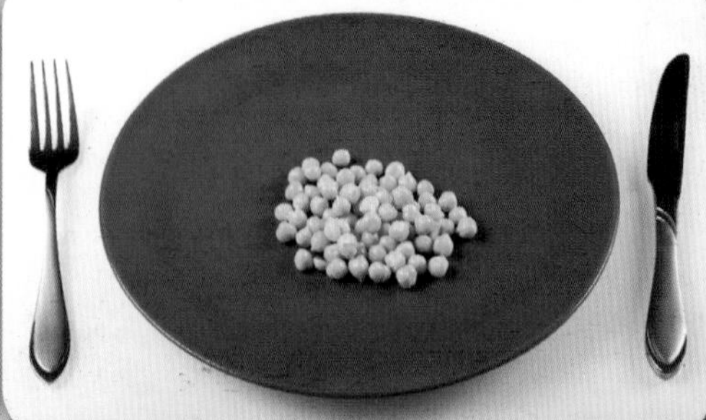

FIBRE	Weight	SAT FAT
2g	Weight: 40g	0g

CARBS	CALS	PROTEIN	FAT
13g	92	6g	2g

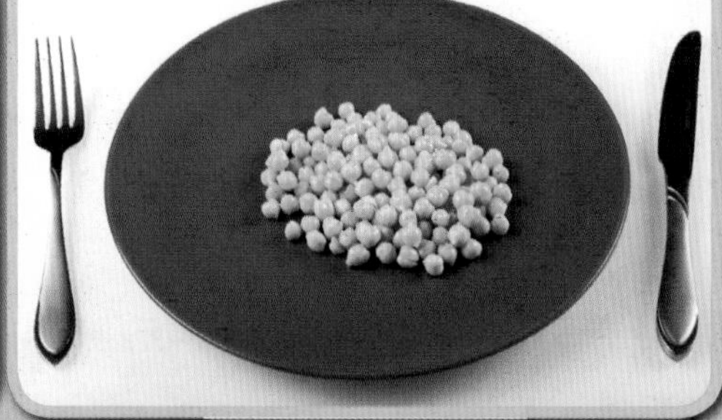

FIBRE	Weight	SAT FAT
4g	Weight: 80g	0g

CARBS	CALS	PROTEIN	FAT
19g	138	9g	4g

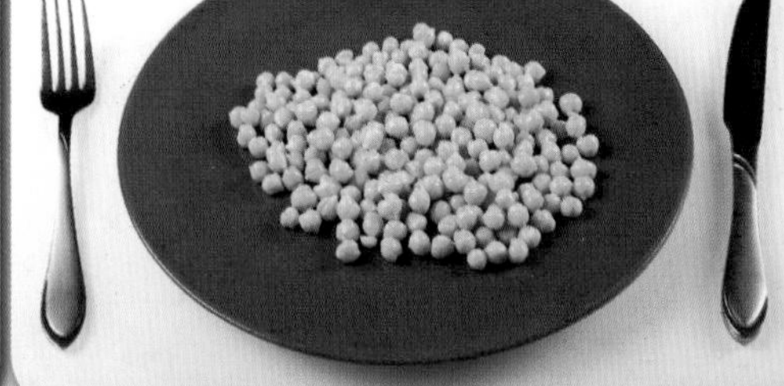

FIBRE	Weight	SAT FAT
7g	Weight: 120g	0g

Courgette (boiled)

1g CARBS	8 CALS	1g PROTEIN	0g FAT

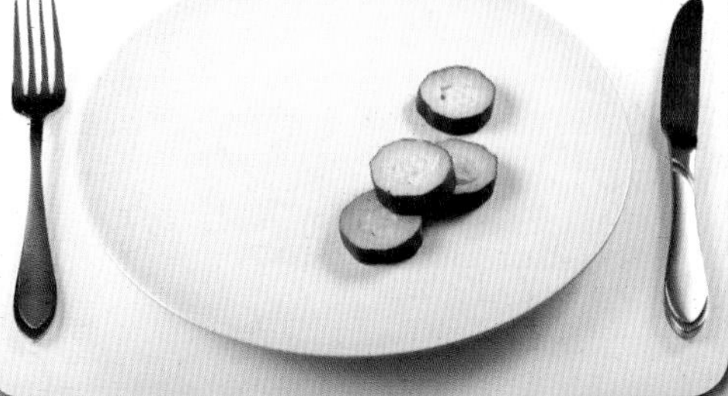

1g FIBRE	Weight: 40g	0g SAT FAT

2g CARBS	15 CALS	2g PROTEIN	0g FAT

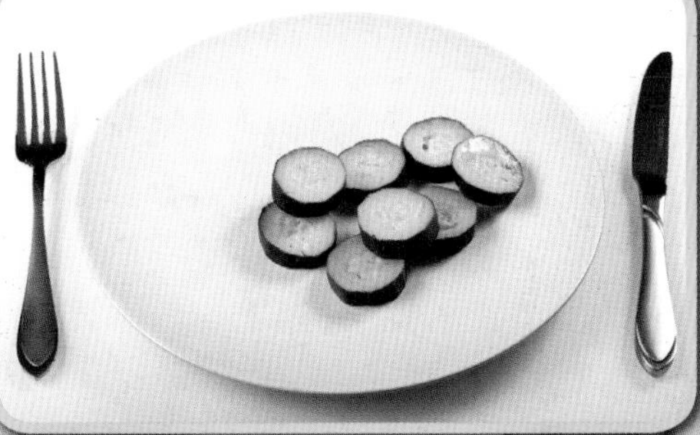

1g FIBRE	Weight: 80g	0g SAT FAT

2g CARBS	23 CALS	2g PROTEIN	1g FAT

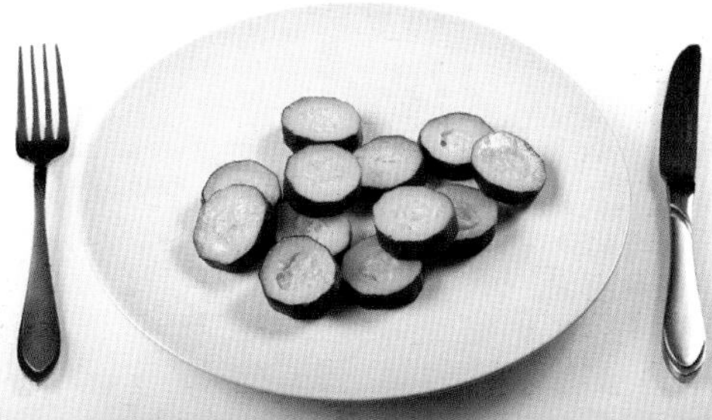

2g FIBRE	Weight: 120g	0g SAT FAT

Cucumber

1g CARBS	4 CALS	0g PROTEIN	0g FAT

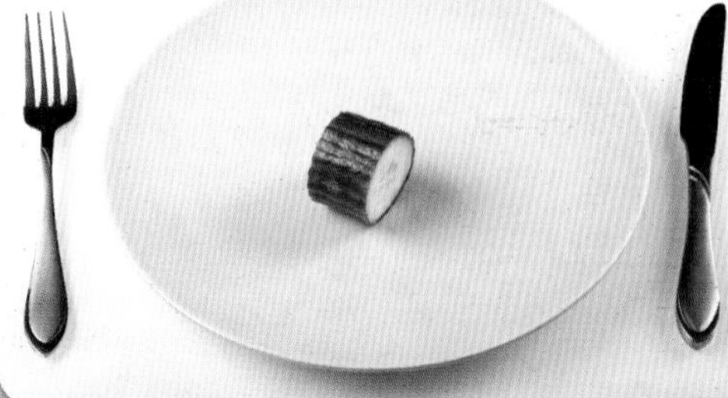

0g FIBRE	Weight: 40g	0g SAT FAT

1g CARBS	8 CALS	1g PROTEIN	0g FAT

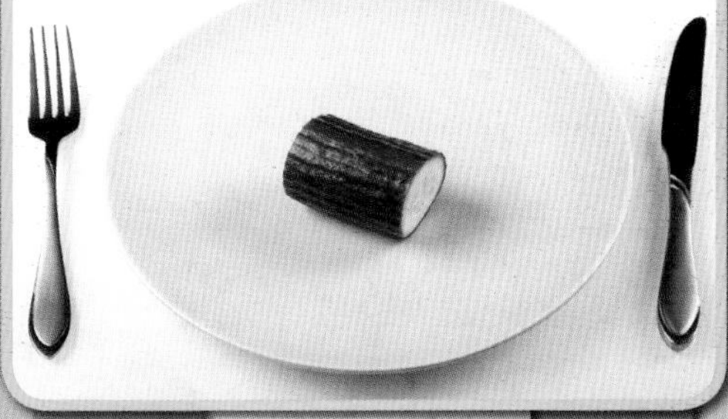

1g FIBRE	Weight: 80g	0g SAT FAT

2g CARBS	12 CALS	1g PROTEIN	0g FAT

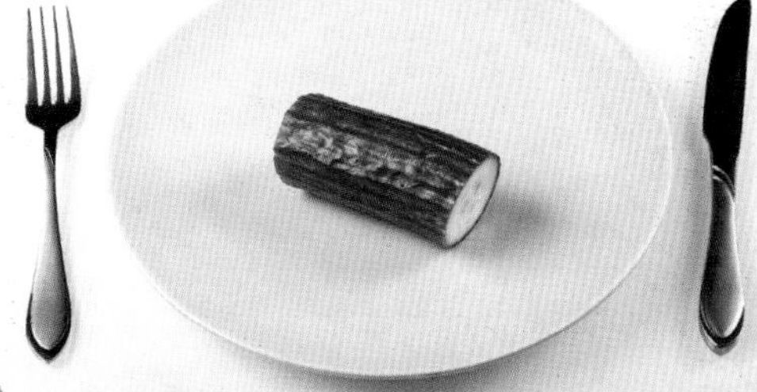

1g FIBRE	Weight: 120g	0g SAT FAT

Edamame Beans

CARBS	CALS	PROTEIN	FAT
1g	17	2g	1g

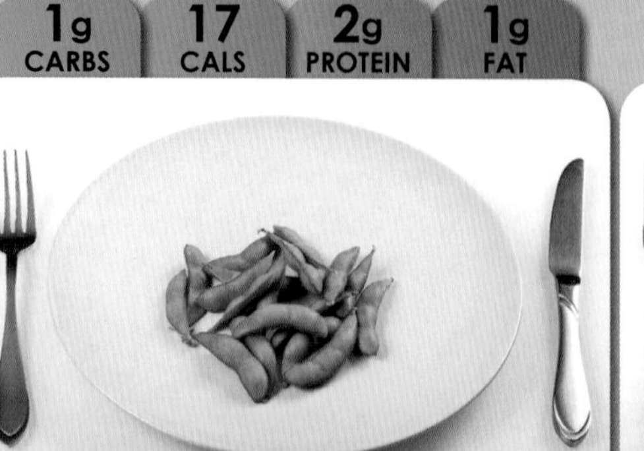

FIBRE	Weight	SAT FAT
1g	Weight: 55g (30g edible)	0g

CARBS	CALS	PROTEIN	FAT
3g	33	3g	1g

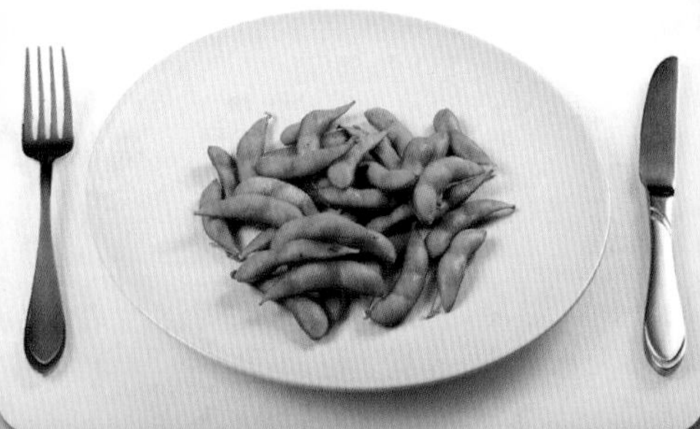

FIBRE	Weight	SAT FAT
1g	Weight: 115g (60g edible)	0g

CARBS	CALS	PROTEIN	FAT
3g	44	4g	2g

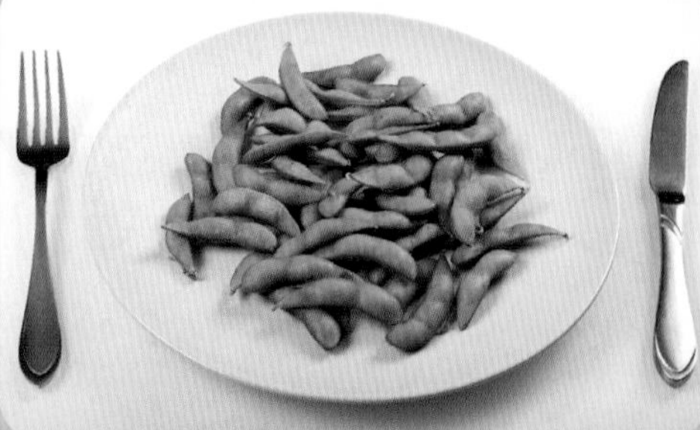

FIBRE	Weight	SAT FAT
2g	Weight: 170g (80g edible)	0g

Green Beans (boiled)

CARBS	CALS	PROTEIN	FAT
1g	9	1g	0g

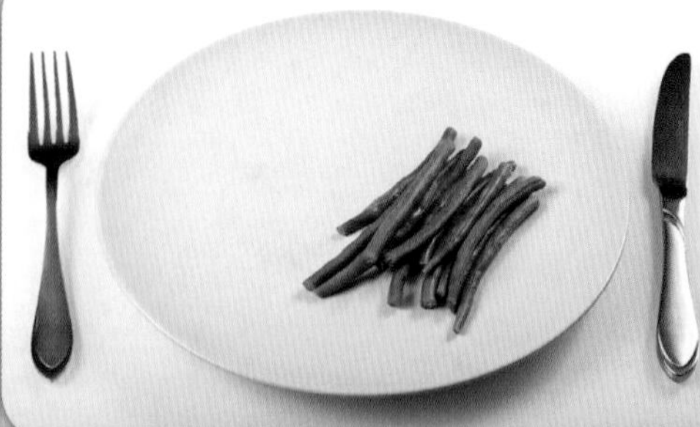

FIBRE	Weight	SAT FAT
1g	Weight: 40g	0g

CARBS	CALS	PROTEIN	FAT
2g	18	1g	0g

FIBRE	Weight	SAT FAT
3g	Weight: 80g	0g

CARBS	CALS	PROTEIN	FAT
4g	26	2g	1g

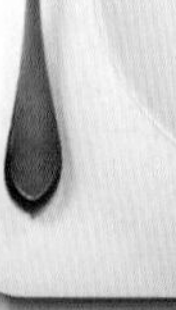

FIBRE	Weight	SAT FAT
4g	Weight: 120g	0g

Kidney Beans (tinned)

CARBS	CALS	PROTEIN	FAT
7g	40	3g	0g

FIBRE	Weight	SAT FAT
3g	Weight: 40g	0g

CARBS	CALS	PROTEIN	FAT
14g	80	6g	1g

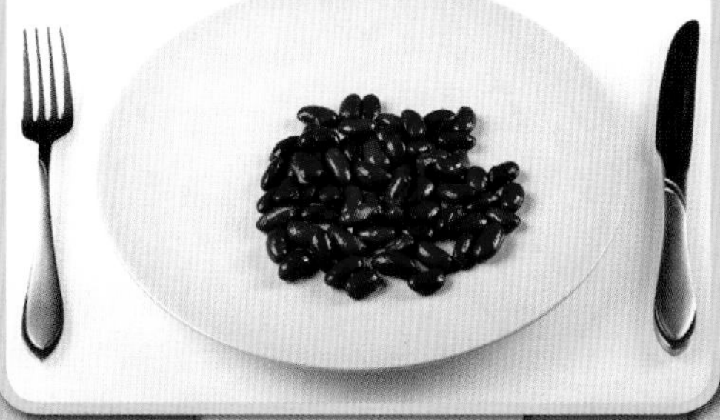

FIBRE	Weight	SAT FAT
7g	Weight: 80g	0g

CARBS	CALS	PROTEIN	FAT
21g	120	8g	1g

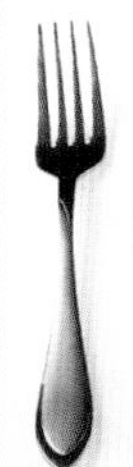
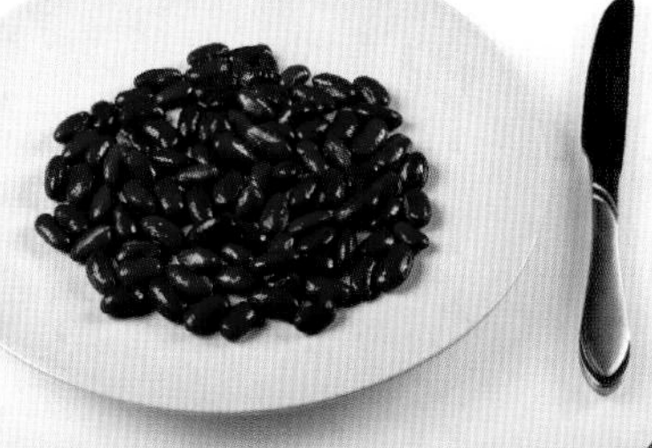
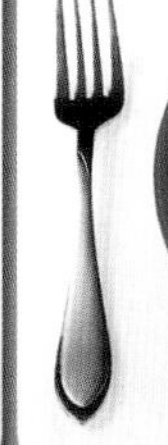

FIBRE	Weight	SAT FAT
10g	Weight: 120g	0g

Leek (boiled)

CARBS	CALS	PROTEIN	FAT
1g	8	1g	0g

FIBRE	Weight	SAT FAT
1g	Weight: 40g	0g

CARBS	CALS	PROTEIN	FAT
2g	17	1g	1g

FIBRE	Weight	SAT FAT
2g	Weight: 80g	0g

CARBS	CALS	PROTEIN	FAT
4g	34	2g	1g

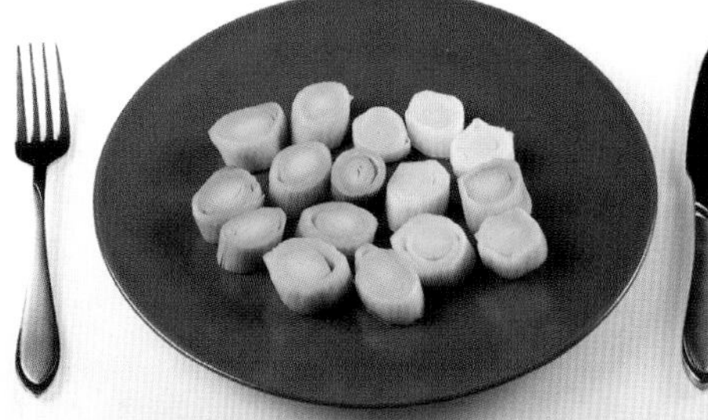

FIBRE	Weight	SAT FAT
4g	Weight: 160g	0g

Lentils (tinned)

CARBS	CALS	PROTEIN	FAT
7g	42	4g	0g

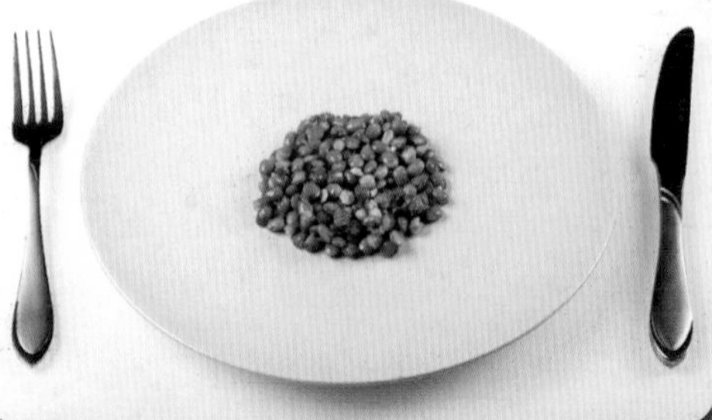

FIBRE	Weight	SAT FAT
2g	Weight: 40g	0g

CARBS	CALS	PROTEIN	FAT
14g	84	7g	1g

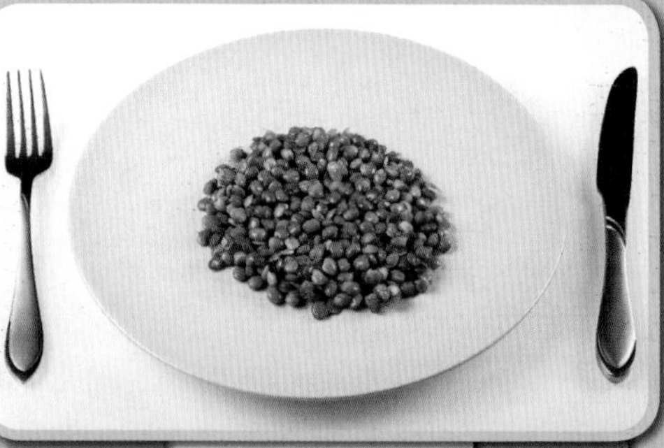

FIBRE	Weight	SAT FAT
4g	Weight: 80g	0g

CARBS	CALS	PROTEIN	FAT
20g	126	11g	1g

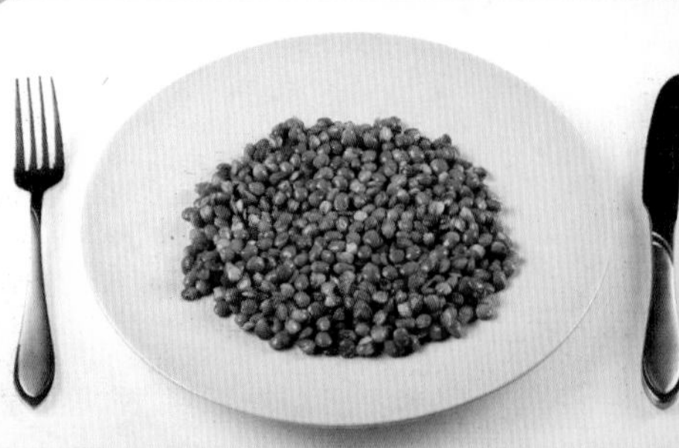

FIBRE	Weight	SAT FAT
6g	Weight: 120g	0g

Lettuce

CARBS	CALS	PROTEIN	FAT
1g	3	0g	0g

FIBRE	Weight	SAT FAT
0g	Weight: 25g	0g

CARBS	CALS	PROTEIN	FAT
1g	7	0g	0g

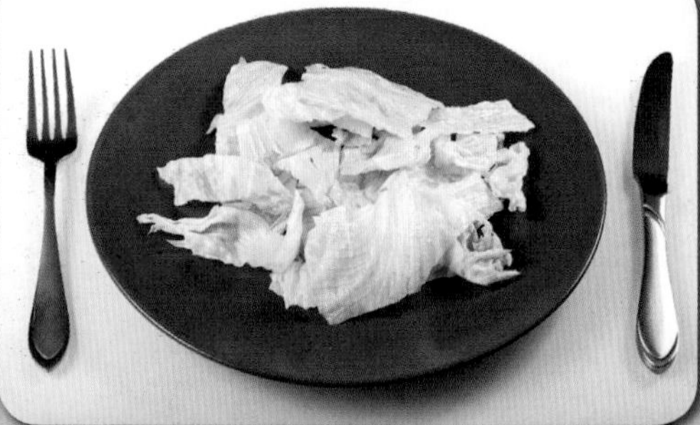

FIBRE	Weight	SAT FAT
0g	Weight: 50g	0g

CARBS	CALS	PROTEIN	FAT
2g	10	1g	0g

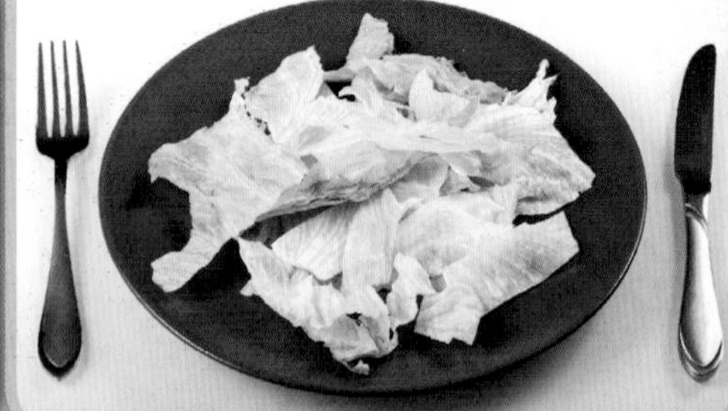

FIBRE	Weight	SAT FAT
1g	Weight: 80g	0g

Mangetout (raw)

1g CARBS	10 CALS	1g PROTEIN	0g FAT

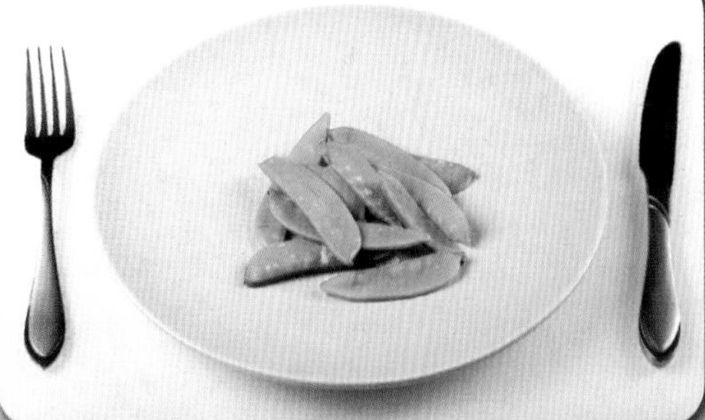

1g FIBRE	Weight: 40g	0g SAT FAT

3g CARBS	21 CALS	3g PROTEIN	0g FAT

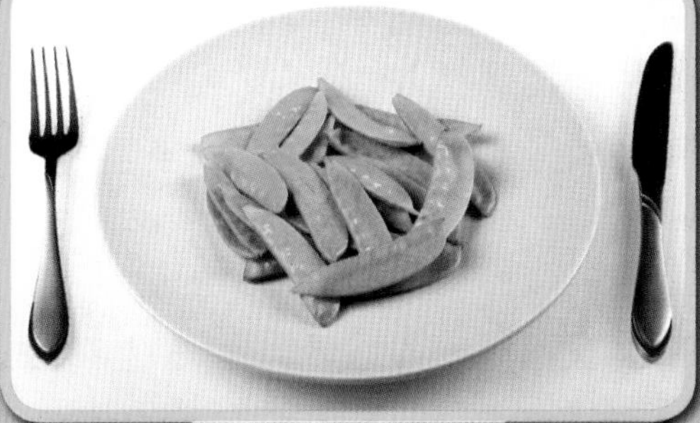

2g FIBRE	Weight: 80g	0g SAT FAT

4g CARBS	31 CALS	4g PROTEIN	0g FAT

4g FIBRE	Weight: 120g	0g SAT FAT

Mixed Salad Leaves

0g CARBS	3 CALS	0g PROTEIN	0g FAT

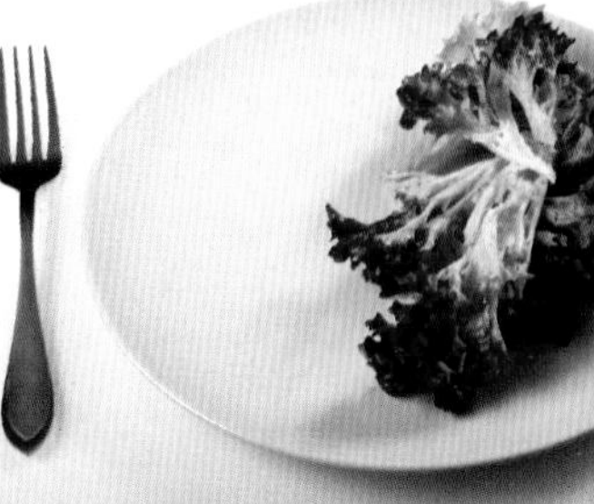

0g FIBRE	Weight: 20g	0g SAT FAT

1g CARBS	6 CALS	0g PROTEIN	0g FAT

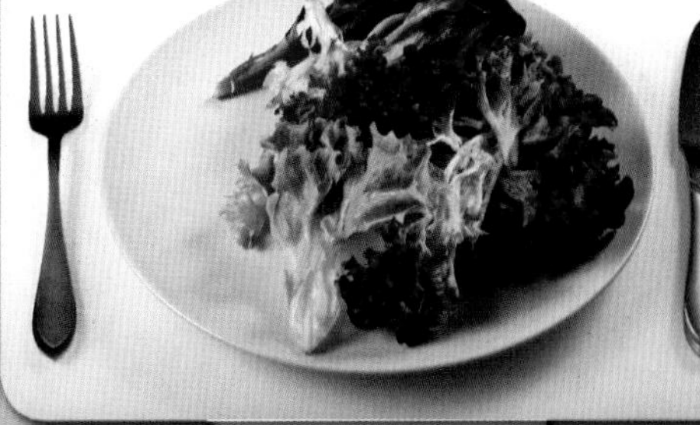

1g FIBRE	Weight: 40g	0g SAT FAT

1g CARBS	8 CALS	1g PROTEIN	0g FAT

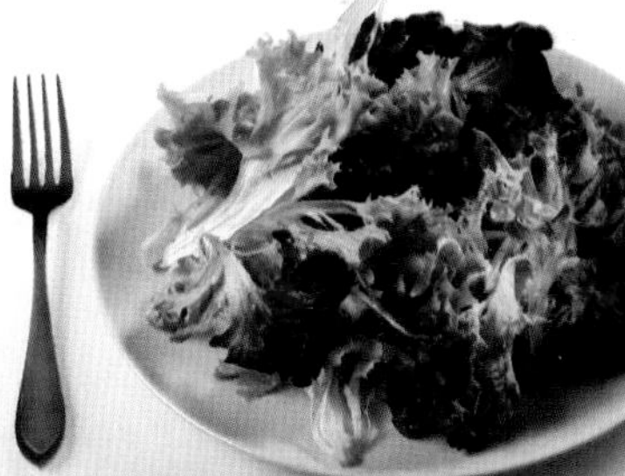

1g FIBRE	Weight: 60g	0g SAT FAT

26cm Dinner Plate

Mushrooms (raw)

CARBS	CALS	PROTEIN	FAT	FIBRE	SAT FAT	Weight
0g	5	1g	0g	1g	0g	40g
0g	10	1g	0g	1g	0g	80g
1g	16	2g	1g	2g	0g	120g

Mushrooms (fried in butter)

CARBS	CALS	PROTEIN	FAT
0g	63	1g	7g

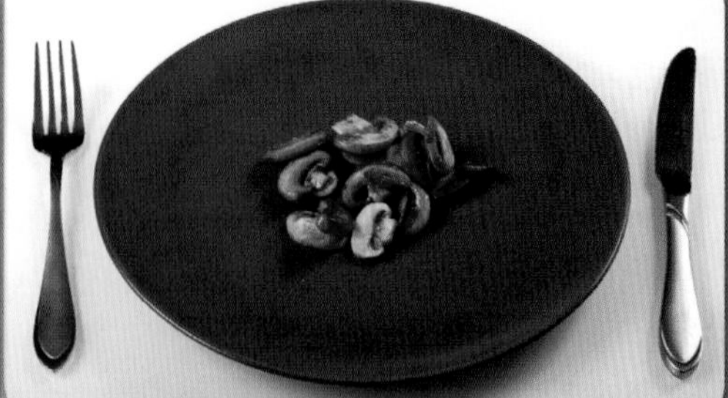

FIBRE	Weight	SAT FAT
1g	Weight: 40g	4g

CARBS	CALS	PROTEIN	FAT
0g	126	2g	13g

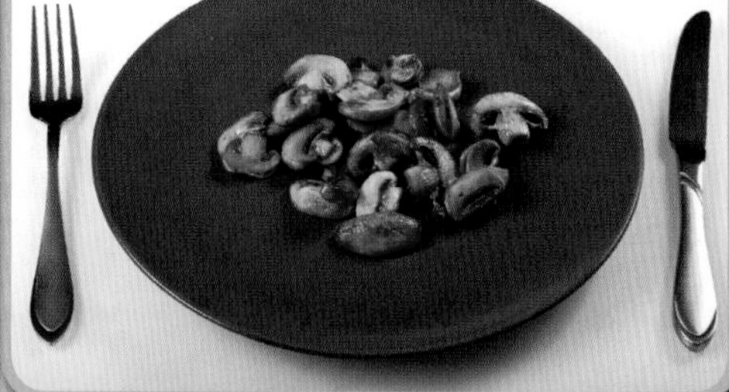

FIBRE	Weight	SAT FAT
2g	Weight: 80g	9g

CARBS	CALS	PROTEIN	FAT
0g	188	3g	19g

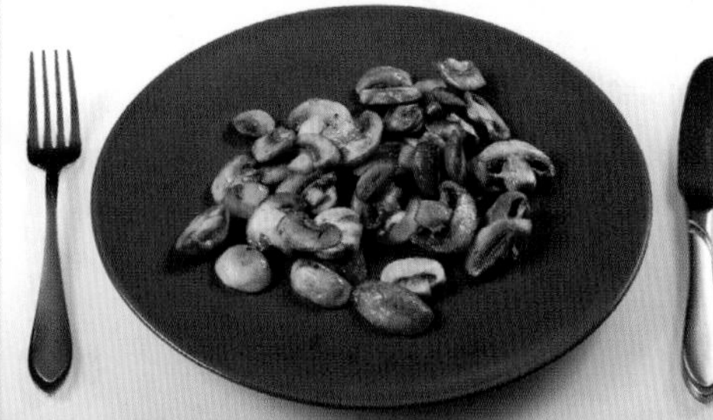

FIBRE	Weight	SAT FAT
2g	Weight: 120g	13g

Onions (raw)

CARBS	CALS	PROTEIN	FAT
3g	14	0g	0g

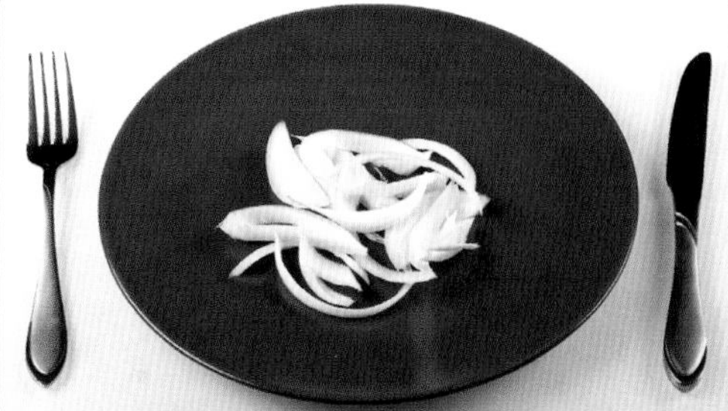

FIBRE	Weight	SAT FAT
1g	Weight: 40g	0g

CARBS	CALS	PROTEIN	FAT
6g	29	1g	0g

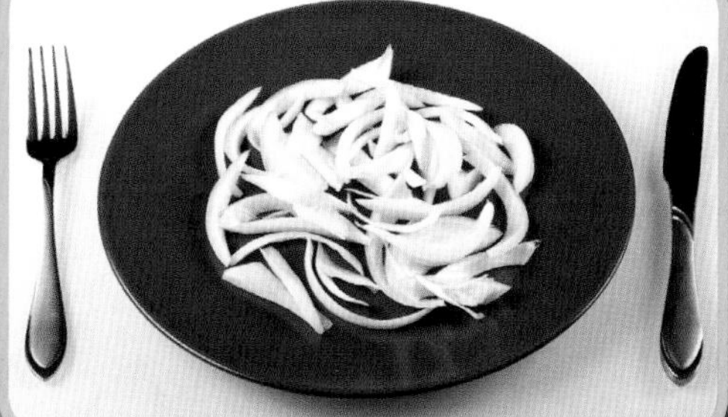

FIBRE	Weight	SAT FAT
2g	Weight: 80g	0g

CARBS	CALS	PROTEIN	FAT
6g	29	1g	0g

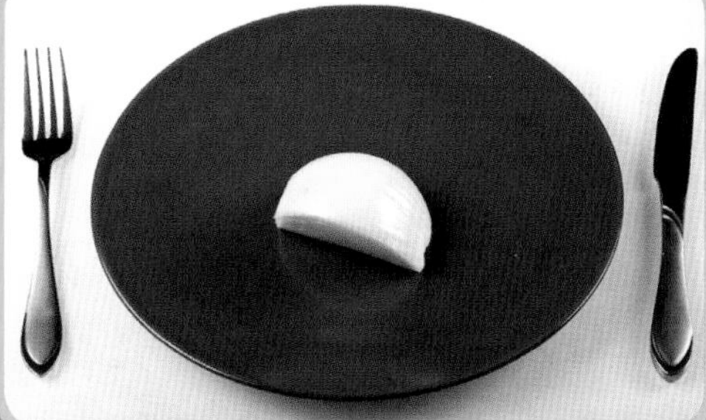

FIBRE	Weight	SAT FAT
2g	Weight: 80g	0g

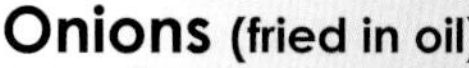

Onions (fried in oil)

CARBS	CALS	PROTEIN	FAT
3g	33	1g	2g

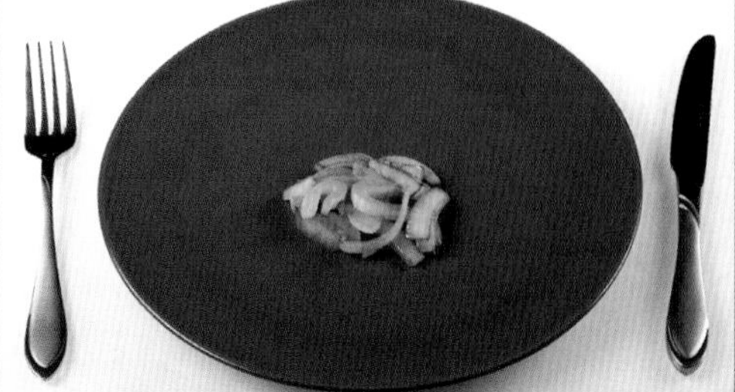

FIBRE	Weight	SAT FAT
1g	Weight: 20g	0g

CARBS	CALS	PROTEIN	FAT
6g	66	1g	5g

FIBRE	Weight	SAT FAT
2g	Weight: 40g	1g

CARBS	CALS	PROTEIN	FAT
11g	131	2g	9g

FIBRE	Weight	SAT FAT
3g	Weight: 80g	1g

Okra (boiled)

CARBS	CALS	PROTEIN	FAT	FIBRE	Weight	SAT FAT
1g	11	1g	0g	2g	40g	0g
2g	22	2g	1g	4g	80g	0g
3g	34	3g	1g	6g	120g	0g

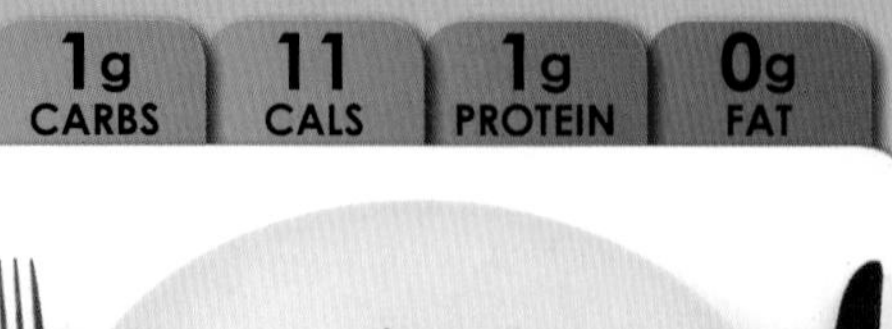
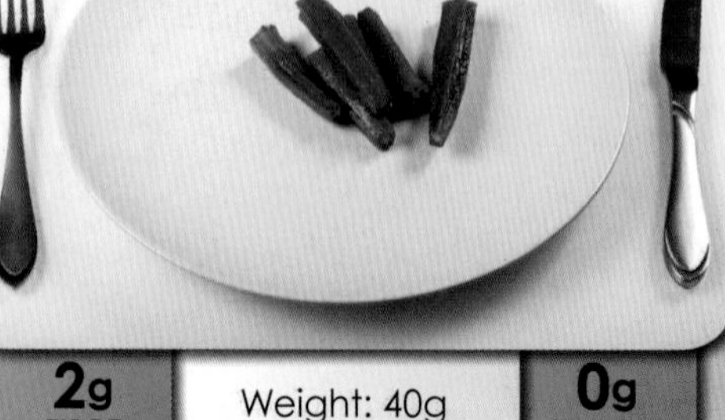
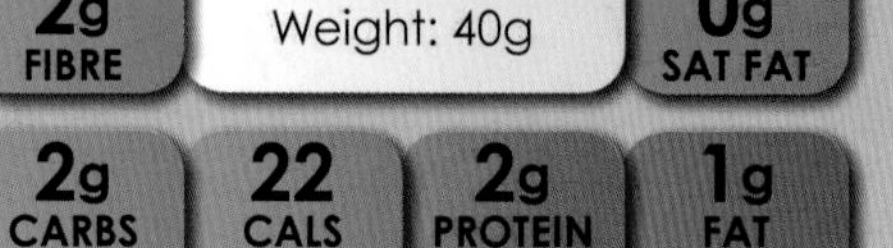
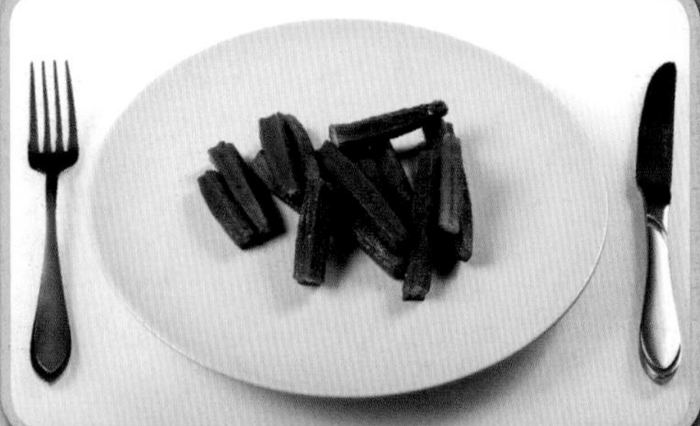
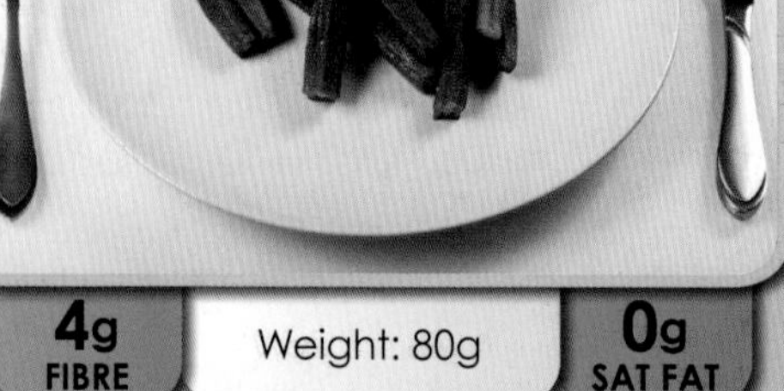
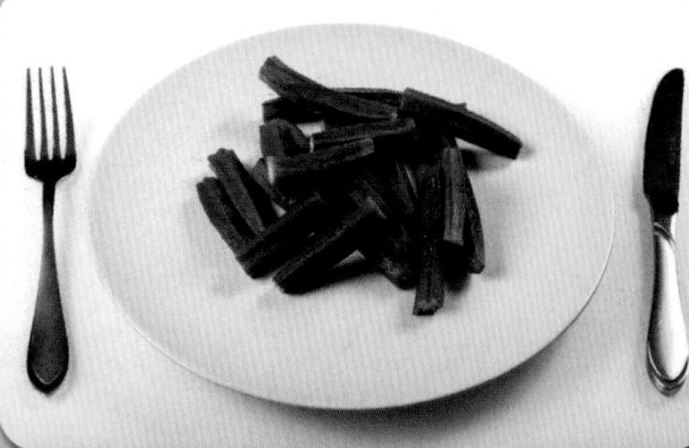
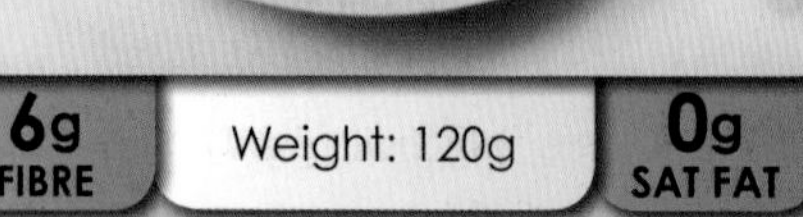

Pak Choi (boiled)

CARBS	CALS	PROTEIN	FAT	FIBRE	Weight	SAT FAT
1g	5	1g	0g	0g	30g	0g
2g	13	1g	0g	1g	80g	0g
3g	22	2g	0g	1g	140g	0g

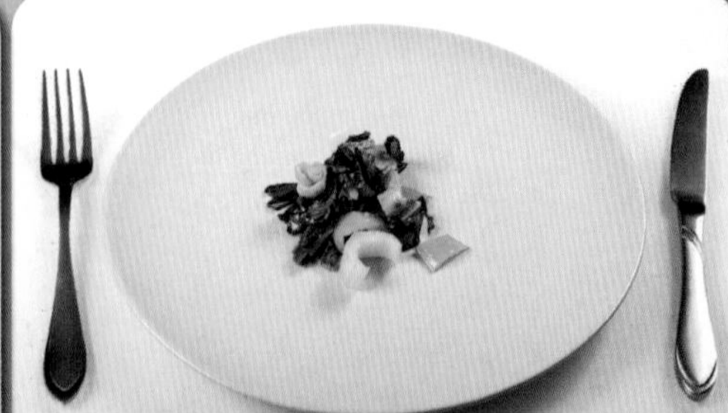
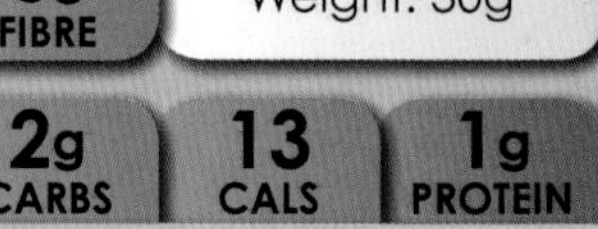
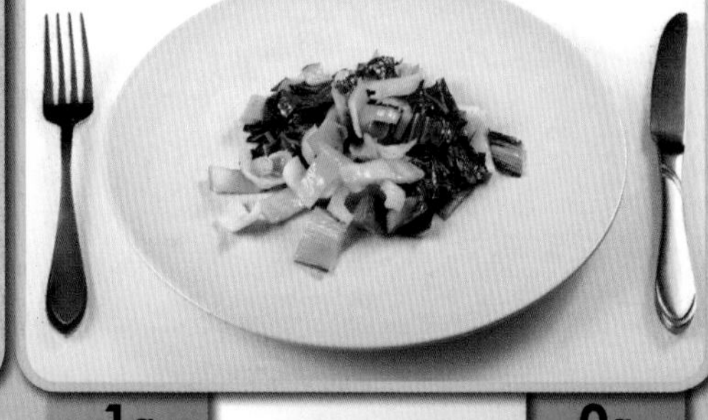
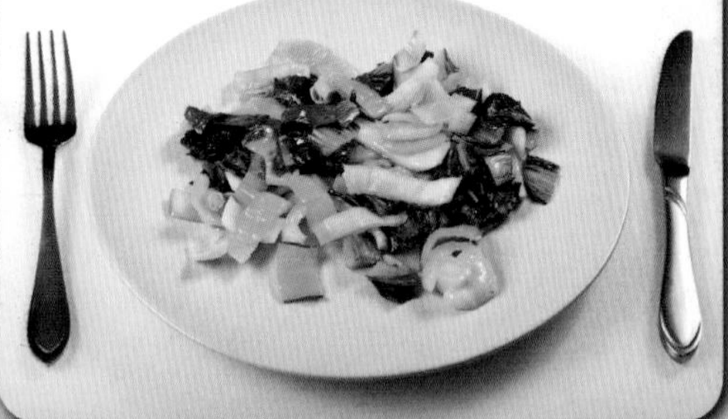
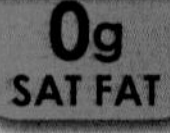

Peas

4g CARBS	28 CALS	2g PROTEIN	0g FAT

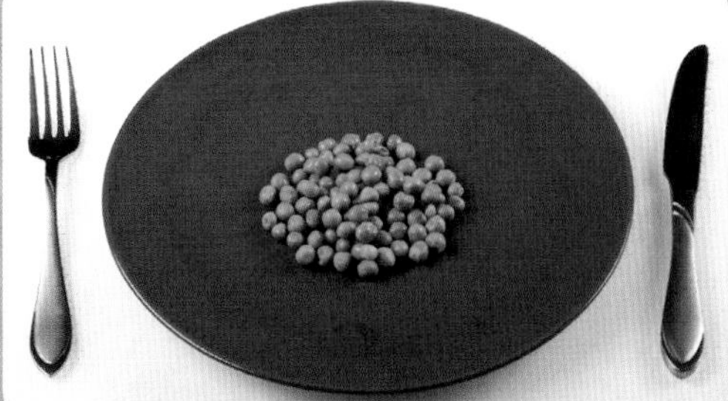

3g FIBRE	Weight: 40g	0g SAT FAT

8g CARBS	55 CALS	5g PROTEIN	1g FAT

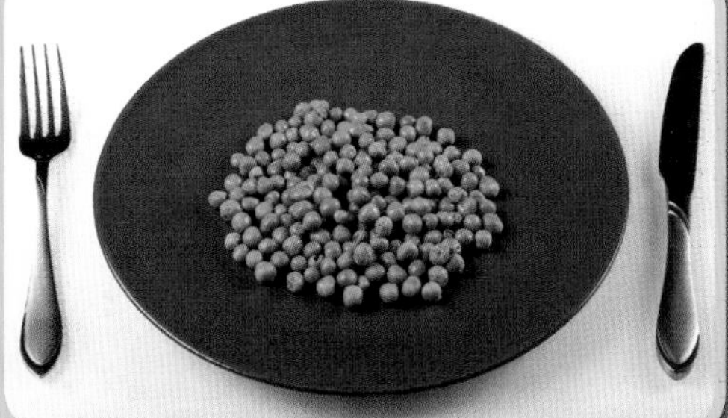

5g FIBRE	Weight: 80g	0g SAT FAT

12g CARBS	83 CALS	7g PROTEIN	1g FAT

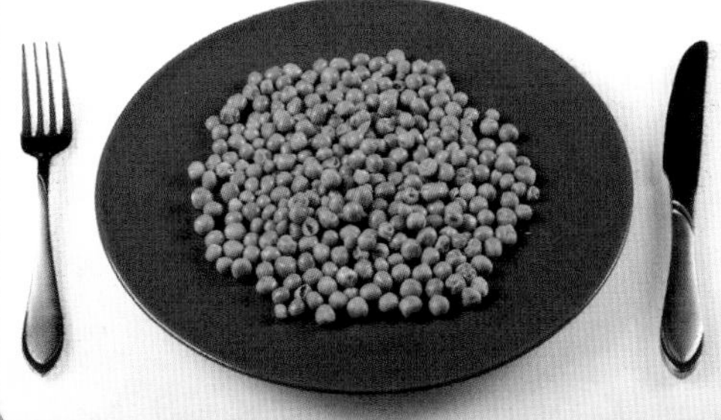

8g FIBRE	Weight: 120g	0g SAT FAT

Mushy Peas

11g CARBS	65 CALS	5g PROTEIN	1g FAT

2g FIBRE	Weight: 80g	0g SAT FAT

21g CARBS	122 CALS	9g PROTEIN	1g FAT

4g FIBRE	Weight: 150g	0g SAT FAT

41g CARBS	243 CALS	17g PROTEIN	2g FAT

7g FIBRE	Weight: 300g	0g SAT FAT

26cm Dinner Plate

Parsnips (roasted)

CARBS	CALS	PROTEIN	FAT	FIBRE	SAT FAT	Weight
8g	62	1g	3g	1g	2g	40g

CARBS	CALS	PROTEIN	FAT	FIBRE	SAT FAT	Weight
15g	125	1g	6g	3g	4g	80g

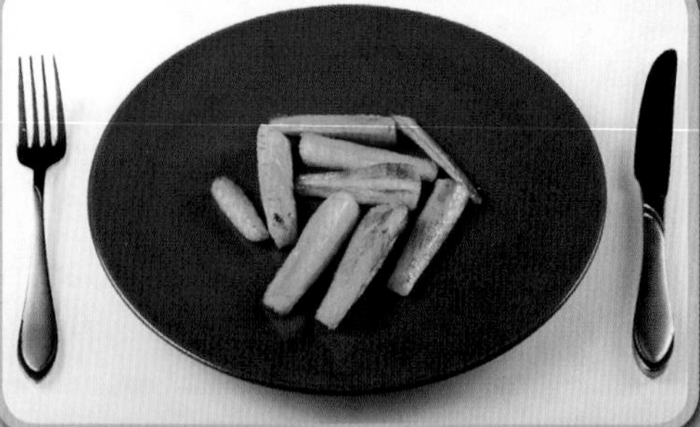

CARBS	CALS	PROTEIN	FAT	FIBRE	SAT FAT	Weight
23g	187	2g	9g	4g	6g	120g

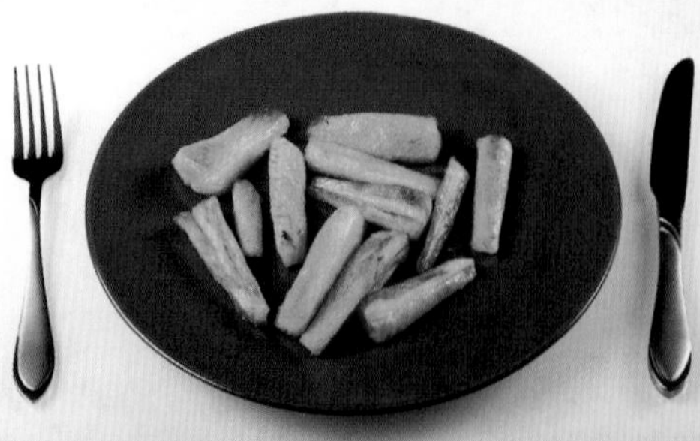

Peppers (raw)

CARBS	CALS	PROTEIN	FAT	FIBRE	SAT FAT	Weight
1g	6	0g	0g	1g	0g	40g

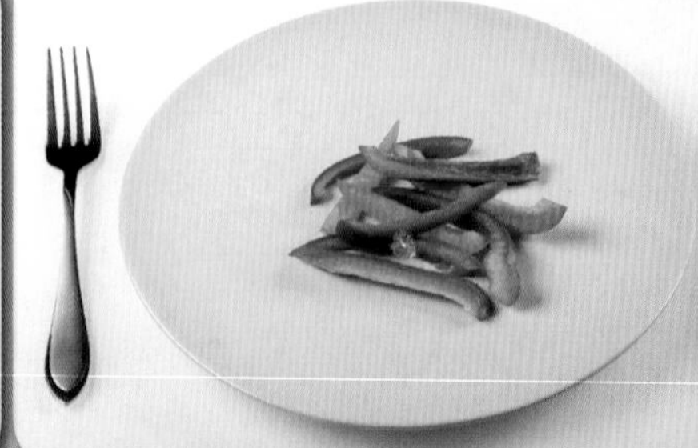

CARBS	CALS	PROTEIN	FAT	FIBRE	SAT FAT	Weight
2g	12	1g	0g	2g	0g	80g

CARBS	CALS	PROTEIN	FAT	FIBRE	SAT FAT	Weight
3g	18	1g	0g	3g	0g	120g

Plantain (boiled)

11g CARBS	45 CALS	0g PROTEIN	0g FAT

1g FIBRE	Weight: 40g	0g SAT FAT

23g CARBS	90 CALS	1g PROTEIN	0g FAT

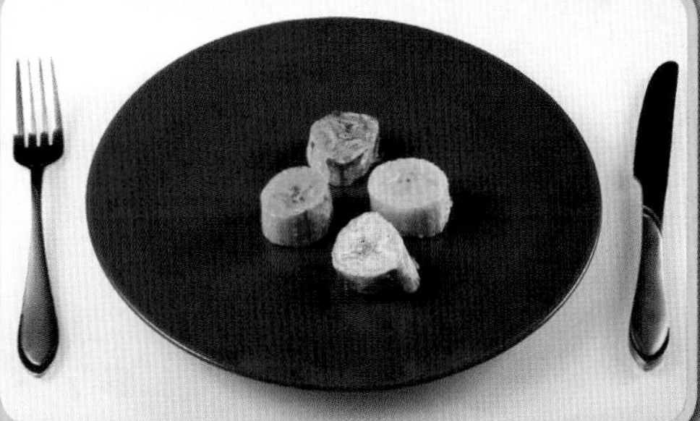

1g FIBRE	Weight: 80g	0g SAT FAT

46g CARBS	179 CALS	1g PROTEIN	0g FAT

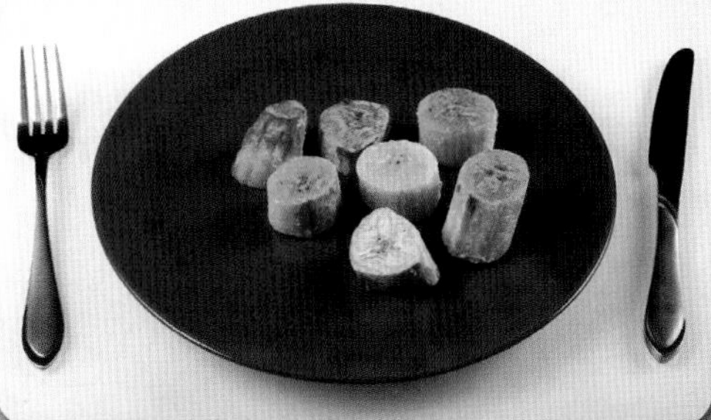

3g FIBRE	Weight: 160g	0g SAT FAT

Plantain (fried)

20g CARBS	112 CALS	1g PROTEIN	4g FAT

1g FIBRE	Weight: 42g	1g SAT FAT

40g CARBS	224 CALS	1g PROTEIN	8g FAT

3g FIBRE	Weight: 84g	1g SAT FAT

60g CARBS	336 CALS	2g PROTEIN	12g FAT

4g FIBRE	Weight: 126g	2g SAT FAT

Radishes

1g CARBS	5 CALS	0g PROTEIN	0g FAT

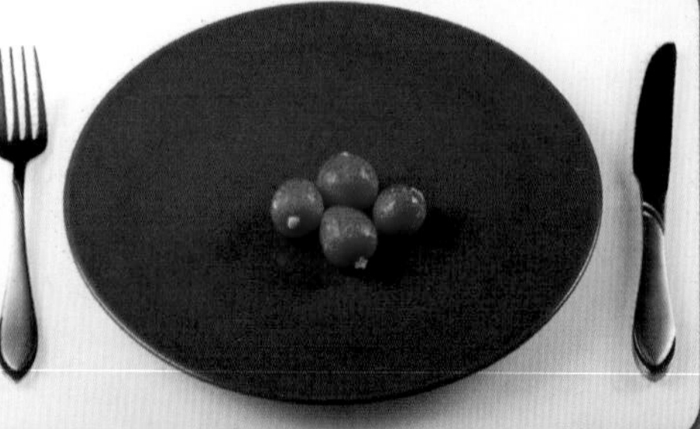

1g FIBRE	Weight: 40g	0g SAT FAT

2g CARBS	10 CALS	1g PROTEIN	0g FAT

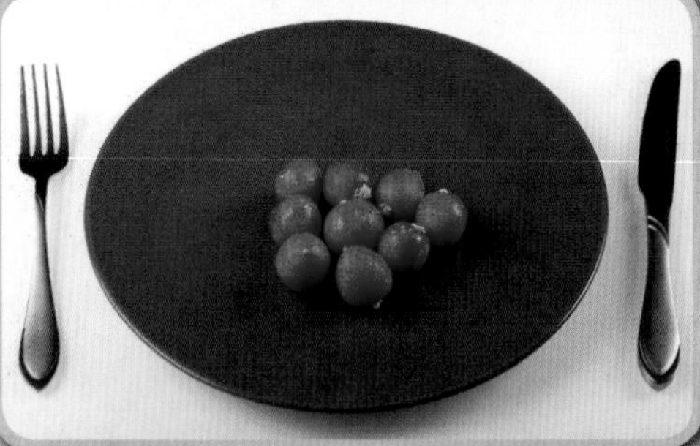

1g FIBRE	Weight: 80g	0g SAT FAT

2g CARBS	14 CALS	1g PROTEIN	0g FAT

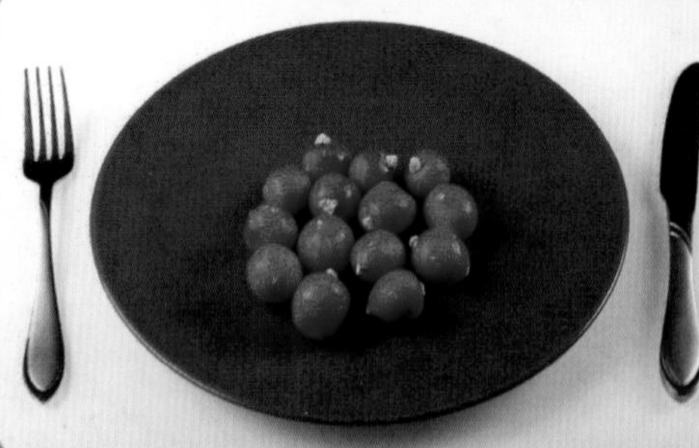

1g FIBRE	Weight: 120g	0g SAT FAT

Rocket

0g CARBS	4 CALS	0g PROTEIN	0g FAT

0g FIBRE	Weight: 20g	0g SAT FAT

1g CARBS	8 CALS	1g PROTEIN	0g FAT

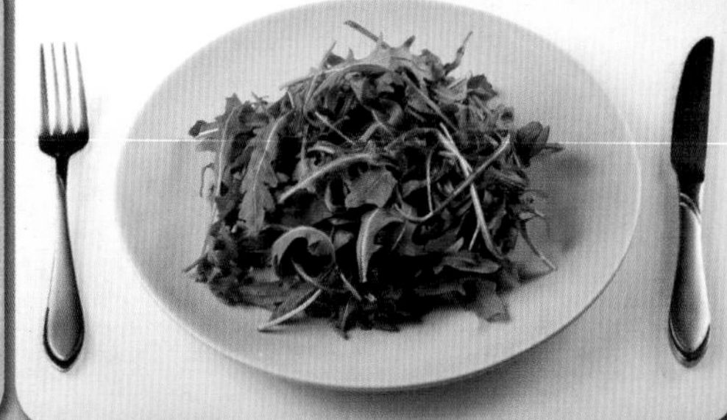

1g FIBRE	Weight: 40g	0g SAT FAT

1g CARBS	16 CALS	2g PROTEIN	0g FAT

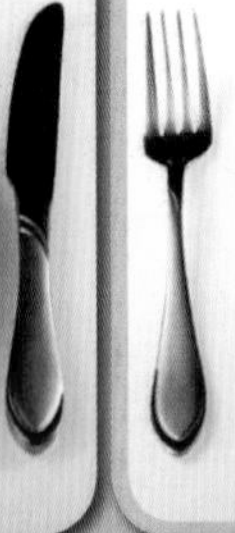

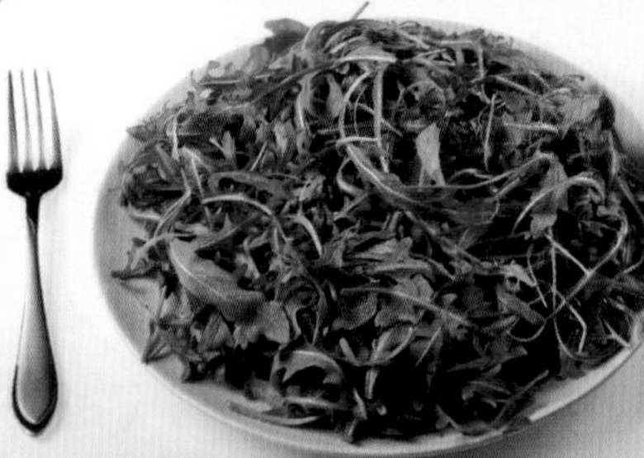

2g FIBRE	Weight: 80g	0g SAT FAT

Spinach (boiled)

CARBS	CALS	PROTEIN	FAT
0g	8	1g	0g

FIBRE	Weight	SAT FAT
1g	Weight: 40g	0g

CARBS	CALS	PROTEIN	FAT
1g	15	2g	1g

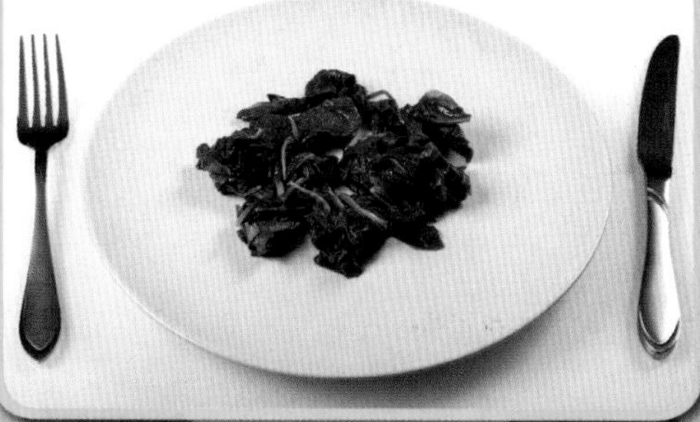
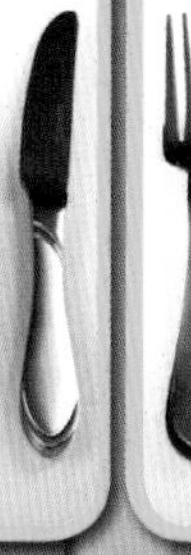

FIBRE	Weight	SAT FAT
2g	Weight: 80g	0g

CARBS	CALS	PROTEIN	FAT
1g	23	3g	1g

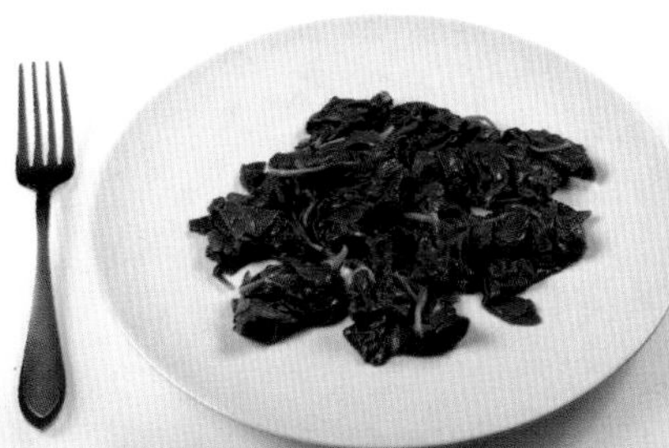
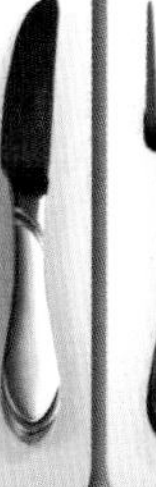

FIBRE	Weight	SAT FAT
3g	Weight: 120g	0g

Spring Greens (boiled)

CARBS	CALS	PROTEIN	FAT
1g	8	1g	0g

FIBRE	Weight	SAT FAT
1g	Weight: 40g	0g

CARBS	CALS	PROTEIN	FAT
1g	16	2g	1g

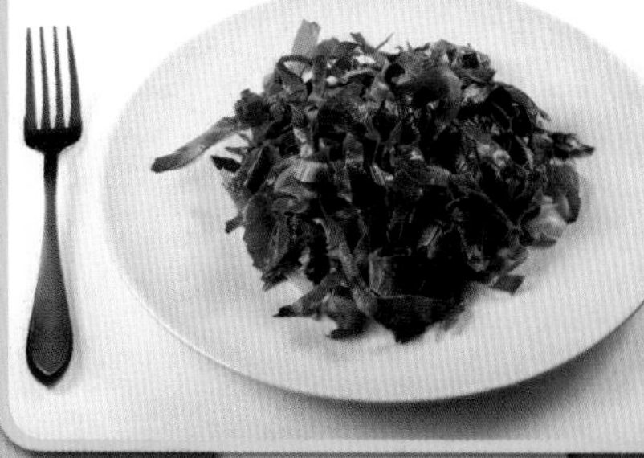

FIBRE	Weight	SAT FAT
3g	Weight: 80g	0g

CARBS	CALS	PROTEIN	FAT
2g	24	2g	1g

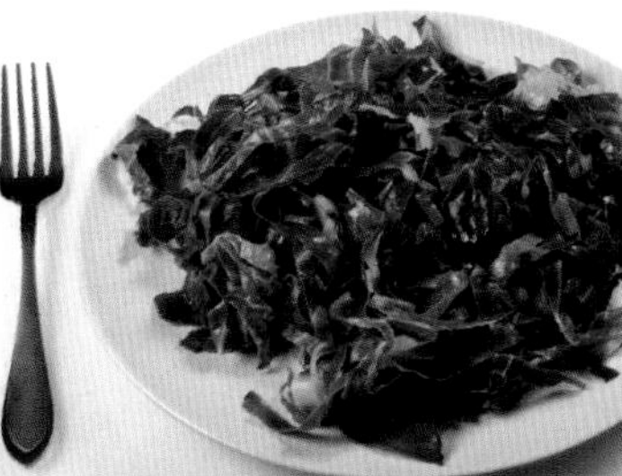

FIBRE	Weight	SAT FAT
4g	Weight: 120g	0g

Sweetcorn

11g CARBS	49 CALS	1g PROTEIN	0g FAT

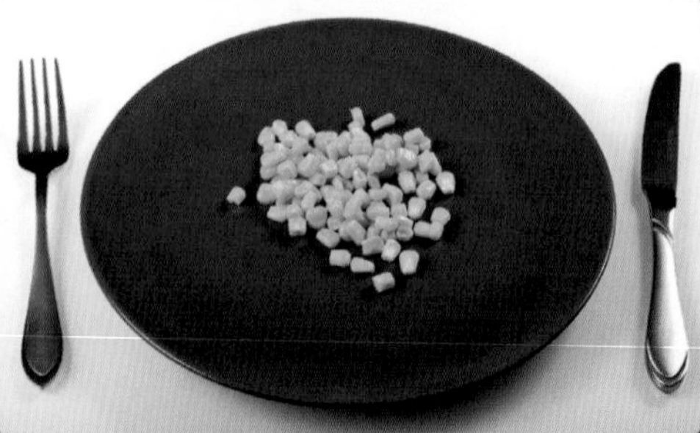

1g FIBRE	Weight: 40g	0g SAT FAT

21g CARBS	98 CALS	2g PROTEIN	1g FAT

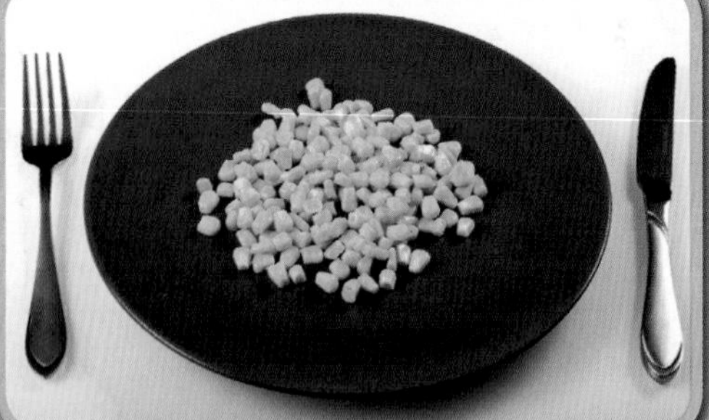

2g FIBRE	Weight: 80g	0g SAT FAT

43g CARBS	195 CALS	5g PROTEIN	2g FAT

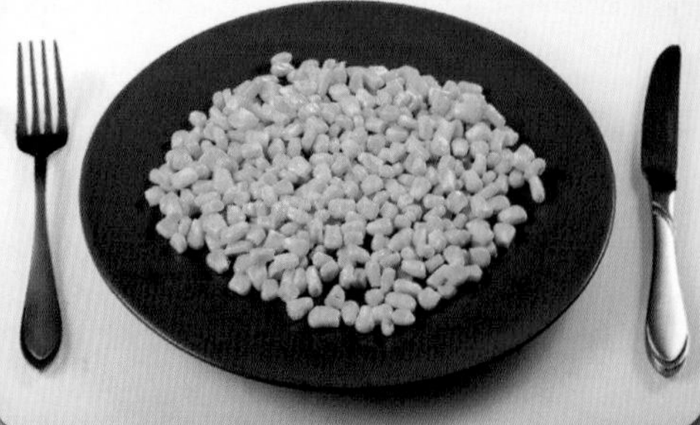

3g FIBRE	Weight: 160g	0g SAT FAT

Corn on the Cob (boiled)

5g CARBS	29 CALS	1g PROTEIN	1g FAT

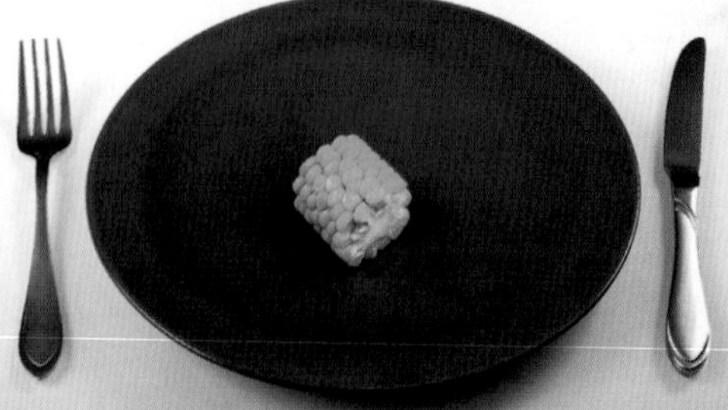

1g FIBRE	Weight: 44g	0g SAT FAT

10g CARBS	56 CALS	2g PROTEIN	1g FAT

1g FIBRE	Weight: 85g	0g SAT FAT

20g CARBS	112 CALS	4g PROTEIN	2g FAT

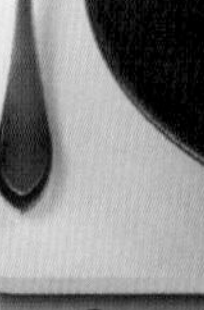

3g FIBRE	Weight: 170g	0g SAT FAT

Sugar Snap Peas (boiled)

2g CARBS	13 CALS	1g PROTEIN	0g FAT

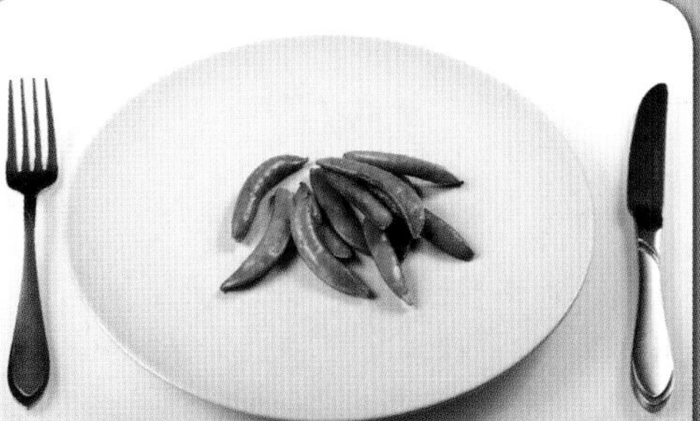

1g FIBRE	Weight: 40g	0g SAT FAT

4g CARBS	26 CALS	3g PROTEIN	0g FAT

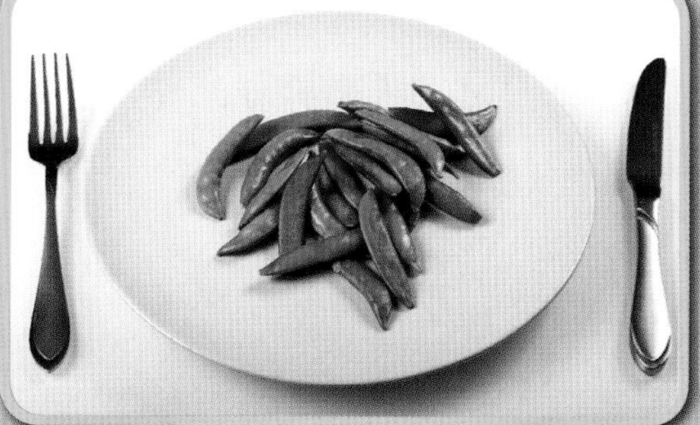

1g FIBRE	Weight: 80g	0g SAT FAT

6g CARBS	40 CALS	4g PROTEIN	0g FAT

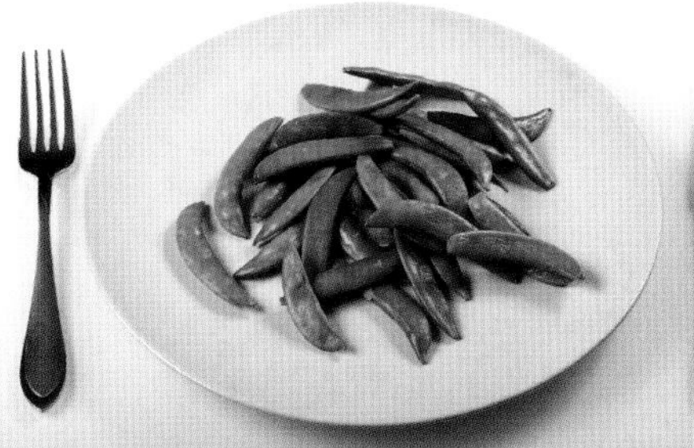

2g FIBRE	Weight: 120g	0g SAT FAT

Tomato

2g CARBS	11 CALS	1g PROTEIN	0g FAT

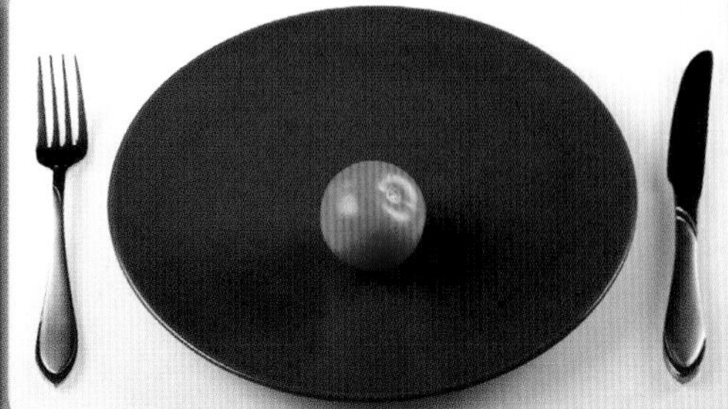

1g FIBRE	Weight: 65g	0g SAT FAT

3g CARBS	14 CALS	1g PROTEIN	0g FAT

1g FIBRE	Weight: 80g	0g SAT FAT

4g CARBS	22 CALS	1g PROTEIN	0g FAT

2g FIBRE	Weight: 130g	0g SAT FAT

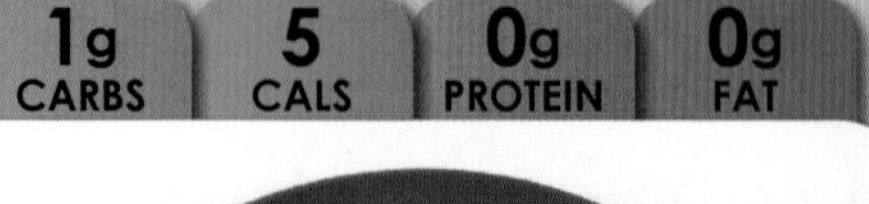

Turnip (boiled)

CARBS	CALS	PROTEIN	FAT
1g	5	0g	0g

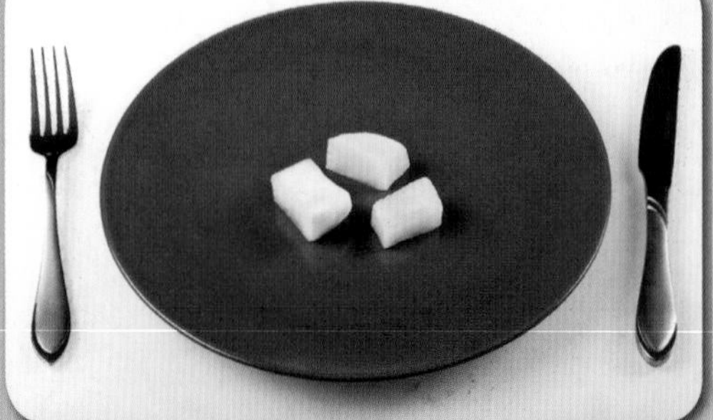

FIBRE		SAT FAT
1g	Weight: 40g	0g

CARBS	CALS	PROTEIN	FAT
2g	10	0g	0g

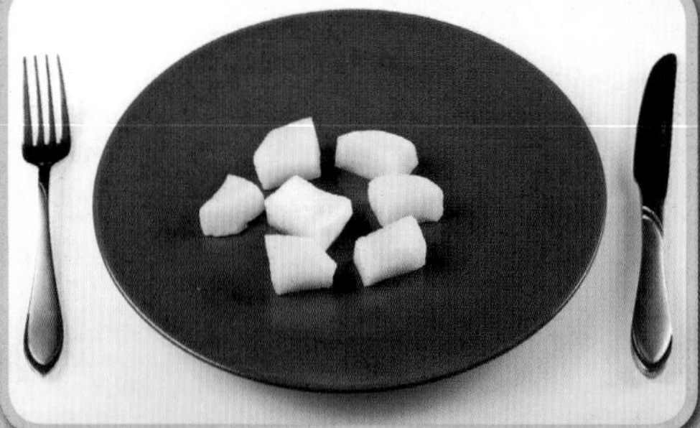

FIBRE		SAT FAT
2g	Weight: 80g	0g

CARBS	CALS	PROTEIN	FAT
3g	19	1g	0g

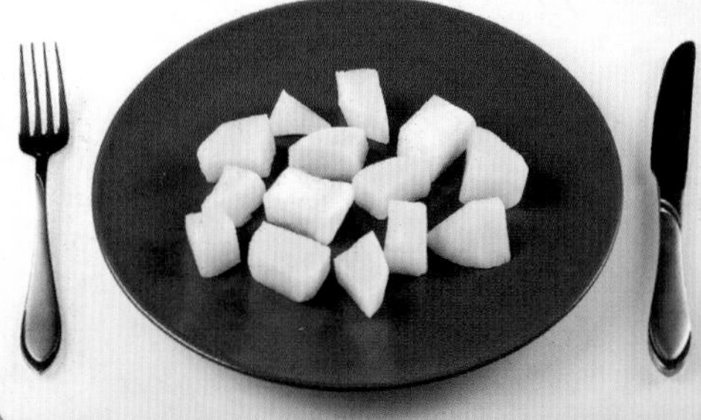

FIBRE		SAT FAT
4g	Weight: 160g	0g

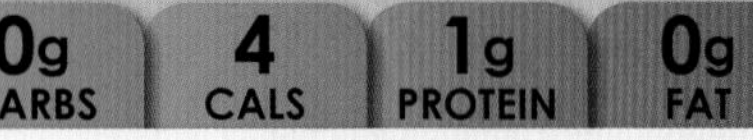

Watercress

CARBS	CALS	PROTEIN	FAT
0g	4	1g	0g

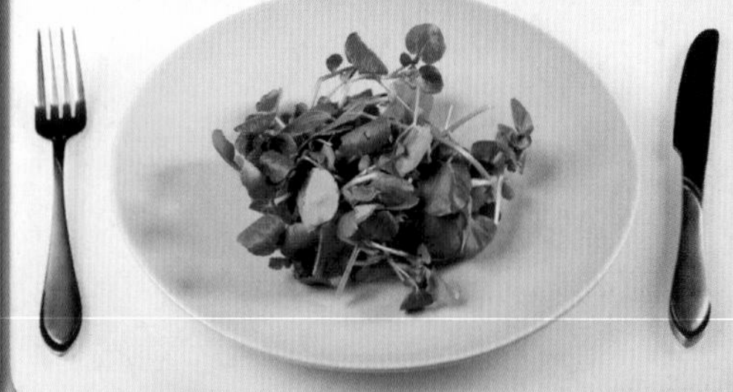

FIBRE		SAT FAT
0g	Weight: 20g	0g

CARBS	CALS	PROTEIN	FAT
0g	9	1g	0g

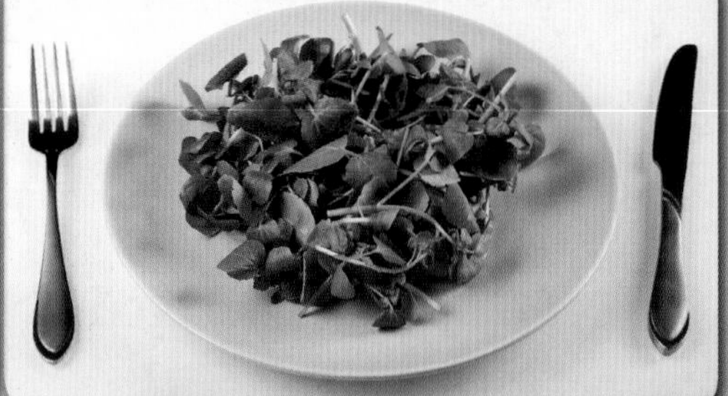

FIBRE		SAT FAT
1g	Weight: 40g	0g

CARBS	CALS	PROTEIN	FAT
0g	18	2g	1g

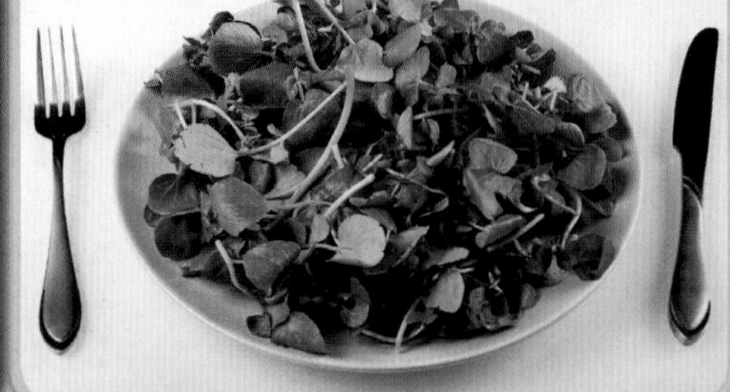

FIBRE		SAT FAT
2g	Weight: 80g	0g

Quorn Chicken Style Pieces

CARBS	CALS	PROTEIN	FAT
3g	52	7g	1g

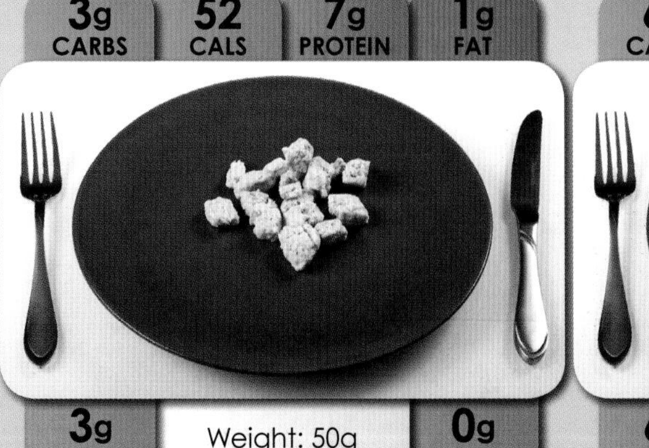

FIBRE	Weight	SAT FAT
3g	Weight: 50g	0g

CARBS	CALS	PROTEIN	FAT
6g	103	14g	3g

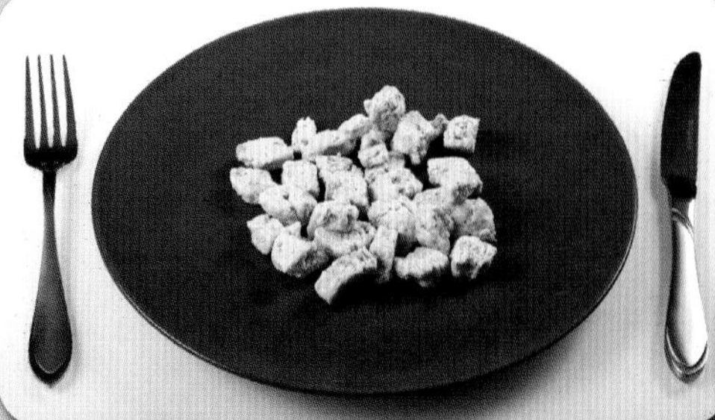

FIBRE	Weight	SAT FAT
6g	Weight: 100g	1g

Quorn Burger (fried)

CARBS	CALS	PROTEIN	FAT
4g	107	7g	7g

FIBRE	Weight	SAT FAT
1g	Weight: 41g	1g

Quorn Burger (grilled)

CARBS	CALS	PROTEIN	FAT
4g	80	7g	4g

FIBRE	Weight	SAT FAT
1g	Weight: 38g	1g

Quorn Sausage (fried)

CARBS	CALS	PROTEIN	FAT
5g	97	5g	6g

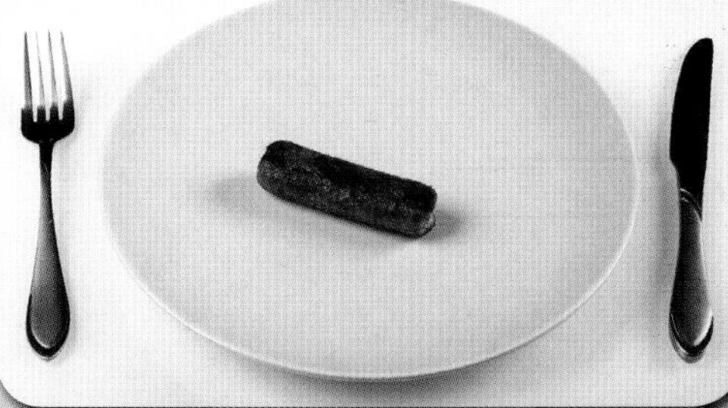

FIBRE	Weight	SAT FAT
2g	Weight: 39g	0g

Quorn Sausage (grilled)

CARBS	CALS	PROTEIN	FAT
5g	70	5g	3g

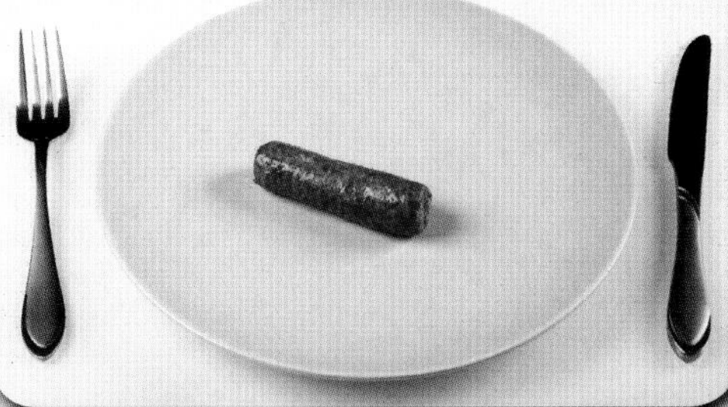

FIBRE	Weight	SAT FAT
2g	Weight: 36g	0g

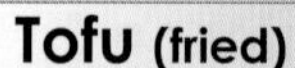

Tofu (fried)

1g CARBS | 85 CALS | 6g PROTEIN | 7g FAT

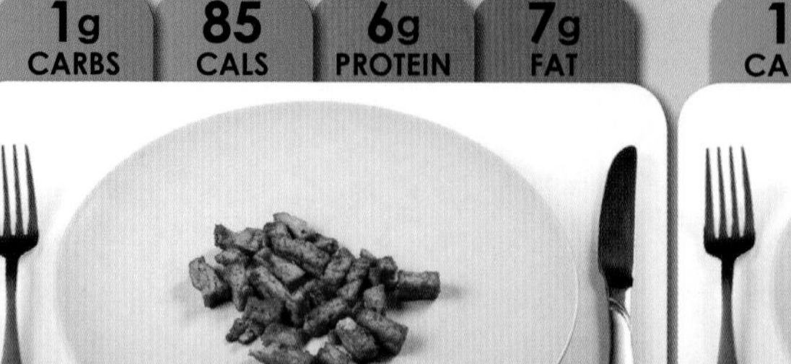

1g FIBRE | Weight: 40g | 1g SAT FAT

1g CARBS | 169 CALS | 12g PROTEIN | 13g FAT

1g FIBRE | Weight: 80g | 2g SAT FAT

Veggie Burger (fried)

28g CARBS | 255 CALS | 5g PROTEIN | 13g FAT

5g FIBRE | Weight: 100g | 2g SAT FAT

Veggie Burger (grilled)

28g CARBS | 228 CALS | 5g PROTEIN | 10g FAT

5g FIBRE | Weight: 100g | 2g SAT FAT

Veggie Sausage (fried)

9g CARBS | 124 CALS | 3g PROTEIN | 8g FAT

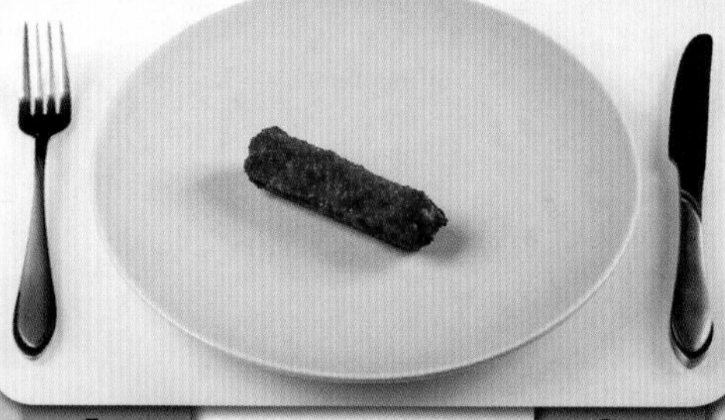

1g FIBRE | Weight: 47g | 2g SAT FAT

Veggie Sausage (grilled)

9g CARBS | 97 CALS | 3g PROTEIN | 5g FAT

1g FIBRE | Weight: 44g | 1g SAT FAT

Fruit Yogurt

CARBS	CALS	PROTEIN	FAT
17g	131	5g	4g

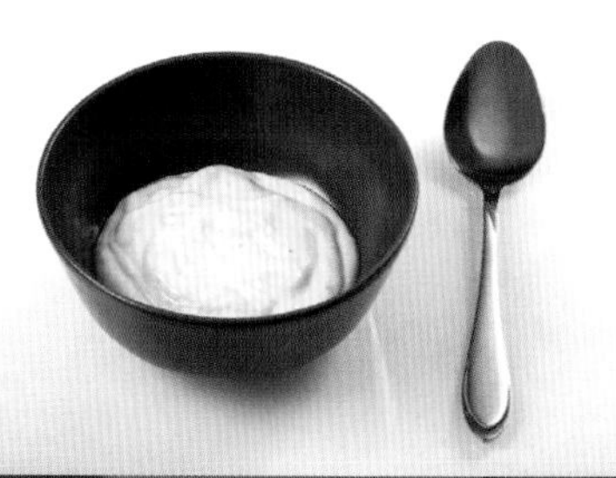

FIBRE	Weight	SAT FAT
0g	Weight: 125g	3g

CARBS	CALS	PROTEIN	FAT
35g	262	11g	9g

FIBRE	Weight	SAT FAT
1g	Weight: 250g	5g

Fruit Yogurt (fat free)

CARBS	CALS	PROTEIN	FAT
11g	72	6g	0g

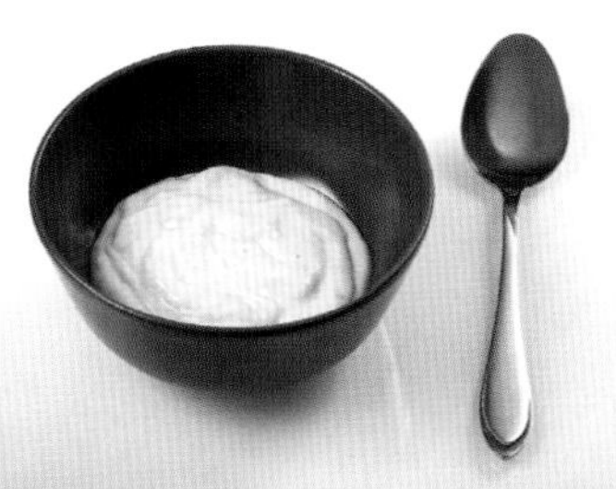

FIBRE	Weight	SAT FAT
0g	Weight: 125g	0g

CARBS	CALS	PROTEIN	FAT
23g	144	12g	0g

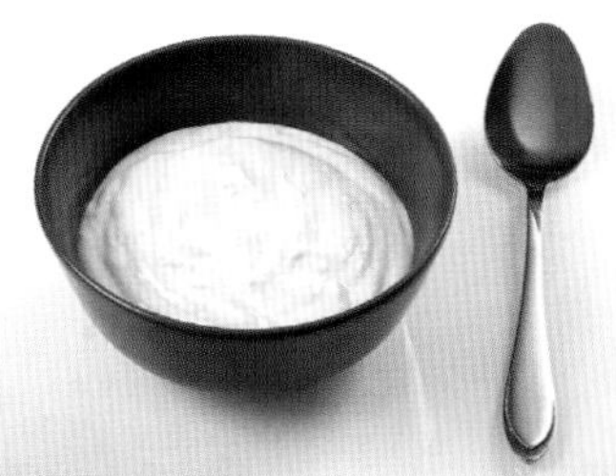

FIBRE	Weight	SAT FAT
1g	Weight: 250g	0g

Fruit Yogurt Pot

CARBS	CALS	PROTEIN	FAT
17g	124	5g	4g

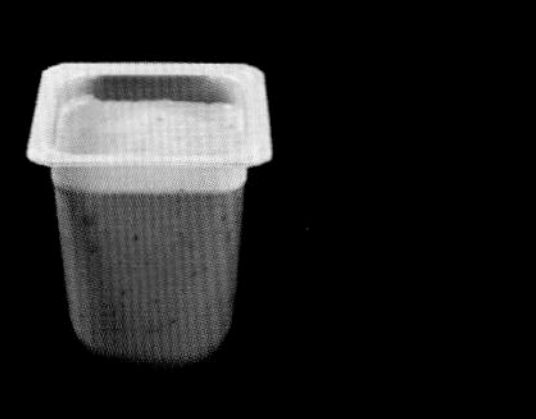

FIBRE	Weight	SAT FAT
1g	Weight: 125g	2g

Fruit Yogurt Pot (fat free)

CARBS	CALS	PROTEIN	FAT
11g	72	6g	0g

FIBRE	Weight	SAT FAT
0g	Weight: 125g	0g

Greek Yogurt

CARBS	CALS	PROTEIN	FAT	FIBRE	Weight	SAT FAT
6g	166	7g	13g	0g	Weight: 125g	9g
12g	333	14g	26g	0g	Weight: 250g	17g

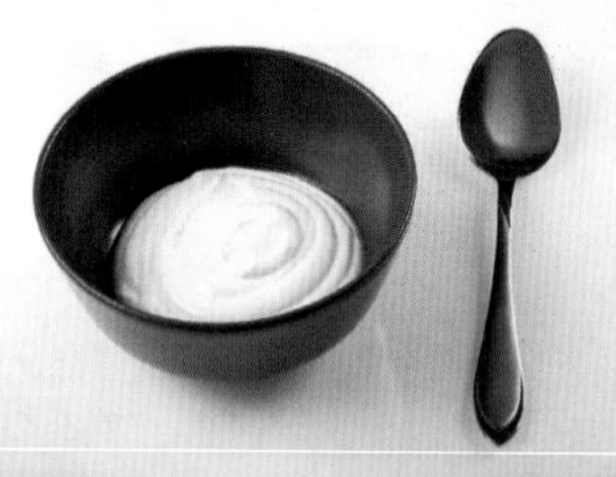

Greek Yogurt (low fat)

CARBS	CALS	PROTEIN	FAT	FIBRE	Weight	SAT FAT
8g	96	9g	3g	0g	Weight: 125g	2g
16g	192	18g	6g	1g	Weight: 250g	4g

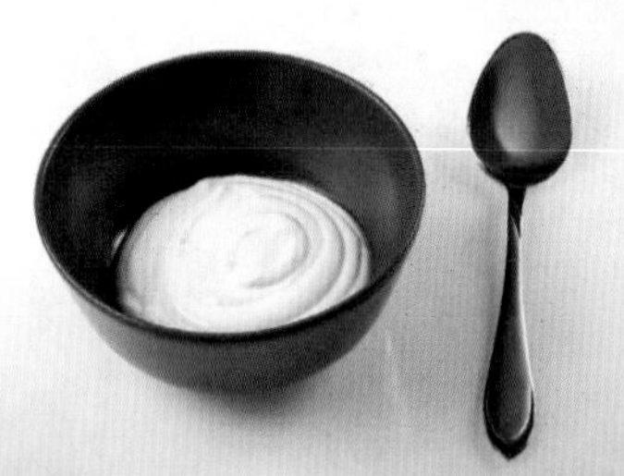

Soya Yogurt

CARBS	CALS	PROTEIN	FAT	FIBRE	Weight	SAT FAT
16g	91	3g	2g	1g	Weight: 125g	0g
32g	183	5g	5g	2g	Weight: 250g	1g

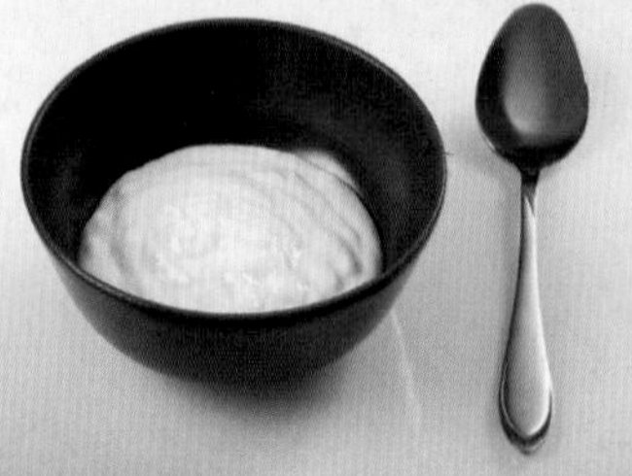

Natural Yogurt

CARBS	CALS	PROTEIN	FAT	FIBRE	Weight	SAT FAT
10g	99	7g	4g	0g	125g	2g
20g	198	14g	8g	0g	250g	5g

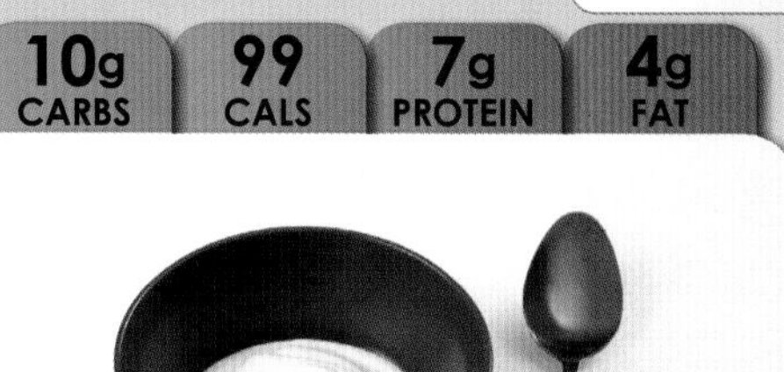

Natural Yogurt (low fat)

CARBS	CALS	PROTEIN	FAT	FIBRE	Weight	SAT FAT
9g	70	6g	1g	0g	125g	1g
19g	140	12g	3g	0g	250g	2g

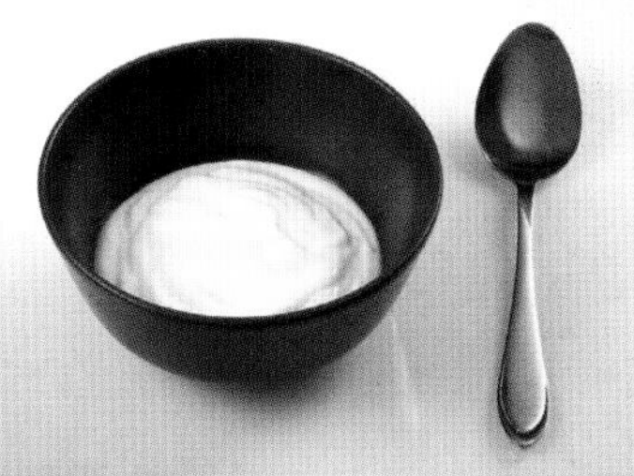

Natural Yogurt (fat free)

CARBS	CALS	PROTEIN	FAT	FIBRE	Weight	SAT FAT
9g	68	7g	0g	0g	125g	0g
18g	135	14g	0g	0g	250g	0g

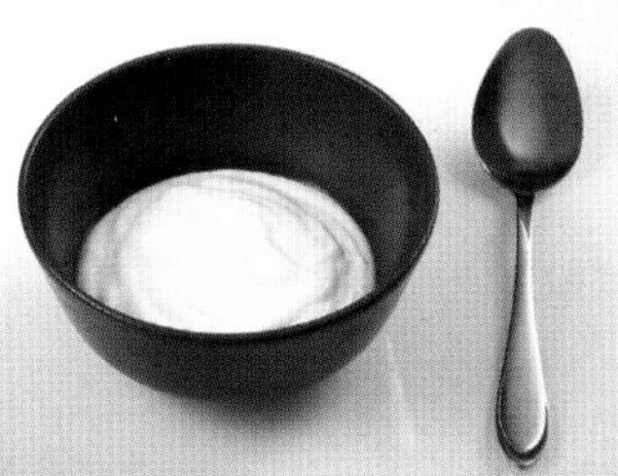

Index

D

N

O

P

T

Acknowledgements

Thank you

We would also like to thank the following people for their advice and support:

Zoë Harrison, the Diabetes Management and Education Group (DMEG) committee of the British Dietetic Association, Helen Hopper, Rachel Kgomotso, Anita Beckwith, Emma Jenkins, Victoria Deprez, Marianne Ouaknin, Jasmine Walton, Paul Robertson, Justine Rose, Chrissi Gray, Ravinder Kundi, Peter Rose, Barry & Joan Cheyette, Pat & Akbar Balolia, Mark Foot, Stu McMillan, Dave Charlton and Sean O'Dell.

Data Sources

Carbohydrate, calorie, protein, fat, saturated fat and fibre values were referenced from:

- Dietplan (version 6.70), Forestfield Software Limited, United Kingdom
- McCance & Widdowson's: The Composition of Foods, Sixth Summary Edition, Food Standards Agency (2002), Cambridge: Royal Society of Chemistry, ISBN 0-85404-428-0
- Kellow J., Costain, L., Beeken, L. The Calorie, Carb and Fat Bible 2012, Weight Loss Resources Limited, United Kingdom, ISBN 978-1-904512-08-0

Other reference values were taken using an average of commercially available products or calculated from recipes. Some values have been estimated based on similar foods. Please note that values in this book are to be used as a guide only. The authors cannot accept any liability for any consequences arising from the use of the information contained within this book. Every effort has been made to ensure figures represent a true and fair value of the carbohydrate, calorie, protein, fat, saturated fat and fibre content of the food and drinks included, but these values can vary between brands, recipes and food preparation methods.

Sustainability Policy

The authors would like to encourage people who read this book to use, where possible, Marine Stewardship Council (MSC) certified sustainable fish. The most commonly available types of fish, such as cod, have been used in this book but we would like to encourage the use of alternative, non-endangered fish such as coley or pollock. For further details, please see the MSC website (**www.msc.org**). We would also like to encourage people to use higher welfare and free-range animal products where possible.